Diabetes and Kidney Disease

Edgar V. Lerma • Vecihi Batuman
Editors

Diabetes and Kidney Disease

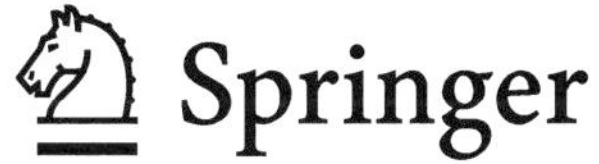

Editors
Edgar V. Lerma
University of Illinois
Chicago, IL, USA

Vecihi Batuman
Nephrology Section
Tulane University Medical School
New Orleans, LA, USA

ISBN 978-1-4939-0792-2 ISBN 978-1-4939-0793-9 (eBook)
DOI 10.1007/978-1-4939-0793-9
Springer New York Heidelberg Dordrecht London

Library of Congress Control Number: 2014937821

© Springer Science+Business Media New York 2014
This work is subject to copyright. All rights are reserved by the Publisher, whether the whole or part of the material is concerned, specifically the rights of translation, reprinting, reuse of illustrations, recitation, broadcasting, reproduction on microfilms or in any other physical way, and transmission or information storage and retrieval, electronic adaptation, computer software, or by similar or dissimilar methodology now known or hereafter developed. Exempted from this legal reservation are brief excerpts in connection with reviews or scholarly analysis or material supplied specifically for the purpose of being entered and executed on a computer system, for exclusive use by the purchaser of the work. Duplication of this publication or parts thereof is permitted only under the provisions of the Copyright Law of the Publisher's location, in its current version, and permission for use must always be obtained from Springer. Permissions for use may be obtained through RightsLink at the Copyright Clearance Center. Violations are liable to prosecution under the respective Copyright Law.
The use of general descriptive names, registered names, trademarks, service marks, etc. in this publication does not imply, even in the absence of a specific statement, that such names are exempt from the relevant protective laws and regulations and therefore free for general use.
While the advice and information in this book are believed to be true and accurate at the date of publication, neither the authors nor the editors nor the publisher can accept any legal responsibility for any errors or omissions that may be made. The publisher makes no warranty, express or implied, with respect to the material contained herein.

Printed on acid-free paper

Springer is part of Springer Science+Business Media (www.springer.com)

To all my mentors and friends, at the University of Santo Tomas Faculty of Medicine and Surgery in Manila, Philippines and Northwestern University Feinberg School of Medicine in Chicago, IL, who have in one way or another influenced and guided me to become the physician that I am.

To all the medical students, interns, and residents at Advocate Christ Medical Center whom I have taught or learned from, especially those who eventually decided to pursue Nephrology as a career.

To my parents and my brothers, without whose unwavering love and support through the good and bad times, I would not have persevered and reached my goals in life.

Most especially, to my two lovely and precious daughters Anastasia Zofia and Isabella Ann, whose smiles and laughter constantly provide me unparalleled joy and happiness; and my very loving and understanding wife Michelle, who has always been supportive of my endeavors both personally and professionally and who sacrificed a lot of time and exhibited unwavering patience as I devoted a significant amount of time and effort to this project. Truly, they provide me with motivation and inspiration.

Edgar V. Lerma

I dedicate this book to my wife Asiye Olcay, my daughter Elif, and my son Gem for their loving support and encouragement.

Vecihi Batuman

Foreword

It gives me great pleasure to write this foreword on this new book about diabetic nephropathy. In the last two decades, we have made tremendous progress in treating diabetes with an improvement in overall glycemic control and better blood pressure control leading to a marked reduction in the microvascular complications of diabetes and their progression. As a result, there has been a significant decline in the rate of end-stage renal disease needing dialysis. However, the diabetes and obesity epidemic continues to take its toll, by increasing the total number of patients with the condition, so that although the rate has declined, the number of patients on dialysis continues to increase. Thus, clinical and societal burden of patients with diabetic nephropathy remains a major public health problem. In addition, certain susceptible individuals either through genetic predisposition or through neglect of their risk factors continued to have accelerated disease with poor long-term prognosis. Therefore, we need to continue to improve our understanding of the condition, its pathophysiology, and current treatment, while developing new treatment strategies, based on the appreciation of novel treatment targets.

This book summarizes the current state of the art in diabetic nephropathy. The first part discusses the fascinating history of the condition and the challenging scope of the problem along with its natural history. It discusses the pathogenesis including hemodynamic alterations related to the renin–angiotensin system and the structural changes that ensue, both in adults and in children as well as in both types of diabetes.

The second and third parts discuss the clinical presentation including strategies for early diagnosis, using novel genetic markers and predictors, as well as clinical pearls to help us to recognize atypical presentations and develop an appropriate differential diagnosis. Important associations are discussed, particularly hypertension, cardiovascular disease, lipid disorders, and eye complications, as well as the special situation of pregnancy. Finally, they discuss transplantation not just to the kidney, but the combined kidney–pancreas transplantation that offers the potential for complete cure of the condition.

This book will serve as an important reference source for the clinician and researcher and help us find ways to eliminate this devastating complication of diabetes.

New Orleans, LA, USA — Vivian Fonseca, M.D.

Preface

Diabetic nephropathy is the most common cause of end-stage kidney disease in the USA and Europe, and its incidence and prevalence continue to rise at a great human and economic cost. Over the past decade there has been literally an explosion of research to all aspects of diabetes and diabetic nephropathy, such as better definition of clinical patterns, i.e., latent autoimmune diabetes of the adult (LADA), maturity onset diabetes of the young (MODY), etc. Novel clinical biomarkers beyond microalbuminuria are being explored, and the implications of proteinuria in diabetes are being reassessed. Recent research continues to discover and characterize new molecular, immunologic, genetic, and epigenetic mechanisms in the pathogenesis of diabetic kidney disease. Advances in the approach to eye disease associated with diabetes in relation to diabetic kidney disease, diabetes during pregnancy, and diabetic kidney disease in children are among the topics covered. The spectrum of histopathology is described in greater detail with focus on pathophysiology. Newer drugs with novel mechanisms of action have been introduced to clinical practice, and additional drugs are likely to follow in the near future. Advances in biotechnology are opening up a whole new vista with an eye to futuristic therapies taking advantage of newer insights into regenerative medicine. There are improvements in transplant medicine, exploring newer protocols in kidney pancreas transplant, islet cell transplant, and even in cross-species transplantation. That diabetes is not a simple lack of glycemic control and it is associated with a broad array of metabolic disorders including lipid abnormalities had been appreciated for sometime, but, again, recent research has contributed new insight into our understanding of these associated metabolic disorders and the consequent cardiovascular morbidity.

The purpose of this book is to provide a convenient single volume to practitioners and investigators, as well as medical students and residents, where an overview of the recent advances in the theory and practice of diabetic kidney disease with an eye on future prospects is available. This, of course, is an ambitious goal; however, we are pleased that we have been able to arrange a coherent collection of chapters authored by prominent experts in their fields making it possible to not only view the current state of the art in diabetic nephropathy but also provide a starting place for additional reading for those who might wish to further investigate a certain aspect of diabetic nephropathy. We are hopeful that the readers of this book, whether clinicians, clinician-scientist, or basic researchers, will find this book a useful compilation, and the reader regardless of her/his level of knowledge in the field will be able to glean some useful information for her/his purpose.

We are thankful to our contributors for preparing their chapters, for their patience and understanding with the editors' suggestions, and making this book a comprehensive review of the current status of diabetic kidney disease. This book would not have been possible without the expert guidance, support, and assistance of our developmental editor Connie Walsh and senior editor Gregory Sutorius, and we wish to thank them for their efforts.

Chicago, IL, USA — Edgar V. Lerma, M.D.
New Orleans, LA, USA — Vecihi Batuman, M.D.

Contents

Contributors

Azin Abazari, M.D. Department of Ophthalmology, Stony Brook University, Stony Brook, NY, USA

Arnold B. Alper Jr., M.D., M.P.H. Department of Internal Medicine, Section of Nephrology, Tulane University School of Medicine, New Orleans, LA, USA

Jeffrey Aufman, M.D. Department of Pathology, Louisiana State University, Shreveport, LA, USA

Vecihi Batuman Tulane University Medical Center, Nephrology Section, New Orleans, LA, USA

Adrian Baudy IV, M.D. Section of Nephrology and Hypertension, Tulane Medical Center, New Orleans, LA, USA

Joumana T. Chaiban, M.D. Internal Medicine, Endocrinology and Metabolic Diseases, Saint Vincent Charity Medical Center, Cleveland, OH, USA

Case Western Reserve University, Cleveland, OH, USA

Jing Chen, M.D., M.M.Sc., M.Sc. Department of Medicine, Tulane University School of Medicine, New Orleans, LA, USA

Eric P. Cohen, M.D. Department of Medicine, Zablocki VA Hospital, Milwaukee, WI, USA

William J. Elliott, M.D., Ph.D. Division of Pharmacology, Pacific Northwest University of Health Sciences, Yakima, WA, USA

Vivian Fonseca, M.D. Department of Medicine, Section of Endocrinology, Tulane University, New Orleans, LA, USA

Nicola G. Ghazi, M.D. King Khaled Eye Specialist Hospital, Riyadh, Saudi Arabia

University of Virginia, Charlottesville, VA, USA

Michelle Haggar, M.D. Department of Medicine, Section of Endocrinology, Tulane University, New Orleans, LA, USA

Allison J. Hahr, M.D. Division of Endocrinology, Metabolism and Molecular Medicine, Medicine Department, Northwestern University Feinberg School of Medicine, Chicago, IL, USA

L. Lee Hamm, M.D. Dean's Office, Tulane Medical School, New Orleans, LA, USA

Kathleen S. Hering-Smith, M.S., Ph.D. Section of Nephrology and Hypertension, Department of Medicine, Tulane University Health Sciences Center, New Orleans, LA, USA

Guillermo A. Herrera, M.D. Department of Pathology, Louisiana State University, Shreveport, LA, USA

Louis J. Imbriano, M.D. Department of Medicine, Winthrop-University Hospital, Mineola, NY, USA

George Jerums, M.D. Austin Health, Endocrine Centre of Excellence, Heidelberg Repatriation Hospital, Heidelberg West, VIC, Australia

Zeynel A. Karcioglu, M.D. Department of Ophthalmology, University of Virginia, Charlottesville, VA, USA

N. Kevin Krane, M.D. Department of Medicine, Section of Nephrology and Hypertension, Tulane University School of Medicine, New Orleans, LA, USA

Armand Krikorian, M.D., F.A.C.E. Internal Medicine, Endocrinology and Metabolism, Advocate Christ Medical Center, Oak Lawn, IL, USA

Jean-Marie Krzesinski, M.D., Ph.D. Unité de Néphrologie, Centre Hospitalier Universitaire, Université de Liège, Liège, Belgium

John K. Maesaka, M.D. Division of Nephrology and Hypertension, Department of Medicine, Winthrop-University Hospital, Mineola, NY, USA

Joseph Mattana, M.D. Division of Nephrology and Hypertension, Department of Medicine, Winthrop University Hospital, Mineola, NY, USA

Mark E. Molitch, M.D. Department of Medicine, Division of Endocrinology, Metabolism and Molecular Medicine, Northwestern University Feinberg School of Medicine, Chicago, IL, USA

Anil Paramesh, M.D., F.A.C.S. Departments of Surgery and Urology, Tulane Abdominal Transplant Institute, Tulane University School of Medicine, New Orleans, LA, USA

Radha Pasala, M.D. Section of Nephrology and Hypertension, Tulane University School of Medicine, New Orleans, LA, USA

Alluru S. Reddi, M.D. Department of Medicine, Division of Nephrology and Hypertension, Rutgers New Jersey Medical School, Newark, NJ, USA

Surya V. Seshan, M.D. Department of Pathology and Laboratory Medicine, Weill Cornell Medical College, New York, NY, USA

Shayan Shirazian, M.D. Department of Medicine, Winthrop-University Hospital, Mineola, NY, USA

Tina K. Thethi, M.D., M.P.H. Department of Medicine, Section of Endocrinology, Tulane University Health Sciences Center, New Orleans, LA, USA

Southeast Louisiana Veterans Health Care, New Orleans, LA, USA

Aileen K. Wang, M.D. Department of Medicine, Section of Endocrinology, Tulane University Health Sciences Center, New Orleans, LA, USA

Ihor V. Yosypiv, M.D. Division of Pediatric Nephrology, Department of Pediatrics, Tulane Hospital for Children, New Orleans, LA, USA

Rubin Zhang, M.D. Department of Medicine, Tulane University School of Medicine, New Orleans, LA, USA

The Background History of Diabetic Nephropathy

1

Michelle Haggar and Vivian Fonseca

Introduction

Symptoms of diabetes are recorded as far back as 400 B.C.; the Indian physician Susruta describes diabetes in an ancient Hindi document as "madhumeha" or the honeyed-urine disease [1]. Around 150 A.D., the Greek physician Aretaeus of Cappadocia wrote:

> Diabetes is a remarkable disorder, and not one very common to man. It consists of a moist and cold wasting of the flesh and limbs into urine… the secretion passes in the usual way, by the kidneys and the bladder. It is not improbable, also, that something pernicious, derived from other disease which attack the bladder and kidneys may sometimes prove the cause of this affliction. The patients never cease making water, but the discharge is as incessant as a sluice let off. This disease is chronic in character, and is slowly engendered, though the patient does not survive long when it is completely established for the marasmus produced is rapid and death is speedy [2]....

For many centuries thereafter, diabetes mellitus was regarded as a disease of the kidney.

The Discovery of Diabetic Nephropathy

Following the now famous paper published by Paul Kimmelstiel and Clifford Wilson in 1936, many incorrectly assume that diabetic renal disease was recently recognized. However, the discovery of diabetic nephropathy has been a gradual process, and the meaning of diabetic renal disease has changed over time [3].

Erasmus Darwin [4] described it as urine that could be coagulated by heat, confirming the observations of Cotunnius [5] and Rollo [6] that the urine of some diabetics contained protein [7]. In the 1830s, research conducted by the "father of nephrology" Richard Bright into the causes of kidney disease led to what became known as Bright's disease. Pierre-François Olive Rayer [8] and Wilhelm Griesinger [9] were the first to hypothesize that diabetes might cause a form of Bright's disease.

In the 1850s, much data on renal histology in patients with diabetes were published. Lionel Beale examined the histology of enlarged diabetic kidneys and analyzed them chemically, showing an excess of fat present in the tubules. Luciano Armanni (1875, cited by Ebstein) and Wilhelm Ebstein [10] described vacuolization of renal tubular epithelium.

The concept of diabetic nephropathy continued to develop, and in 1883, Ehrlich confirmed glycogen infiltration—a common postmortem finding in the pre-insulin era. For the next 50 years, these tubular deposits of glycogen were the only lesion believed to be specifically associated with diabetes, later called "nephropathia diabetic" by Aschoff in 1911.

Kenzo Waku [11] published a description of diffuse capillary wall thickening studied by silver staining in 8 of 13 diabetic patients, in a Japanese journal written in German. No clinical details of the patients were provided, and the study gained little attention. It was not until 1936, when Kimmelsteil and Wilson published their paper "Intercapillary lesions in glomeruli of kidney" in the American Journal of Pathology, that interest intensified in the study of diabetic vascular complications.

The Pathology of Diabetic Renal Disease

Paul Kimmelstiel (1900–1970), a native of Hamburg, Germany, came to the USA in 1933. Clifford Wilson (1906–1997), a relatively unknown British clinician, went to Harvard University as a Rockefeller travelling fellow and met Kimmelstiel. Their first paper [12] described glomerular lesions in eight patients who died of renal failure. The lesions

M. Haggar, M.D. (✉) • V. Fonseca, M.D.
Department of Medicine, Section of Endocrinology, Tulane University, 930 Poydras Street, Apt 1709, New Orleans, LA 70112, USA
e-mail: mhaggar@tulane.edu

E.V. Lerma and V. Batuman (eds.), *Diabetes and Kidney Disease*,
DOI 10.1007/978-1-4939-0793-9_1, © Springer Science+Business Media New York 2014

were attributed to diabetes mellitus because seven of the eight patients were known to have the disease. Most of the patients had hypertension, heavy albuminuria, and edema, and were aged 48–68 years. The diabetic patients had diabetes from a range of 10 months to 10 years. Their glomeruli showed uniform lesions involving large expansion of the intercapillary space. This expansion was shown to be continuous with the hyaline lesions of the afferent glomerular arteriole. Kimmelstiel and Wilson did not emphasize the association of these lesions with diabetes, but suggested that the appearance was an acceleration of senile glomerulosclerosis. They noted that it was a rare finding and that it could complicate glomerulonephritis.

Although Kimmelstiel and Wilson's observations were received initially with uncertainty, they stimulated interest in diabetic vascular pathology. After their publication, the eponym "Kimmelstiel–Wilson nodules" began to be applied to diabetic renal lesions. However, it was Arthur Allen (1941) who clarified the link with diabetes [13]. He studied autopsies of 105 patients with diabetes (all of which were over age 40), 100 patients with hypertension, 100 patients without hypertension or diabetes, and 34 patients with glomerulonephritis. Thirty four percent of the diabetics showed the lesion, but otherwise it was seen in only three other patients.

Initial Studies of Renal Biopsies

Before 1950, renal histology samples were mostly obtained from autopsied patients. The only way of analyzing kidney tissue from a live person was through an open operation. In 1951, Danish physicians Poul Iversen and Claus Brun described a method involving needle biopsy [14]. It became possible to obtain renal specimens of diabetic patients in all stages of disease. By the end of the 1950s, there were a large amount of data collected such as those published by Robert Kark in Chicago [15]. These data revealed that patients with mild glomerular disease may have heavy proteinuria, and patients with less renal involvement may have complex lesions of nodular glomerulosclerosis.

In 1957 the electron microscope [16] and in 1959 immunofluorescent protein tracing [15] were used to study glomerular lesions in patients with diabetes mellitus. Using these techniques, the hypothesis of a diffuse thickening of the basement membrane in diabetics was proven. In 1956, Ruth Østerby-Hansen published a study [17], which showed that there was no thickening of the peripheral glomerular basement membrane in early diabetic patients. This finding brought forth the possibility of treatment through modifying whatever was causing subsequent changes.

Radioimmunoassay and the Concept of Microalbuminuria

In New York in the 1950s, Rosalyn Yalow and Solomon Aaron Berson developed the technique of radioimmunoassay, and they later published their findings [18]. The technique allowed for the precise measurement of minute amounts of proteins and hormones. In 1960, Harry Keen and associates from Guy's Hospital used the technique to detect small amounts of albumin in the urine of diabetics. Their paper [19] was published in the Lancet in 1963. Keen studied diabetics at all stages of disease, including those who had no proteinuria on conventional testing. Keen realized that elevated albumin excretion below the proteinuric level might be important in the natural history of diabetic renal disease, and the concept of microalbuminuria was developed.

In 1982, GianCarlo Viberti published findings that confirmed that microalbuminuria could predict the subsequent evolution of overt nephropathy with proteinuria in type 1 diabetics [20], and in 1984, Carl-Erik Mogensen showed the same finding in type 2 diabetics [21]. Concurrently, it became apparent that the reduction of blood pressure could postpone renal failure [22].

The Discovery of the Renin–Angiotensin–Aldosterone System

In the 1950s, Mann et al. documented the natural history of diabetic renal disease. Death from renal failure that resulted from diabetic nephropathy usually occurred in patients who had longstanding type 1 diabetes. However, after the 1970s with improved treatments, much larger number of patients with type 2 diabetes began to survive and develop end-stage renal disease. Attention began to shift from the treatment to the prevention of diabetic nephropathy.

Pharmacologic blockade of the renin–angiotensin–aldosterone system (RAAS) has become the standard of care for patients with type 2 diabetes mellitus and renal involvement [23]. The history of the discovery of the RAAS began in 1898 with the studies by Tigerstedt and Bergman, who reported the pressor effect of renal extracts; they named the renal substance renin based on its origin [24]. Angiotensin-converting enzyme inhibitors (ACE-i) were the first class of clinically applicable drugs that specifically block the RAAS. Originally, ACE-i were developed as antihypertensives, in particular aimed at the treatment of high renin hypertension. The first proposals [25, 26] that the outcome of diabetic nephropathy could be improved using RAAS blockade with ACE-i drugs began in the early 1980s. Brenner and Zatz showed that rats with diabetes that were treated with ACE-i were protected against nephropathy; however, conventional blood pressure lowering agents did not [27]. The first controlled trial [28] of ACE-i in humans with diabetes appeared in 1987.

In 1993, the landmark study using captopril was published [29]. The trial demonstrated that captopril protected against deterioration of renal function in patients with type 1 diabetes and diabetic nephropathy and was significantly more effective than blood pressure control alone. Captopril reduced the risk of doubling of the serum creatinine by 48 % when compared with standard antihypertensive therapy. Both treatment groups had similar blood pressures; thus, the effect of captopril on progression was determined to be independent of its antihypertensive properties, an effect termed "renoprotection."

In 2001, the Irbesartan Diabetic Nephropathy Trial [30], designed to ascertain whether the use of the angiotensin-II receptor blocker Irbesartan or the calcium channel blocker amlodipine provided similar renoprotection in overt nephropathy associated with type 2 diabetes, was published. Irbesartan was shown to reduce the risk of doubling the serum creatinine by 33 % when compared with standard antihypertensive therapy and by 37 % when compared with treatment with amlodipine. Blood pressures were again similar across groups, indicating that these salutary effects were a result of renoprotection. Similar results were reported using losartan in the Reduction of End Points in NIDDM with the Angiotensin II Antagonist Losartan (RENAAL) trial [31].

Results of the Irbesartan in Patients with Type 2 Diabetes and Microalbuminuria (IRMA II) trial were also published in 2001. IRMA II studied the effects of the use of Irbesartan (300 or 150 mg/day versus placebo) to prevent progression from the earlier stage of microalbuminuria to the later stage of overt nephropathy in patients with hypertension and type 2 diabetes. The study demonstrated that patients receiving Irbesartan (300 mg/day) had about one third the risk of developing overt nephropathy compared with the patients not receiving (adjusted risk reduction 68 % at 300 mg/day) [32].

Value of Glycemic Control

Diabetes is the most common cause of ESRD in Western countries, and glycemic control is correlated with the development and progression of diabetic nephropathy (DN). Epidemiologic studies have demonstrated that DN risk is higher in patients with poor metabolic control [26, 33, 34]. Although genetic factors modulate DN risk and some patients do not develop this complication despite several years of poor glycemic control, there is evidence that hyperglycemia is a necessary precondition for DN lesions. Two major early glomerular lesions, glomerular basement membrane thickening and mesangial expansion, are not present at diagnosis of diabetes but are found 2–5 years after onset of hyperglycemia [33].

Studies in identical twins who are discordant for type 1 diabetes support the concept that hyperglycemia is necessary for the development of diabetic glomerulopathy. Twin studies show that the nondiabetic siblings had structurally normal kidneys, while their diabetic twin pair had glomerular lesions [35]. Moreover, normal kidneys from nondiabetic donors that are transplanted into patients with diabetes develop lesions of DN [36, 37].

A number of articles now suggest a long-term survival advantage with simultaneous pancreas kidney (SPK) transplantation, compared with single kidney transplantation alone for patients with end-stage renal disease caused by diabetic nephropathy [38]. SPK offers the opportunity to test the ability of pancreas transplantation to prevent the development of diabetic glomerular lesions, because the renal graft has never been exposed to hyperglycemia. Patients who have dual-organ operation almost always normalize their glycemic values afterward, and this is partly why these patients live longer than those who get a kidney alone. In 1985, Bohman et al. were the first to demonstrate that the development of diabetic glomerulopathy was prevented in the recipients of SPK [39]. In 1993, the same group confirmed prior observations when they reported data on a cohort of 20 SPK patients who were followed for up to 6 years, compared with a group of 34 kidney transplant recipients with diabetes [40]. More recent studies support the same observation [41, 42].

Treatment of Hyperglycemia

In type 1 diabetes, the Diabetes Control and Complications (DCCT) Research Group trial demonstrated that intensive treatment was associated with decreased incidence of microalbuminuria and reduced progression to macroalbuminuria as compared with conventional treatment [43]. In type 2 diabetes, the UK Prospective Diabetes Study (UKPDS) Group trial demonstrated a reduced incidence of microalbuminuria in the intensively treated group as compared with conventional treatment, but a parallel finding in macroalbuminuria was not significant [44]. However, the Kumamoto study [45] and the Veterans Affairs Cooperative study [46] both showed that intensive treatment was effective for primary prevention (decreased incidence of microalbuminuria) and secondary prevention (reduced progression to macroalbuminuria).

The Epidemiology of Diabetes Interventions and Complications (EDIC)/DCCT follow-up study [47] and the UKPDS study also found that lowering HbA1c reduced decline in GFR in type 1 and type 2 diabetes, respectively.

Intensive Glycemic Control

The benefit of intensive glycemic control for nephropathy is currently under debate. Intensive treatment of hyperglycemia may prevent DN, including development of microalbuminuria, but there is little evidence that it slows the progression of chronic kidney disease [48].

In the Action to Control Cardiovascular Risk in Diabetes (ACCORD) trial, assignment of the treatment group to an HbA1c goal of less than 6 % led to increased mortality and cessation of the trial [49]. Furthermore, in one analysis of data from the ACCORD study, combined intensive glycemic and blood pressure control did not produce an additive benefit on microvascular outcomes in patients with type 2 diabetes. This differs from the findings of the ADVANCE study [50], which showed that intensive glucose and BP controls were independently beneficial and their combination produced synergistic benefits in nephropathy, new-onset microalbuminuria, and new-onset macroalbuminuria.

Current Status

The rate of diabetes-related ESRD incidence among individuals with diabetes is decreasing [51]. However, the overall prevalence of diabetes-related ESRD in the general population continues to increase because of the growing number of individuals with diabetes. Therefore, diabetic nephropathy continues to be a major public health problem.

References

1. Krall LP, Levine R, Barnett D. The history of diabetes. In: Kahn CR, Weir GC, editors. Joslin's diabetes mellitus. Philadelphia: Lea & Febiger; 1994.
2. Aretaeus, De causis et signis acutorum morborum (lib. 2) Francis Adams LL.D., Ed.
3. Stewart Cameron J. The discovery of diabetic nephropathy: from small print to centre stage. J Nephrol. 2006;10:S75.
4. Darwin E. Zoonomia (The Laws of Organic Life). 1801.
5. Cotunnius D. De Ischiade Nervosa. Vienna, 1770.
6. Rollo J. Cases of the diabetes mellitus. 2nd ed. London: Dilly; 1798.
7. Cameron JS, Ireland JT, Watkins PJ. The kidney and renal tract. In: Keen HF, Jarrett J, editors. Complications of diabetes. London: Edward Arnold Ltd.; 1975. p. 99.
8. Rayer P. In: Traite des Maladies du Rein, Vol. 2. Baillere, Tindall, and. Cox, editors. Paris; 1840.
9. Griesinger W. Studien uber diabetes. Archiv Physiologie Heilkunde. 1859;3:1–75.
10. Ebstein W. Weiteres über Diabetes mellitus, insbesondere über die Complicationdesselben mit Typhus abdominalis. Deutsch Arch f klin Med 1882;30:1–44.
11. Waku K. Ueber die Verunderung der Glomeruli der Diabetesniere. Tr Jap Path Soc. 1928;18:413–6.
12. Kimmelstiel P, Wilson C. Intercapillary lesions in glomeruli of kidney. Am J Pathol. 1936;12:83.
13. Allen AC. So-called intercapillary glomerulosclerois—a lesion associated with diabetes. Arch Pathol. 1941;32:33–51.
14. Iversen P, Brun C. Aspiration biopsy of the kidney. Am J Med. 1951;11(3):324–30.
15. Gellman DD, Pirani CL, Soothill JF, Muehrcke RC, Kark RM. Diabetic nephropathy. A clinical and pathologic study based on renal biopsies. Medicine (Baltimore). 1959;38:321–67.
16. Irvine E, Rinehart JF, Mortimore GE, Hopper JJ. The ultrastructure of the renal glomerulus in intercapillary glomerulosclerosis. Am J Pathol. 1956;32:647–53.
17. Østerby-Hansen R. A quantitative estimate of the peripheral glomerular basement membrane in recent juvenile diabetes. Diabetologia. 1965;1:97–100.
18. Yalow RS, Berson SA. Immunoassay of endogenous plasma insulin in man. J Clin Invest. 1960;39:1157–75.
19. Keen H, Chlouverakis C. An immunoassay method for urinary albumin in low concentrations. Lancet. 1963;ii:913–6.
20. Viberti GC, Hill RD, Argyropoulos A, Mahmud U, Keen H. Microalbuminuria as a predictor of clinical nephropathy in insulin-dependent diabetics. Lancet. 1982;i:1430–2.
21. Mogensen DE. Microabluminuria predicts clinical proteinuria and early mortality in maturity-onset diabetes. N Engl J Med. 1984;310:356–60.
22. Mogensen CE. Long-term antihypertensive treatment inhibiting progression of diabetic nephropathy. Br Med J. 1982;285:685–8.
23. American Diabetes Association. Hypertension management in adults with diabetes. Diabetes Care. 2004;27 Suppl 1:S65–7.
24. Basso N, Terragno NA. History about the discovery of the renin-angiotensin system. Hypertension. 2001;38:1246–9.
25. Kofoed-Enevoldsen A, Borch-Johnsen K, Kreiner S, Nerup J, Deckert T. Declining incidence of persistent proteinuria in type I (insulin-dependent) diabetics. Diabetes. 1987;36:205–9.
26. Krolewski AS, Warram JH, Chriestleib AR, Busick EJ, Kathan CR. The changing natural history of nephropathy in type I diabetes. Am J Med. 1985;78:785–94.
27. Zatz R, Brenner BM. Pathogenesis of diabetic nephropathy. The hemodynamic view. Am J Med. 1985;80:443–53.
28. Marre M, Chatellier G, Leblanc H, Guyene TT, Menard J, Passa P. Prevention of diabetic nephropathy with enalapril in normotensive diabetics with microalbuminuria. Br Med J. 1988;297:1092–5.
29. Lewis EJ, Hunsicker LG, Bain RP, Rohde RD, for the Collaborative Study Group. The effect of angiotensin-converting enzyme inhibition on diabetic nephropathy. N Engl J Med. 1993;329:1456–62.
30. Lewis EJ, Hunsicker LG, Clarke WR, et al., for the Collaborative Study Group. Renoprotective effect of the angiotensin-receptor antagonist irbesartan in patients with nephropathy due to type 2 diabetes. N Engl J Med. 2001;345:851–60.
31. Brenner BM, Cooper ME, de Zeeuw D, et al., for the RENAAL Study Investigators. Effects of Losartan on renal and cardiovascular outcomes in patients with type 2 diabetes and nephropathy. N Engl J Med. 2001;345:861–69.
32. Barnett AH. Inhibition of the renin-angiotensin system in diabetic patients—beyond HOPE. Br J Cardiol. 2004;11:123–7.
33. Parving H-H, Mauer M, Ritz E. Diabetic nephropathy. In: Brenner BM, editor. Brenner and rector's the kidney. 7th ed. Philadelphia: WB Saunders; 2004. p. 1777–818.
34. The EURODIAB IDDM Complications Study Group. Microvascular and acute complications in insulin dependent diabetes mellitus: The EURODIAB IDDM Complications Study. Diabetologia. 1994;37: 278–85.
35. Steffes MW, Sutherland DER, Goetz FC, Rich SS, Mauer SM. Studies of kidney and muscle biopsy specimens from identical twins discordant for type I diabetes mellitus. N Engl J Med. 1985;312:1282–7.
36. Mauer SM, Goetz FC, McHugh LE, Sutherland DE, Barbosa J, Najarian JS, Steffes MW. Long-term study of normal kidneys transplanted into patients with type I diabetes. Diabetes. 1989;38: 516–23.

37. Mauer SM, Steffes MW, Connett J, Najarian JS, Sutherland DE, Barbosa J. The development of lesions in the glomerular basement membrane and mesangium after transplantation of normal kidneys into diabetic patients. Diabetes. 1983;32:948–52.
38. Wiseman AC. Pancreas transplant options for patients with type 1 diabetes mellitus and chronic kidney disease: simultaneous pancreas kidney or pancreas after kidney? Curr Opin Organ Transplant. 2012;17(1):80–6.
39. Bohman S-O, Tyden G, Wilczek H, Lundgren G, Jaremko G, Gunnarsson R, Ostman J, Groth G. Prevention of kidney graft diabetic nephropathy by pancreas transplantation in man. Diabetes. 1985;34:306–8.
40. Wilczek HE, Jaremko G, Tyden G, Groth CG. Pancreatic graft protects a simultaneously transplanted kidney from developing diabetic nephropathy: a 1 to 6 year follow-up study. Transplant Proc. 1993;1:1314–5.
41. Young BY, Gill J, Huang E, et al. Living donor kidney versus simultaneous pancreas-kidney transplant in type I diabetics: an analysis of the OPTN/UNOS database. Clin J Am Soc Nephrol. 2009;4:845–52.
42. European Association for the Study of Diabetes (EASD) 48th Annual Meeting: Abstract 149. Presented October 4, 2012.
43. Diabetes Complications and Control Trial Research Group. The effect of intensive treatment of diabetes on the development and progression of long-term complications of insulin dependent diabetes mellitus. N Engl J Med. 1993;329:977–86.
44. UKPDS Group. Intensive blood-glucose control with sulphonylureas or insulin compared with conventional treatment and risk of complications in patients with type 2 diabetes. Lancet. 1998;352:837–53.
45. Ohkubo Y, Kishikawa H, Araki E, Miyata T, Isami S, Motoyoshi S, Kojima Y, Furuyoshi N, Shichiri M. Intensive insulin therapy prevents the progression of diabetic microvascular complications in Japanese patients with non-insulin-dependent diabetes mellitus: a randomized prospective 6-year study. Diabetes Res Clin Pract. 1995;28:103–17.
46. Levin SR, Coburn JW, et al. Effect of intensive glycemic control on microalbuminuria in type 2 diabetes. Veterans Affairs Cooperative Study on Glycemic Control and Complications in Type 2 Diabetes Feasibility Trial Investigators. Diabetes Care. 2000;23(10):1478–85.
47. Epidemiology of Diabetes Interventions and Complications (EDIC). Design, implementation, and preliminary results of a long-term follow-up of the Diabetes Control and Complications Trial cohort. Diabetes Care. 1999;22(1):99–111.
48. Coca SG, Ismail-Beigi F, Haq N, Krumholz HM, Parikh CR. Role of intensive glucose control in development of renal end points in type 2 diabetes mellitus systematic review and meta-analysis. Arch Intern Med. 2012;172(10):761–9.
49. Gerstein HC, Miller ME, Byington RP, et al. Effects of intensive glucose lowering in diabetes study group. type 2 diabetes. N Engl J Med. 2008;358:2545–59.
50. Patel A, MacMahon S, Chalmers J, Neal B, Billot L, Woodward M, Marre M, Cooper M, Glasziou P, Grobbee D, Hamet P, Harrap S, Heller S, Liu L, Mancia G, Mogensen CE, Pan C, Poulter N, Rodgers A, Williams B, Bompoint S, de Galan BE, Joshi R, Travert F. Intensive blood glucose control and vascular outcomes in patients with type 2 diabetes. N Engl J Med. 2008;358: 2560–72.
51. Burrows NR, Li Y, Geiss LS. Incidence of treatment for end-stage renal disease among individuals with diabetes in the U.S. continues to decline. Diabetes Care. 2010;33(1):73–7.

Part I

Natural Course, Pathogenesis, Morphology and Genetics

2 Diabetic Nephropathy: Scope of the Problem

Jing Chen

Diabetic nephropathy is a common complication of diabetes and the leading cause of chronic kidney disease in the developed world. Approximately 40 % of persons with diabetes develop diabetic nephropathy, manifested as albuminuria and/or decreased glomerular filtration rate. Even mild degrees of albuminuria and decrease in glomerular filtration rate are associated with significantly increased risks of cardiovascular disease, end-stage renal disease, and premature deaths.

Epidemiology of Diabetic Nephropathy

Prevalence of diabetes has reached epidemic proportions in the world. According to the International Diabetes Federation, there were 366 million people with diabetes in 2011, and this is expected to rise to 552 million by 2030 [1]. Most people with diabetes live in low- and middle-income countries, and these countries are anticipated the greatest increase in diabetes over the next decades. In the USA, 11.3 % or 25.6 million adults aged 20 years or older had diabetes in 2011, with prevalence increasing in older age groups (26.9 % of people aged ≥65 years) [2].

With the global epidemic of diabetes, diabetic nephropathy has become an important clinical and public health challenge. IH de Boer and colleagues estimated the disease burden of diabetic nephropathy in the US adult population aged 20 years or older using data from the National Health and Nutrition Examination Survey [3]. Diabetic nephropathy was defined as diabetes with the presence of albuminuria, impaired glomerular filtration rate, or both. The prevalence of diabetic nephropathy in the US adult population aged 20 years and older was 3.3 % (95 % confidence interval, 2.8–3.7 %) (Table 2.1). The estimated number of persons with diabetic nephropathy in the USA was 6.9 million (95 % CI, 6.0–7.9 million) during 2005–2008 [3]. Among the US adults with diabetes, the prevalence of any diabetic nephropathy was 34.5 %, the prevalence of albuminuria (with or without impaired glomerular filtration rate) was 23.7 %, and the prevalence of impaired glomerular filtration rate (with or without albuminuria) was 17.7 % in 2005–2008 (Table 2.1).

The prevalence of diabetic nephropathy in the general population was not available from other countries. However, the prevalence of albuminuria in diabetes patients was reported in various populations. Parving HH et al. reported the prevalence of micro-/macroalbuminuria in a cross-sectional study among 32,208 type 2 diabetes patients from 33 countries [4]. The overall prevalence of microalbuminuria and macroalbuminuria was 38.8 % and 9.8 %, respectively, in the study population. Asian and Hispanic patients had the highest prevalence of microalbuminuria (43.2 % and 43.8 %) and macroalbuminuria (12.3 % and 10.3 %) while Caucasians had the lowest microalbuminuria (33.3 %) and macroalbuminuria (7.6 %). Twenty-two percent of patients had impaired renal function (glomerular filtration rate <60 mL/min/1.73 m^2). Unnikrishnan RI and colleagues reported that the prevalence of overt nephropathy and microalbuminuria was 2.2 % and 26.9 %, respectively, among type 2 diabetes patients in urban Asian Indians [5]. Among 8,897 Japanese type 2 diabetes patients from 29 medical clinics (i.e., general practitioners) or general/university-affiliated hospitals from different areas, the prevalence of microalbuminuria and decreased glomerular filtration rate (<60 mL/min per 1.73 m^2) was 31.6 % and 10.5 %, respectively [6].

The prevalence of diabetic nephropathy varied among ethnic groups in the US population. The Pathways Study, a cross-sectional analysis among 2,969 primary care diabetic patients of a large regional health maintenance organization observed the racial/ethnic differences in early diabetic nephropathy despite comparable access to diabetes care [7]. Among those without hypertension, microalbuminuria was two-fold greater (odds ratio 2.01; 95 % confidence interval 1.14–3.53)

J. Chen, M.D., M.M.Sc., M.Sc. (✉)
Department of Medicine, Tulane University School of Medicine, 1430 Tulane Avenue, SL45, New Orleans, LA, USA
e-mail: jchen@tulane.edu

E.V. Lerma and V. Batuman (eds.), *Diabetes and Kidney Disease*,
DOI 10.1007/978-1-4939-0793-9_2, © Springer Science+Business Media New York 2014

Table 2.1 Prevalence (95 % confidence interval) of diabetic nephropathy in the US population, NHANES 2005–2008

		Persons with diabetes		
	Overall US population	Total	Albuminuria	Impaired GFR
Age ≥20 years	3.3 (2.8, 3.7)	34.5 (30.5, 38.5)	23.7 (19.3, 28.0)	17.7 (15.2, 20.2)
Age 20–64 years	1.8 (1.4, 2.1)	24.6 (19.9, 29.3)	20.7 (16.3, 25.1)	6.0 (3.9, 8.2)
Age ≥65 years	10.7 (9.3, 12.2)	51.2 (45.7, 56.7)	28.7 (23.5, 33.8)	37.4 (3.5, 43.3)

Data are adopted from de Boer IH et al. JAMA. 2011;305(24):2532–9

and macroalbuminuria was threefold greater (odds ratio 3.17; 95 % confidence interval 1.09–9.26) for Asians as compared with whites. Among those with hypertension, adjusted odds of microalbuminuria were greater for Hispanics (odds ratio 3.82; 95 % confidence interval 1.16–12.57) than whites, whereas adjusted odds of macroalbuminuria were threefold greater for blacks (odds ratio 3.32; 95 % confidence interval 1.26–8.76) than for whites [7].

The prevalence of diabetic nephropathy has been increasing in the US population. For example, de Boer and colleagues reported that the diabetic nephropathy prevalence increased 18 % from 1988–1994 to 1999–2004 and 34 % from 1988–1994 to 2005–2008 ($p=0.003$ for trend). Increase in the prevalence of diabetic nephropathy was directly related to the increased prevalence of diabetes, without a change in the prevalence of diabetic nephropathy among those with diabetes [3]. Increases in diabetic nephropathy prevalence were largest for persons aged 65 years or older among whom diabetic nephropathy was most common.

Diabetic nephropathy is the single leading cause of end-stage renal disease, accounting for nearly half of all end-stage renal disease cases [8]. The US Renal Data System reported that the incidence rates (per million population) of end-stage renal disease due to diabetes, hypertension, glomerulonephritis, and cystic kidney disease in 2010 were 152, 99, 22.7, and 8.1, respectively [8]. The prevalence of end-stage renal disease due to diabetes, hypertension, glomerulonephritis, and cystic kidney disease in 2010 were 656, 437, 263, and 85, respectively. Diabetic nephropathy is also the major cause of end-stage renal disease in other western populations [9, 10].

The costs for diabetic nephropathy to individual and society are considerable [8, 11, 12]. In the USA, total Medicare spending in 2010 was $522.8 billion and expenditure for end-stage renal disease was $32.9 billion [8]. This number did not include expenditure for non-Medicare patients, which was additionally estimated to be $14.5 billion [8]. In 2010, overall per person per year costs for patients with chronic kidney disease reached $22,323 for Medicare patients aged 65 and older and $13,395 for non-Medicare patients aged 50–64 in the MarketScan database [8]. Among Medicare patients with both chronic kidney disease and diabetes, per person per year costs for African-Americans reached $28,651 and $24,593 in whites in 2010 [8]. The cost of diabetic nephropathy progression was recently analyzed using information from the Kaiser Permanente Northwest health maintenance organization [12]. Among patients who progressed, annual medical costs were 37 % higher following progression from normoalbuminuria to microalbuminuria ($10,188 vs. $7,424) and 41 % higher following progression from microalbuminuria to macroalbuminuria ($12,371 vs. $8,753).

In summary, the prevalence of diabetic nephropathy is high and increasing in the US and other populations. Diabetic nephropathy accounts for nearly half of all incident cases of end-stage renal disease in the USA. In addition, diabetic nephropathy is associated with increased mortality from cardiovascular disease and all causes. Medicare and non-Medicare spending on diabetic nephropathy and consequent end-stage renal disease is substantial in the USA. Therefore, the prevention of diabetic nephropathy is important to improve health outcomes of persons with diabetes and to reduce the societal burden of chronic kidney disease.

Obesity, Metabolic Syndrome, and Diabetic Nephropathy

The growing prevalence of obesity and metabolic syndrome (the cluster of risk factors including hypertension, insulin resistance and dyslipidemia) is the major driving force for the continued increase in the prevalence of type 2 diabetes [13]. These disorders likely interact to exacerbate the kidney damage (Fig. 2.1).

Hypertension associated with obesity, metabolic syndrome, and diabetes may play an important role in the pathogenesis of diabetic nephropathy. Previous studies indicate that central obesity, metabolic syndrome, and diabetes lead to increase of blood pressure [14–17]. Clinical trials also indicate that weight loss reduces blood pressure in most hypertensive subjects and is effective in primary prevention of hypertension [15].

Central obesity induces hypertension initially by increasing renal tubular reabsorption of sodium and causing a hypertensive shift of renal-pressure natriuresis through multiple mechanisms including activation of the sympathetic nervous system and renin–angiotensin–aldosterone system, as well as physical compression of the kidneys [18, 19]. The hypertension, as well as the increases in intraglomerular capillary

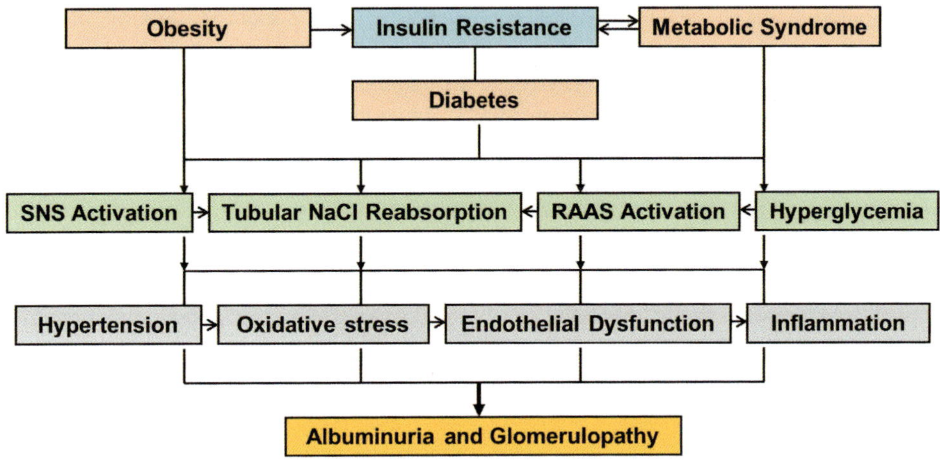

Fig. 2.1 Interaction of obesity-, metabolic syndrome-, and diabetes-related kidney disease. *SNS* sympathetic nervous system, *RAAS* renin–angiotensin–aldosterone system

pressure, and the metabolic abnormalities (e.g., dyslipidemia, hyperglycemia) likely interact to accelerate renal injury. Similar to obesity-associated glomerular hyperfiltration, renal vasodilation and increases in glomerular filtration rate and intraglomerular capillary pressure, and increased blood pressure also are characteristics of diabetic nephropathy [20]. Increased systolic blood pressure further exacerbates the disease progression to proteinuria and a decline in glomerular filtration rate leading to end-stage renal disease [21]. Multiple studies have clearly shown the protective effect on the kidneys of reducing blood pressure in diabetes. Furthermore, tight blood pressure control in diabetic patients may slow progression of nephropathy to a greater extent than tight control of blood glucose [22].

Hyperfiltration and increased glomerular filtration rate are the common early renal changes associated obesity and diabetes [20, 23]. The underlying mechanism may include increased salt reabsorption by the proximal tubule or loop of Henle, leading to tubuloglomerular feedback-mediated reduction in afferent arteriolar resistance, increased intraglomerular capillary pressure, and increased glomerular filtration rate [24]. The increased glomerular filtration rate initially serves as a compensatory response that permits restoration of salt balance but eventually contributes to renal injury, especially when blood pressure is elevated. Tubuloglomerular feedback-mediated dilation of afferent arterioles and attendant impairment of renal autoregulation permit increases in blood pressure to be transmitted to the glomerular capillaries causing even greater increases in intraglomerular capillary pressure and glomerular injury than would occur with comparable increases in blood pressure in kidneys of non-obese, nondiabetic subjects [25]. In addition, hyperglycemia may also contribute to the development of glomerular hyperfiltration through mechanisms similar to those occurring in obesity. Reduced delivery of salt to the macula densa, as a consequence of increased proximal reabsorption of glucose and sodium, may reduce afferent arteriolar resistance and increase intraglomerular capillary pressure and glomerular filtration rate via attenuated tubuloglomerular feedback [26–28]. Also, afferent vasodilation and efferent vasoconstriction in response to circulating or locally formed vasoactive factors (e.g., angiotensin II) produced in response to hyperglycemia or shear stress may promote diabetic glomerular hyperfiltration [29, 30]. Even though the mechanisms explaining the increase in glomerular filtration rate in diabetes and obesity uncomplicated by diabetes may be similar, the factors that trigger tubuloglomerular feedback-mediated renal vasodilation and glomerular hyperfiltration are different. Some studies suggest that hyperglycemia, obesity, and hypertension may have at least partially additive effects on glomerular hemodynamics [25]. For example, mice lacking the gene for the melanocortin-4 receptor are obese, hyperinsulinemic, and hyperleptinemic but normotensive at 55 weeks of age [32]. These animals have moderately increased glomerular filtration rate and only modest albuminuria compared with WT mice; however, their glomerular filtration rate and albuminuria increased further when rendered hypertensive following treatment with N(G)-nitro-L-arginine methyl ester. These data suggest that elevations in blood pressure exacerbate obesity-related glomerular hyperfiltration and albuminuria, further supporting the concept of an additive, or perhaps synergistic, effect of various components of obesity, metabolic syndrome, diabetes, and hypertension on glomerular hemodynamics. In addition, obesity, metabolic syndrome and diabetes are states of low-grade inflammation and oxidative stress, all of which may lead to kidney damage, progressive loss of nephrons, and decline in glomerular filtration rate over time. Another element of the metabolic syndrome, hyperlipidemia, has been linked to reductions in glomerular filtration rate in diabetic nephropathy, especially in the latter stages of the disease. Numerous clinical trials have pointed to the importance of lipid control in preserving glomerular filtration rate in patients with diabetes [33]. However, further studies are needed to determine if the beneficial effects of lipid-lowering agents in diabetic nephropathy are due to improvement in the lipid profile or if there are other renoprotective effects.

Diabetic nephropathy and elements of the metabolic syndrome including insulin resistance and hyperinsulinemia are associated with the development of microalbuminuria early in the disease process [34, 35]. The development of microalbuminuria in diabetic nephropathy was traditionally thought to stem from damage to the glomerular filtration barrier as a consequence of increases in blood pressure which are transmitted to the glomeruli, raising intraglomerular capillary pressure and glomerular filtration rate, and/or hyperglycemia-associated inflammation and oxidative stress [34]. An alternative explanation is that diabetes also impairs proximal tubular reabsorption of albumin which filters across the glomerular barrier [36]. Hyperlipidemia is known to be a risk factor for the development of albuminuria in patients with diabetes [37].

Diabetes and obesity are both states of low-grade inflammation associated with macrophage infiltration into the adipose tissue and the kidney. The infiltrating macrophages become a source of a whole host of proinflammatory cytokines including tumor necrosis factor-α, interleukin-6, and monocyte chemoattractant protein-1 [38]. Furthermore, increased adiposity triggers the release of adipokines into the circulation that in turn may cause renal injury via production of reactive oxygen species. Persistent hyperglycemia also activates vasoactive hormonal pathways including the renin–angiotensin system and endothelin. These in turn activate common second messenger signaling pathways such as protein kinase C and mitogen-activated protein kinase and transcription factors such as nuclear factor-κB that lead to the alteration in gene expression of a plethora of growth factors and cytokines such as transforming growth factor-β. Transforming growth factor-β is a key player in promoting podocyte apoptosis, mesangial cell proliferation and extracellular matrix synthesis, and cellular events that are important in the development of diabetes and obesity-associated glomerular injury [39]. Hyperglycemia and associated metabolic disturbances also cause mitochondrial dysfunction and enhanced generation of reactive oxygen species, which directly alter the expression of key proteins and cytokines causing renal injury. Kidneys of obese individuals often have glomerular/mesangial lipid deposits (foam cells) present, which supports the concept of lipotoxicity, i.e., lipid-induced renal injury [25]. One of the mechanisms by which hyperlipidemia promotes glomerular injury is through renal upregulation of sterol-regulatory element-binding proteins, which in turn promotes podocyte apoptosis and mesangial cell proliferation and cytokine synthesis.

In summary, data from basic and clinical studies suggest that obesity, hypertension, hyperglycemia, hyperlipidemia, and other elements of the metabolic syndrome are highly interrelated and contribute to the development and progression of diabetic nephropathy. Therefore spontaneously targeting at prevention and treatment of obesity, metabolic syndrome, and diabetes may help to maximize the reduction of associated kidney damage.

Geriatrics and Diabetic Nephropathy

Increase in the prevalence of diabetic nephropathy also derives directly from the growth in the prevalence of diabetic nephropathy among individuals aged 65 years and older. Individuals older than 65 years are disproportionately affected by diabetes and related end-stage renal disease. According to data from the National Health and Nutrition Examination Survey, diabetes prevalence was 26.9 % among people aged ≥65 years [2, 40]. The prevalence of diabetic nephropathy was increased from 7.1 % in 1988–1994 to 8.6 % in 1999–2004 and 10.7 % in 2005–2008 among individuals aged 65 years and older [3, 41]. Recent data also revealed that the adjusted point prevalence rates per million population of reported diabetes-related end-stage renal disease for individuals aged 60–69 and ≥70 years were 410.3 and 475.7 in whites and 1439.9 and 1471.5 in African-Americans [8, 42].

Although diabetic nephropathy represents a major health threat for the aging American population, chronic kidney disease care in elderly subjects with diabetes is suboptimal. Patel and colleagues [43] reported that only 7.2 % of 6,033 veterans (mean age 66 ± 11 years) with diabetes and chronic kidney disease underwent evaluation by a nephrologist during a 5-year study period. Furthermore, clinical guidelines developed by the American Geriatrics Society Panel on Improving Care for Elders with Diabetes have not specifically focused on the subject of advanced chronic kidney disease in older patients with diabetes [44].

One of the challenges of managing the elderly with diabetic nephropathy is that they may develop more complications, especially heart, eye, and peripheral vascular diseases. In its 2011 National Diabetes Fact Sheet, the Centers for Disease Control reported that in 2004, heart disease and prior stroke were, respectively, noted on 68 % and 16 % of diabetes-related death certificates among people aged 65 years or older [2]. Moreover, the CDC indicated that, in 2005, 27 % of adults with diabetes who were 75 years or older reported some degree of visual impairment compared with 15 % of diabetic patients who were between 18 and

44 years of age [2]. Individuals aged 65 years or older account for 55 % of diabetic subjects who had nontraumatic lower extremity amputations [45]. Caring for elderly patients with diabetic renal disease imposes a huge financial burden on governments and family members. For example, the American Diabetes Association indicated that the total estimated cost of diabetes in 2007 was $174 billion, including $58 billion to treat diabetes-related chronic complications [46].

Diabetic nephropathy in the elderly is mainly due to type 2 diabetes and its distribution is uneven among racial groups. American-Indians, African-Americans, and Mexican-Americans have a greater incidence than Caucasians by as much as three to one depending on the minority cohort selected for comparison [42]. Genetic susceptibility, suboptimal care in minority groups, delayed diagnosis of type 2 diabetes, and environmental factors are reasons proposed to explain such disparity.

The histologic diagnosis of diabetic nephropathy in older patients may be challenging because mesangial matrix expansion and thickening of the glomerular basement membrane have also been attributed to kidney senescence [47]. Likewise, tubular atrophy and interstitial fibrosis may be aging related or due to chronic inflammation or vascular disease [48]. Elderly patients with type 2 diabetes may have renal ischemia due to renal artery stenosis. Sawicki and colleagues [49] reported that the prevalence of renal artery stenosis in subjects with type 2 diabetes and hypertension was greater than 10 %. Bilateral artery stenosis was found in 43 % of these cases.

Nearly all studies demonstrating beneficial effects of metabolic and blood pressure controls on diabetic kidney disease have been performed in young to middle-aged cohorts. Importantly, the management of diabetic kidney disease in older people is frequently based on extrapolations of data gathered in selected and motivated younger people. Moreover, people older than 70 years have been virtually excluded in trials supporting major US practice guidelines for the use of angiotensin-converting enzyme inhibitors and angiotensin receptor blockers in chronic kidney disease. In managing diabetes and diabetic nephropathy in the elderly, clinicians should keep in mind several key points. (1) Elderly diabetic patients constitute a diverse group expressing various clinical and functional situations. (2) The American Geriatric Society Panel on Improving Care for Elders with Diabetes recommends that treatment of elderly patients with diabetes focus on specific problems and priorities [50]. (3) The American Geriatric Society has also introduced the concept of time horizon for the benefits of certain treatments. Glycemic control may take as long as 8 years to have positive results on microvascular complications. Benefits of good blood pressure and lipid control may not be noticeable before 2 or 3 years [51]. (4) Many elderly patients with diabetes are frail and are also at greater risk for developing several common geriatric syndromes, such as depression, cognitive impairment, urinary incontinence, injurious falls, and persistent pain. The Assessing Care of Vulnerable Elders (ACOVE) project defines a frail elderly patient as a vulnerable person who is older than 65 years and is at increased risk of death or functional decline within 2 years [51]. (5) In consequence, renoprotection in a geriatric population should be tailored according to patients' autonomy, degree of frailty, life expectancy, comorbidity index, and the stage of diabetic nephropathy. (6) Elderly diabetic patients may be susceptible to nephrotoxic agents such as radiocontrast; specific caution should be taken in preventing and monitoring radiocontrast-induced nephropathy.

Caring for geriatric patients afflicted by diabetic nephropathy requires a long-term commitment by patients and health care professionals. This care is better accomplished by a team consisting of a primary care physician or geriatrician, an endocrinologist, a nephrologist, a cardiologist, an ophthalmologist, a podiatrist, a nutritionist, and a nurse educator. Much effort should be made to diagnose type 2 diabetes early and educate diabetic subjects and primary care providers about the effectiveness of glycemic control and blood pressure lowering to prevent or delay diabetic nephropathy and end-stage renal disease.

References

1. Whiting D, Guariguata L, Weil C, et al. IDF diabetes atlas: global estimates of the prevalence of diabetes for 2011 and 2030. Diabetes Res Clin Pract. 2011;94:311–21.
2. Centers for Disease Control and Prevention. National diabetes fact sheet: national estimates and general information on diabetes and prediabetes in the United States, 2011. US Department of Health and Human Services. Atlanta, GA: Centers for Disease Control and Prevention; 2011.
3. de Boer IH, Rue TC, Hall YN, Heagerty PJ, Weiss NS, Himmelfarb J. Temporal trends in the prevalence of diabetic kidney disease in the United States. JAMA. 2011;305(24):2532–9.
4. Parving H, Lewis J, Ravid M, et al. Prevalence and risk factors for microalbuminuria in a referred cohort of type II diabetic patients: a global perspective. Kidney Int. 2006;69:2057–63.
5. Unnikrishnan R, Rema M, Pradeepa R, et al. Prevalence and risk factors of diabetic nephropathy in an urban South Indian population: the Chennai Urban Rural Epidemiology Study (CURES 45). Diabetes Care. 2007;30:2019–24.
6. Yokoyama H, Sone H, Oishi M, Kawai K, Fukumoto Y, Kobayashi M. Japan Diabetes Clinical Data Management Study Group. Prevalence of albuminuria and renal insufficiency and associated clinical factors in type 2 diabetes: the Japan Diabetes Clinical Data Management study (JDDM15). Nephrol Dial Transplant. 2009; 24(4):1212–9.
7. Young B, Katon W, Von Korff M, et al. Racial and ethnic differences in microalbuminuria prevalence in a diabetes population: the pathways study. J Am Soc Nephrol. 2005;16:219–28.
8. US Renal Data System. USRDS 2012 Annual Data Report: Atlas of Chronic Kidney Disease and End-Stage Renal Disease in the United States. National Institutes of Health, National Institute of Diabetes and Digestive and Kidney Diseases. Bethesda, MD; 2012.

9. Hill CJ, Fogarty DG. Changing trends in end-stage renal disease due to diabetes in the United Kingdom. J Ren Care. 2012;38 Suppl 1:12–22.
10. Grace B, Clayton P, McDonald S. Increases in renal replacement therapy in Australia and New Zealand: understanding trends in diabetic nephropathy. Nephrology (Carlton). 2012;17:76–84.
11. Deloitte Access Economics. Two of a KinD (Kidneys in Diabetes): the burden of diabetic kidney disease and the cost effectiveness of screening people with type 2 diabetes for chronic kidney disease. Kidney Health Australia. Melbourne, VIC: Kidney Health Australia; 2011.
12. Nichols G, Vupputuri S, Lau H. Medical care costs associated with progression of diabetic nephropathy. Diabetes Care. 2011;34:2374–8.
13. Ogden CL, Carroll MD, Curtin LR, McDowell MA, Tabak CJ, Flegal KM. Prevalence of overweight and obesity in the United States, 1999–2004. JAMA. 2006;295:1549–55.
14. Hall JE, Jones DW, Kuo JJ, da Silva A, Tallam LS, Liu J. Impact of the obesity epidemic on hypertension and renal disease. Curr Hypertens Rep. 2003;5:386–92.
15. Neter JE, Stam BE, Kok FJ, Grobbee DE, Geleijnse JM. Influence of weight reduction on blood pressure: a meta-analysis of randomized controlled trials. Hypertension. 2003;42:878–84.
16. Garrison RJ, Kannel WB, Stokes III J, Castelli WP. Incidence and precursors of hypertension in young adults: the Framingham Offspring Study. Prev Med. 1987;16:235–51.
17. Maric-Bilkan C. Obesity and diabetic kidney disease. Med Clin North Am. 2013;97(1):59–74.
18. Hall JE, Henegar JR, Dwyer TM, Liu J, Da Silva AA, Kuo JJ, Tallam L. Is obesity a major cause of chronic kidney disease? Adv Ren Replace Ther. 2004;11:41–54.
19. Henegar JR, Bigler SA, Henegar LK, Tyagi SC, Hall JE. Functional and structural changes in the kidney in the early stages of obesity. J Am Soc Nephrol. 2001;12:1211–7.
20. Yip JW, Jones SL, Wiseman MJ, Hill C, Viberti G. Glomerular hyperfiltration in the prediction of nephropathy in IDDM: a 10-year follow-up study. Diabetes. 1996;45:1729–33.
21. Van Buren PN, Toto R. Hypertension in diabetic nephropathy: epidemiology, mechanisms, and management. Adv Chronic Kidney Dis. 2011;18:28–41.
22. Mancia G. Effects of intensive blood pressure control in the management of patients with type 2 diabetes mellitus in the Action to Control Cardiovascular Risk in Diabetes (ACCORD) trial. Circulation. 2010;122:847–9.
23. Chagnac A, Weinstein T, Herman M, Hirsh J, Gafter U, Ori Y. The effects of weight loss on renal function in patients with severe obesity. J Am Soc Nephrol. 2003;14:1480–6.
24. Hall JE. The kidney, hypertension, and obesity. Hypertension. 2003;41:625–33.
25. Griffin KA, Kramer H, Bidani AK. Adverse renal consequences of obesity. Am J Physiol Renal Physiol. 2008;294:F685–96.
26. Vallon V, Schroth J, Satriano J, Blantz RC, Thomson SC, Rieg T. Adenosine A(1) receptors determine glomerular hyperfiltration and the salt paradox in early streptozotocin diabetes mellitus. Nephron Physiol. 2009;111:30–8.
27. Woods LL, Mizelle HL, Hall JE. Control of renal hemodynamics in hyperglycemia: possible role of tubuloglomerular feedback. Am J Physiol. 1987;252:F65–73.
28. Persson P, Hansell P, Palm F. Tubular reabsorption and diabetes-induced glomerular hyperfiltration. Acta Physiol (Oxf). 2010;200:3–10.
29. Cherney DZ, Scholey JW, Miller JA. Insights into the regulation of renal hemodynamic function in diabetic mellitus. Curr Diabetes Rev. 2008;4:280–90.
30. Carmines PK. The renal vascular response to diabetes. Curr Opin Nephrol Hypertens. 2010;19:85–90.
31. Jauregui A, Mintz DH, Mundel P, Fornoni A. Role of altered insulin signaling pathways in the pathogenesis of podocyte malfunction and microalbuminuria. Curr Opin Nephrol Hypertens. 2009;18:539–45.
32. do Carmo JM, Tallam LS, Roberts JV, Brandon EL, Biglane J, da Silva AA, Hall JE. Impact of obesity on renal structure and function in the presence and absence of hypertension: evidence from melanocortin-4 receptor-deficient mice. Am J Physiol Regul Integr Comp Physiol. 2009;297:R803–12.
33. Fried LF, Orchard TJ, Kasiske BL. Effect of lipid reduction on the progression of renal disease: a meta-analysis. Kidney Int. 2001;59:260–9.
34. Jauregui A, Mintz DH, Mundel P, Fornoni A. Role of altered insulin signaling pathways in the pathogenesis of podocyte malfunction and microalbuminuria. Curr Opin Nephrol Hypertens. 2009;18:539–45.
35. de Boer IH, Sibley SD, Kestenbaum B, Sampson JN, Young B, Cleary PA, Steffes MW, Weiss NS, Brunzell JD. Central obesity, incident microalbuminuria, and change in creatinine clearance in the epidemiology of diabetes interventions and complications study. J Am Soc Nephrol. 2007;18:235–43.
36. Comper WD, Russo LM. The glomerular filter: an imperfect barrier is required for perfect renal function. Curr Opin Nephrol Hypertens. 2009;18:336–42.
37. Rutledge JC, Ng KF, Aung HH, Wilson DW. Role of triglyceride-rich lipoproteins in diabetic nephropathy. Nat Rev Nephrol. 2010;6:361–70.
38. King GL. The role of inflammatory cytokines in diabetes and its complications. J Periodontol. 2008;79:1527–34.
39. Ziyadeh FN. Mediators of diabetic renal disease: the case for tgf-Beta as the major mediator. J Am Soc Nephrol. 2004;15:S55–7.
40. McDonald M, Hertz RP, Unger AN, et al. Prevalence, awareness, and management of hypertension, dyslipidemia, and diabetes among United States adults aged 65 and older. J Gerontol A Biol Sci Med Sci. 2009;64(2):256–63.
41. Coresh J, Selvin E, Stevens LA, et al. Prevalence of chronic kidney disease in the United States. JAMA. 2007;298(17):2038–47.
42. United States Renal Data System. USRDS 2008 annual data report. Bethesda, MD: National Institutes of Health, National Institute of Diabetes and Digestive and Kidney Diseases; 2008.
43. Patel UD, Young EW, Ojo AO, et al. CKD progression and mortality among older patients with diabetes. Am J Kidney Dis. 2005;46(3):406–14.
44. Abaterusso C, Lupo A, Ortalda V, et al. Treating elderly people with diabetes and stages 3 and 4 chronic kidney disease. Clin J Am Soc Nephrol. 2008;3:1185–94.
45. Sugarman JR, Reiber GE, Baumgardner G, et al. Use of therapeutic footwear benefit among diabetic medicare beneficiaries in three states, 1995. Diabetes Care. 1998;21:777–81.
46. American Diabetes Association. Economic costs of diabetes in the U.S. in 2007. Diabetes Care. 2008;31(3):596–615.
47. Zhou XJ, Laszik ZG, Silva FG. Anatomical changes in the aging kidney. In: Macias-Nunez JF, Cameron JS, Oreopoulos DG, editors. The aging kidney in health and disease. New York: Springer; 2007. p. 39–54.
48. Nadasdy T, Laszik ZG, Blick KE. Tubular atrophy in the end-stage kidney: a lectin and immunohistochemical study. Hum Pathol. 1994;25:22–8.
49. Sawicki P, Kaiser S, Heinemann L, et al. Prevalence of renal artery stenosis in diabetes mellitus: an autopsy study. J Intern Med. 1991;229:489–92.
50. Brown SF, Mangione CM, Saliba D, et al. California Healthcare Foundation/American Geriatrics Society Panel Improving Care for Elders with Diabetes. Guidelines for improving the care of older persons with diabetes mellitus. J Am Geriatr Soc. 2003;51 Suppl 5:S265–80.
51. Wenger NS, Shekelle PG, Roth CP. The ACOVE investigators: introduction to the assessing care of vulnerable elders-3 quality indicator measurement set. J Am Geriatr Soc. 2007;55 Suppl 2:S247–52.

3 Natural Course (Stages/Evidence-Based Discussion)

Aileen K. Wang and Tina K. Thethi

Introduction

Diabetic kidney disease (DKD) has historically been called diabetic nephropathy if there is macroalbuminuria or proteinuria [1, 2]. DKD is a progressive kidney disease as a complication of prolonged hyperglycemia that occurs in both type 1 (T1) and type 2 (T2) diabetes mellitus (DM). Some of the secondary causes of DM include medications, pancreatic disorder, and excess of hormones such as cortisol, catecholamine, or growth hormone, and genetic predisposition [3]. According to national diabetes fact sheet of 2011, DM is the most common cause of renal failure in 2008 in the United States (USA), making about 44 % of all new cases [4]. Another survey among US adults collected by National Health and Nutrition Examination Survey (NHANES) in 2010 showed that prevalence of end stage renal disease (ESRD) due to diabetes increased 1.8 % to 656 million per population [5]. The incidence of ESRD secondary to diabetes is the most common accounting for 152 per million population in 2010 [5]. T2DM accounts for about 90 % of diabetes; thus it is a more common cause of DKD including ESRD [5]. ESRD secondary to T2DM varies among countries and racial group from 43 % in Europe to 61 % in Australia [6]. Similarly among patients with T1DM, ESRD from initial diagnosis has occurred 2.2 % at 20 years and 7.8 % at 30 years in Finland [7] and 4 % at 10 years and 7 % at 20 years after development of persistent microalbuminuria in Diabetes Control and Complication Trial (DCCT) and Epidemiology of Diabetes Interventions and Complications (EDIC) Study [8].

The use of terminology for DKD has been introduced for consistent classification of chronic kidney disease (CKD) by Diabetes and CKD guidelines and its use has been endorsed by Kidney Disease Outcomes Quality Initiative (KDOQI) Clinical Practice Guidelines and Clinical Practice Recommendations (CPGCPR) for Diabetes and CKD [9]. It has been suggested to use the term DKD as "presumptive diagnosis of kidney disease caused by diabetes" in place of diabetic nephropathy [9]. KDOQI CPGCPR recommends using the term diabetic glomerulopathy for kidney disease due to diabetes diagnosed by kidney biopsy [9].

Natural History of DKD in T1DM

Studies in the 1960s to 1980s have recognized that at diagnosis of T1DM changes occur in kidneys' function, structure and biochemical parameters and have laid the groundwork to characterization of the natural course of DKD, which occurs in series of five stages [10–15]. As the clinical onset of T1DM is well known compared to T2DM, where diagnosis may have been delayed, much of our understanding of DKD has been delineated mainly from experimental animal models and partly from patients with T1DM. However, not all animal models resemble the actual human disease process and thus the knowledge of the course of kidney disease comes with limitations. Approximately 25–40 % of patients with T1DM and 5–40 % with T2DM develop diabetic nephropathy [10]. Numerous factors have been associated with the development of DKD such as hypertension, cardiovascular disease (CVD), hyperlipidemia, and obesity (BMI ≥ 30) [9]. This chapter will discuss the current understanding of the etiology, disease course, different stages of and modification related to DKD.

A.K. Wang, M.D. (✉)
Department of Medicine, Section of Endocrinology, Tulane University Health Sciences Center, 1430 Tulane Avenue, SL-53, 1601 Perdido Street, New Orleans, LA 70112, USA
e-mail: awang7@tulane.edu

T.K. Thethi, M.D., M.P.H.
Department of Medicine, Section of Endocrinology, Tulane University Health Sciences Center, 1430 Tulane Avenue, SL-53, 1601 Perdido Street, New Orleans, LA 70112, USA

Southeast Louisiana Veterans Health Care, New Orleans, LA, USA

E.V. Lerma and V. Batuman (eds.), *Diabetes and Kidney Disease*,
DOI 10.1007/978-1-4939-0793-9_3, © Springer Science+Business Media New York 2014

Associated metabolic abnormalities resulting from DM lead to alterations in hemodynamics, structural, and biochemical parameters within kidneys [1, 10]. Many investigative studies have paved the way in identification of different stages that occur in DKD. Nephropathy is preceded by microalbuminuria. DKD (also been previously known as diabetic nephropathy) can be described in five stages in relation to changes at function such as urinary albumin excretion (UAE) and glomerular filtration rate (GFR), and structure in terms of renal morphology. The majority of changes in different stages have been best delineated by Mogensen in 1983 [1, 10, 16]. In this chapter, we will discuss the various stages of DKD, which are summarized in Table 3.1 including the unique characteristics at each stage.

The natural history of DKD in T1DM and T2DM is not quite the same but the stages have more similarities than differences, which will be discussed later in this chapter under the stages for T2DM. The differences can be seen in various ethnicities and age groups between the two types of diabetes. For example, patients with T1DM are younger at diagnosis compared to T2DM [8, 15, 17–19]. The DKD utilizes the same UAE values for classification of microalbuminuria and macroalbuminuria, and GFR value for both T1DM and T2DM and CKD stages.

The National Kidney Foundation (NKF) classifies CKD based on GFR, which is different from staging by UAE level in other systems. NKF defines CKD as "kidney damage or GFR less than 60 mL/min/1.73 m^2 for 3 or more months" [20]. It also defines "kidney damage" as "pathologic abnormalities or markers of damage, including abnormalities in blood or urine tests or imaging studies" [20, 21]. There can be coexistence of DKD and CKD as not all CKD are due to DKD [9]. NKF recommends utilizing Modification of Diet in Renal Disease (MDRD) equation for estimation of GFR [9]. The stages of CKD classified by GFR in relation to UAE value are shown in Table 3.2. Some cases of CKD may need kidney biopsy to confirm the diagnosis of DKD [9].

Stage 1: Hypertrophy-Hyperfiltration

The initial stage is known as hypertrophy-hyperfiltration or -hyperfunction. At diagnosis of T1DM the changes in function, morphology, and biochemical profile occur within diabetic kidneys. The experimental models of animals and humans with DM have displayed initial structural changes of growth in kidney size and function [16, 22–24]. The functional changes such as increase in GFR [11, 17, 24], renal plasma flow (RPF) [11, 15, 24, 25], and filtration fraction (FF) [11, 24] occur in subjects with diabetes in the initial stage [22]. At diagnosis and less than 1-year duration of DM, these changes have been shown to be present [11]. Structural alteration of increased kidney volume [15, 24, 26] can be seen within days to weeks of T1DM diagnosis and may contribute to increased GFR [22, 27]. Biochemical or hormonal alterations in DM includes hyperglycemia, hypoinsulinemia, hyperglucagonemia, normal to elevated growth hormone, and increased UAE, which may also contribute to increased GFR [14, 22, 24, 28]. The changes occurring in stage 1 may be completely or partially reversible [27].

The increased GFR demonstrated in animal models of T1DM [29] as well as in most human cases of T1DM [24, 26] as a consequence of renal hypertrophy [30] and intrarenal hemodynamic abnormalities due to hyperglycemia is responsible for hyperfiltration [1, 10, 31]. This in turn leads to glomerular hypertension [32].

The streptozotocin-induced diabetes rat model in the early stage has shown kidney hypertrophy [14, 33] and altered renal metabolism of pyrimidine nucleotide metabolism especially uridine triphosphate (UTP) with greater RNA content and increased transforming growth factor-beta (TGF-β) receptor in the renal cortex [33, 34]. In the diabetic kidney cortex, as a result of altered UTP metabolism, there is increased glycogen content leading to formation of Armanni-Ebstein lesion (subnuclear vacuolation in the proximal tubules) and thickening of glomerular basement membrane (GBM) and deposition of basement membrane like material in the mesangium [33, 35, 36]. These early changes including increased renal weight and hypertrophy can be prevented or reversed with insulin therapy [14] if it is started at diagnosis of diabetes and dosed continuously [37]. The changes may not be reversible if insulin is initiated after 3 weeks of onset of diabetes even if the therapy is continued [14]. However, diabetic kidneys in humans may return to normal size when hyperglycemia is controlled for 3 months [31].

The short-term study by Christiansen et al. in nine humans newly diagnosed with T1DM has evaluated the changes in GFR, RPF, FF, and kidney size before and after 8 days of insulin treatment [24]. The study found that before insulin therapy there is a statistically significant elevation in GFR by 44 %, RPF by 18 %, and increased kidney size by 29 % compared to subjects without diabetes [24]. After insulin therapy GFR, RPF, and FF had decreased significantly but GFR remained 20 % above normal value and kidney size did not change compared to control group [24]. This study showed that subjects with T1DM have statistically significantly bigger kidney size and increased GFR at diagnosis but there was no significant change in kidney size after insulin treatment [24]. After improvement of hyperglycemia over 1–2 weeks, approximately 20 % reduction in GFR was found in other studies [17, 38]. However, GFR in T1DM did not decrease to a similar value compared to subjects without DM, as complete normalization of glycemic control was not obtained in T1DM group [17, 24, 38]. This study and some of the earlier

Table 3.1 Classification and characteristics of diabetic nephropathy stages in T1DM

Stages	UAE values	Characteristics
1: Hypertrophy-hyperfiltration (at diagnosis)	Normal UAE: <20 µg/min, <30 mg/24 h, <30 mg mg/g	• Kidneys have increased size and weight, hypertrophy of glomerulus, increased intraglomerular pressure, increased TGF-β receptors, hyperfunction, may have normal BM
		• GFR can be normal or increased usually greater than 150 mL/min
		• BP is usually normal or but can be increased (especially if there is coexisting essential hypertension)
		• The changes in kidney function are reversible
2: Silent stage normoalbuminuria	Normal UAE as above: <20 µg/min, <30 mg/24 h, <30 mg mg/g	• Kidneys have increased GBM width, expansion of mesangium, and increased tubular BM width. Possible accumulation of BM like material and membrane
	UAE can be increased during stressful situation	• GFR can be normal, decreased, or high (greater than 150 mL/min)
		• BP starting to increase
3: Incipient diabetic nephropathy	Microalbuminuria: 20–200 µg/min, 30–300 mg/24 h, 30–300 mg/g[a] (USA), 2.5–25 mg/mmol (men) and 3.5–35 mg/mmol (women) in Europe & elsewhere	• Kidney lesions can range from stage 2 to 4 with some starting glomerular closure and elevated intraglomerular pressure
		• Renal function is well preserved but hyperfiltration maybe present
		• GFR can be well preserved but can be increased or decreased (from 70 to greater than 150 mL/min)
		• BP is usually higher compared to nondiabetic patients with exaggerated rise during exercise. Loss of nocturnal dip in BP
		• With strict glycemic, BP, and lipid control this stage can be reversible
		• Without treatment approximately 80 % of patients will progress to stage 4
		• Retinopathy is often present in most T1DM
4: Overt diabetic nephropathy	Macroalbuminuria[b]: 200 µg/min, ≥300 mg/24 h, >300 mg/g[a]	• Kidneys have advanced lesions including diffuse or nodular glomerulosclerosis, increased mesangial volume, additional increase in GBM width, mesangial expansion, more frequent glomerular closure, and tubulointerstitial lesions
		• GFR usually starts to decline (can range from 70 to 15 mL/min) but can be normal
		• BP is usually high in majority of patients
		• Renal changes are usually not reversible
		• In a few T1DM UAE can regress
5: End stage renal disease (uremia)	Decreased UAE as closure of nephron	• Kidneys have advanced lesions with hypertrophy of the rest of glomeruli, and generalized closure of glomeruli
		• GFR is usually decreased and typically <15 mL/min requiring renal replacement therapy
		• BP is further increasing
		• Renal lesions can recur after kidney transplant

Modified and adapted from [6, 9, 16, 33, 96, 100]

BM basement membrane, *UAE* urinary albumin excretion, *GBM* glomerular basement membrane, *BP* blood pressure, *GFR* glomerular filtration rate, *TGF-β* transforming growth factor-beta

[a]ACR on spot urine sample

[b]Measurement of total proteinuria (≥500 mg/24 h or ≥430 mg/L in a spot urine sample) can also define this stage

Table 3.2 CKD stages by GFR in relation to UAE value

GFR (mL/min/1.73 m² BSA)	CKD stages	Description
≥90	1	GFR may be normal or increased. Changes in kidney function and structure can be detected
		DKD if UAE is in macroalbuminuria range
		Possible DKD if UAE is in microalbuminuria range
		At risk for DKD if UAE is in normoalbuminuria range[a]
60–89	2	GFR is mildly decreased. There are changes in kidney function and structure
		The rest for possibility of DKD in relation to UAE range is the same as in Stage I
30–59	3	GFR is moderately decreased
		DKD if UAE is in macroalbuminuria range
		Possible DKD if UAE is in microalbuminuria range
		Less likely DKD if UAE is in normoalbuminuria range[b]
15–29	4	GFR is severely decreased
		DKD if UAE is in macroalbuminuria range
		Less likely DKD if UAE is in microalbuminuria range[b]
		Less likely DKD if UAE is in normoalbuminuria range[b]
<15 or dialysis	5	End stage renal failure
		The rest for possibility of DKD in relation to UAE range is the same as in Stage IV

Modified and adapted from [9, 20, 21, 69]

BSA body surface area, *CKD* chronic kidney disease, *DKD* diabetic kidney disease, *GFR* glomerular filtration rate, *UAE* urinary albumin excretion

[a]There may be significant loss of kidney function if GFR less than 90 mL/min. Risk of DKD includes DM, poor glycemic control, hypertension, CVD, UAE in high normal range, nonwhite race, family history of hypertension, or CKD, retinopathy, and DM [9, 21]

[b]If kidney biopsy does not show glomerulopathy, consider CKD and diabetes coexistence and will require further investigation as described in NKQI guidelines

studies do not mention hemoglobin A1C (HbA1C) level. Similar findings have been demonstrated by other short-term studies [15, 17, 26, 31].

Mogensen et al. in their short-term study of six newly diagnosed T1DM have evaluated whether a reduction of kidney size and GFR occurs after 3 months of insulin treatment [31]. The mean GFR before insulin therapy decreased from 142.7 ± 9.7 mL/min (range 137–159) to 129 ± 10.2 mL/min (range 118–147) after 3 months of insulin therapy, which was a significant fall by 12 % and at the same time the kidney size as well as the kidney weight decreased by 13 % [26]. The kidney size was enlarged to a similar degree in both newly diagnosed T1DM patients before treatment compared to those patients with previously treated 1–12 years of T1DM [26]. This study showed that after strict glycemic control to near or normal value anatomical and functional abnormalities can be reversed as both the GFR and the kidney size fell to normal or near normal values [17, 26, 31]. It was also noted that easier glycemic control close to normal values was attained in short to moderate duration of DM. No significant change was found on RPF of newly diagnosed T1DM [31] and of T1DM duration of 1–12 years [26].

Hyperfiltration secondary to renal hypertrophy occurs as a result of both glomerular and tubular hypertrophy [1]. Tubular hypertrophy results in increased kidney weight [39]. Proximal tubular hypertrophy is associated with increased salt reabsorption, which can affect glomerular hyperfiltration [30]. In early diabetes, increased GFR is accompanied by glomerular hypertrophy with enlargement of capillary surface area, indicating a positive correlation between the two [13]. GFR elevation is affected by glycemic state, thus near normal metabolic control can reverse GFR to normal levels [13].

Early in the course of T1DM in humans and animal models showed hemodynamic changes and elevated GFR, however the exact mechanisms are not fully understood. GFR is affected by RPF, transglomerular pressure, and ultrafiltration coefficient (Kf) [24, 40]. The hemodynamic changes within the kidney leading to increased GFR have been demonstrated in micropuncture studies of animal models. In the rat model with early stage of diabetes, studies showed that in moderately hyperglycemic rats there is glomerular hyperfiltration [confirmed by elevated single nephron GFR (SNGFR) measurements], increased effective RPF, and increased intraglomerular capillary pressure [32]. However, in severely hyperglycemic rats SNGFR was reduced [32]. Other rat models showed increased GFR, RFP, and transglomerular pressure, and normal or increased Kf [41, 42]. The increased intraglomerular capillary pressure stimulates intrarenal renin-angiotensin system (RAS) [1].

Poorly controlled T1DM is associated with abnormal growth hormone (GH) level, and infusion of GH results in statistically significant elevations in GFR and RPF but no change in FF [40, 43]. Another study by Christensen et al. demonstrated that normal subjects who received human GH for 1 week to the level comparable to that seen in patients with T1DM showed a statistically significant rise in GFR and RPF but no significant change in kidney size, UAE, or urine beta 2-microglobulin excretion [40]. The author concluded that increased RPF due to elevated GH contributes to elevated GFR [40].

Glycemic control affects GFR and RPF in some studies but not in others. Hyperglycemia induced by infusion of glucose to well-controlled T1DM and normal subjects to blood glucose level of greater than 140–250 mg/dL in two studies caused an elevation in GFR and RPF, and decreased sodium excretion [44–46]. However, another study in T1DM patients did not find a consistent increase in GFR and RPF after glucose administration [47].

Not all studies showed the link between early hyperfiltration and later progression to proteinuria stage [2]. The interrelation among hemodynamic, structural, and functional changes within the diabetic kidneys has been implicated in the development and progression of nephropathy.

Glomerular hyperfiltration means elevated GFR and is usually defined as two standard deviations above the mean GFR of healthy person although there is no definite agreed value; some studies used GFR greater than 125 mL/min/1.73 m^2 [48]. In a study by Mogensen et al. in subjects with T1DM diagnosed at age 20 or younger with a follow up to 14–16 years, patients who progressed to diabetic nephropathy had GFR greater than 150 mL/min/1.73 m^2 and renal hyperfiltration was defined as GFR greater than 150 mL/min/1.73 m^2 [49]. Short duration of diabetes with GFR greater than 150 mL/min/1.73 m^2 with concurrent microalbuminuria has greater risk of late diabetic nephropathy [2, 50–52].

The correlation between the GFR, RPF, FF, UAE, and the duration of T1DM merits further discussion. In patients with newly diagnosed T1DM, mean GFR was 156 ± 25 mL/min before insulin treatment and mean GFR decreased to 124 mL/min $\pm$ 11, within first 1–4 weeks of insulin treatment [17]. Similarly FF was increased before, and showed a significant fall after the first few weeks of insulin treatment. However, RPF was within the normal range before and did not change after treatment [17]. In terms of duration of DM, GFR was significantly increased in DM with duration of 1–6 and 7–12 years, with mean values of 140 ± 20 and 137 ± 15 mL/min respectively. GFR started to fall after a duration of 13–18 years and more than 18 years of DM, with mean values of 123 ± 19 and 110 ± 31 mL/min respectively [17]. RPF and FF increased significantly with respect to 1–12 years duration of T1DM and both started to decline after 13–18 or more than 18 years of DM [17]. As for UAE, it remained within the normal range even after 19 or more years of T1DM and thus was independent of the duration of DM in patients without proteinuria though UAE rate fell significantly with insulin treatment [17].

Stage 2: The Silent Stage

The second phase of DKD is known as the silent stage with normoalbuminuria. This stage lacks clinical signs and has normal to near normal UAE regardless of duration of T1DM [16]. This stage can occur from 1 to more than 15 years duration of T1DM [16]. GFR is usually normal to elevated [10]. The increased GFR can range between 20 and 30 % higher above normal in treated, and even higher, 30–44 %, in those with untreated diabetes [10, 24]. However, in some T1DM patients there are significant structural changes in the kidney such as thickening of basement membrane and expansion of mesangium, which may develop after 2 years of DM [1, 27]. Although the kidney function may be well preserved in many patients with normal UAE, the structural changes may or may not be detected on renal biopsy [53]. Once these lesions develop the changes may not be reversible and may progress over time [27]. The studies did not show consistent data for RPF as some showed increased [24] while others demonstrated normal or depressed values [47].

Caramori et al. conducted a study in patients with T1DM with normoalbuminuria who had T1DM for at least 10 years and they were compared for differences in renal structures (by renal biopsies) and clinical features to another group with normal and low GFR (<90 mL/min/1.73 m^2) [54]. The study found that patients with low GFR had more advanced diabetic glomerular lesions such as higher GBM width, fractional volume of the glomerulus occupied by mesangium, fractional volume of the glomerulus occupied by mesangial cells, fractional volume of the glomerulus occupied by mesangial matrix, but lower surface density of the peripheral GBM per glomerulus compared to those with normal GFR. Low GFR was more common in females than males, if retinopathy and/or hypertension were present [54]. Retinopathy was present in 64 % of total patients; 58 % in normal GFR group and 91 % in low GFR group. Thus retinopathy was more common in the low GFR group with more of proliferative type. Hypertension was present in 36 % of patients and 20.9 % were receiving antihypertensive and 6 % were receiving angiotensin converting enzyme inhibitors (ACEIs) or angiotensin receptor blockers (ARBs). Prevalence of hypertension was similar in both groups but use of antihypertensive medication was statistically significantly higher in the low GFR group. There was no statistically significant difference between mean HbA1C levels between two groups [54].

However, the study conducted by Hansel et al. did find reduced GFR in normoalbuminuric T1DM patients who were not on antihypertensive medications and in microalbuminuric T1DM patients [55]. Impaired renal function may be present in T1DM patients despite normal UAE values. These results showed that normoalbuminuric group had significantly lower HbA1C (mean 7.9 %), GFR, and mean arterial blood pressure (BP) compared to microalbuminuric patients (mean HbA1C was 8.9 %) [55]. BP in normoalbuminuric subjects was not significantly different from BP of the control group. The author concluded that normal UAE is a reliable indicator of well-preserved renal function. Glomerular hyperfiltration, elevated BP, and poor metabolic control can be seen in microalbuminuric patients [55, 56].

When changes in kidney function are not readily detectible at baseline, use of provocation tests such as exercise test has been suggested [10]. Vittinghus et al. demonstrated that in normal subjects without diabetes, extreme exercise can lead to protein excretion in urine [57]. As UAE is more common at moderately high workload in patients with 3–17 years of T1DM, it was concluded that GBM was not able to retain albumin during higher filtration pressure that occurs during exercise [58]. It has been postulated that the albumin excretion is from glomerular area in diabetic subjects as high intensity exercise resulted in only a small increase in beta-2-microglobulin excretion [10]. The exercise test done by Mogensen et al. showed that patients with T1DM achieving 55–65 % of maximal heart rate (HR) had higher urinary albumin [10]. The studies by Koivisto et al. [59] and Viberti et al. [60] demonstrated that insulin treatment results in normalization of albuminuria after exercise in patients with T1DM. The post-exercise albuminuria was likely a reflection of hemodynamic changes in kidneys [10, 57].

Less than 40 % of T1DM patients will progress to microalbuminuria; thus it is prudent to prevent ESRD with early detection in susceptible patients in this stage [1]. In this stage when there is poor glycemic control, UAE can increase during exercise and at rest. Ambulatory blood pressure (AMBP) monitoring studies have shown a modest rise in BP in this phase up to 5 years before UAE increases [56]. No significant difference in the increased systolic BP (SBP) and no correlation between increased albuminuria and BP rise have been shown [57]. At the start of the study the patients with T1DM who progressed from normoalbuminuria to microalbuminuria stage have clinical characteristics of higher HbA1C (mean > 9 %) and higher diastolic BP (DBP) at the start of the study, male sex, history of smoking and more severe retinopathy [63].

Detection of kidney disease in this phase is limited. Investigators have tried to identify specific biomarkers as predictors associated with this phase but studies are still in progress. Some of the studies include plasma markers such as prorenin [62] level, which was shown to be elevated in T1DM patients and may have genetic predisposition among siblings of T1DM people. Another study suggested that detection of immune-unreactive and immune-reactive albumin fragments in urine by high-performance liquid chromatography (HPLC) [63] may provide earlier detection of those who will progress to next stage, microalbuminuria. An additional study used serum cystatin C to estimate GFR to detect changes in renal function in T1DM [64]. Another showed that total renin [61] can be increased up to 5 years before the onset of microalbuminuria. It should be noted that long-standing T1DM patients with normoalbuminuria are at substantial risk of progressing to diabetic nephropathy stage.

Stage 3: Microalbuminuria or Incipient Diabetic Nephropathy (IDN)

The third stage is known as microalbuminuria or IDN. Depending on the population the prevalence of microalbuminuria varies from 7 to 22 % in T1DM and the annual incidence is about 1 to 2 % in both T1DM and T2DM [9, 65–67]. In subjects with T1DM, it often occurs after 5–15 years after the initial diagnosis and has increased UAE rate to microalbuminuria range of 20–200 μg/min or 30–300 mg/24 h [9, 49]. Microalbuminuria is also defined as albumin-to-creatinine ratio (ACR) of 30–300 mg/g in the USA and 2.5–25 mg/mmol in Europe and elsewhere, and it is also a marker of CKD [49]. The urine should be collected at rest or as an outpatient procedure and two of three urine samples are required to be in the microalbuminuria range within 3–6 months at least 1 month apart to confirm classification [9, 68, 69]. Excluding other causes for increased UAE especially if duration of diabetes is less than 6 years is advised [9]. The UAE range in this category is above normal but below overt diabetic nephropathy (ODN) value. Hyperfiltration can also occur in this stage in T1DM [2]. GFR is usually preserved but it can be increased or decreased. Regression of microalbuminuria [70] or progression to ODN can occur in stage 3 [71]. Uncontrolled or untreated hypertension worsens DKD. Kidney structural lesions in this stage are detectable on renal biopsy.

It is important to note that UAE measurements can be affected by hydration status, recent vigorous exercise, urinary tract infection, hematuria, fever, and other kidney disease, and prolonged erect posture at the time of collection especially during 24 h urine collections [9, 20, 21]. Current radioimmunoassay methods can detect urinary albumin in microgram concentration and are sensitive, and thus the American Diabetes Association (ADA) and KDOQI clinical practice guidelines recommend using spot urine ACR preferably in the first morning void to avoid 24 h urine collection and conditions that can cause variability of UAE value [9, 69]. Urine ACR approximates 24 h UAE as it is not affected by various ways of urine collection and 24-h and timed urine collections are not as accurate or convenient [9].

Results from a study of 43 T1DM patients by Mogensen et al. [2] showed that of 4 patients (9.2 %) with initial UAE < 15 μg/min, who have progressed to microalbuminuria range (mean UAE of 41.1 ± 17.4), had their GFR increased to >150 mL/min/1.73 m^2. Of the 12 patients (27.9 %) with initial UAE < 70 μg/min, 9 patients (20 %)

had statistically significant progression of UAE to 2,373 ± 2,488 range and GFR had decreased to 93 ± 47 mL/min/1.73 m^2 at mean follow up of 7 years [16]. Those patients had higher initial mean SBP and DBP and even higher mean SBP and DBP at follow up. Initial SBP was 10 mmHg higher compared to those that remained normoalbuminuric. Thus those that progressed to macroalbuminuria range had a tendency to have declining GFR and RPF, and higher SBP (means were >11 mmHg) at follow up compared to normoalbuminuric or microalbuminuric groups. No difference in BP was noted from initial examination to follow up in those who remained normoalbuminuric and progressed to microalbuminuria range. The patients who remained normoalbuminuric (27 patients) at follow up had stable UAE (their initial UAE was <15 μg/min) and BP and a statistically significantly decreased RPF. In short, findings from this study showed that T1DM patients with UAE between 20 and 70 μg/min had higher GFR >150 mL/min/1.73 m^2 on initial exam compared to patients with UAE>70 μg/min. In patients with UAE >70 μg/min and less than 200, GFR starts to decline during this stage [16]. This long-term study showed that hyperfiltration contributed to the pathogenesis of late DKD [2, 16].

In DCCT/EDIC study the cumulative incidences of persistent microalbuminuria in the conventional therapy group at 10, 20, and 30 years duration of T1DM were 14 %, 33 %, and 38 %, respectively [8]. Persistent microalbuminuria occurred more frequently after 20 years of diagnosis of diabetes. In the intensive therapy group the cumulative incidence of persistent microalbuminuria at 10, 20, 30 years duration of T1DM were 10 %, 21 %, 25 %, respectively and persistent microalbuminuria occurring after 20 years of diagnosis of diabetes were lower than conventional group [8]. Progression to macroalbuminuria, impaired GFR, and ESRD occurred at 10 year cumulative incidence of 28 %, 15 %, and 4 % respectively and regression to normoalbuminuria occurred at 40 %. Among patients with regression to normoalbuminuria after 10 years of initial persistent microalbuminuria diagnosis, the prevalence of them on ACE inhibitors and angiotensin receptor blockers (ACEIs and ARBs, respectively) were 47 %, on lipid-lowering medications were 12 %, mean HbA1C at the time of regression was 7.7 %, and mean BP was 121/77 mmHg [8]. Even if they progress to macroalbuminuria stage, the regression to normoalbuminuria has occurred in a minority of patients if GFR was not impaired [8].

Clinically in this phase there is an increase of both SBP and DBP and a loss of nocturnal dip in BP before progressing to microalbuminuria stage [72]. Renal function may be increased, normal, or decreased. Effective intervention in this phase may prevent further decline in renal function.

The study by Mogensen et al. of 28 T1DM patients found that there is a correlation with an increase in BP and albuminuria [10]. Other studies have similar findings showing that intervention during IDN helps in preserving renal function more effectively than in ODN [73]. There was no increase in urinary beta-2 microglobulin, which implied that tubular function was not affected and the increased UAE indicated progressive glomerular changes [10]. During this stage renal function is still preserved but GFR was elevated at the entry and during follow up. There was a significant decline in RPF and significant rise in DBP during this period, thus it is speculated that RPF changes may reflect modifications of glomeruli and possible rise in BP in this stage [10].

There is a significant correlation between the rise in exercise-induced albuminuria and SBP during exercise but not with HR, leading to speculation that microcirculatory and structural changes in glomeruli may exist [74]. There is a decline in creatinine excretion noted after insulin treatment in subjects with diabetes with early nephropathy suggesting impaired renovascular auto-regulation contributing to higher SBP during exercise [75]. It has been postulated that elevated BP may worsen diabetic nephropathy after appearance of microalbuminuria.

Studies in human T1DM have shown that microalbuminuria can be transient and can regress to normoalbuminuria [70]. A study by Perkins et al. showed that there was a 58 % regression of microalbuminuria in subjects with T1DM [70] but the study by Hovind et al. showed lower rates [71]. Notably, in the study by Perkins et al., microalbuminuria of short duration, HbA1c <8 %, low SBP (<115 mmHg), and low levels of both cholesterol and triglycerides had positive association with the regression of microalbuminuria [70].

Poor metabolic control can also contribute to elevated BP. Both poor glycemic and BP management may contribute to progression of DKD as observed in interventional studies to treat hypertension in diabetes [76]. Early antihypertensive treatment with goal BP less than 135/85 mmHg can reverse microalbuminuria and preserve GFR [16, 76, 77]. Improved metabolic control also prevents progression of microalbuminuria [78].

Microalbuminuria is a clinical manifestation of DKD and renal morphologic studies have demonstrated that microalbuminuric phase can be associated with advanced glomerular structural changes [79]. Untreated persistent microalbuminuria will lead to ODN [2]. Thus it is beneficial to repeat spot urinary microalbumin if there is isolated elevation in urinary microalbumin to confirm diagnosis. Current recommendations to screen for diabetic nephropathy in T1DM includes biannual urinary albumin, assessment of GFR by obtaining creatinine, and appropriate staging [9, 69]. This stage clearly indicates that effective blood pressure, lipid, and glycemic control will help prevent progression to macroalbuminuria stage and may facilitate regression to normoalbuminuria stage [9].

Stage 4: Macroalbuminuria

This stage is known as macroalbuminuria or ODN. It is defined by increased UAE rate ≥300 mg/24 h or >200 μg/min, on at least two of three urine samples collected within 6 months while excluding other causes of elevated UAE [1, 9, 10, 49, 68]. It is also characterized as persistent proteinuria greater than 0.5 g/24 h in total protein excretion [16]. In patients with T1DM, this stage usually occurs after 10–15 years but in some patients it can also appear 40–50 years later [23]. In Denmark T1DM patients have 31 % risk of developing persistent proteinuria and the risk was higher in males than females and with early onset under age 10 [80]. In the same study 6 % developed persistent proteinuria after 10 years of T1DM and prevalence of 18 % during first 20 years of T1DM with most occurring after duration of 12–25 years [80]. The prevalence of persistent proteinuria after 35 or 40 years of T1DM was low and about 70 % of T1DM will not develop ODN [80]. If patients do not receive adequate treatment during the macroalbuminuria phase, there is a high probability that they will develop subsequent renal failure [23].

In early course of ODN, most patients' GFR and serum creatinine can be within the normal ranges but some people will have hyperfiltration [16]. As ODN stage progresses there is a decline in GFR [6]. Further progression in the kidney structural changes can be detected in early and intermediate course of ODN, such as additional increase in thickening of GBM, expansion of mesangium, and rate of glomerular closure [16]. In advanced stage 4 the remaining glomeruli hypertrophy more [16]. Proteinuria is a clinical sign of future deterioration of renal function and it implies poor prognosis and shorter life expectancy [81]. The mean time of survival was 7 years after inception of proteinuria, and approximately 2–7 years after serum creatinine rises [80].

There are at least two peaks of incidence in ODN with no definite clear contributors although poor glycemic or BP control, genetic, molecular, and environmental factors have been proposed in predisposition [71]. More than two-thirds of patients with macroalbuminuria have uncontrolled systemic hypertension and this has been associated with increase in proteinuria [82, 83]. Untreated macroalbuminuria leads to progressive elevation of BP and declining GFR with eventual progression to ESRD [71]. In the study by Parving et al. patients with T1DM and persistent proteinuria before treatment have mean decline in GFR with mean value of 0.9 mL/min/month with further elevation in BP and UAE values and during antihypertensive treatment mean GFR decline rate decreased to 0.39 mL/min/month [84]. The study by Mogensen et al. during this stage demonstrated that the mean decline in GFR was 1.24 mL/min/month before antihypertensive treatment and it decreased to 0.45 mL/min/month during antihypertensive treatment with decreased yearly UAE to −7 % with improved SBP and DBP [73]. Viberti et al. showed that strict glycemic control may have beneficial effect on slowing the rate of GFR decline in this stage [85].

The trials have shown that controlling BP slows the GFR decline rate [51, 73]. Long-term antihypertensive medications during this stage have shown to decelerate the progression of albuminuria and declining GFR by 60 % and significantly reduced both SBP and DBP [10]. However the filtration rate continues to decrease despite treatment in patients with difficulty achieving BP goal of 140/90 or lower during that period [51].

Stage 5: Uremia

This most advanced phase is called uremic stage or end stage renal failure. It is common in both T1DM and T2DM and occurs in 30–40 % of T1DM and 10–35 % of T2DM [1, 16]. It is characterized by uremia and often has decreasing UAE due to closure of nephrons [16]. There are advanced kidney lesions and generalized glomerular obliteration. BP in this stage is usually high. Patients with DM and ESRD require renal replacement therapy (RRT), which includes dialysis or renal transplantation, which has better outcomes. Diabetes-associated renal lesions have been shown to recur in transplanted kidney [1]. ESRD is associated with high cardiovascular mortality [9] (Table 3.1).

Natural History of Diabetic Kidney Disease in T2DM

The natural history of DKD in T2DM patients has been less well delineated compared to T1DM patients. This could be partly because most T2DM patients are older and have unknown duration of diabetes prior to diagnosis and concurrent obesity, hypertension, hyperlipidemia and higher rates of CVD that limit the expression of DKD [9]. Microalbuminuria occurs in approximately 7 % at the time of diagnosis and up to 18 % within 5 years of T2DM diagnosis, suggesting existence of 10 years of undiagnosed T2DM [1].

The study in Pima Indians has provided valuable insight about DKD in T2DM. Pima Indians have the highest prevalence of T2DM, with prevalence of 40–45 % in adults over age 35 years, and they have low incidence of T2DM during childhood to peak incidence at 40 years for male and 50 years for female [86]. Most are obese subjects with diabetes and insulin resistance [6, 87]. The kidney structural and functional changes in T1DM are similar in T2DM for most part [9]. Among Pima Indians with kidney disease the highest mortality occurs in subjects with T2DM on RRT and mortality rate increases with duration of diabetes and from CVD, infection, and malignancy [88].

Stage 1: Initial Stage in T2DM

At initial diagnosis of T2DM and early stage 1 of DKD, hyperfiltration may or may not occur. If hyperfiltration does occur in T2DM, it is less frequent, at rates of 15–45 % compared to 90–95 % in T1DM [6, 89–91]. In a study of 16 recently diagnosed non-proteinuric T2DM patients, hyperfiltration (elevated GFR) was present in 44 % of patients, with median GFR (133 mL/min/1.73 m^2; range, 95–165) in the group with T2DM, which was significantly higher than obese nondiabetic controls (median, 118; range, 95–139) [90]. Vora et al. studied 110 Caucasian patients newly presenting with T2DM showed significantly elevated GFR, effective RPF, and FF compared to nondiabetic control group [91]. These patients have BP in the normal range and did not have prior treatment for diabetes. The mean age was 52.5 ± 10.1 years, GFR was above 140 mL/min in 16 % and above mean ±2 SD of the normal in 45 %, and microalbuminuria was noted in 7 % of T2DM patients [91]. In 20 Pima Indians with T2DM mean GFR (140 ± 6 mL/min) was 15 % higher than patients without diabetes (122 ± 5 mL/min) [87]. However, this study found normal GFR in newly diagnosed T2DM [92]. As GFR typically declines with age, it is possible to have hyperfiltration while GFR remains within normal adult range [1]. The interpretation of GFR and hyperfiltration must be carefully analyzed.

There may be elevated BP at diagnosis of T2DM, and most patients require treatment [16]. This is different from T1DM where most people during normoalbuminuric range have normal BP, and elevation in BP is obviously linked to renal disease with higher BP corresponding to greater UAE level [16]. The T2DM patients often display hyperinsulinemia and insulin increases renal sodium reabsorption. Thus high insulin may indirectly play a role in hypertension by sodium retention [16, 93]. During the initial stage, not all T2DM patients have increased glomerular volume [94].

Stage 2: Normoalbuminuria

T2DM patients with normoalbuminuria comparable to stage 2 in T1DM may or may not have hyperfiltration and usually have normal renal size and may have diabetic glomerulopathy [16]. The GFR has positive correction with UAE, borderline correlation with renal size but none with glycated hemoglobin, which is different from the finding in T1DM patients [16]. The annual CVD death risk in patients without nephropathy (urinary albumin concentration (UAC) less than microalbuminuria range) was 0.7 % in the United Kingdom Prospective Disease Study (UKPDS) [19].

Schmitz et al. studied 19 normoalbuminuric T2DM patients with light microscopy to determine the relationship between glomerular morphology and UAE showed that there was no increase in glomerular volume and no significant frequency in occlusion of glomeruli [94]. These patients were only on oral hypoglycemics or diet controlled. In this study the fraction of red-stained material (periodic-acid Schiff positive substance) in open glomeruli was increased by 14 % signifying the existence of glomerulopathy in T2DM subjects, but also indicating that high UAC did not reflect more advanced glomerulopathy [94]. The finding of increased glomerular size in both early and late T1DM was not demonstrated in this study in T2DM. In addition, hyperfiltration was not a precursor to the finding of glomerulopathy as suggested by the same study [94]. Higher DBP was seen in T2DM patients who progress from normoalbuminuria to microalbuminuria and there was no difference in HbA1C but mean value was 8.8 % [63].

Stage 3: Microalbuminuria or Incipient Diabetic Nephropathy

The prevalence of microalbuminuria in T2DM varies from 6.5 to 42 % and it may be present at or before diagnosis of T2DM, which is different from T1DM [1, 65–67]. The presence of microalbuminuria in T2DM increases the CVD risks such as MI or stroke and it may not be a specific indicator for diabetic renal disease as in T1DM patients as other factors such as incipient or overt cardiac insufficiency, urinary tract infection, and urinary obstruction can contribute to it [9]. In hypertensive T2DM patients BP levels tend to increase as UAE progresses to microalbuminuric range [16]. In T2DM, GFR is reduced especially in patients with microalbuminuria or in older patients with normoalbuminuria [6].

Regression of microalbuminuria or remission to normoalbuminuria can occur in T2DM. In a study that included 216 T2DM Japanese patients with microalbuminuria, Araki et al. defined regression as a 50 % decrease in UAE values over a 2-year period [95]. Six year cumulative incidence of remission was at 51 %, regression was at 54 %, and progression to ODN was at 28 % [95]. The factors associated with regression or remission were short duration of microalbuminuria, use of ACEIs or ARBs, lower HbA1C (less than 6.95 %), and SBP less than 129 mmHg [95].

The data from UKPDS of 5,097 newly diagnosed T2DM patients describe the progression of DKD through the stages from microalbuminuria, macroalbuminuria (UAC values used in the study were 50–299 and ≥300 mg/L, respectively), persistently elevated plasma creatinine (EPC) (creatinine ≥175 μmol/L [96]) or RRT, and death [19]. From the time of diagnosis of T2DM development of microalbuminuria occurred at 2.0 % per year. The prevalence of microalbuminuria 10 years after diagnosis of diabetes was 24.9 % with increasing annual CVD death risk of 2.0 % in microalbuminuria group [19]. Many patients with T2DM with microalbuminuria also progress to overt proteinuria [1].

Table 3.3 Stages of diabetic nephropathy in Type 1 DM and T2 DM in comparison

Stages	Type 1 DM	Type 2 DM
1: Hyperfiltration and hypertrophy	• Younger mean age at diagnosis	• Older mean age at diagnosis
	• GFR and capillary glomerular pressure are increased	• Occur less common than in T1DM and GFR needs careful interpretation as it declines with age
	• BP is usually normal or increased	• BP is often high at diagnosis and requires treatment
2: Silent stage (normoalbuminuria)	• GFR is increased or decreased	• May or may not have hyperfiltration and GFR could be within normal range
	• BP is increased (+)	
3: Microalbuminuria (incipient nephropathy)	• GFR is preserved but it can be increased or decreased	• Microalbuminuria may be present at diagnosis and is not specific indicator for T2DM
	• BP is further increased (++); Increased SBP and DBP. Hypertension is an important prognostic factor for early mortality [16]	• Hypertension has not been identified as markers for early mortality
	• Occur 5–10 years after diagnosis	• UAE can regress to normoalbuminuria range
	• Increased UAE can be reversible	
4: Macroalbuminuria or overt nephropathy	• GFR is normal or decreased	• May progress to overt proteinuria
	• Increased BP (++)	• Some studies have described both T1DM and T2DM who develop renal impairment without significant proteinuria (mechanism not known)
	• Usually occurs after 10–15 years of T1DM but can appear after 40–50 years	
	• Predicts progression to renal failure if untreated and this stage is not reversible and majority will progress to ESRD	
5: End stage renal disease or uremia	• GFR is decreased	• Similar risks for ESRD in T1DM and T2DM
	• Further rise of BP (+++)	• T2DM is more common than T1DM so majority of ESRD patients have T2DM
	• Occurs in 40 % of T1DM and requires RRT	

Adapted from [1, 16]
T1DM type 1 diabetes mellitus, *T2DM* type 2 diabetes mellitus, *GFR* glomerular filtration rate, *BP* blood pressure, *SBP* systolic blood pressure, *DBP* diastolic blood pressure, *UAE* urinary albumin excretion, *ESRD* end stage renal failure, *RRT* renal replacement therapy

Substantial renal impairment without significant proteinuria has also been described in both T1DM [97] and T2DM [98] patients. As the risk of ESRD in T2DM patients and renal impairment is similar with or without microalbuminuria, it is important to assess serum creatinine and estimated GFR as recommended by ADA and NKDQI guidelines [9, 69].

Stage 4: Overt Diabetic Nephropathy

This stage in T2DM may appear 5 years earlier compared to in T1DM as time to diagnosis is delayed [6]. The results from UKPDS showed that progression from microalbuminuria to macroalbuminuria was 2.8 % per year [19]. The prevalence of macroalbuminuria was less with 5.3 % 10 years after T2DM diagnosis, and these patients had higher annual CVD death risk of 3.5 %, which was higher than transitioning to renal failure [19].

Stage 5: End Stage Renal Disease

Cumulative incidence of ESRD is 10–35 % among T2DM patients [6]. Generally Nelson et al. reported the cumulative incidence of ESRD development in Pima Indians with T2DM was 40 % after 10 years and 61 % after 15 years of detected proteinuria (protein-to-creatinine ratio ≥0.5 g/g) [99]. GFR decline rate is similar among T2DM patients who develop diabetes at young age (like Pima Indian) compared to T1DM [6]. From UKPDS study the transition from macroalbuminuria to EPC or RRT was at 2.3 % per year and with a prevalence of EPC or RRT was at 0.8 % 10 years following T2DM diagnosis. The patients with EPC or on RRT have annual risk of cardiovascular death at 12.1 % and annual death rate of 19.2 %, both of which were much higher than in stages 1–4 [19]. Thus CVD death risk increases with progressive UAE elevation and DKD stages [19]. This stage has higher CVD risk and patients eventually need RRT for survival. Antihypertensive medications and improved glycemic control are beneficial in this stage [9] (Table 3.3).

References

1. Brownlee M, Aiello LP, Cooper ME, Vinik AI, Nesto RW, Boulton AJM. Complications of diabetes mellitus. In: Melmed S, Polonsky K, Larsen PR, Kronenberg KM, editors. Williams textbook of endocrinology. 12th ed. Philadelphia: Saunders (Elsevier); 2011. p. 1462–551.
2. Mogensen CE, Christensen CK. Predicting diabetic nephropathy in insulin-dependent patients. N Engl J Med. 1984;311(2):89–93.

3. Masharani U, German M. Pancreatic hormones and diabetes mellitus. In: Gardner DG, Shoback D, editors. Greenspan's basic & clinical endocrinology. 9th ed. New York: The McGraw-Hill Companies; 2011. p. 573.
4. CDC National Center for Health Statistics-Homepage. National diabetes fact sheet: national estimates and general information on diabetes and prediabetes in the United States, 2011. 2013. http://www.cdc.gov/nchs/nhanes.htm. Accessed 26 Apr 2013.
5. National Institutes of Health, National Institute of Diabetes and Digestive and Kidney Diseases. U S Renal Data System, USRDS 2012 Annual Data Report: Atlas of Chronic Kidney Disease and End-Stage Renal Disease in the United States. 2012. http://www.usrds.org/atlas.aspx. Accessed 26 Apr 2013.
6. Ismail N, Becker B, Strzelczyk P, Ritz E. Renal disease and hypertension in non-insulin-dependent diabetes mellitus. Kidney Int. 1999;55(1):1–28.
7. Finne P, Reunanen A, Stenman S, Groop PH, Gronhagen-Riska C. Incidence of end-stage renal disease in patients with type 1 diabetes. JAMA. 2005;294(14):1782–7.
8. de Boer IH, Rue TC, Cleary PA, Lachin JM, Molitch ME, Steffes MW, et al. Long-term renal outcomes of patients with type 1 diabetes mellitus and microalbuminuria: an analysis of the Diabetes Control and Complications Trial/Epidemiology of Diabetes Interventions and Complications cohort. Arch Intern Med. 2011;171(5):412–20.
9. KDOQI. KDOQI clinical practice guidelines and clinical practice recommendations for diabetes and chronic kidney disease. Am J Kidney Dis. 2007;49(2 Suppl 2):S12–154.
10. Mogensen CE, Christensen CK, Vittinghus E. The stages in diabetic renal disease. With emphasis on the stage of incipient diabetic nephropathy. Diabetes. 1983;32 Suppl 2:64–78.
11. Ditzel J, Junker K. Abnormal glomerular filtration rate, renal plasma flow, and renal protein excretion in recent and short-term diabetics. Br Med J. 1972;2(5804):13–9.
12. Osterby R. Early phases in the development of diabetic glomerulopathy. Acta Med Scand Suppl. 1974;574:3–82.
13. Osterby R, Gundersen HJ, Horlyck A, Kroustrup JP, Nyberg G, Westberg G. Diabetic glomerulopathy. Structural characteristics of the early and advanced stages. Diabetes. 1983;32 Suppl 2:79–82.
14. Seyer-Hansen K. Renal hypertrophy in streptozotocin-diabetic rats. Clin Sci Mol Med Suppl. 1976;51(6):551–5.
15. Christiansen JS, Gammelgaard J, Frandsen M, Parving HH. Increased kidney size, glomerular filtration rate and renal plasma flow in short-term insulin-dependent diabetics. Diabetologia. 1981;20(4):451–6.
16. Mogensen CE, Schmitz A, Christensen CK. Comparative renal pathophysiology relevant to IDDM and NIDDM patients. Diabetes Metab Rev. 1988;4(5):453–83.
17. Mogensen CE. Kidney function and glomerular permeability to macromolecules in juvenile diabetes with special reference to early changes. Dan Med Bull. 1972;19 Suppl 3:1–40.
18. Schmitz A, Christensen T, Taagehoej JF. Glomerular filtration rate and kidney volume in normoalbuminuric non-insulin-dependent diabetics—lack of glomerular hyperfiltration and renal hypertrophy in uncomplicated NIDDM. Scand J Clin Lab Invest. 1989;49(2):103–8.
19. Adler AI, Stevens RJ, Manley SE, Bilous RW, Cull CA, Holman RR, et al. Development and progression of nephropathy in type 2 diabetes: the United Kingdom Prospective Diabetes Study (UKPDS 64). Kidney Int. 2003;63(1):225–32.
20. National Kidney Foundation. K/DOQI clinical practice guidelines for chronic kidney disease: evaluation, classification, and stratification. Am J Kidney Dis. 2002;39(2 Suppl 1):S1–266.
21. Levey AS, Coresh J, Balk E, Kausz AT, Levin A, Steffes MW, et al. National Kidney Foundation practice guidelines for chronic kidney disease: evaluation, classification, and stratification. Ann Intern Med. 2003;139(2):137–47.
22. Mogensen CE, Steffes MW, Deckert T, Christiansen JS. Functional and morphological renal manifestations in diabetes mellitus. Diabetologia. 1981;21(2):89–93.
23. Brown DM, Andres GA, Hostetter TH, Mauer SM, Price R, Venkatachalam MA. Kidney complications. Diabetes. 1982;31(Suppl 1 Pt 2):71–81.
24. Christiansen JS, Gammelgaard J, Tronier B, Svendsen PA, Parving HH. Kidney function and size in diabetics before and during initial insulin treatment. Kidney Int. 1982;21(5):683–8.
25. Mogensen CE. Glomerular filtration rate and renal plasma flow in short-term and long-term juvenile diabetes mellitus. Scand J Clin Lab Invest. 1971;28(1):91–100.
26. Mogensen CE, Andersen MJ. Increased kidney size and glomerular filtration rate in early juvenile diabetes. Diabetes. 1973;22(9):706–12.
27. Mogensen CE. Diabetes mellitus and the kidney. Kidney Int. 1982;21(5):673–5.
28. Gerich JE, Tsalikian E, Lorenzi M, Schneider V, Bohannon NV, Gustafson G, et al. Normalization of fasting hyperglucagonemia and excessive glucagon responses to intravenous arginine in human diabetes mellitus by prolonged infusion of insulin. J Clin Endocrinol Metab. 1975;41(06):1178–80.
29. Allen TJ, Cooper ME, Lan HY. Use of genetic mouse models in the study of diabetic nephropathy. Curr Diab Rep. 2004;4(6):435–40.
30. Thomson SC, Vallon V, Blantz RC. Kidney function in early diabetes: the tubular hypothesis of glomerular filtration. Am J Physiol Renal Physiol. 2004;286(1):F8–15.
31. Mogensen CE, Andersen MJ. Increased kidney size and glomerular filtration rate in untreated juvenile diabetes: normalization by insulin-treatment. Diabetologia. 1975;11(3):221–4.
32. Hostetter TH, Troy JL, Brenner BM. Glomerular hemodynamics in experimental diabetes mellitus. Kidney Int. 1981;19(3):410–5.
33. Sharma K, Jin Y, Guo J, Ziyadeh FN. Neutralization of TGF-beta by anti-TGF-beta antibody attenuates kidney hypertrophy and the enhanced extracellular matrix gene expression in STZ-induced diabetic mice. Diabetes. 1996;45(4):522–30.
34. Cortes P, Dumler F, Venkatachalam KK, Levin NW. Effect of diabetes mellitus on renal metabolism. Miner Electrolyte Metab. 1983;9(4–6):306–16.
35. Arison RN, Ciaccio EI, Glitzer MS, Cassaro JA, Pruss MP. Light and electron microscopy of lesions in rats rendered diabetic with streptozotocin. Diabetes. 1967;16(1):51–6.
36. Cortes P, Dumler F, Venkatachalam KK, Goldman J, Sastry KS, Venkatachalam H, et al. Alterations in glomerular RNA in diabetic rats: roles of glucagon and insulin. Kidney Int. 1981;20(4):491–9.
37. Cortes P, Levin NW, Dumler F, Rubenstein AH, Verghese CP, Venkatachalam KK. Uridine triphosphate and RNA synthesis during diabetes-induced renal growth. Am J Physiol. 1980;238(4):E349–57.
38. Parving HH, Rutili F, Granath K, Noer I, Deckert T, Lyngsoe J, et al. Effect of metabolic regulation on renal leakiness to dextran molecules in short-term insulin-dependent diabetics. Diabetologia. 1979;17(3):157–60.
39. Thomas MC, Burns WC, Cooper ME. Tubular changes in early diabetic nephropathy. Adv Chronic Kidney Dis. 2005;12(2):177–86.
40. Christiansen JS, Gammelgaard J, Orskov H, Andersen AR, Telmer S, Parving HH. Kidney function and size in normal subjects before and during growth hormone administration for one week. Eur J Clin Invest. 1981;11(6):487–90.
41. Hostetter TH. Renal microcirculation in diabetes mellitus. Acta Endocrinol Suppl (Copenh). 1981;242:22–4.

42. Jensen PK, Christiansen JS, Steven K, Parving HH. Renal function in diabetic rats. Acta Endocrinol Suppl (Copenh). 1981;242:25.
43. CORVILAIN J, ABRAMOW M, BERGANS A. Some effects of human growth hormone on renal hemodynamics and on tubular phosphate transport in man. J Clin Invest. 1962;41:1230–5.
44. FOX M, THIER S, ROSENBERG L, SEGAL S. Impaired renal tubular function induced by sugar infusion in man. J Clin Endocrinol Metab. 1964;24:1318–27.
45. Brochner-Mortensen J. The glomerular filtration rate during moderate hyperglycemia in normal man. Acta Med Scand. 1973;1–2(1):31–7.
46. Christiansen JS, Frandsen M, Parving HH. Effect of intravenous glucose infusion on renal function in normal man and in insulin-dependent diabetics. Diabetologia. 1981;21(4):368–73.
47. Mogensen CE, Christensen NJ, Gundersen HJ. The acute effect of insulin on renal haemodynamics and protein excretion in diabetics. Diabetologia. 1978;15(3):153–7.
48. Palatini P. Glomerular hyperfiltration: a marker of early renal damage in pre-diabetes and pre-hypertension. Nephrol Dial Transplant. 2012;27(5):1708–14.
49. Mogensen CE, Keane WF, Bennett PH, Jerums G, Parving HH, Passa P, et al. Prevention of diabetic renal disease with special reference to microalbuminuria. Lancet. 1995;346(8982):1080–4.
50. Mogensen CE, Christensen CK, Pedersen MM, Alberti KG, Boye N, Christensen T, et al. Renal and glycemic determinants of glomerular hyperfiltration in normoalbuminuric diabetics. J Diabet Complications. 1990;4(4):159–65.
51. Mogensen CE. Long-term antihypertensive treatment inhibiting progression of diabetic nephropathy. Br Med J (Clin Res Ed). 1982;285(6343):685–8.
52. Christiansen JS. On the pathogenesis of the increased glomerular filtration rate in short-term insulin-dependent diabetes. Dan Med Bull. 1984;31(5):349–61.
53. Mauer SM, Steffes MW, Ellis EN, Sutherland DE, Brown DM, Goetz FC. Structural-functional relationships in diabetic nephropathy. J Clin Invest. 1984;74(4):1143–55.
54. Caramori ML, Fioretto P, Mauer M. Low glomerular filtration rate in normoalbuminuric type 1 diabetic patients: an indicator of more advanced glomerular lesions. Diabetes. 2003;52(4):1036–40.
55. Hansen KW, Mau Pedersen M, Christensen CK, Schmitz A, Christiansen JS, Mogensen CE. Normoalbuminuria ensures no reduction of renal function in type 1 (insulin-dependent) diabetic patients. J Intern Med. 1992;232(2):161–7.
56. Poulsen PL, Hansen KW, Mogensen CE. Ambulatory blood pressure in the transition from normo- to microalbuminuria. A longitudinal study in IDDM patients. Diabetes. 1994;43(10):1248–53.
57. Vittinghus E, Mogensen CE. Graded exercise and protein excretion in diabetic man and the effect of insulin treatment. Kidney Int. 1982;21(5):725–9.
58. Vittinghus E, Mogensen CE. Albumin excretion and renal haemodynamic response to physical exercise in normal and diabetic man. Scand J Clin Lab Invest. 1981;41(7):627–32.
59. Koivisto VA, Huttunen NP, Vierikko P. Continuous subcutaneous insulin infusion corrects exercise-induced albuminuria in juvenile diabetes. Br Med J (Clin Res Ed). 1981;282(6266):778–9.
60. Viberti G, Pickup JC, Bilous RW, Keen H, Mackintosh D. Correction of exercise-induced microalbuminuria in insulin-dependent diabetics after 3 weeks of subcutaneous insulin infusion. Diabetes. 1981;30(10):818–23.
61. Allen TJ, Cooper ME, Gilbert RE, Winikoff J, Skinni SL, Jerums G. Serum total renin is increased before microalbuminuria in diabetes. Kidney Int. 1996;50(3):902–7.
62. Daneman D, Crompton CH, Balfe JW, Sochett EB, Chatzilias A, Cotter BR, et al. Plasma prorenin as an early marker of nephropathy in diabetic (IDDM) adolescents. Kidney Int. 1994;46(4):1154–9.
63. Comper WD, Osicka TM, Clark M, MacIsaac RJ, Jerums G. Earlier detection of microalbuminuria in diabetic patients using a new urinary albumin assay. Kidney Int. 2004;65(5):1850–5.
64. Cherney DZ, Sochett EB, Dekker MG, Perkins BA. Ability of cystatin C to detect acute changes in glomerular filtration rate provoked by hyperglycaemia in uncomplicated Type 1 diabetes. Diabet Med. 2010;27(12):1358–65.
65. Lloyd CE, Stephenson J, Fuller JH, Orchard TJ. A comparison of renal disease across two continents; the epidemiology of diabetes complications study and the EURODIAB IDDM Complications Study. Diabetes Care. 1996;19(3):219–25.
66. Microvascular and acute complications in IDDM patients: the EURODIAB IDDM Complications Study. Diabetologia. 1994; 37(3):278–85.
67. Marshall SM, Alberti KG. Comparison of the prevalence and associated features of abnormal albumin excretion in insulin-dependent and non-insulin-dependent diabetes. Q J Med. 1989; 70(261):61–71.
68. Mogensen CE. Microalbuminuria and hypertension with focus on type 1 and type 2 diabetes. J Intern Med. 2003;254(1):45–66.
69. American Diabetes Association. Standards of medical care in diabetes-2013. Diabetes Care. 2013;36:S11–65.
70. Perkins BA, Ficociello LH, Silva KH, Finkelstein DM, Warram JH, Krolewski AS. Regression of microalbuminuria in type 1 diabetes. N Engl J Med. 2003;348(23):2285–93.
71. Hovind P, Tarnow L, Rossing P, Jensen BR, Graae M, Torp I, et al. Predictors for the development of microalbuminuria and macroalbuminuria in patients with type 1 diabetes: inception cohort study. BMJ. 2004;328(7448):1105.
72. Lurbe E, Redon J, Kesani A, Pascual JM, Tacons J, Alvarez V, et al. Increase in nocturnal blood pressure and progression to microalbuminuria in type 1 diabetes. N Engl J Med. 2002;347(11): 797–805.
73. Mogensen CE. Antihypertensive treatment inhibiting the progression of diabetic nephropathy. Acta Endocrinol Suppl (Copenh). 1980;238:103–8.
74. Kitzmiller JL, Brown ER, Phillippe M, Stark AR, Acker D, Kaldany A, et al. Diabetic nephropathy and perinatal outcome. Am J Obstet Gynecol. 1981;141(7):741–51.
75. Christensen NJ, Gundersen HJ, Mogensen CE, Vittinghus E. Intravenous insulin decreases urinary albumin excretion in long-term diabetics with nephropathy. Diabetologia. 1980;18(4): 285–8.
76. Marre M, Bernadet P, Gallois Y, Savagner F, Guyene TT, Hallab M, et al. Relationships between angiotensin I converting enzyme gene polymorphism, plasma levels, and diabetic retinal and renal complications. Diabetes. 1994;43(3):384–8.
77. Christensen CK, Mogensen CE. Antihypertensive treatment: long-term reversal of progression of albuminuria in incipient diabetic nephropathy. A longitudinal study of renal function. J Diabet Complications. 1987;1(2):45–52.
78. Feldt-Rasmussen B, Mathiesen ER, Deckert T. Effect of two years of strict metabolic control on progression of incipient nephropathy in insulin-dependent diabetes. Lancet. 1986;2(8519):1300–4.
79. Steinke JM, Sinaiko AR, Kramer MS, Suissa S, Chavers BM, Mauer M, et al. The early natural history of nephropathy in Type 1 Diabetes: III. Predictors of 5-year urinary albumin excretion rate patterns in initially normoalbuminuric patients. Diabetes. 2005; 54(7):2164–71.
80. Deckert T, Andersen AR, Christiansen JS, Andersen JK. Course of diabetic nephropathy. Factors related to development. Acta Endocrinol Suppl (Copenh). 1981;242:14–5.
81. Turin TC, Tonelli M, Manns BJ, Ahmed SB, Ravani P, James M, et al. Proteinuria and life expectancy. Am J Kidney Dis. 2013; 61(4):646–8.
82. Bilous RW, Mauer SM, Sutherland DE, Steffes MW. Mean glomerular volume and rate of development of diabetic nephropathy. Diabetes. 1989;38(9):1142–7.
83. Parving HH, Andersen AR, Smidt UM, Christiansen JS, Oxenboll B, Svendsen PA. Diabetic nephropathy and arterial hypertension.

The effect of antihypertensive treatment. Diabetes. 1983;32 Suppl 2:83–7.
84. Parving HH, Andersen AR, Smidt UM, Svendsen PA. Early aggressive antihypertensive treatment reduces rate of decline in kidney function in diabetic nephropathy. Lancet. 1983;1(8335):1175–9.
85. Viberti GC, Bilous RW, Mackintosh D, Bending JJ, Keen H. Long term correction of hyperglycaemia and progression of renal failure in insulin dependent diabetes. Br Med J (Clin Res Ed). 1983;286(6365):598–602.
86. Knowler WC, Bennett PH, Hamman RF, Miller M. Diabetes incidence and prevalence in Pima Indians: a 19-fold greater incidence than in Rochester, Minnesota. Am J Epidemiol. 1978;108(6):497–505.
87. Myers BD, Nelson RG, Williams GW, Bennett PH, Hardy SA, Berg RL, et al. Glomerular function in Pima Indians with noninsulin-dependent diabetes mellitus of recent onset. J Clin Invest. 1991;88(2):524–30.
88. Pavkov ME, Bennett PH, Sievers ML, Krakoff J, Williams DE, Knowler WC, et al. Predominant effect of kidney disease on mortality in Pima Indians with or without type 2 diabetes. Kidney Int. 2005;68(3):1267–74.
89. Vora JP, Leese GP, Peters JR, Owens DR. Longitudinal evaluation of renal function in non-insulin-dependent diabetic patients with early nephropathy: effects of angiotensin-converting enzyme inhibition. J Diabetes Complications. 1996;10(2):88–93.
90. Nowack R, Raum E, Blum W, Ritz E. Renal hemodynamics in recent-onset type II diabetes. Am J Kidney Dis. 1992;20(4):342–7.
91. Vora JP, Dolben J, Dean JD, Thomas D, Williams JD, Owens DR, et al. Renal hemodynamics in newly presenting non-insulin dependent diabetes mellitus. Kidney Int. 1992;41(4):829–35.
92. Schmitz A, Hansen HH, Christensen T. Kidney function in newly diagnosed type 2 (non-insulin-dependent) diabetic patients, before and during treatment. Diabetologia. 1989;32(7):434–9.
93. Weidmann P, Trost BN. Pathogenesis and treatment of hypertension associated with diabetes. Horm Metab Res Suppl. 1985;15:51–8.
94. Schmitz A, Gundersen HJ, Osterby R. Glomerular morphology by light microscopy in non-insulin-dependent diabetes mellitus. Lack of glomerular hypertrophy. Diabetes. 1988;37(1):38–43.
95. Araki S, Haneda M, Sugimoto T, Isono M, Isshiki K, Kashiwagi A, et al. Factors associated with frequent remission of microalbuminuria in patients with type 2 diabetes. Diabetes. 2005;54(10):2983–7.
96. Caramori ML, Kim Y, Fioretto P, Huang C, Rich SS, Miller ME, et al. Cellular basis of diabetic nephropathy: IV. Antioxidant enzyme mRNA expression levels in skin fibroblasts of type 1 diabetic sibling pairs. Nephrol Dial Transplant. 2006;21(11):3122–6.
97. Lane PH, Steffes MW, Mauer SM. Glomerular structure in IDDM women with low glomerular filtration rate and normal urinary albumin excretion. Diabetes. 1992;41(5):581–6.
98. Tsalamandris C, Allen TJ, Gilbert RE, Sinha A, Panagiotopoulos S, Cooper ME, et al. Progressive decline in renal function in diabetic patients with and without albuminuria. Diabetes. 1994;43(5):649–55.
99. Nelson RG, Knowler WC, McCance DR, Sievers ML, Pettitt DJ, Charles MA, et al. Determinants of end-stage renal disease in Pima Indians with type 2 (non-insulin-dependent) diabetes mellitus and proteinuria. Diabetologia. 1993;36(10):1087–93.
100. Brito PL, Fioretto P, Drummond K, Kim Y, Steffes MW, Basgen JM, et al. Proximal tubular basement membrane width in insulin-dependent diabetes mellitus. Kidney Int. 1998;53(3):754–61.

Pathogenesis of Diabetic Nephropathy: Hemodynamic Alterations/Renin Angiotensin System

4

Arnold B. Alper Jr.

Introduction

Diabetic nephropathy, a microvascular complication of diabetes, is clinically characterized by an initial increase in glomerular filtration rate (GFR) and microalbuminuria [1]. If left untreated, these early pathophysiologic changes will progress to renal fibrosis and tubulointerstitial damage along with a decline in GFR, ultimately leading to kidney failure [2, 3].

Diabetic nephropathy and its related pathophysiologic alterations in renal microcirculation is thought to develop as a result of the interaction between metabolic and hemodynamic factors that together activate common intracellular pathways that trigger the production of various cytokines and growth factors leading to kidney disease. Persistent elevations in blood glucose alter renal hemodynamics through activation of several vasoactive hormonal pathways, including the renin-angiotensin-aldosterone system (RAS), endothelin, and urotensin [4, 5]. These hormones then in turn can activate second messenger signaling pathways, including protein kinase C, transcription factors, including NK-κB, and cytokines, including TGF-β, VEGF, and PDGF, all of which can lead to the development of albuminuria, glomerulosclerosis, and tubulointerstitial fibrosis characteristic of diabetic nephropathy [6, 7]. This chapter will provide a detailed review of these hemodynamic and hormonal mechanisms that underlie the development of diabetic nephropathy.

Renin-Angiotensin-Aldosterone System

The role of the RAAS in the pathophysiology of diabetic nephropathy (diabetic nephropathy) is well established. Whereas older studies focused on the systemic RAS and provided controversial and contradictory results, more recent advances have examined the role of the local intrarenal RAS that acts independently of the systemic RAS and has been shown to be activated in both experimental and human diabetes [8, 9]. While classically angiotensin II (Ang II) was regarded as the single effector molecule of the RAS, in recent years studies have demonstrated that aldosterone, renin, and prorenin have direct effects in the diabetic kidney [10]. Further, more recent studies have shown that metabolites of Ang II, including angiotensin 1-7 (Ang (1-7)) and angiotensin 1-9 (Ang (1-9)), may play an important role in the development and progression of diabetic nephropathy [11, 12].

Indeed, the renal RAS is unique among local RAS systems because all of the necessary components for intrarenal Ang II are present along the nephron in both intratubular and interstitial compartments [13, 14]. AT II formation is dependent on the availability of the substrates angiotensinogen (AGT), angiotensin I (Ang I), and the enzymatic activities of renin, angiotensin converting enzyme (ACE), angiotensin converting enzyme 2 (ACE 2), and ACE-independent enzymatic pathways including the serine proteases, such as chymase. Angiotensin 1-7, Ang (1-7), a metabolite of Ang II, can be formed directly from ANG II via hydrolysis from ACE2 or indirectly from Ang I via ACE [15, 16] (Fig. 4.1). The study of the evolving and complex interactions between these various hormones and their receptors has led to a much greater understanding of the pathophysiology of diabetic nephropathy.

Angiotensin II (Ang II)

Ang II, the most potent effector hormone of the RAS, has diverse actions in many different renal cell types. While there are conflicting data regarding increased activation of the systemic RAS in type 1 or type 2 diabetes, it is well established that the intrarenal RAS is up-regulated in diabetic nephropathy, contributing to much of the pathophysiology of this condition [17, 18]. Further, most recent studies have demonstrated that cell-specific RAS exists, for example

A.B. Alper Jr., M.D., M.P.H. (✉)
Department of Internal Medicine, Section of Nephrology, Tulane University School of Medicine, 1430 Tulane Avenue, New Orleans, LA 70112, USA
e-mail: aalper2@tulane.edu

E.V. Lerma and V. Batuman (eds.), *Diabetes and Kidney Disease*,
DOI 10.1007/978-1-4939-0793-9_4, © Springer Science+Business Media New York 2014

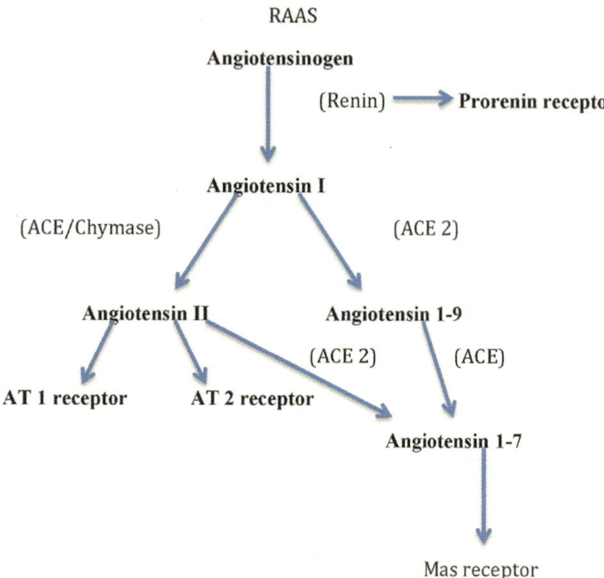

Fig. 4.1 Evolving view of the RAAS

in the proximal tubule, and is up regulated in the diabetic kidney [9]. Although the intrarenal RAS is activated early in diabetes, the exact mechanism remains unknown. The discovery of GR91, a G-protein-coupled receptor that is activated by succinate, may provide a link between hyperglycemia and RAS activation [19]. In rat models, infusion of succinate increases PRA and blood pressure, both of which are abolished by angiotensin-converting enzyme (ACE) inhibition or bilateral nephrectomy [19]. High levels of glucose stimulate succinate accumulation, and this directly increases renin release from isolated juxtaglomerular apparatus in vitro [20].

Data concerning intrarenal RAS states in diabetic nephropathy are inconsistent. Direct measurements have failed to establish that intrarenal RAS Ang II is consistently elevated diabetes [21]. On the other hand, urinary AGT levels have been shown to be consistently elevated in both experimental models and human forms of diabetic nephropathy [22, 23]. The localization of renin in the collecting tubule and the delivery of proximally produced AGT, along with ACE in the tubular fluid, allows for the local formation of both Ang I and Ang II, despite suppression of juxtaglomerular renin [24].

Recent studies in type 2 diabetes mellitus have shown that there is a major role for ACE-independent formation of Ang II. There have been several reports that chymase is markedly unregulated in mesangial cells, mast cells, and vascular smooth muscle cells in experimental models of diabetic nephropathy and that chymase inhibitors, such as chymostatin, significantly block Ang II formation [25, 26]. Park et al. reported that afferent arteriole vasoconstriction in control kidneys that is produced by Ang I was significantly blunted by ACE inhibition, but not by serine protease inhibition [27]. On the other hand, afferent arteriole vasoconstriction produced by intrarenal conversion of Ang I to Ang II was significantly blunted by serine protease inhibition but not ACE inhibition in diabetic kidneys [27]. These data suggest that there appears to be a switch from ACE-dependent to serine-protease dependent Ang II formation in the diabetic kidney.

In the kidney, Ang II acts via signaling through its two receptor subtypes, the AT-1 and AT-2 receptors. The AT-1 receptor is thought to be widely distributed throughout the kidney, while the AT-2 receptor is only found in glomerular endothelial cells and tubular epithelial cells in the cortex, interstitial, and tubular cells in the outer medulla, and inner medullary collecting duct cells [28, 29]. It is generally accepted that these receptors mediate the opposing effects of Ang II such that activation of AT-1 receptors leads to vasoconstriction, sodium retention, and cell proliferation, while activation of the AT-2 receptors leads to vasodilation, natriuresis, and inhibition of cell proliferation [30, 31]. Interestingly, several reports have demonstrated that the expression of renal AT-1 receptors is decreased in diabetic nephropathy, suggesting that it may be the sensitivity of the AT-1 receptors to Ang II, rather than the level of its expression, that mediates the harmful effects of Ang II activation of the AT-1 receptor [18, 32]. Further, both the early hyperfiltration and later decline in GFR seen with diabetic nephropathy is thought to be associated with AT-1 receptor-mediated alterations in vascular responsiveness to Ang II [33, 34].

In addition to hemodynamic effects, it is becoming increasingly well documented that Ang II via the AT-1 receptor contributes significantly to the development and progression of diabetic renal structural injury. These deleterious actions of Ang II have been mainly attributed to the stimulation of profibrotic cytokines such as TGF-β, VEGF, PDGF, and also to the downstream activation of signaling pathways involving PKC and NF-κB [35, 36]. The net result of all of these actions is the formulation of tubulointerstitial fibrosis and glomerulosclerosis. Ang II has also been shown to be a potent inflammatory agent in the kidney, activating the differentiation and proliferation of monocytes and macrophages [37]. Further, Ang II has been reported to increase accumulation of advanced glycation end-products, which in turn also contributes to renal injury.

In mesangial cells, AII induces hypertrophy and hyperplasia and promotes extracellular matrix accumulation by both increasing the synthesis of and decreasing the degradation of extracellular matrix components [37]. In podocytes, AII exerts effects that alter the permselectivity of the glomerular filtration barrier. In vitro studies have demonstrated that exposure of podocytes to AII results in the redistribution and loss of nephrin as well as changes in the cytoskeleton distribution, including loss of stress fibers, cortical accumulation of F-actin, and cell retraction [38]. Also, AII can induce reorganization of F-actin fibers paralleled by increased albumin permeability across the podocyte monolayers [39]. AII stimulates production of alpha3(IV) collagen and promotes both hypertrophy and apoptosis of the podocyte [40]. In tubular cells, AII induces cell hypertrophy, apoptosis, and epithelial-myofibroblast transdifferentiation. It also promotes extracellular matrix accumulation by upregulating TGFβ receptor type 2 expression, thus amplifying the effects of TGFβ1 on the tubule [41].

The role of the AT-2 receptor in the pathobiology of the diabetic kidney is much less well understood and there is much conflicting data regarding these receptors. Indeed, experimental models of diabetic nephropathy have reported both increased and decreased expression of the AT-2 receptor [29, 31]. The decrease in the AT-2 receptors expression supports the concept that AT-2 receptors may mediate beneficial effects of Ang II, such as cell differentiation and apoptosis protecting against glomerulosclerosis and that these beneficial effects are lost through downregulation of AT-2 receptor expression. Further support for the important role of the AT-2 receptor in diabetic nephropathy comes from a report of an AT-2 receptor gene polymorphism that is associated with the decline in renal function and premature aging in the arterial system of type 1 diabetics [42]. However, the effects of AT-2 receptor activation are certainly not uniform and there is much debate regarding the role of the AT-2 receptor in diabetic renal damage. Several recent studies have shown that blockage of the AT-2 receptor may confer some renal protection in certain settings [43, 44]. Further, the AT-2 receptor has been implicated in promoting renal damage through generation of reactive oxygen species. Additionally, it has been shown that the blockade of both AT-1 and AT-2 receptors is necessary to completely block the inflammatory process in a model of diabetic kidney damage [44]. Obviously, further study and investigation of the role of the AT-2 receptor in diabetic nephropathy is much needed, particularly in view of the importance of the RAS in the pathology of diabetic nephropathy.

It is important to note that not all studies are in agreement with regard to the level of expression of not only the AT-1 and AT-2 receptors but other components of the RAS as well. This likely explanation for these divergent findings is the different experimental animal models of diabetic nephropathy used in the various studies, duration of diabetes, as well as the techniques used to measure the levels of expression of the RAS. In addition, diabetes may not only alter the level of expression of various RAS components but may also alter the distribution of these components in various kidney compartments. These observations once again stress the importance of not only an intrarenal RAS but also cell-specific expression of RAS in the pathology of diabetic nephropathy.

ACE2

The complexity of the intrarenal RAS continues to evolve with discovery of new enzymes and receptors. One such enzyme is ACE2, a novel enzyme of the RAS, that leads to generation of angiotensin degradation products, such as A1-7, a peptide which is antiangiogeneic and has vasodilatory properties that can antagonize the effects of AII [45] (see Fig. 4.1). Many experts now consider this enzyme to be part of a counter-regulatory mechanism to the classical RAS. Since its initial discovery, ACE2 has been identified in a number of human tissues including the heart, kidneys, and testes, suggesting that this enzyme may play an important role in both renal and cardiovascular homeostasis [46].

ACE2 is the first ACE homologue with 42 % sequence homology and this metalloprotease contains only one HEXXH consensus sequence, resulting in monocarboxypeptidase activity [46]. Also, ACE2 has a 48 % sequence homology with collectrin, a newly discovered protein responsible for regulation of renal amino acid transport and maintenance of collecting duct morphology [47]. It exists as both membrane bound and soluble forms. While ACE2 is capable of cleaving the terminal leucine from Ang I to generate Ang(1-9), it has a 400-fold affinity for Ang II, cleaving the terminal phenylalanine residue from ANG II to generate Ang(1-7) [47]. While Ang II, has well known vasoconstrictor, proinflammatory, and prooxidant effects, mediated largely through the AT-1 receptor, Ang(1-7), the primary product of AT II degradation via ACE2, acts through the Mas receptor, to produce vasodilation by means of increased bradykinin and nitric oxide, to increase release of prostaglandins, and to inhibit norepinephrine release [48, 49].

ACE2 expression has been identified in multiple compartments of the kidney including the renal cortical tubules (predominantly) and the apical border of the proximal convoluted tubule, where ACE2 co-localizes with podocyte specific markers such as nephrin, podocin, and synaptopodin [50, 51].

ACE2 expression in the kidney has been studied in diabetes mellitus type 1 and type 2 models. In a study of 8-week-old db/db mice, a model of early type 2 diabetes, ACE2 mRNA and expression are elevated, while ACE expression is decreased in both glomeruli and cortex prior to the development of diabetic nephropathy [50]. Thus, it appears that in early stages of diabetic kidney disease, ACE2 is upregulated, probably as a protective mechanism against the ACE-dependent Ang II formation. As a result of prolonged hyperglycemia and consequent activation of proinflammatory and profibrotic pathways, ACE2 expression becomes downregulated and this may contribute to kidney disease progression. Further, in diabetic kidney models, decreased ACE2 expression is associated with increased albuminuria and inhibition of ACE2 by MLN-4760 increased urinary albumin excretion three to fourfold [53]. ACE2 inhibition also has been reported to cause increased mesangial matrix expansion, increased vascular thickness, and focal loss of podocytes, indicating that ACE2 may be necessary for podocyte maintenance. Finally, in two models of type 1 diabetes, ACE2 gene deletion caused accelerated development of diabetic kidney disease [54]. Additionally, human studies have shown that ACE expression is increased while ACE2 expression is decreased in the tubules of diabetic nephropathy [52]. These current findings suggest that ACE2 likely participates in a compensatory mechanism in the diabetic kidney prior to the onset of diabetic nephropathy while protecting against podocyte loss, thus preventing the worsening glomerular injury.

Metabolites of Ang II: Ang(1-7) and Ang(1-9)

Angiotensin (1-7) is a heptapeptide member of the RAS and can be formed as a result of the metabolism of Ang(1-9) by ACE and metabolism of Ang II by ACE2 (see Fig. 4.1). In the kidney, Ang(1-7) appears to be generated from its precursor Ang I by neprilysin, thimet oligopeptidase, or prolyl oligopeptidase that are located either on the brush border or in the cytoplasm [12, 57]. However, studies in rat kidney cortex have shown that Ang(1-7) is primarily generated via ACE2-dependent degradation of Ang II [50]. Ang(1-7), through its binding to the Mas receptor is a potent vasodilator that also has been shown to have antihypertensive, anti-inflammatory, and antiproliferative properties in the kidney [15, 55]. These actions, therefore, essentially antagonize the actions of Ang II mediated via the AT-1 receptor. To date, however, there is limited information regarding the direct effects of Ang(1-7) in the diabetic kidney. In streptozotocin-induced Wistar rats, there is a downregulation in the expression of Ang(1-7) mRNA compared with the nondiabetic rat, but differences in renal Ang(1-7) levels were not detected [56]. In this same experimental model, treatment with Ang(1-7) and/or the Ang(1-7) receptor Mas agonist AVE-00991 reduced albuminuria and prevented diabetes-induced abnormal vascular responsiveness to norepinephrine, endothelin-1, and Ang II [11]. Similarly, treatment of streptozotocin-induced diabetic rats with Ang(1-7) attenuated NADPH oxidase activation, diminished proteinuria, and decreased diabetes-induced increase in renal vascular responsive to AT II [58]. These observations support the paradigm that Ang(1-7) is a renoprotective agent in diabetes.

In the nonrenal vasculature, Ang(1-7) exerts a vasodilatory effect that involves increased production of nitric oxide, prostaglandins, or endothelium-dependent hyperpolarizing relaxing factor [59, 60]. These effects are blocked by the Ang(1-7) Mas receptor antagonist, suggesting involvement of Mas receptor signaling pathways.

However, the role in Ang(1-7) in the regulation of renal hemodynamics is incompletely understood and the data are conflicting. In rat renal vasculature, in vitro studies have been performed showing that although Ang(1-7) did not affect vascular function, it prevented Ang II-induced vasoconstriction of isolated renal arteries in vitro. In Wistar Kyoto rats and SHR rats, Ang (1-7) increases renal blood flow and inhibits Ang II pressor responses [61, 62]. The latter effect is blocked by antagonism of the Mas receptor, cyclo-oxygenase inhibition, or NOS inhibition, suggesting a role for Mas-mediated release of prostaglandins and nitric oxide in the vasodilatory response to Ang(1-7).

Ang I can be degraded into Ang (1-9) by ACE2 [63]. The role of Ang(1-9) in the kidney remains poorly understood and has not been properly evaluated. Some investigators believe Ang (1-9) may have a beneficial role as Ang(1-9) can be converted into a potential vasodilator Ang(1-7). However, increased conversion of exogenous Ang(1-9) into Ang II in glomerular extracts from diabetic rats has been reported with the reaction catalyzed by an unknown carboxypeptidase [12]. This observation suggests that Ang(1-9) may have a detrimental role in kidney function at it may provide an additional pathway for Ang II formation in the diabetic kidney. Conversion of Ang I to Ang(1-9) is thought to be of significance only under conditions that raise Ang II levels such as treatment with an angiotensin receptor blocker [64]. Further studies are definitely needed to determine the role of Ang (1-9) in the diabetic kidney.

Recent studies have identified the importance of Ang IV, a N-terminal angiotensin degradation product, in cardiovascular disease [65]. Ang IV is generated in response to tissue injury and binds to the AT-4 receptor. In the kidney, Ang IV has been shown to have both vasoconstrictor and vasodilatory effects and induces PAI-1 expression in models of hypertension [66]. However, there is no significant data regarding the role of Ang IV in the diabetic kidney.

Renin and Prorenin

It is well established that ACE inhibition is only partially effective in attenuating the progression of diabetic nephropathy. It has been speculated that this may be due to local kidney tissue renin accumulation, which, in turn, may lead to higher renal Ang II levels via renin-dependent, but ACE independent pathways [67]. However, plasma renin activity is generally decreased in diabetics, while renal levels are elevated, especially in the tubules [68]. Unlike the juxtaglomerular cells where Ang II inhibits renin release via the AT-1 receptor, in the collecting duct Ang II stimulates renin expression via the AT-1 receptor [69]. In animal models of diabetes and hypertension, collecting duct prorenin and renin are upregulated. The elevated levels of prorenin observed in diabetes may come from the epithelial cells of the collecting duct [70]. Thus, whereas the juxtaglomerular apparatus may suppress renin production in the diabetic, upregulated renin production produced in the distal nephron may be able to support continued intrarenal Ang II formation and amplify or maintain the hypertensive state as well as renal damage [69]. The increase in local tubular renin has been thought to be responsible for increased local formation of Ang II that subsequently leads to increased tubulointerstitial fibrosis and injury.

Prorenin is a precursor of renin that under normal physiologic conditions lacks renin enzymatic activity. Plasma prorenin levels have been shown to be elevated in patients with type 2 diabetes, especially those with microalbuminuria [71]. Both prorenin and renin have been demonstrated to have direct action in the kidney via binding to the membrane-associated protein called the prorenin/renin receptor, (pro) renin receptor [72]. This receptor, which is expressed in the heart, brain, placenta, liver, and kidney tissue, binds prorenin and, with a lesser affinity, renin. When bound to this receptor, prorenin undergoes a conformational change and becomes enzymatically active without undergoing proteolysis. This mechanism may contribute to local Ang II formation, especially in tissues that lack the renin gene. This receptor has been localized predominantly to mesangial cells, distal tubules, glomeruli, and the macula densa [72, 73]. Activation of the (pro)renin receptor in cultured mesangial via binding of prorenin/renin to this receptor has been shown to activate the mitogen-activated protein kinase (MAPK)-extracellular signal-regulated kinase (ERK) pathway as well as increase profibrotic mediators such as TGF-β, PAI-1, fibronectin, and collagen 1 [73, 74] even in the presence of an angiotensin receptor blocker or ACE inhibitor [73]. These findings suggest that activation of the (pro)renin receptor in mesangial cells by elevated levels of prorenin as occurs in diabetes, may lead to significant glomerulosclerosis, independent of Ang II formation.

The (pro)renin receptor has been found in human podocytes where prorenin infusion leads to an increase in intracellular Ang II that is blocked by the direct renin inhibitor, aliskiren [75]. As seen with mesangial cells, stimulation of the (pro)renin receptor in podocytes results in the activation of the MAPK-ERK pathway but does not lead to increased levels of PAI-1 or TGF-β [75]. It should be noted that excessive stimulation of the (pro)renin receptor by high levels of prorenin is self-limiting.

A site-specific binding protein, a so-called *decoy protein* has been found and it prevents prorenin activation on binding to the (pro)receptor [73]. In an experimental model of diabetic nephropathy, the "decoy protein" has been demonstrated to lessen glomerulosclerosis and tubulointerstitial fibrosis, both directly and indirectly [76, 77]. These findings support the concept of the role for renin and prorenin in the pathophysiology of diabetic nephropathy, either alone, or in concert together with Ang II. However, more studies are needed to determine if blockade of the (pro)renin receptor will provide significant renoprotective effects in diabetic nephropathy in humans.

Aldosterone

Aldosterone has become increasingly recognized as an important mediator of kidney damage in diabetic nephropathy. Long-term ACE inhibition is associated with increases in plasma aldosterone levels in many patients after an initial reduction or unchanged levels, so-called *aldosterone escape* [81]. Whereas aldosterone was previously believed to be involved in just water and electrolyte balance, there is emerging evidence for it having direct action on target cells leading to renal injury via oxidative stress, inflammation, and fibrosis. These findings led to the belief that one of the reasons for incomplete renal protection offered by ACE inhibition is elevation in aldosterone levels. In experimental animal models of diabetes, the administration of spironolactone, a mineralocorticoid receptor antagonist, lead to decreased albuminuria, glomerulosclerosis, macrophage infiltration, renal MCP-1 synthesis, and expression of NF-β [78]. In patients with type 2 diabetes mellitus and diabetic nephropathy, spironolactone usage has been shown to decrease albuminuria and PAI-1 [79]. A more recent study showed that the use of a more selective mineralocorticoid receptor antagonist, eplerenone, reduced proteinuria in hypertensive diabetic patients to a similar extent to that seen with ACE inhibitors [80]. Additionally, clinical studies have also demonstrated a relationship between increased serum levels of aldosterone and deterioration in kidney function.

With the exception of the brain, extra-adrenal synthesis of aldosterone is controversial. However, the enzyme responsible for aldosterone synthesis from deoxycorticosteroid, P450 11β2 (CYP11β2) has been reported to be present in the rat kidney, mainly in the glomerulus and podocytes [82]. Upregulation of this enzyme was observed in a rat model of type 1 diabetes [82]. It is unknown if such a system exists in the human kidney and further study is needed in this area.

Renal Vascular Response to Diabetes

Both hemodynamic and non-hemodynamic pathogenic pathways contribute to the development of glomerulosclerosis and, subsequent, tubulointerstitial fibrosis in diabetic nephropathy. The hemodynamic changes involve changes in arteriolar function that ultimately cause hyperfiltration early during the course of diabetes. In addition to the RAS, several other hormone systems and electrolytes may play a key role in this process.

9C-Peptide

C-peptide is a 31-residue cleavage product of insulin synthesis that is secreted from the pancreas along with insulin. Thus, type 1 diabetics with impaired insulin secretion have decreased C-peptide levels. Although originally thought to be biologically inert, C-peptide is now recognized to exert renoprotective effects in patients and animals with type 1 diabetes [83]. C-peptide administration has been shown to attenuate hyperfiltration, hypertrophy, and albuminuria presumably through the effects on the Na+/K+ ATPase, but the precise mechanism has remained speculative [84]. A study from Nordquist and colleagues showed that C-peptide exerts a direct vasoconstrictor effect on isolated perfused afferent arterioles from mice with alloxan-induced type 1 diabetes, while having minimal effect on afferent arterioles from nondiabetic mice [85]. This finding suggests that reduced endogenous C-peptide levels may contribute to the afferent arteriolar vasodilation associated with diabetic hyperfiltration. Further, as C-peptide has been shown to be a vasodilator in most vascular beds, its vasoconstrictor effect on the afferent arteriole in type 1 diabetes underscores the likelihood that novel mechanisms control afferent arteriolar function under these conditions.

COX-2

New evidence is also increasing regarding the role of arachadonic acid metabolites, specifically COX-2, in the renal vascular dysfunction seen with diabetic nephropathy. Although altered metabolism of arachadonic acid has been linked to diabetic hyperfiltration based on the effects of nonsteroidal anti-inflammatory drugs, only recently has evidence emerged of specific involvement. In streptozotocin-induced diabetic rat kidneys there is evidence for increased expression of COX-2 and reversal of hyperfiltration with COX-2 inhibition whereas in normal rats there was no effect on GFR [86]. Subsequent studies have confirmed these findings and suggested that peroxynitrite as a contributing stimulus for the upregulation of COX-2 [87, 88]. In adolescents and young adults with diabetes and hyperfiltration, COX-2 inhibition has been shown to blunt hyperfiltration while in those diabetics with a normal GFR and no hyperfiltration, COX-2 inhibition increased the GFR [89]. Obviously, these divergent findings attest to the complexity of COX-2-dependent influences on glomerular function in type 1 diabetics. Further, it appears as though the renal hemodynamic response to COX-2 inhibition is sex specific, such that the dependence on vasodilator prostaglandins is greater in women than men, suggesting that sex hormones may contribute to the pathogenesis of diabetic nephropathy through renal vascular events that occur early in diabetes [90].

In a study in type 1 diabetics, a chronic infusion of the somatostatin analog, octreotide, was able to partially reverse the early hyperfiltration and increase in renal size, seen in these patients [96]. Although plasma glucose, plasma glucagon, and growth hormone levels were unchanged, there was a decrease in the plasma concentration of insulin-like growth factor 1 (IGF-1). Interestingly, an infusion of IGF-1 in normal subjects has been shown to similar hemodynamic findings to that seen in early diabetic patients, renal vasodilation, and an elevation in GFR [97]. These results have also been replicated in animal models [98].

Another important effect of hyperglycemia may be the accumulation of sorbitol and the formation of glycosylated proteins. Excess glucose can be converted intracellularly, via aldose reductase, to sorbitol that then accumulates in the cell. Studies in human type 1 diabetics with microalbuminuria demonstrated that the infusion of tolrestat, an aldose reductase inhibitor, lowers the GFR toward normal and reduces albumin excretion [99].

Chronic hyperglycemia induces some of the excess circulating glucose to combine with free amino acids on circulating and tissue proteins. This process initially forms reversible glycation products that later transform into irreversible advance glycation end products. In rat models, the infusion of glycation products to the level seen in diabetic rats can increase real plasma flow, GFR, and intraglomerular pressure typical of untreated diabetes [100]. Infusion of advanced glycation products in vivo results in significant increases in expression of various components of the RAS [103]. Further, infusion of Ang II increases both serum and renal accumulation of glycation products, highlighting the complex interaction of events underlying the pathology of diabetic nephropathy.

Diabetes and Renal Autoregulation

Glomerular hyperfiltration and glomerular capillary hypertension are generally thought to play a significant role in the pathology of diabetic nephropathy, especially glomerulosclerosis. These conditions are often exacerbated by even mild elevations in systemic arterial pressure that is transmitted to the glomerulus through vasodilated preglomerular microvasculature. Even mild reductions in systemic blood pressure have been demonstrated to produce significantly less glomerular damage. In order for systemic arterial pressure to be transmitted to the glomerulus there would be need for impairment of renal autoregulatory capability.

This would imply that hyperglycemia impairs autoregulation of local glomerular microcirculation with dilation of arterioles, more so of the afferent arteriole, thus affecting the transcapillary hydraulic pressure difference [91]. A number of different factors may contribute to the altered autoregulation seen in diabetes, including hormones such as IGF-1 and sex hormones, sorbitol, and increased sodium reabsorption and tubuloglomerular feedback.

Enhanced tubular sodium reabsorption, due to increased sodium glucose transport in the proximal tubule, has also been demonstrated to play an important role in renal blood flow autoregulation. Hyperinsulinemia and high glucose concentration in the ultrafiltrate stimulate sodium-glucose transport in the proximal tubule leading to increased sodium reabsorption [101]. This rise in proximal sodium reabsorption decreases solute and fluid delivery to the macula densa, thereby activating the tubuloglomerular feedback-dependent afferent arteriolar vasodilation and increase in GFR.

It has also been postulated that hyperglycemia sensitizes the target organs to blood pressure-induced damage, most likely by activation of the local RAS with local Ang II production. High glucose levels have been shown to increase the expression of renin and AGT in mesangial and tubular cells, which could increase intrarenal Ang II levels, and then activate various cytokines, leading to extracellular matrix accumulation. Indeed, diabetes mellitus has been demonstrated to affect both mechanisms of autoregulation, the myogenic response as well as tubuloglomerular feedback. Thus, it is not surprising to find studies demonstrating that renal autoregulation is impaired in diabetes. In a micropuncture study of a rat model of type 2 diabetes, renal autoregulation was shown to be impaired early in the diabetic rats, but not in non-diabetic controls [92]. These changes were noted prior to the development of overt hyperglycemia, consistent with the notion that an autoregulatory defect is an early event in diabetes and can contribute significantly to the development of diabetes nephropathy. However, a study by Lau et al. in rats with streptozotocin-induced diabetes revealed that these rats have significantly augmented renal blood flow and autoregulatory capability at low perfusion pressures, compared with non-diabetic rats [93]. Thus, there is a lack of consensus regarding the autoregulatory capability of the renal vasculature early in diabetes. The complexity of this situation is likely due, at least in part, to the gradual impairment of glomerular autoregulation that occurs with increasing duration of diabetes in both humans and rodents [94, 95].

Recent studies have suggested that primary changes in preglomerular microvascular smooth muscle play a key role in the afferent arteriolar vasodilation seen in the hyperfiltration present early in diabetic nephropathy. Pharmacologic blockade of ATP-sensitive K+ channels causes contraction of afferent arterioles from rats with streptozotocin-induced diabetes, while having minimal impact on afferent arterioles from normal rats [102]. This observation suggests that open K+ channels contribute to tonic afferent arteriolar vasodilation during diabetes. It is felt that these K+ channels likely contribute to afferent arteriolar dilation in diabetes by promoting vascular smooth muscle membrane hyperpolarization thereby reducing calcium influx through voltage-gated channels and ultimately decreasing intracellular calcium concentration. This impaired electromechanical coupling would be expected to impair vasoactive responses to multiple humoral agents, the myogenic response, tubuloglomerular feedback, and ultimately autoregulation, all of which are present in diabetic nephropathy.

References

1. Hostetter TH. Hyperfiltration and glomerulosclerosis. Semin Nephrol. 2003;23(2):194–9.
2. Caramori ML, Mauer M. Diabetes and nephropathy. Curr Opin Nephrol Hypertens. 2007;12(3):273–82.
3. Leon CA, Raij L. Interaction of haemodynamic and metabolic pathways in the genesis of diabetic nephropathy. J Hypertens. 2005;23(11):1931–7.
4. Cooper M, Boner G. Dual Blockade of the renin-angiotensin-aldosterone system in diabetic nephropathy. Diabet Med. 2004;21 Suppl 1:15–8.
5. Hanes DS, Nahar A, Weir MR. The tissue renin-angiotensin-aldosterone system in diabetic mellitus. Curr Hypertens Rep. 2004;6(2):98–105.
6. Noh H, King GL. The role of protein kinase C activation in diabetic nephropathy. Kidney Int Suppl. 2007;106:S49–53.
7. Zhu Y, Usui HK, Sharma K. Regulation of transforming growth factor beta in diabetic nephropathy: implications for treatment. Semin Nephrol. 2007;27(2):153–60.
8. Hollenberg NK, Price DA, Fisher ND, Lansang MC, Perkins B, Gordon MS, Williams GH, Laffel LM. Glomerular hemodynamics and renin-angiotensin system in patients with type I diabetes mellitus. Kidney Int. 2003;63:172–8.
9. Zimpelmann J, Kumar D, Levine DZ, Wehbi G, Imig JD, Navar LG, Burns KD. Early diabetes mellitus stimulates proximal tubule renin mRNA expression in the rat. Kidney Int. 2000;58(6):2320–30.
10. Schmieder RE. The potential role of prorenin in diabetic nephropathy. J Hypertens. 2007;25(7):1323–6.
11. Benter IF, Yousif MH, Anim JT, Cojocel C, Diz DI. Angiotensin (1-7) prevents the development of severe hypertension and end-organ damage in spontaneously hypertensive rats treated with L-NAME. Am J Physiol Heart Circ Physiol. 2006;290(2):H684–91.
12. Singh R, Singh AK, Leehey DJ. A novel mechanism for angiotensin II formation in streptozotocin-diabetic rat glomeruli. Am J Physiol Renal Physiol. 2005;288(6):F1183–90.
13. Kobori H, Nangaku M, Navar LG, Nishiyama A. The intrarenal renin-angiotensin system: from physiology to the pathobiology of hypertension and the kidney disease. Pharmacol Rev. 2007;59(3):251–87.
14. Dzau VJ, Re R. Tissue angiotensin system in cardiovascular medicine. A paradigm shift? Circulation. 1994;89(1):493–8.
15. Trask AJ, Ferraio CM. Angiotensin (1-7): pharmacology and new perspectives in cardiovascular treatments. Cardiovasc Drug Rev. 2007;25(2):162–74.
16. Hamming I, Cooper ME, Haagmans BL, Hooper NM, Korstanje R, Osterhaus AD, Tiemens W, Turner AJ, Navis G, van Goor H. The emerging role of ACE2 in physiology and disease. J Pathol. 2007;212(1):1–11.

17. Wolf G, Ziyadeh FN. The role of angiotensin II in diabetic nephropathy: an emphasis on nonhemodynamic mechanisms. Am J Kidney Dis. 1997;29(1):153–63.
18. Kennefick TM, Oyama TT, Thompson MM, Vora JP, Anderson S. Enhanced renal sensitivity to angiotensin actions in diabetes mellitus in the rat. Am J Physiol. 1996;271(3):F595–602.
19. He W, Miao FJ, Lin DC, Schwander RT, Wang Z, Gao J, Chen JL, Tian H, Ling L. Citric acid cycle intermediates as ligands for orphan G-protein-coupled receptors. Nature. 2004;429(6988):1881–93.
20. Toma I, Kang JJ, Sipos A, Vargas S, Bansal E, Hanner F, Meer E, Peti-Pterdi J. Succinate receptor GPR91 provides a direct link between high glucose levels and renin release in murine and rabbit kidney. J Clin Invest. 2008;118(7):2526–34.
21. Anderson S. Physiologic actions and molecular expression of the renin-angiotensin system in the diabetic rat. Miner Electrolyte Metab. 1998;24(6):406–11.
22. Kobori H, Katsurada A, Miyata K, Ohashi N, Satou R, Saito T, Hagiwara Y, Miyashita K, Navar LG. Determination of plasma and urinary angiotensinogen levels in rodents by newly developed ELISA. Am J Physiol Renal Physiol. 2008;294(5):F1257–63.
23. Yamamoto T, Nakagawa T, Suzuki H, Ohashi N, Fukusawa H, Fujigaki Y, Kato A, Nakamura Y, Suzuki F, Hishida A. Urinary angiotensinogen as a marker of intrarenal angiotensin II activity associated with deterioration of renal function in patients with chronic kidney disease. J Am Soc Nephrol. 2007;18(5):1558–65.
24. Kobori H, Ozawa Y, Suzaki Y, Prieto-Carrasquero MC, Nishiyama A, Shoji T, Cohen EP, Navar LG. Young scholars award lecture: intratubular angiotensinogen in hypertension and kidney disease. Am J Hypertens. 2006;19(5):541–50.
25. Huang XR, Chen WY, Truong LD, Lan HY. Chymase is upregulated in diabetic nephropathy: implications for an alternative pathway of angiotensin II-mediated diabetic renal and vascular disease. J Am Soc Nephrol. 2003;14(7):1738–47.
26. Jones SE, Gilbert RE, Kelly DJ. Tranilast reduces mesenteric vascular collagen deposition and chymase-positive mast cells in experimental diabetes. J Diab Comp. 2004;18(10):309–15.
27. Park S, Bivona BJ, Kobori H, Seth DM, Chappell MC, Lazartigues C, Harrison-Bernard LM. Major role for ACE-independent intrarenal ANG II formation in type II diabetes. Am J Physiol Renal Physiol. 2010;298(1):F37–48.
28. Zhuo JL, Li XC. Novel roles of intracrine angiotensin II and signaling mechanisms in kidney cells. J Renin Angiotensin Aldosterone Syst. 2007;8(1):23–33.
29. Wehbi GJ, Zippelmann J, Carey RM, Levine DZ, Burns KD. Early streptozotocin-diabetes mellitus downregulates rat kidney AT2 receptors. Am J Physiol Renal Physiol. 2001;280(2):F254–65.
30. Griffin KA, Bidani AK. Progression of renal disease: renoprotective specificity of the renin-angiotensin system blockade. Clin J Am Soc Nephrol. 2006;1(5):1054–65.
31. Hakam AC, Siddiqui AH, Hussain T. Renal angiotensin II AT2 receptors promote natriuresis in streptozotocin-induced diabetic rats. Am J Physiol Renal Physiol. 2006;290(2):F503–8.
32. Bonnet F, Candido R, Carey RM, Casley D, Russo LM, Osicka TM, Cooper ME, Cao Z. Renal expression of angiotensin receptors in long-term diabetes and the effects of angiotensin type I receptor blockade. J Hypertens. 2002;20(8):1615–24.
33. Gurley SB, Coffman TM. The renin-angiotensin system and diabetic nephropathy. Semin Nephrol. 2007;27(2):144–52.
34. Carmines PK, Ohishi K. Renal arteriolar contractile responses to angiotensin II in rats with poorly controlled diabetes. Clin Exp Pharmacol Physiol. 1999;26(11):877–82.
35. Maric C, Zheng W, Walther T. Interactions between angiotensin II and atrial natriuretic peptide in renomedullary interstitial cells: the role of neutral endopeptidase. Nephron Physiol. 2006;103(3):149–56.
36. Ruiz-Ortega M, Lorenzo O, Rupurez M, Konig S, Wittig B, Egido J. Angiotensin II activates nuclear transcription factor kappaB through AT(1) and AT(2) in vascular smooth muscle cells: molecular mechanisms. Circ Res. 2000;86(12):1266–72.
37. Ruiz-Ortega M, Bustos C, Hernandez-Presa MA, Lorenzo O, Plaza JJ, Egido J. Angiotensin II participates in mononuclear cell recruitment in experimental immune complex nephritis through nuclear factor-kappa B activation and monocyte chemoattractant protein-J synthesis. J Immunol. 1998;161(1):430–9.
38. Doublier S, Salvidio G, Lupia E, Ruotsalainen V, Verzola D, Defarri G, Camussi G. Nephrin expression is reduced in human diabetic nephropathy: evidence for a distinct role for glycated albumin and angiotensin II. Diabetes. 2003;52(4):1023–30.
39. Macconi D, Abbate M, Morigi M, Angioletti S, Mister M, Buelli S, Bonomelli M, Mundel P, Endlich K, Remuzzi A, Remuzzi G. Permselective dysfunction of podocyte-podocyte contact upon angiotensin II unravels the molecular target for renoprotective intervention. Am J Pathol. 2006;168(4):1073–85.
40. Chen S, Lee JS, Iglesias-de la Cruz MC, Wang A, Izquierdo-Lahuerta A, Gandhi NK, Danesh FR, Wolf G, Ziyadeh FN. Angiotensin II stimulates alpha3(IV) collagen production in mouse podocytes via TGF-beta and VEGF signaling: implications for diabetic glomerulopathy. Nephrol Dial Transplant. 2005;20(7):1320–8.
41. Wolf G, Ziyadeh FN. Renal tubular hypertrophy induced by angiotensin II. Semin Nephrol. 1997;17(5):448–54.
42. Pettersson-Fernholm K, Frojdo S, Fagerudd J, Thomas MC, Forsblom C, Wessman M, Groop PH. The AT2 gene may have a gender-specific effect on kidney function and pulse pressure in type I diabetic patients. Kidney Int. 2006;69(10):1880–4.
43. Cao Z, Bonnet F, Candido R, Nesteroff SP, Burns WC, Kawachi H, Shimizu F, Carey RM, DeGasparo M, Cooper ME. Angiotensin type 2 receptor antagonism confers renal protection in a rat model of progressive renal injury. J Am Soc Nephrol. 2002;13(7):1773–87.
44. Esteban V, Lorenzo O, Ruperez M, Suzuki Y, Mezzano S, Blanco J, Kretzler M, Sugaya T, Egido J, Ruiz-Ortega M. Angiotensin II, via AT1 and AT2 receptors and NF-kappaB pathway, regulates the inflammatory response in unilateral ureteral obstruction. J Am Soc Nephrol. 2004;15(6):1514–29.
45. Ferrario CM, Chappell MC. Novel angiotensin peptides. Cell Mol Life Sci. 2004;61(21):2720–7.
46. Tipnis SR, Hooper NM, Hyde R, Karran E, Chrisitie G, Turner AJ. A human homolog angiotensin-converting enzyme. Cloning and functional expression as a captopril-insensitive carboxypeptidase. J Biol Chem. 2000;275(43):33238–43.
47. Danilczyk U, Sarao R, Remy C, Benabbas C, Stange G, Richter A, Arya S, Pospisilik JA, Singer D, Camargo SMR, Makrides V, Ramadan T, Verrey F, Wagner CA, Penninger JM. Essential role of collectrin in renal acid transport. Nature. 2006;444(7122):1088–91.
48. Santos RAS, e Silva ACS, Maric C, Silva DMR, Machado RP, de Buhr I, Heringer-Walther S, Pinheiro SVB, Lopes MT, Bader M, Mendes EP, Lemos VS, Campagnole-Santos MJ, Schultheiss HP, Speth R, Walther T. Angiotensin(1-7) is an endogenous ligand for the G protein-coupled receptor Mas. Proc Natl Acad Sci. 2003;100(14):8258–63.
49. Paula RD, Lima CV, Khosla MC, Santo RAS. Angiotensin(1-7) potentiated the hypotensive effect of bradykinin in conscious rats. Hypertension. 1995;26(6 Pt 2):1154–9.
50. Tikellis C, Johnston CI, Forbes JM, Burns WC, Burrell LM, Risvanis J, Cooper ME. Characterization of renal angiotensin-converting enzyme 2 in diabetic nephropathy. Hypertension. 2003;41(3):392–7.
51. Ye M, Wysocki J, William J, Soler MJ, Cokic I, Batlle D. Glomerular localization and expression of angiotensin-converting enzyme 2 and angiotensin converting enzyme: implications for albuminuria in diabetes. J Am Soc Nephrol. 2006;17(11):3067–75.
52. Mizuiri S, Hemmi H, Arita M, Ohashi Y, Tanaka Y, Miyagi M, Sakai K, Ishikawa Y, Shibuya K, Hase H, Aikawa A. Expression of ACE and ACE2 in individuals with diabetic kidney disease and healthy controls. Am J Kidney Dis. 2008;51(4):613–23.

53. Soler MJ, Wysocki J, Ye M, Lloveras J, Kanwar Y, Batlle D. ACE2 inhibition worsens glomerular injury in association with increased ACE expression in streptozotocin-induced diabetic mice. Kidney Int. 2007;72(8):614–23.
54. Wong DW, Oudit GY, Reich H, Kassiri Z, Zhou J, Liu QC, Backx PH, Penninger JM, Herzenberg AM, Schlet JW. Loss of angiotensin-converting enzyme-2 (Ace2) accelerate diabetic kidney injury. Am J Pathol. 2007;171(2):439–51.
55. Ferrario CM. Angiotensin(1-7) and antihypertensive mechanisms. J Nephrol. 1998;11(6):278–83.
56. Ronchi FA, Irigoyen MC, Casarini DE. Association of somatic and N-domain angiotensin-converting enzymes from Wistar rat tissue with renal dysfunction in diabetes mellitus. J Renin Angiotensin Aldosterone Syst. 2007;8(1):34–41.
57. Ward PE, Sheridan MS. Converting enzyme, kininase, and angiotensinase of renal and intestinal brush border. Exp Med Biol. 1983;156(Pt B):835–44.
58. Benter IF, Yousif MH, Dhaunsi GS, Kaur J, Chappell MC, Diz DI. Angiotensin(1-7) prevents activation of NADPH oxidase and renal vascular dysfunction in diabetic hypertensive rats. Am J Nephrol. 2008;28(1):25–33.
59. Heitsch H, Brovkovych S, Malinski T, Wiemer G. Angiotensin(1-7) stimulated nitric oxide and superoxide release from endothelial cells. Hypertension. 2001;37:72–6.
60. Brosnihan KB, Li P, Ferrario CM. Angiotensin(1-7) dilates canine coronary through kinins and nitric oxide. Hypertension. 1996;27(3 pt 2):523–8.
61. Sampaio WO, Nascimento AA, Santos RA. Systemic and regional hemodynamic effects of angiotensin(1-7) in rats. Am J Physiol Heart Circ Physiol. 2003;284(6):H1985–94.
62. Dharmani M, Mustafa MR, Achike FI, Sim MK. Effects of angiotensin(1-7) on the action of angiotensin II in the renal and mesenteric vasculature of hypertensive and streptozotocin-induced diabetic rats. Eur J Pharmacol. 2007;561(1–3):144–50.
63. Ferrario CM, Iyer SN. Angiotensin(1-7): a bioactive fragment of the renin-angiotensin system. Regul Pept. 1998;78(1–3):13–8.
64. Ocaranza MP, Godoy I, Jalil JE, Varas M, Collantes P, Pinto M, Roman M, Ramirez C, Copaja M, Diaz-Araya G, Castro P, Lavandero S. Enalapril attenuates downregulation of angiotensin-converting enzyme 2 in the late phase of ventricular dysfunction in the myocardial infarcted rat. Hypertension. 2006;48(4):572–8.
65. Ruiz-Ortega M, Esteban V, Egido J. The regulation of the inflammatory response through nuclear-factor kappaB pathway by angiotensin IV extends the role of the renin angiotensin system in cardiovascular diseases. Trends Cardiovasc Med. 2007;17(1):19–25.
66. Abrahamsen CT, Pullen MA, Schnackenberg CG, Grygielko ET, Edwards RM, Laping NJ, Brooks DP. Effects of angiotensin II and IV on blood pressure, renal function, and PAI-1 expression in the heart and kidney of the rat. Pharmacology. 2002;66(1):26–30.
67. Athyros VG, Mikhaildis DP, Kakafika AI, Tziomalos K, Karagiannis A. Angiotensin II reactivation and aldosterone escape phenomena in renin-angiotensin-aldosterone system blockade: is oral renin inhibition the solution? Expert Opin Pharmacother. 2007;8(5):529–35.
68. Kelly DJ, Skinner SL, Gilbert RE, Cox AJ, Cooper ME, Wilkinson-Berka JL. Effects of endothelin or angiotensin II receptor blockade on diabetes in transgenic (mRen-2)27 rat. Kidney Int. 2000;57(5):1882–94.
69. Prieto-Carrasquero MC, Kobori H, Ozawa Y, Guiterrez A, Seth D, Navar LG. AT1 receptor-mediated enhancement of collecting duct renin in angiotensin I-dependent hypertensive rats. Am J Physiol Renal Physiol. 2005;289(3):F632–7.
70. Kang JJ, Toma I, Sipos A, Meer EJ, Vargas SL, Peti-Peterdi J. The collecting duct is the major source of prorenin in diabetes. Hypertension. 2008;51(6):1597–604.
71. Daneman D, Crompton CH, Balfe JW, Sochett EB, Chatzilias A, Cotter BR, Osmond DH. Plasma prorenin as an early marker of nephropathy in diabetic (IDDM) adolescents. Kidney Int. 1994;46(4):1154–9.
72. Danser AH, Deinum J. Renin, prorenin, and the putative (pro)renin receptor. J Renin Angiotensin Aldosterone Syst. 2005;6(3):163–5.
73. Nguyen G, Delarue F, Burckle C, Bouzhir L, Giller T, Sraer JD. Pivotal role of the renin/prorenin receptor in angiotensin II production and cellular responses to renin. J Clin Invest. 2002;109(11):1417–27.
74. Huang Y, Wongamorntham S, Kasting J, McQuilan D, Owens RT, Yu L, Noble NA, Border W. Renin increases mesangial cell transforming growth factor-β1 and matrix proteins through receptor-mediated, angiotensin II-mediated independent mechanisms. Kidney Int. 2006;69(1):105–13.
75. Sakoda M, Ichihara A, Kurauchi-Mito A, Narita T, Kinouchi K, Murohashi-Bokuda K, Saleem MA, Nishiyama A, Suzuki F, Itoh H. Aliskiren inhibits intracellular angiotensin II levels without affecting (pro)renin receptor signals in human podocytes. Am J Hypertens. 2010;23(5):575–80.
76. Ichihara A, Hayashi M, Kaneshiro Y, Suzuki F, Nakagawa T, Tada Y, Koura Y, Nishiyama A, Okada H, Uddin MN, Nabi AH, Ishida Y, Inagami T, Saruta T. Inhibition of diabetic nephropathy by a decoy peptide corresponding to the "handle" region for nonproteolytic activation of prorenin. J Clin Invest. 2004;114(8):1128–35.
77. Ichihara A, Kaneshiro Y, Suzuki F. Prorenin receptor blockers: effects on cardiovascular complications of diabetes and hypertension. Expert Opin Investig Drugs. 2006;15(10):1137–9.
78. Han SY, Kim CH, Kim HS, Jee YH, Song HK, Lee MH, Han KH, Kim HK, Kang YS, Han JY, Kim YS, Cha DR. Spironolactone prevents diabetic nephropathy through an anti-inflammatory mechanism in type II diabetic rats. J Am Soc Nephrol. 2006;17(5):1362–72.
79. Matsumoto S, Takebayashi K, Aso Y. The effect of spironolactone on circulating adipocytokines in patients with type 2 diabetes complicated by diabetic nephropathy. Metabolism. 2006;55(12):1645–52.
80. Epstein M, Williams GH, Weinberger M, Lewin A, Krause S, Mukherjee R, Patni R, Beckerman B. Selective aldosterone blockade with eplerenone reduces albuminuria in patients with type 2 diabetes. Clin J Am Soc Nephrol. 2006;1(5):940–51.
81. Sato A, Hayashi K, Naruse M, Saruta T. Effectiveness of aldosterone blockade in patients with diabetic nephropathy. Hypertension. 2003;41(1):64–8.
82. Xue C, Siragy HM. Local renal aldosterone system and its regulation by salt, diabetes, and angiotensin II type-1 receptor. Hypertension. 2005;46(3):584–90.
83. Rebsomen L, Khammar A, Raccah D, Tsimaratos M. C-peptide effects on renal physiology and diabetes. Exp Diabetes Res. 2008;2008:281536.
84. Vague P, Coste TC, Jannot MF. C-peptide, Na+, K+ ATPase and diabetes. Exp Diabesity Res. 2004;5(1):37–50.
85. Nordquist L, Lai EY, Sjoquist M, Patzak A, Persson AE. Proinsulin C-peptide constricts glomerular afferent arterioles in diabetic mice. A potential renoprotective mechanism. Am J Physiol Regul Integ Comp Physiol. 2008;294(3):R836–41.
86. Komers R, Lindsley JN, Oyama TT, Schutzer WE, Reed JF, Mader SL, Anderon S. Immunohistochemical and functional correlations of renal cyclooxygenase-2 in experimental diabetes. J Clin Invest. 2001;107(7):889–98.
87. Li H, Chen YJ, Quilley J. Effect of tempol on renal cyclooxygenase expression and activity in experimental diabetes in the rat. J Pharmacol Exp Ther. 2005;314(2):818–24.
88. Chen YJ, Li J, Quiley J. Effect of inhibition of nitric oxide synthase on renal cyclooxygenase in the diabetic rat. Eur J Pharmacol. 2006;541(1–2):80–6.

89. Cherney DZ, Miller JA, Scholey JW, Bradley TJ, Slorach C, Curtis JR, Dekker MG, Nassallah R, Hebert RL, Sochett EB. The effect of cyclooxygenase-2 inhibition on renal hemodynamic function in humans with type I diabetes. Diabetes. 2008;57(3):688–95.
90. Cherney DZI, Scholey JW, Nasrallah R, Dekker MG, Slorach C, Bradley TJ, Hebert RL, Sochett EB, Miller JA. Renal hemodynamic effect of cyclooxygenase 2 inhibition in young men and women with uncomplicated type I diabetes mellitus. Am J Physiol Renal Physiol. 2008;294(6):F1336–41.
91. Hostetter TH, Renke HG, Brenner BM. Case for intrarenal hypertension in initiation and progression of diabetic and other glomerulopathies. Am J Med. 1982;72(3):375–80.
92. Hashimoto S, Yamada K, Kawata T, Mochizuki T, Schnermann J, Koike T. Abnormal autoregulation and tubuloglomerular feedback in prediabetic and diabetic OLETF rats. Am J Physiol Renal Physiol. 2009;296(3):F598–604.
93. Lau C, Sudbury I, Thomson M, Howard PL, Magil AB, Cupples WA. Salt-resistant blood pressure and salt-sensitive renal autoregulation in chronic streptozotocin diabetes. Am J Physiol Reg Integ Comp Physiol. 2009;296(6):R1761–70.
94. Hashimoto Y, Ideura T, Yoshimura A, Koshikawa S. Autoregulation of renal blood flow in streptozotocin-induced diabetic rats. Diabetes. 1989;38(9):1109–13.
95. Schjoedt KJ, Christensen PK, Jorsal A, Boomsma F, Rossing P, Parving HH. Autoregulation of glomerular filtration rate during spironolactone treatment in hypertensive patients with type I diabetes: a randomized crossover trial. Nephrol Dial Transplant. 2009;24(11):3343–9.
96. Serri O, Beauregard H, Brazeau P, Abribat T, Lambert J, Harris A, Vachon L. Somatostatin analog, octreotide, reduces increased intraglomerular filtration rate and kidney size in insulin-dependent diabetes. JAMA. 1991;265(7):888–92.
97. Hirschberg R, Brunori G, Kopple JD, Guler HP. Effects of insulin-like growth factor 1 on renal function in normal men. Kidney Int. 1993;43(2):387–97.
98. Hirschberg R, Kopple JD. The growth hormone-insulin-like growth factor axis and renal glomerular function. J Am Soc Nephrol. 1992;9:1417–22.
99. Passariello N, Sepe J, Marrazzo G, De Cicco A, Peluso A, Pisano MC, Sgambato S, Tesauro P, D'Onoforio F. Effect of aldose reductase inhibitor (tolrestat) on urinary albumin excretion rate and glomerular filtration rate in IDDM subjects with nephropathy. Diabetes Care. 1993;16(5):789–95.
100. Sabbatini M, Sansone G, Uccello F, Giliberti A, Conte G, Andreucci VE. Early glycosylation products induce glomerular hyperfiltration in normal rats. Kidney Int. 1992;42(4):875–81.
101. Thomson SC, Vallon V, Blantz RC. Kidney function in early diabetes: the tubular hypothesis of glomerular filtration. Am J Physiol Renal Physiol. 2004;286(1):F8–15.
102. Ikenaga H, Bast JP, Fallet RW. Exaggerated impact of ATP-sensitive K+ channels on afferent arteriolar diameter in diabetes mellitus. J Am Soc Nephrol. 2000;11(7):1199–206.
103. Thomas MC, Tikellis C, Burns WM, Biakowski K, Cao Z, Coughlin MT, Jandeleit-Dahm K, Cooper ME, Forbes JM. Interaction between renin angiotensin system and advanced glycation in the kidney. J Am Soc Nephrol. 2005;16(10):2976–84.

5 Renal Structural Changes in Type 1 and 2 Diabetes Mellitus: Pathology, Pathogenesis, and Clinical Correlations

Jeffrey Aufman and Guillermo A. Herrera

Introduction

In 1936 Kimmelstiel and Wilson [1] reported a series of eight autopsies from patients in which they observed thickening of the intercapillary regions of the glomerular capillaries with the formation of nodules in autopsies and suggested that a combination of diabetes mellitus and arteriosclerosis was responsible for the findings. Seven of the patients he described had diabetes mellitus for years preceding their death and one patient had no information available as he died 3 h after admission with no previous history. The authors concluded that the lesion identified represented the typical changes in the glomerulus that occurred in patients with long-standing diabetes mellitus and termed this lesion diffuse intercapillary glomerulosclerosis. Because of their seminal contribution pointing out the structural changes in glomeruli of diabetic patients, the most salient finding in this lesion, the mesangial nodules are still referred to as Kimmelstiel–Wilson nodules. At about the same time, another diabetic patient was reported by Murakami in Japan [2] with similar histological picture. Since the life span of patients with diabetes mellitus was quite compromised until insulin became available, the renal lesions did not fully develop in many patients.

Gellman et al. in 1959 for the first time reported an overview and clinical correlation of findings in renal biopsies from patients with diabetes mellitus [3]. The only material available prior to this manuscript was descriptions based on kidneys examined at autopsy.

There have been attempts to separate typical from atypical diabetic nephropathy using various parameters including concomitant superimposed glomerular conditions and other tubular interstitial and vascular alterations, either directly related to diabetes or superimposed conditions.

J. Aufman, M.D. • G.A. Herrera, M.D. (✉)
Department of Pathology, Louisiana State University, 1501 Kings Highway, Shreveport, LA 71 130, USA
e-mail: gherr1@lsuhsc.edu

The morphological findings in diabetic nephropathy occurring in patients with type 1 and 2 diabetes overlap significantly to a point that it is virtually of no value to separate them. In general patients with type 2 diabetic nephropathy reveal more significant vascular alterations and more heterogeneity in their glomerular lesions which can be morphologically altered by the effects of a number of comorbid disorders such as hypertension [4].

The alterations that take place in the kidneys of patients with diabetic nephropathy can be generically conceptualized as expansion of the extracellular matrices which include glomerular basement membrane and mesangial matrix, and segmental glomerular collapse, generally a more advanced change, characterized by focal and segmental glomerulosclerosis/hyalinosis.

Morphologic Findings in Diabetic Nephropathy and Related Physiopathology

The clinically latent period between the onset of clinical detection of diabetes and specific morphological findings that can be related to it generally lasts for more than 10 years. This period is usually manifested in the kidney by hyperperfusion, increased kidney size, enlarged glomeruli, and hyperfiltration [5]. The glomerular hemodynamic changes take place as a consequence of increased plasma flow and elevated glomerular transcapillary hydrostatic pressure resulting from a decrease in both afferent and efferent arteriolar resistances with the efferent arterioles being more dilated than the afferent ones. Many factors have been implicated in this phenomenon including prostanoids, nitric oxide (NO), atrial natriuretic factor, growth hormone, glucagon, insulin, and angiotensin II, making this situation a difficult one to sort out. Elevated intraglomerular pressure has been linked to mesangial matrix overproduction and podocyte injury [6].

Other factors of importance in the diabetic milieu which also alter hemodynamics include vascular endothelial growth factor (VEGF) likely mediated through production

E.V. Lerma and V. Batuman (eds.), *Diabetes and Kidney Disease*,
DOI 10.1007/978-1-4939-0793-9_5, © Springer Science+Business Media New York 2014

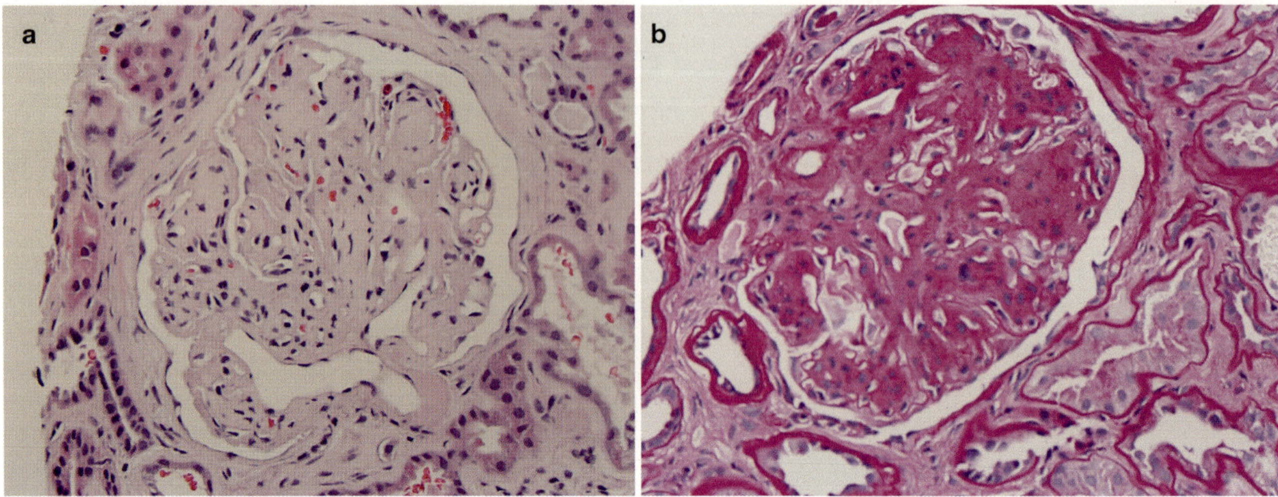

Fig. 5.1 (**a**) Hematoxylin and eosin (H&E) stain-X500; (**b**) periodic acid Schiff (PAS) stain-X500. Nodular glomerulosclerosis. Diabetic nephropathy. The hallmark of diabetic nephropathy, nodular glomerulosclerosis. Well-defined mesangial nodules of variable size, and thickening of peripheral capillary walls. Note that the mesangial cells that remain are at the periphery of the mesangial nodules

of NO and the effect of transforming growth factor-β (TGF-β) leading also to hyperfiltration by producing dilatation of the afferent arterioles via inhibiting calcium transients. Shear stress and mechanical stretch caused by hemodynamic alterations represent yet additional factors inducing release of pertinent cytokine and growth factors. The local activation of local cytokines and growth factors mechanistically associate hemodynamic stress to structural changes in the diabetic glomerulus [7–13]. Other researchers have attempted to link glomerular hyperfiltration to a primary defect in tubular sodium reabsorption such that diabetic-induced hypertrophy of tubules mediates stimulation of sodium chloride reabsorption, again linking renal structural changes with the hemodynamic adaptations that take place in diabetic renal disease [3, 13, 14].

In the 30 % or so of diabetic patients that will develop overt nephropathy, microalbuminuria is the earliest clinical manifestation which may progress over several years to nephrotic range proteinuria and decreased renal function. However, there are significant numbers of patients with diabetic nephropathy that progress into renal failure without ever developing nephrotic range proteinuria.

There are morphological correlates associated with this progression. The great majority of patients that are biopsied are, as expected, those that have developed clinical manifestations beyond microalbuminuria. The development of nephrotic range proteinuria, in some cases massive proteinuria, is an indication for renal biopsy to attempt to identify if any concomitant glomerulopathies may be responsible for these changes, as therapeutic interventions are needed if that is the case. However, more often than not that is not the case.

Glomerular basement membrane thickening represents the earliest specific change in the diabetic glomerulus in type 1 and 2 diabetic patients and increases with duration of disease [6, 8, 15]. The overlap that is seen in glomerular diabetic lesions in type 1 and 2 patients has been recognized. The initial finding detectable ultrastructurally is subepithelial lamellation of the lamina densa as a manifestation of early deposition of additional basement membrane material which is responsible for the increase in thickness.

Upper limits for normal glomerular basement membrane thickness vary according to the methods used and in some instances, fixation and processing of tissues for electron microscopy. If the orthogonal intercept method is employed to measure the glomerular basement membranes, the upper limit of thickness is 520 nm (0.52 μm) for adult men and 471 nm for women [16]. Using cutoff levels based on variations in thickness from normal glomerular basement membrane thickness of more than two standard deviations, Haas et al. published data that indicates that in males over 9 years of age, glomerular basement membranes thicker than 430 nm (0.43 μm) are abnormal and this number reflects the upper limit of acceptable thickness and in females 399 nm (0.399 μm) is the corresponding cutoff [17]. For children younger than 9 years of age a table provides guidance. The thickness of the glomerular basement membranes may change with fixation and processing protocols used in the various laboratories. It is also markedly altered if material is taken from paraffin for ultrastructural assessment [18]. Each renal pathology laboratory should establish its own reference values to determine normal range of thickness for the glomerular basement membranes using an approach that has been accepted such as the ones mentioned. This will avoid incorrect assessments of the glomerular basement membranes.

Concomitantly with the increased thickness in the glomerular basement membranes, there is deposition of mesangial

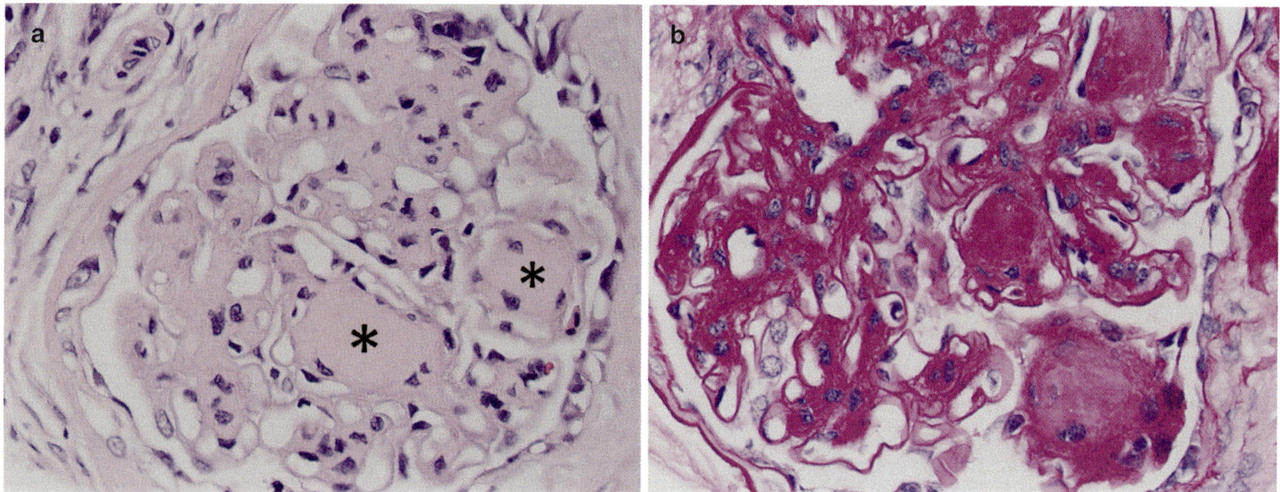

Fig. 5.2 (**a**) H&E stain-X750; (**b**) PAS-X750. Nodular glomerulosclerosis. Diabetic nephropathy. Details of mesangial nodules (*asterisks*) which are PAS positive

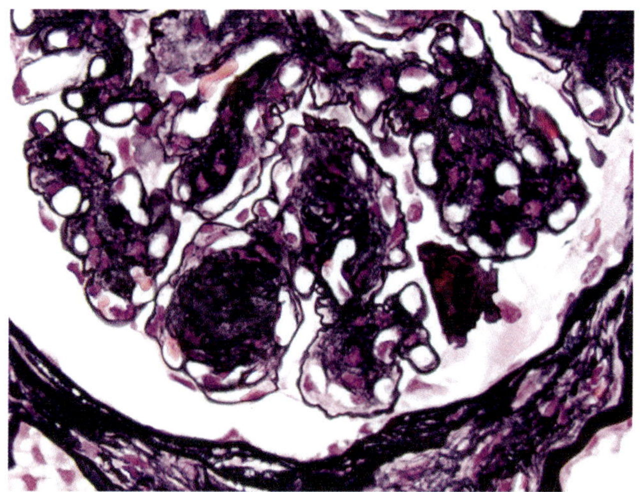

Fig. 5.3 Silver methenamine-X750. Nodular glomerulosclerosis. Diabetic nephropathy. Mesangial nodules are silver positive indicating increased mesangial matrix as their main component. Lamellation of mesangial nodule (*circle*). Few mesangial cells at the periphery

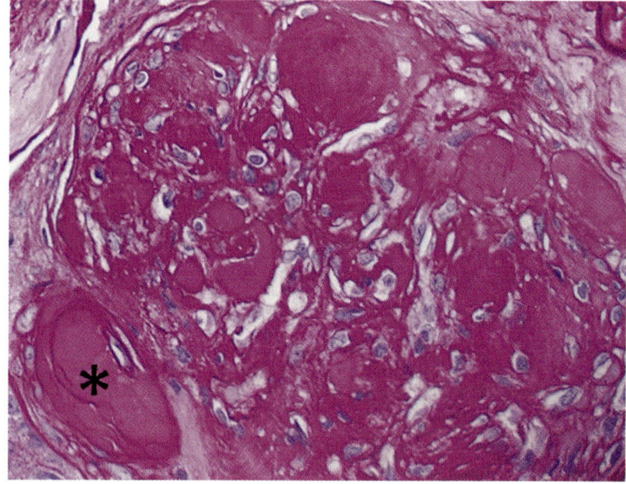

Fig. 5.4 PAS-X750. Hyaline arteriolosclerosis. Diabetic nephropathy. Hyaline material in the wall of arteriole is PAS positive, somewhat more glassy than the staining of mesangial nodules

matrix leading to mesangial expansion [4, 6, 14, 19]. However, this finding by itself is rather nonspecific and can be seen in virtually any primary glomerular disease in its early stages and even as a reactive change in glomeruli in patients with primary tubular interstitial or vascular diseases. Therefore, the diagnostic value of this finding is rather limited. Once the expanded mesangium becomes nodular, then nodular glomerulosclerosis is recognized and this finding is far more specific for diabetic nephropathy (Figs. 5.1, 5.2, 5.3, 5.4, 5.5, 5.6, 5.7, 5.8, and 5.9). It is not exclusively seen in diabetic nephropathy but it is a good marker in the proper clinical setting.

The molecular mechanism responsible for the mesangial matrix expansion is secretion and activation of TGF-β by mesangial cells [4, 20]. Mesangial nodules vary in number and size from glomerulus to glomerulus and they vary from slightly hypercellular at the beginning to eventually paucicellular or even almost acellular with remaining mesangial cells generally located at the periphery surrounding the acellular center with increased matrix [19]. Mesangial nodules are positive with the PAS (periodic acid Schiff) and silver methenamine stains (Figs. 5.1b, 5.2b, 5.3, and 5.4) and stain blue with the trichrome stain. In some nodules lamellation is appreciable, most noticeable in the silver methenamine stained sections.

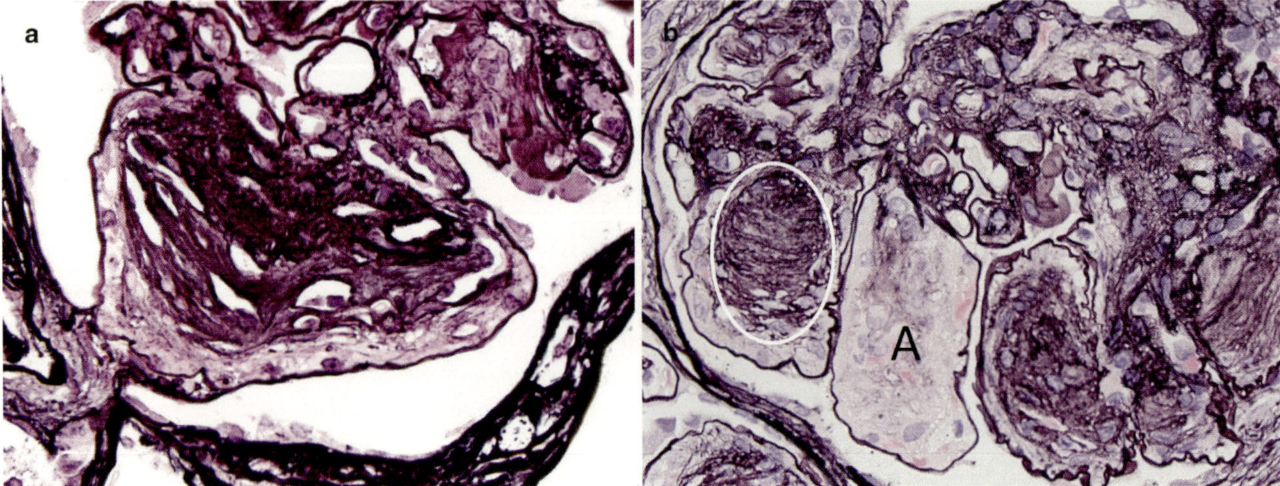

Fig. 5.5 (**a**, **b**) Silver methenamine stain-X750. Microaneurysm formation. Diabetic nephropathy. Process of microaneurysm formation (early events) with mesangiolysis in (**a**) and aneurysm (A) already formed in (**b**). Note that peripheral capillary walls are thinner than normal outlining the aneurysm. Also note mesangiolysis in adjacent mesangial nodules

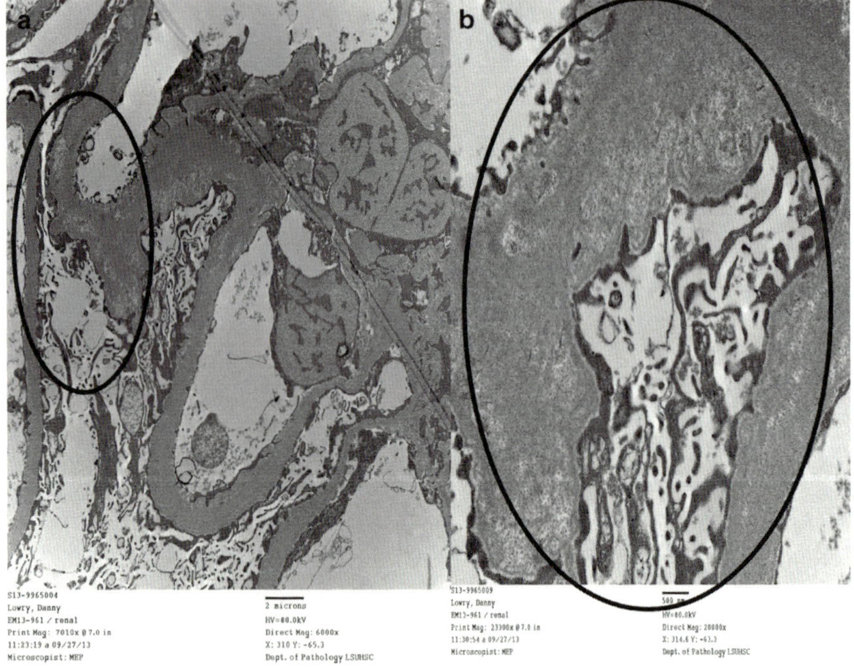

Fig. 5.6 (**a**, **b**) Transmission electron microscopy, uranyl acetate and lead citrate-AX15500, BX13500. Diabetic nephropathy. Thickening of glomerular basement membranes accompanied by subepithelial lamellation (**a**), the latter best seen on (**b**) (*circled areas*)

Mesangiolysis is a key injury in the development and progression of nodular glomerulosclerosis, the most characteristic advanced lesion in diabetic nephropathy [19, 21–23]. Experimental studies by Matsusaka et al. [24] have shown that podocyte death is inducible and that if the degree of such injury is sufficient, mesangiolysis ensues. The loss of podocytes early in the process of diabetic nephropathy represents a significant contributory factor to mesangiolysis and resultant mesangial matrix accumulation. Mesangiolysis is associated with formation of microaneurysms. In aneurysmal areas, the surrounding glomerular basement membrane becomes thin. So the process has been delineated by some authors as occurring as follows: repetitive mesangiolysis (destruction/dissolution of mesangial matrix) resulting in formation of microaneurysms, capillary collapse, and matrix deposition leading to the formation of mesangial nodules (Fig. 5.5) [21].

Other glomerular findings include insudative and exudative deposits. In 1994, Stout defined "insudative lesions" as consisting of intramural accumulations of presumably

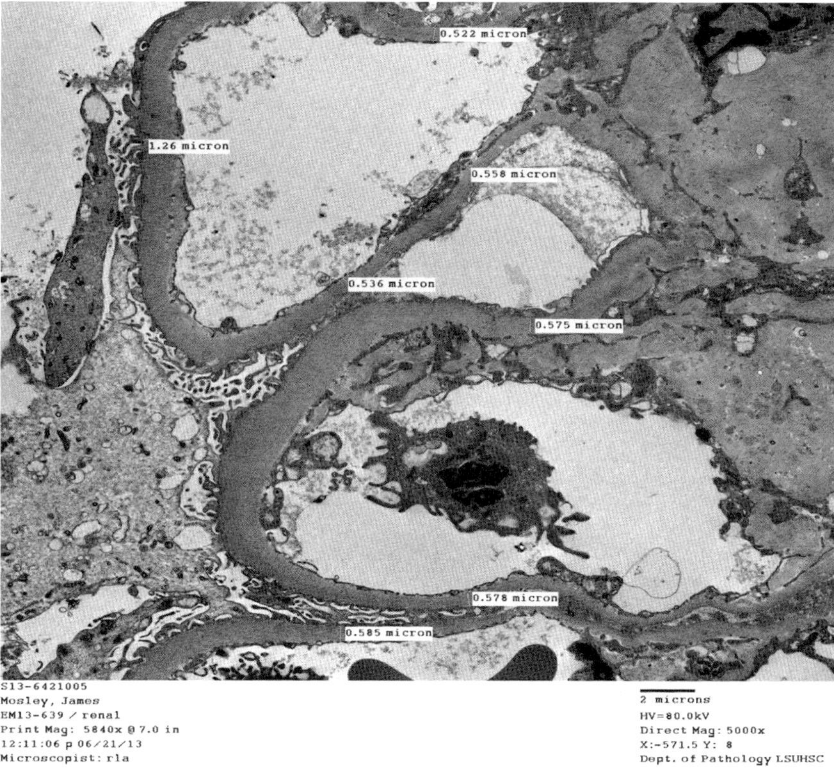

Fig. 5.7 Transmission electron microscopy, uranyl acetate and lead citrate-X8500. Diabetic nephropathy. Uniform thickening of the glomerular basement membranes (all measuring more than 520 nm to 0.52 μm) in thickness

imbibed plasma proteins and lipids within renal arterioles, glomerular capillaries, Bowman's capsule, or proximal convoluted tubules [25]. These deposits are eosinophilic and acellular, thus described as "hyaline." If they are seen "hanging" from or within Bowman's capsule they are referred to capsular drops (Fig. 5.10). They are typically found between parietal epithelial cells and Bowman's capsule. Stout pointed out that these lesions can be identified in 5.3 % of biopsies from patients with glomerular pathology other than diabetic nephropathy [19]. These lesions are rather suggestive of diabetic nephropathy but not entirely specific for it, although some believe that the capsular drops are specific, but not entirely pathognomonic of diabetic nephropathy [26]. If in turn, they protrude from or are intimately related to the peripheral capillary walls, they are called hyaline of "fibrin" caps. However, the term fibrin cap is considered obsolete as they contain no fibrin. Hyalinosis is a much better term.

Associated lesions are observed in the vasculature (Figs. 5.4 and 5.11). Hyaline arteriolosclerosis of both afferent and efferent arterioles is a characteristic diabetic finding. In fact, according to Stout, hyalinosis of the efferent arteriole is rather specific for diabetic nephropathy [25]. In contrast, hyalinosis of the afferent arteriole occurs in a number of other conditions, most notably vascular nephrosclerosis and cyclosporine nephrotoxicity. Identifying efferent arterioles in renal samples cannot be done reliably which makes this finding a difficult one to confirm and the dogma has been to determine the presence of hyalinosis in both arterioles at the vascular pole in glomeruli as the finding to be trusted as a typical finding in diabetic nephropathy.

In regard to atherosclerosis, lesions found in the arterioles and arteries are relatively nonspecific (Figs. 5.12 and 5.13) [25]. However, accelerated atherosclerosis represents a rather common alteration appreciated in renal biopsies from patients with diabetes, predominantly in those with advanced renal disease (Fig. 5.13). Bohle and associates found that the accelerated atherosclerosis was most common in those patients with advanced diabetic nephropathy [27]. Intimal fibrous thickening is the most characteristic finding; however, thickening of the media can also be seen.

Tubular interstitial manifestations characterized by interstitial fibrosis, tubular atrophy, and dropout (Fig. 5.14) typically occur associated with and as a direct result of the glomerular and vascular changes and, as expected, these changes parallel in degree the findings seen in the other two renal compartments [19, 23]. Tubular basement membranes thicken in parallel to similar alterations in the glomerular basement membranes. Interstitial inflammation generally with mononuclear cells occurs and also leads to interstitial fibrosis, tubular atrophy, and dropout. Many studies show

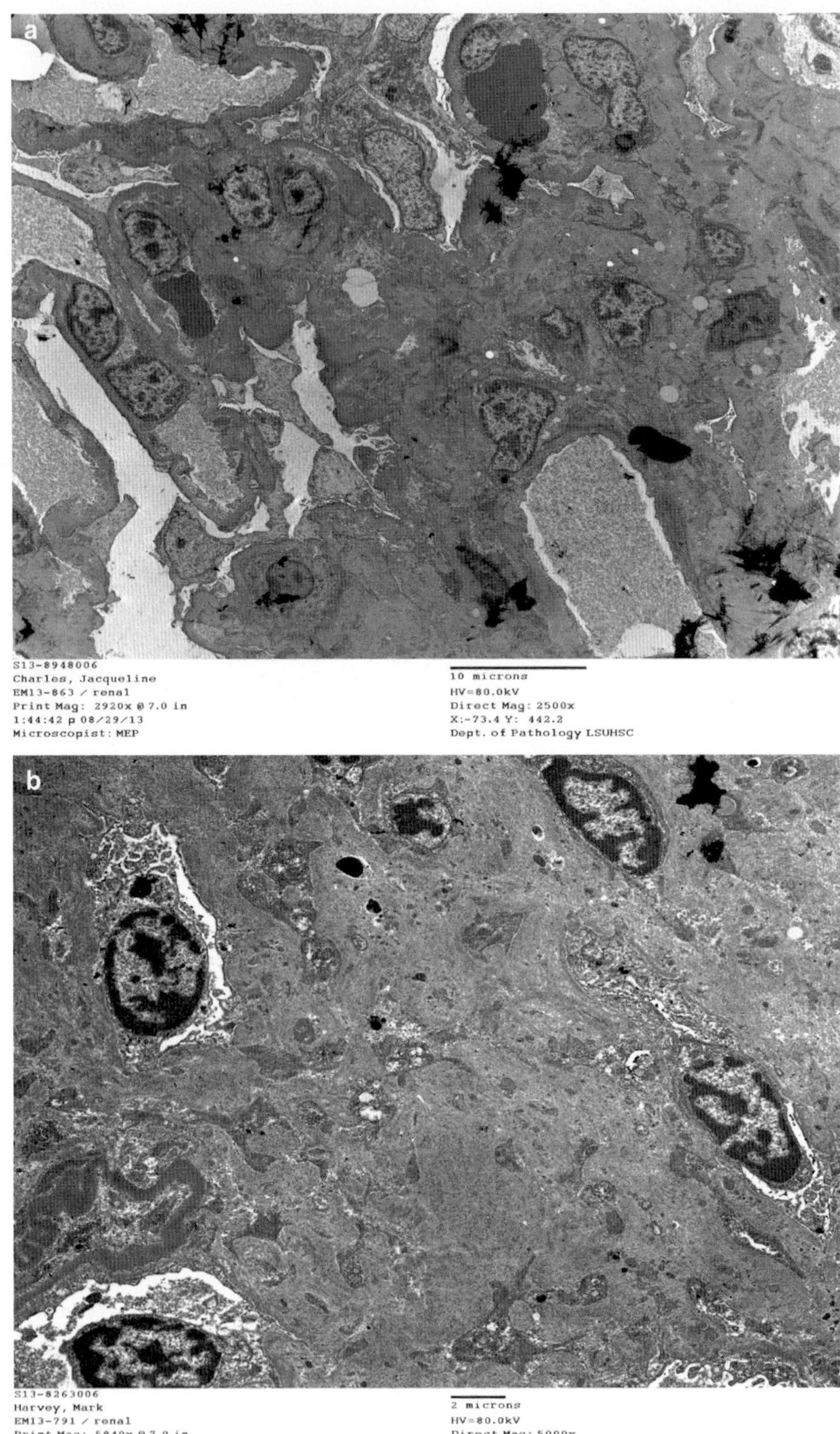

Fig. 5.8 (**a**, **b**) Transmission electron microscopy, uranyl acetate and lead citrate-AX7500; BX12500. Diabetic nephropathy. Mesangial expansion in (**a**) with increased matrix clearly seen in (**b**) associated with formation of obvious mesangial nodule

that the severity of chronic glomerular and tubular interstitial pathology is closely related [27].

Focal, segmental glomerulosclerosis has been shown to be also an important component of the glomerular lesions in some diabetic patients, usually occurring in the more advanced stages of the disease. The implications for this finding are significant in the prognosis and management of these patients and will be discussed later.

Comparison of Diabetic Nephropathy in Type 1 and 2 Diabetic Patients

Most of our knowledge of diabetic nephropathy has come from studying the disease in type 2 diabetic patients since they are much more common than type 1 only (about 20 % of all diabetic patients) but there has been a significant number

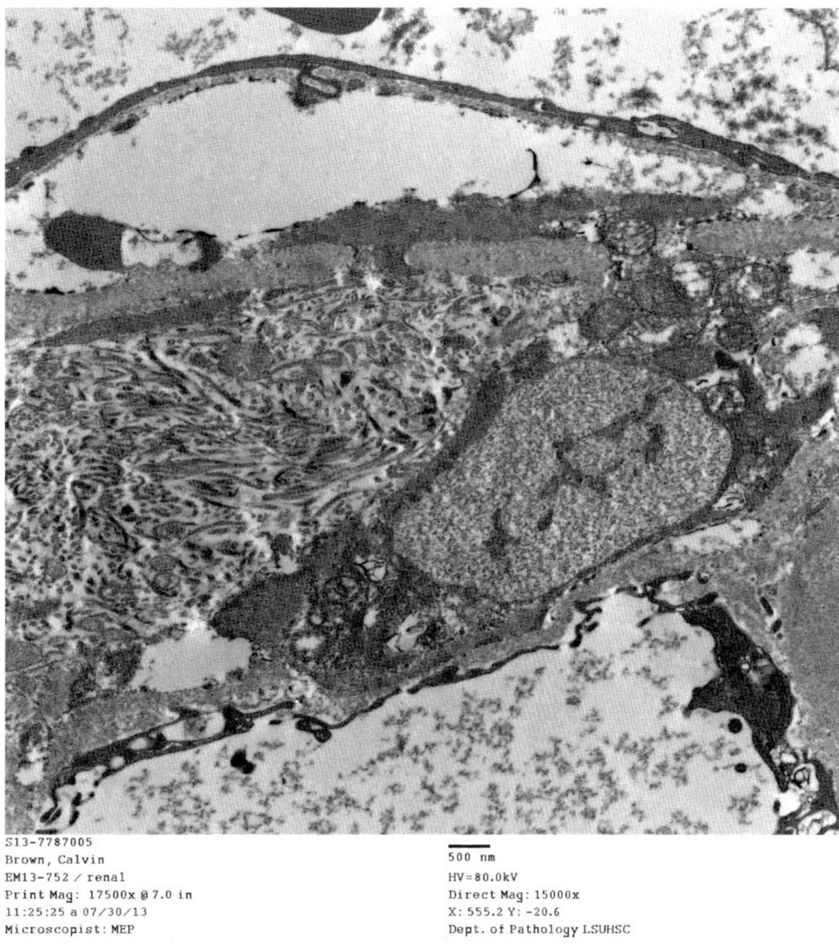

Fig. 5.9 Transmission electron microscopy, uranyl acetate and lead citrate-X12500. Diabetic nephropathy. Fibrillary collagen in mesangial nodule. Note parallel disposition of collagen fibers and periodicity in fibers

of studies focusing on the renal pathology in type I diabetic patients. As previously stated, much overlap exists in the renal structural changes that occur in both conditions.

About 40 % of patients with long-standing type 1 diabetes mellitus develop overt renal disease progressing to significant renal insufficiency [19]. The decline in glomerular filtration rate, hypertension, and proteinuria in general seem to correlate with a number of renal structural abnormalities, including increased mesangial fractional volume [Vv(mes/glom)], decreased glomerular filtration surface, interstitial expansion, increased numbers of globally sclerosed glomeruli, and arteriolar hyalinosis. However since all these appear to correlate, it has been impossible to determine if one of these findings is more closely related to progressive renal functional impairment in diabetic nephropathy in cross-sectional studies [28–31].

However, the correlation of structural changes with renal functional findings is difficult in some instances, especially in type 1 diabetic patients, in some specific aspects. It has been shown that severe glomerular lesions may be seen in normoalbuminuric patients with type I diabetes and also that normoalbuminuric patients with decreased glomerular filtration rate have more advanced lesions than expected. Glomerular basement membrane width after long type 1 diabetes duration is a strong independent predictor of diabetic nephropathy risk in normoalbuminuric type 1 diabetes patients [32].

A study by Fioretto et al. attempted to relate structural renal changes to functional alterations in insulin-dependent diabetic patients [29]. It was found in a 5-year follow-up study that increasing mesangial fractional volume was closely linked to the development of albuminuria and early overt nephropathy, while interstitial expansion and glomerular glomerulosclerosis did not progress this time period as anticipated would happen. In addition, the structural changes of diabetic nephropathy were progressive, even in patients with stable renal function [31].

Perrin also evaluated the course of diabetic nephropathy in normoalbuminuric patients with type I diabetes mellitus for 6 years with sequential renal biopsies. The study consisted of a cohort of six patients who had hypertension and were treated with antihypertensive medications for 2 years or

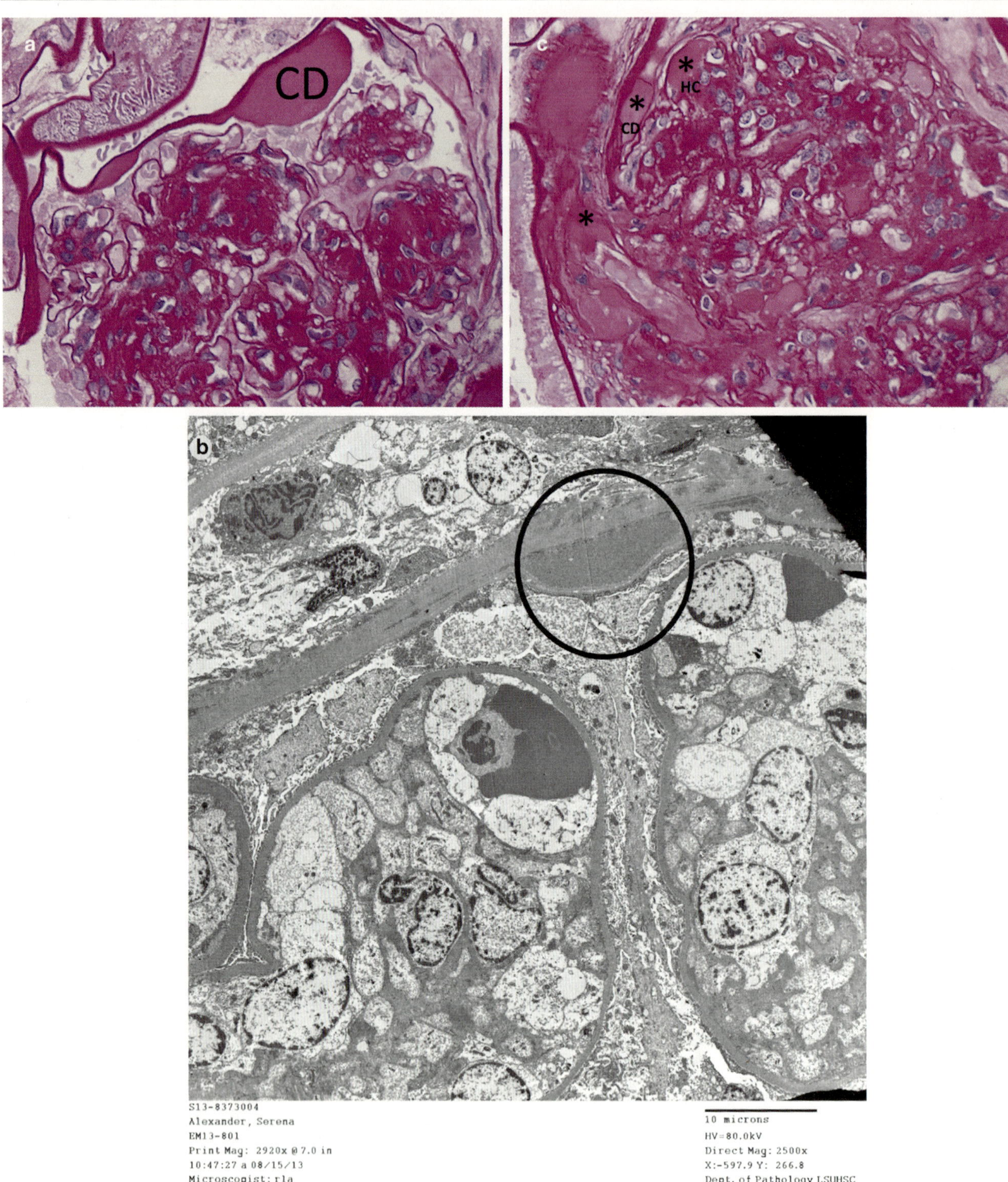

Fig. 5.10 (**a**, **c**) PAS stain; (**b**) transmission electron microscopy, uranyl acetate and lead citrate-AX750, BX5800, CX750. Diabetic nephropathy. In (**a**) capsular drop (PAS positive) (CD) hanging from Bowman's capsule with corresponding ultrastructural appearance in (**b**) (*circled*). In (**c**) capsular drop (*CD) and hyaline cap (*HC)

more, and this group was compared with an untreated group composed of four similar additional patients. The study demonstrated that no progression occurred in the treated patients who also improved their metabolic control, but morphologic parameters deteriorated in the untreated patients. Glomerular and mesangial volume, mesangial matrix volume fraction, and foot process width of visceral epithelial cells increased significantly [31].

The role of hypertension in the progression of diabetic nephropathy has been a subject of debate. Initially it was felt that the development of serious diabetic nephropathy was independent of hypertension. More recently, studies have indicated that the presence of hypertension in patients with overt diabetic nephropathy is associated with a more rapid decline of glomerular filtration rate and that effective treatment of the hypertension has resulted in slowing the rate of decline of the glomerular filtration rate in these patients, who are far more commonly patients with type 2 diabetes [31].

Podocytes are reduced in nephropathy associated with both type 1 and 2 diabetes mellitus [20]. Podocyte reduction has also been demonstrated in animal models of diabetic nephropathy [33, 34]. This reduction in podocytes may precede and in some studies predict the appearance of clinically detectable. It does not appear that podocytopathy is more common in patients with either type 1 or 2 diabetic nephropathy.

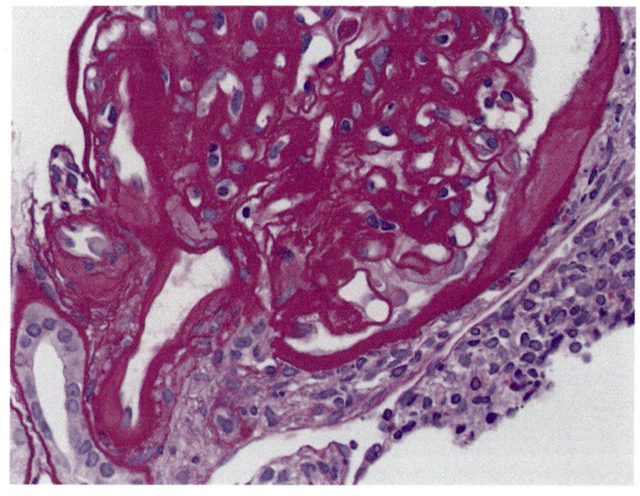

Fig. 5.11 PAS stain-X750. Diabetic nephropathy. Hyaline arteriolosclerosis in afferent and efferent arterioles

The information available in the literature supports that glomerular, predominantly mesangial, structural changes are important in the clinical transition to microalbuminuria or overt nephropathy (rather than glomerular basement membrane thickening), at least in insulin-dependent diabetic patients, while interstitial pathology does not seem to have a pathogenetic role at this stage of the disease [23, 35]. Interstitial fibrosis is more likely directly implicated in the progression of the diabetic nephropathy to end-stage renal disease.

More heterogeneity is seen in biopsies from patients with nephropathy and type 2 diabetes when compared with those with type 1 [19]. This is probably a result of aging, hypertension, and atherosclerosis, conditions that are usually present in these cases in a more florid manner, but the possibility that this may be at least partly inherent to the disease process in this subset of diabetic patients cannot be completely excluded at this time.

If type 2 diabetic patients with similar renal function are compared with type 1 patients, structural changes related to diabetic nephropathy are less severe and the correlations between renal function and glomerular structural alterations are less precise, probably because there are a number of factors playing a role related to vascular pathology and other conditions that are not integral parts of the nephropathy in type 1 diabetic patients [19].

Finally, some researchers have noted that by the time renal function abnormalities become manifest, renal structural lesions are quite advanced [8].

Pathologic Classification of Diabetic Nephropathy

In order to better understand diabetic nephropathy, a unifying pathologic classification has been proposed to encompass renal lesions seen in type 1 and 2 diabetes mellitus to be able to relate them to structural kidney alterations and

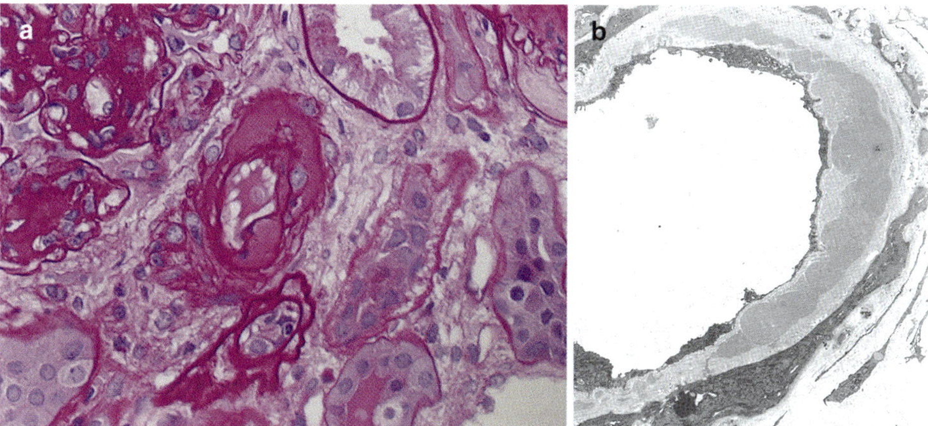

Fig. 5.12 (**a**) PAS stain; (**b**) transmission electron microscopy, uranyl acetate and lead citrate-AX7500, B-X350. Diabetic nephropathy. Hyalinosis in the wall of small size artery in (**a**). Electron dense material in vessel wall in (**b**) corresponds to the area with hyalinosis

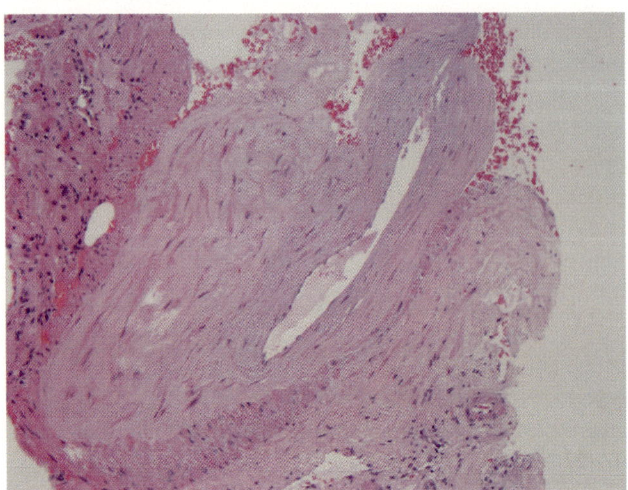

Fig. 5.13 (**a**) H&E-X350. Diabetic nephropathy. Atherosclerosis in medium to large size arteries

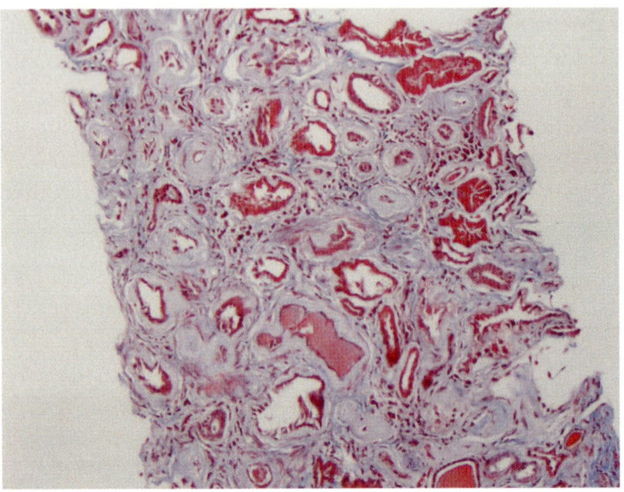

Fig. 5.14 Trichrome stain-X350. Diabetic nephropathy. Interstitial fibrosis (blue staining) associated with tubular atrophy/dropout and thickening of tubular basement membranes

consequently, clinical manifestations [23]. The glomerular alterations that may occur in diabetic patients with glomerular alterations are divided into four classes:

Class I is characterized by glomerular basement membrane thickening proven by electron microscopy and only, mild nonspecific changes by light microscopy that do not meet criteria for any of the other classes. Class II encompasses mesangial expansion which is divided into mild (IIa) or severe (IIb) but without identifiable mesangial nodularity. This category is analogous to what has been referred to as "diffuse diabetic glomerulosclerosis." If the mesangial matrix is more than 25 % of the total mesangium it should be classified as Class IIb, but without mesangial nodularity in more than 50 % of the glomeruli. Class III is referred to as nodular glomerulosclerosis. At least one convincing mesangial nodule should be present in a glomerulus to be included in this category. No more than 50 % globally sclerosed glomeruli should be present in the specimen examined. Class IV represents a more advanced form of nodular glomerulosclerosis with more than 50 % globally sclerosed glomeruli in the sample. This classification has been tested with good interobserver reproducibility (intraclass correlation coefficient=0.84).

This classification serves several purposes including: (1) improves communication between renal pathologists among themselves and with clinicians, (2) provides structural criteria to be used for prognostic and interventional studies, and (3) improves ability to manage patients clinically using morphologic parameters to evaluate efficacy of various interventions in delaying progression or renal disease and aids in determining the need for other therapeutic maneuvers. According to the authors, this classification is based on glomerular pathology only because these are relatively easy to recognize with good interobserver agreement and also because glomerular lesions best reflect the natural course of progressive diabetic nephropathy [19].

Tubular interstitial and vascular pathology are not incorporated into this categorization of renal lesions in samples from diabetic nephropathy but are encouraged to be tabulated in a scoring format for a more comprehensive evaluation of the findings.

This classification ignores focal, segmental glomerulosclerosis, an important lesion that may carry with it clinical and prognostic significance, especially as it directly relates to podocyte injury and related issues addressed later in the chapter.

Structural Abnormalities of the Thickened Glomerular Basement Membranes and Expanded Mesangium in Diabetic Nephropathy: Light, Ultrastructural and Immunofluorescence Microscopy Data

Although there is a tendency to consider diabetic nephropathy a progressive disease as patients live longer with the disease, there is evidence that functional abnormalities are not always progressive and regression from one state to a better one occurs [4, 36, 37]. Renal biopsies have shown that glomerular changes reflect and correlated with renal dysfunction but interstitial fibrosis is the best indicator of prognosis/progression to end-stage renal disease [19].

Seminal studies carried out by several ways led to the concept that the structural and functional architecture and composition of the glomerular basement membranes consists of a backbone of collagen IV that forms a compacted meshwork and plays a crucial role in the size and charge-selective sieving properties of the ultrafiltration unit in the kidney. The proteoglycan-containing layer provides a negatively

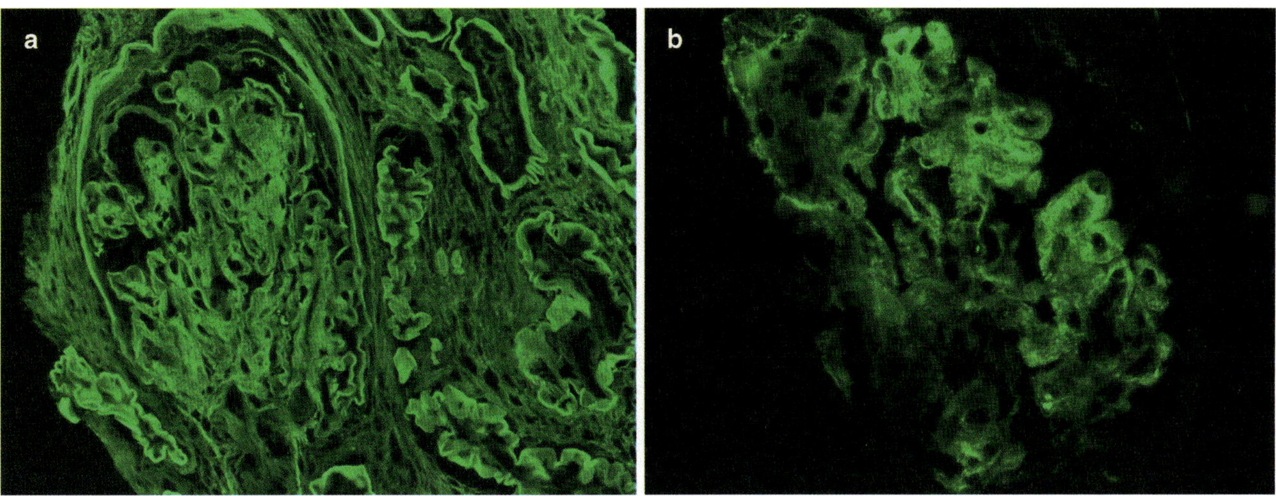

Fig. 5.15 Direct immunofluorescence for albumin and IgM, respectively, AX350, BX500. Diabetic nephropathy. Linear staining along peripheral capillary walls in glomeruli and along tubular basement membranes for IgG in (**a**). Granular, predominantly mesangial staining for IgM in (**b**)

charged screen which is placed in front of the lamina densa with a major role in filtration of macromolecules. Glomerular basement membranes undergo fundamental alterations in diabetes that impair the filtration barrier. Biochemical alterations of the glomerular basement membranes occur along with the thickening of the lamina densa that typically occurs in diabetic nephropathy. It has been proposed that there is increased synthesis of basement membrane components and decreased incorporation of heparan sulfates into glycosaminoglycans resulting in decreased amounts of heparan sulfate proteoglycans (HSGP) in the diabetic glomerular basement membranes in relation to total protein [38]. However, the contribution of HSPG to early albuminuria has been challenged. In vivo rat studies removing HSGP from the glomerular basement membranes did not result in proteinuria [39], suggesting that heparan sulfate is not a major determinant for the charge-selective characteristics of the capillary wall. Also recent studies using antibodies for heparan sulfate in renal biopsies with type I diabetic nephropathy have demonstrated that the staining is not different in intensity to that detected in controls [40]. This last study convincingly demonstrated a lack of scientific evidence to support those changes in heparin sulfate expression, structure, or sulfation played a role in the early proteinuria in patients with diabetic nephropathy.

In the normal glomerulus, the mesangium predominantly contains collagen IV, though many other extracellular matrix proteins and glycoproteins are also typically observed. In diabetic nephropathy there is increased mesangial staining for collagen IV, laminin, and fibronectin while staining for HSPG in the glomerular basement membranes has recently been found to be similar than in control glomeruli. As mesangial nodules became bigger, it has been shown that the staining for interstitial collagens such as V and III (but not collagen I) increased, while the corresponding staining for collagen IV decreased [41, 42]. However, it has been shown that the amount of collagen IV in mesangial nodules actually is increased and its decreased staining is due to decreased density of collagen IV in relation to other extracellular matrix proteins. This also correlates with the focal deposition of fibrillary collagen in some mesangial nodules, typically observed in advanced diabetic nephropathy [35]. Another protein that accumulates in the mesangial nodules is tenascin which makes the restructuring of the mesangium a challenge as destruction of tenascin by metalloproteinases is difficult [43].

Mesangial expansion represents the first noticeable finding by light microscopy in patients with diabetic nephropathy but is often considered nonspecific and of questionable value in making a definitive diagnosis of diabetic nephropathy. Mesangial matrix expansion has been documented in renal biopsies within 5 years of the diagnosis of diabetes mellitus.

Immunofluorescence features of diabetic nephropathy are rather constant. Linear staining for IgG and albumin (Fig. 5.15a) along peripheral capillary walls in glomeruli and along tubular basement membranes represents the most characteristic findings. In some cases there is also linearity with similar pattern for both light chains. This pattern of linear staining in diabetic glomeruli has been thought to be due to stickiness of the glomerular basement membranes to antibodies used for immunofluorescence and is not related to immune complex-mediated processes or circulating cytotoxic antibodies. Granular deposition of C3 and IgM (Fig. 5.15b) is also seen with some frequency, especially in the more advanced cases. If segmental glomerulosclerosis/hyalinosis is present in addition to trapping of C3 and IgM there is also variable granular C1q staining, also attributed to trapping.

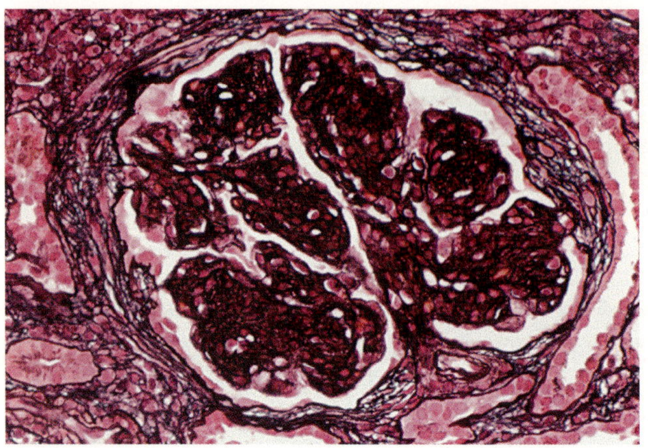

Fig. 5.16 Silver methenamine stain-X500. Diabetic fibrillosis. Note increased staining in mesangial nodules alternating with empty appearing (nonstaining areas) where the fibrillary material (which does not take the silver) accumulates

Ultrastructurally the light microscopic findings are confirmed. Thickening of the glomerular basement membranes and expansion of mesangial areas eventually leading to the formation of well-defined nodules with increased extracellular matrix are observed (Fig. 5.8). These changes are diffuse and generalized but can vary considerably from one glomerulus to the next. In the early stages of diabetic nephropathy when glomerular basement membrane thickening represents an early development, light microscopy is limited in terms of assessing this finding unequivocally making it a must to rely on ultrastructural evaluation to determine that the glomerular basement membranes are indeed thickened. Glomerular basement membrane thickening detected ultrastructurally may be seen as early as 2 years after the diagnosis of diabetes mellitus in some patients and increased thickness of the glomerular basement membranes occurs with time [15, 19, 44].

In addition, there is effacement of the foot processes of the visceral epithelial cells and sometimes these are detached from the glomerular basement membranes, most commonly in advanced lesions. The glomerular basement membranes sometimes exhibit subepithelial lamellation, predominantly in early cases (Fig. 5.6). Mesangial expansion with increased matrix and focal hyalinotic foci is seen in mesangial nodules [19]. There is also cellular debris and in some cases, mostly those with advanced alterations, fibrillary collagen is seen (Fig. 5.9). Hyaline deposits, represented by electron dense areas, containing plasma proteins can be seen in various glomerular locations corresponding the already described "capsular drops and/or hyaline caps." Similar hyaline deposits are confirmed predominantly in arterioles and small arteries (Fig. 5.12).

In a small number of patients with diabetic nodular glomerulosclerosis, there is deposition of randomly disposed fibrillary material composed of 10–25 nm in diameter nonbranching fibrils (Figs. 5.16 and 5.17) [45]. This could be a confusing finding for pathologists who will need to exclude a number of conditions, but diabetic patients with diabetic fibrillosis behave clinically identical to those patients with similar degree of structural renal abnormalities. Microaneurysms can be detected. There are no immune complexes, monoclonal protein deposits, or fibrils with characteristics of amyloid, all of these finding of importance when a differential diagnosis with some other entities that may have similar morphological glomerular findings is being considered.

Understanding the Pathology in Diabetic Nephropathy: From the Research Laboratory to the Evaluation of Renal Samples

In the last 30–35 years, extensive research has been conducted dealing with the pathogenesis of diabetic nephropathy and addressing issues such as progression to end-stage renal disease. Emphasis has been placed on understanding the pathogenesis of diabetic nephropathy in an effort to decipher new therapeutic protocols aimed at ameliorating and/or stopping the development and/or progression of diabetic nephropathy.

Diabetic renal lesions develop for at least one decade before they result in detectable renal functional alterations, so there is plenty of time to work on reversing initial changes that may take place heralding the more deleterious structural effects more difficult to control and ameliorate/stop.

While many different pathobiological pathways have been considered to play a role in the genesis of the renal lesions in diabetes mellitus, some have gained more acceptability over the years. In particular, there are three pathways that appear to be the most important in diabetic nephropathy, for all of which hyperglycemia appears to be the main driving force: (1) The myo-inositol/polyol pathway, (2) the pathways associated with formation of advanced glycation end products (AGEs) and generation of reactive oxygen species (ROS), and (3) hyperfiltration. The cyclohexanehexol myo-inositol (also called polyol) pathway remains at the center of most hypotheses [20, 46].

Chronic hyperglycemia is postulated to be associated with impaired myo-inositol metabolism and end organ damage. Diabetes mellitus has been shown to cause increased polyol pathway activity generating decreased tissue myo-inositol by depleting tissue stores of myo-inositol, paving the way to the genesis of pathological changes. Reduced intracellular myo-inositol is thought to result in abnormal phospholipid metabolism and decreased Na+-K+-ATPase activity leading to abnormal cellular function. Investigators have substantiated that myo-inositol is decreased in the diabetic kidney. Another important event in this pathway is activation of protein kinase C-β (PCK-β). The sequence of events that occur in this pathway has been described in an animal model of STZ-induced diabetic rats (model of type 1 diabetes) and

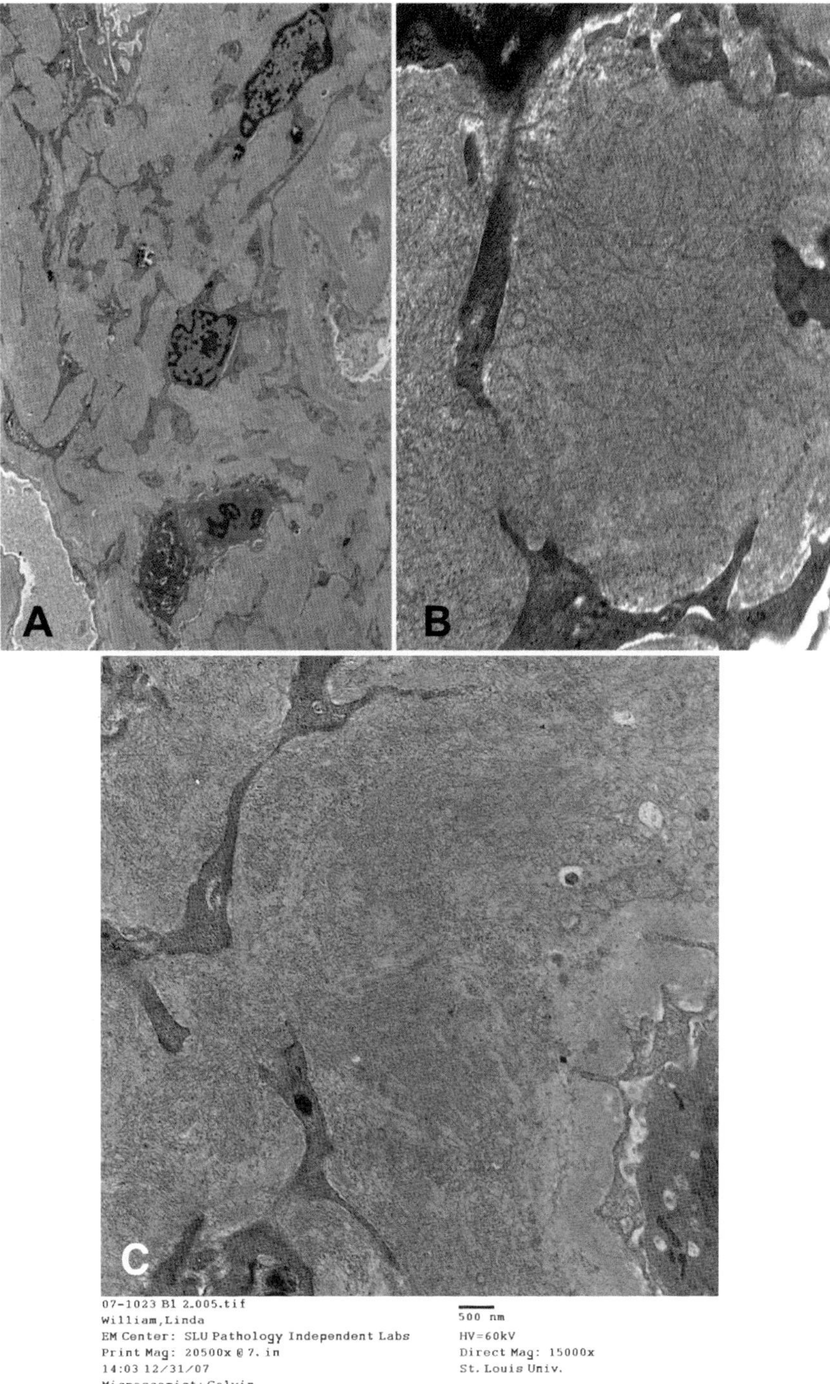

Fig. 5.17 (**a–c**) Transmission electron microscopy, uranyl acetate and lead citrate-AX9500, BX12500, CX17500. Diabetic fibrillosis. Fibrils measuring 15–25 nm in diameter in mesangial nodules

db/db mice (model of type 2 diabetes—leptin deficiency) [47, 48]. When these animals are treated with inhibitors of PCK-β or inhibitors of the polyol pathway (i.e., aldose reductase), amelioration of the disease was noted. This suggests that therapeutic interventions aiming at this pathway may be attractive as treatments to ameliorate the progression of diabetic nephropathy.

The second pathway is characterized by the interaction of AGEs with their receptor, RAGE, to lead to a complex series of events that culminate in cellular dysfunction thus generating an inflammatory response and ROS leading to oxidative stress. Both in vitro and in vivo animal studies have shown the relevance of this pathway in diabetic nephropathy. It remains to demonstrate that the same is true in humans.

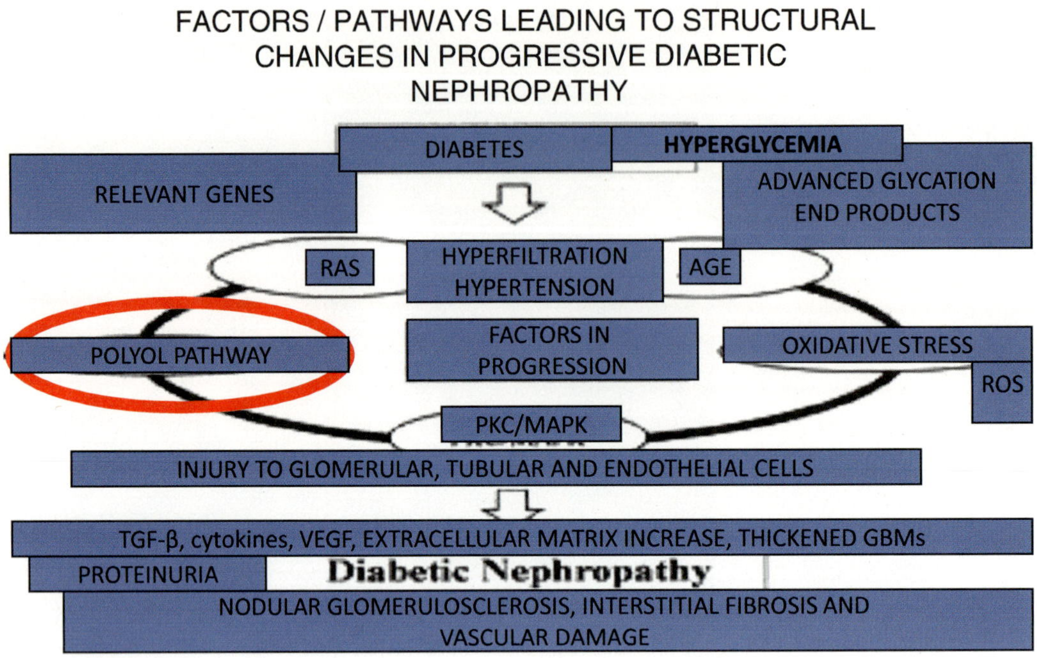

Fig. 5.18 Schematic representation of factors/pathways leading to structural changes in progressive diabetic nephropathy

The ROS generated also results in cellular dysfunction affecting both the glomerular and tubular cells, compounding the negative effects on renal function. ROS is generated predominantly via the NADPH oxidase system or at the level of the mitochondria. NADPH oxidase inhibitors work well in ameliorating the effects of this pathway in animal studies, representing additional possible therapeutic avenues to address diabetic nephropathy and its progression [30].

The third pathway relates to the hyperfiltration that is present in patients with diabetic nephropathy and has proven to have an adverse effect on the course of diabetic nephropathy promoting progression to renal failure. Reduction of glomerular hyperfiltration using angiotensin system inhibitors has had remarkable beneficial effects in the decrease of proteinuria and progression of diabetic nephropathy in animal studies and in human trials of patients with diabetic nephropathy.

The three pathways converge and produce simultaneous damage to glomerular, tubular, interstitial, and endothelial cells acting as the axis of renal structural damage in diabetic nephropathy (Fig. 5.18) [30].

Expansion of the glomerular mesangium at the expense of glomerular capillary filtration surface area represents a crucial and well-established mechanism leading to progressive loss of renal function in diabetic nephropathy.

Pathogenetic events involved in the creation of the characteristic glomerular lesion have been delineated. Though much work still remains to be done, the evidence available points toward initial glomerular basement membrane and peripheral capillary wall alterations, namely thickening and biochemical changes of the glomerular basement membranes followed by mesangial changes leading to the formation of mesangial nodules. The role that TGF-β plays in the generation of mesangial nodules has been well established.

In vitro studies have allowed detailed examination of the mechanisms involved when mesangial cells are cultured in high ambient glucose concentrations with emphasis on cell function [30]. Extension of these studies to in vivo situations has confirmed that most of the in vitro findings reflect reality as it occurs in humans. Studies of diabetic mice indicate that like in humans there is variable susceptibility to developing diabetic nephropathy [45, 47, 48]. In contrast, unlike in humans, each inbred mouse strain represents a genetically homogeneous and easily replenishable resource that is amenable to be used in repeated experimental studies providing an excellent platform to gain insights into the pathogenesis of diabetic nephropathy. Mice provide unparalleled flexibility for studying diabetic nephropathy. There are many mice models modified by strain and genetic mutations that have been used and these are reviewed in a recent publication, highlighting their value and pitfalls for various applications [47]. Obviously the most useful ones recapitulate morphological changes in humans, including glomerular basement membrane thickening and mesangial expansion. These are the db/db and Akita mice models. Some of these mice recapitulate early and late morphologic manifestations of diabetic nephropathy (mice with eNOS deficiency, OVE26 FVB mice, and BTBR ob/ob mice). Unfortunately all animal models of diabetic nephropathy also have important limitations.

The in vitro studies have shown increased mesangial cell proliferation driven by PDFG-beta followed by TGF-β secretion and/or activation leading to mesangial matrix deposition; however, the rats do not progress to renal failure. In contrast, prolonged mild type 2 diabetes mellitus results in morphological changes typical of preclinical diabetic nephropathy in GK (Goto-Kakizaki)-rats but does not lead to albuminuria or progressive renal disease. Finally, the association of type 2 diabetes with hyperlipidemia in obese Zucker rats results in early podocyte damage and subsequent progression to sequential glomerulosclerosis suggesting that in at least a subset of patients with diabetic nephropathy, a concomitant podocytopathy occurs [49]. In clinical practice, there are diabetic patients that develop massive proteinuria and show in their biopsies segmental glomerulosclerosis; this subset of patients with diabetic nephropathy may be the ones with the concomitant podocytopathy [20, 45]. It remains to be deciphered whether the podocyte dysfunction is directly related to the diabetic nephropathy or a secondary pathological process.

Experimental studies have shown that the damage to the podocytes results from modification of the podocytes themselves [33]. Podocyte loss but not necessarily injury likely occurs late in the course of diabetic nephropathy and appears to correlate best with progression of the diabetic nephropathy [50]. Morphological alterations have been noted that appear to be of importance in characterizing and understanding this lesion in diabetes. Podocytes detach from the glomerular basement membranes and bulge exposing endocytotic vesicles rich in albumin. The detachment of the podocytes from the glomerular basement membranes appears to be a key initial finding that initiates the cascade of events that follow. This detachment has been suggested to be linked to the disappearance of the α3β1 integrin, a key molecule which is likely bound to the laminin in the glomerular basement membranes and anchors the visceral epithelial cells to the glomerular basement membranes [51]. Collapse of the glomerular capillary walls follows with progressive disappearance of capillary walls and accumulation of hyaline and lipidic material together with synthesis of extracellular matrix components, including some that are not part of the normal glomerular composition. As a result of the above, the glomerular basement membranes and the basement membranes of the Bowman's capsule form attachments and this interaction further fosters generation and eventual deposition of additional extracellular matrix.

Interestingly, pathophysiological alterations in mesangial cells have been traditionally considered to be the essence of diabetic kidney disease, in terms of initiation, development, and progression of this disorder. Recent evidence implicates the podocyte as a likely player in early disease initiation. Furthermore, insulin resistance appears to contribute to endothelial dysfunction suggesting some role also for glomerular endothelial cell damage in the pathogenesis of diabetic nephropathy [20]. Insulin resistance very likely contributes to endothelial dysfunction [20].

The additional understanding of how podocyte damage can participate in the initiation and/or progression of diabetic nephropathy represents an important contribution to the understanding of how diabetic patients progress into renal failure and why some of these patient do so rapidly after years of stable renal function. Regoli and Bendayan have suggested that a decrease of α3β1 at the podocyte basal membrane facing the glomerular basement membrane may be an important biochemical alteration leading to dysfunction of the capillary walls [51]. This change occurs before morphological alterations are detectable in the glomerular basement membranes and appears to be, therefore, an early (and perhaps key initiating) event preceding overt diabetic nephropathy.

Progression of diabetic nephropathy has been addressed in the research laboratory using cell culture and animal models [52]. For example, exposure of glomerular mesangial cells and proximal tubular cells to hyperglycemic conditions may alter cell proliferation and/or extracellular matrix turnover by means of modulating cytokine production. Mechanisms involved in these processes have been elucidated. Extension of these studies to experimental in vivo situations has confirmed a significant number of these findings but has also shown some unexpected results. Increased glomerular cellular proliferation and mesangial matrix accumulation driven by the combined effects of PDGF-β and TGF-β occur in streptocotocin-induced diabetes but this is not accompanied by the development of the nephropathy to renal failure. Furthermore, although prolonged mild type 2 diabetes induces morphological changes characteristic of preclinical diabetic nephropathy in GK-rats it does not result in albuminuria or in progressive renal disease [52].

Endothelial cell injury is extremely important in diabetic nephropathy. Injury to the renal vasculature via damage to endothelial cells leads to increased expression of adhesion molecules and chemokines, resulting in macrophage influx into the renal parenchyma, and establishes a microenvironment of constant "low-grade inflammation" [20].

Finally, the association of type 2 diabetes with hyperlipidemia in obese Zucker rats results in early podocyte damage and subsequent progression to glomerulosclerosis, tubular interstitial damage, and renal insufficiency emphasis after the role of podocyte injury [38, 53]. There is much work left to be done to identify specific mediators involved in the genesis and development of the above mentioned processes, including defining conditions/mechanisms that will determine progression of subclinical morphological changes to overt nephropathy. This area remains as one of the most important to focus on in future novel developments of therapeutic interventions in diabetes.

Another approach that has been taken to further enhance our understanding of events that participate in the progression of diabetic nephropathy is to study genes that can be involved in this progression. High-throughput and genome-wide approaches in animal models have been used to detect relevant genes. Several genes such as Tim44 (translocase of inner mitochondrial membrane-44), RSOR/MIOX (renal-specific oxidoreductase-inositol oxygenase), UbA52 (ubiquitin A), Rap1b (Ras-related GTPase), gremlin, osteopontin, hydroxysteroid dehydrogenase-3β isotype 4, and those in the Wnt signaling pathway have been identified as differentially expressed in kidneys of diabetic rodents. Functional analysis of those genes and translational research efforts to determine the impact of these genes in humans will be of potential value in the prevention and treatment of diabetic nephropathy. Identification of other pertinent biomarkers and therapeutic target genes will soon follow [54].

Papillary necrosis occurs with some frequency in patients with diabetic nephropathy and deserves a few comments. It is more common in females. A common risk for developing papillary necrosis is recurrent urinary tract infections, which tend to occur with some frequency in patients with diabetes mellitus. Clinical presentation is typically pyuria and microscopic hematuria, though there are cases, which present with acute renal failure, if there is bilateral ureteral obstruction due to sloughing of papillae. The presence of papillary necrosis is usually a poor prognostic sign for patients with diabetes mellitus and most times accompany other manifestations of diabetic nephropathy.

Reversibility of Structural and Functional Damage in Advanced Diabetic Nephropathy

Reversibility of the structural changes that occur in diabetic nephropathy remains controversial [4, 36, 50]. The mainstay of current therapy for diabetic nephropathy includes control of hyperglycemia and blood pressure, and inhibition of the renin-angiotensin-aldosterone system (RAAS). While these therapies can be effective in slowing progression they have had no proven effect on reversing structural or functional damage and their efficacy is indeed limited. The paradigm to be deciphered poses the question whether restoration of a normal metabolic milieu or direct effects of given molecules such as leptin represent the best avenue toward attempting to reverse the changes attributed to the diabetic nephropathy.

In order to evaluate possible therapeutic interventions that can be aimed at reversing lesions, there is a need to use effective in vitro and in vivo platforms in the research laboratory. No relevant animal models exist in which reversibility can be tested. One of the issues that have become important is the role of podocytes in the advancement and irreversibility of diabetic nephropathy. As diabetic nephropathy advances, podocytes are lost in at least a subset of these patients, mostly those with advanced nephropathy. Podocytes are nonreplicating cells which make reversibility by means of regeneration of visceral epithelial cells not possible. Some investigators defend the opinion that the restoration of functional podocytes abrogates the injury process in diabetic nephropathy and allows reversal of the structural changes during the reparative phase. Therefore, conceptually speaking, while reconstitution of a normal glomerulus after podocyte loss may be a significant challenge, it has been shown that this problem can be overcome, at least experimentally. Some believe that podocytes in diabetic nephropathy can regenerate so that reversal of diabetic nephropathy is attainable.

In a murine model of type 2 diabetic nephropathy, BTbR ob/ob leptin-deficient mice with diabetic nephropathy were administered leptin. The identification of leptin receptors within isolated glomeruli from BTBR mice established the possibility that leptin can exert a direct effect in reversing alterations. In fact, leptin replacement, but not inhibition of the renin-angiotensin-aldosterone system (RAAS), resulted in near complete reversal of structural and functional alterations. Mesangial matrix expansion, mesangiolysis, basement membrane thickening, and podocyte loss were all reversed along with proteinuria and accumulation of ROS. This model closely resembles diabetic nephropathy (much better than other animal models available) which emphasizes the importance of these studies and their relevance to humans [55].

Some studies have shown to a limited but yet important degree that reversal of nephropathy is governed by leptin signaling rather than by restoration of a normal metabolic milieu in the mesangium [36]. The demonstration that pStat3, a key downstream molecule in the leptin signaling pathway, provides strong evidence that leptin signaling in the kidney contributes, though to an unknown degree, to reversal of nephropathy, although it is recognized that the pStat3 could be the result of other signaling pathways. Studies to address these two possibilities will provide the final answer to this question [36].

Differential Diagnosis of Diabetic Nephropathy

From a structural point of view the lesions in diabetic nephropathy are not specific. Therefore, there is a differential diagnosis to be considered depending on which findings are present.

Isolated glomerular basement membrane thickening can be a nonspecific alteration in vascular nephrosclerosis. This is accompanied by alterations in the renal vasculature that can support such diagnosis; however, vascular changes are also common in diabetic nephropathy, sometimes preceding detectable characteristic glomerular changes. The combination of the typical glomerular alterations and the accompanying vascular changes, most notably hyalinosis in afferent and efferent

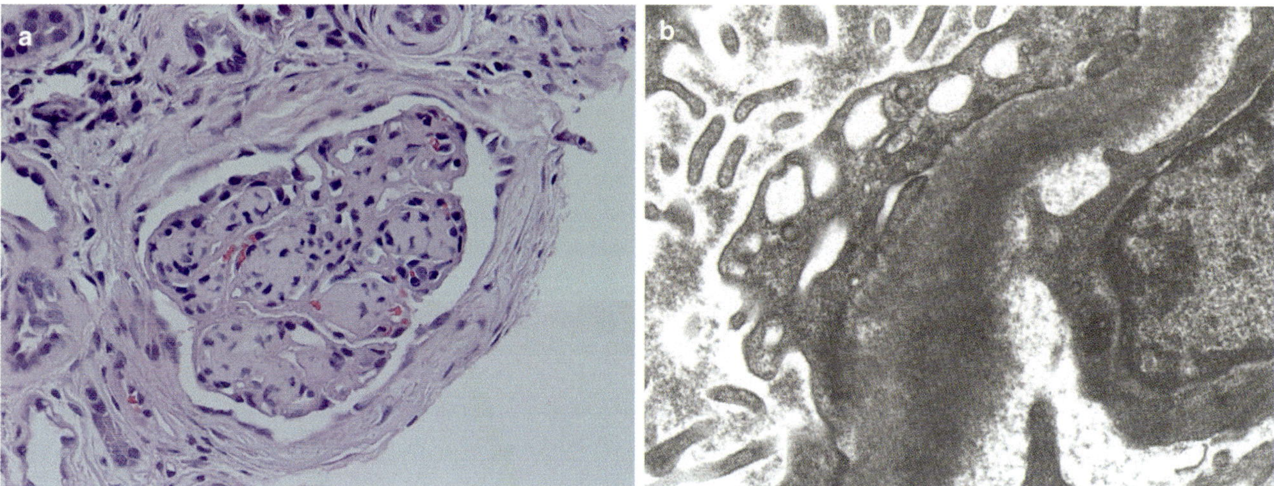

Fig. 5.19 (**a**) H&E-X500; (**b**) transmission electron microscopy, uranyl acetate and lead citrate-X18500. Nodular glomerulosclerosis. Light chain deposition disease. In (**a**) note pattern of nodular glomerulosclerosis similar to what is seen in diabetic nephropathy. Punctate electron dense material (light chains) in subendothelial zones making possible a diagnosis of light chain deposition disease

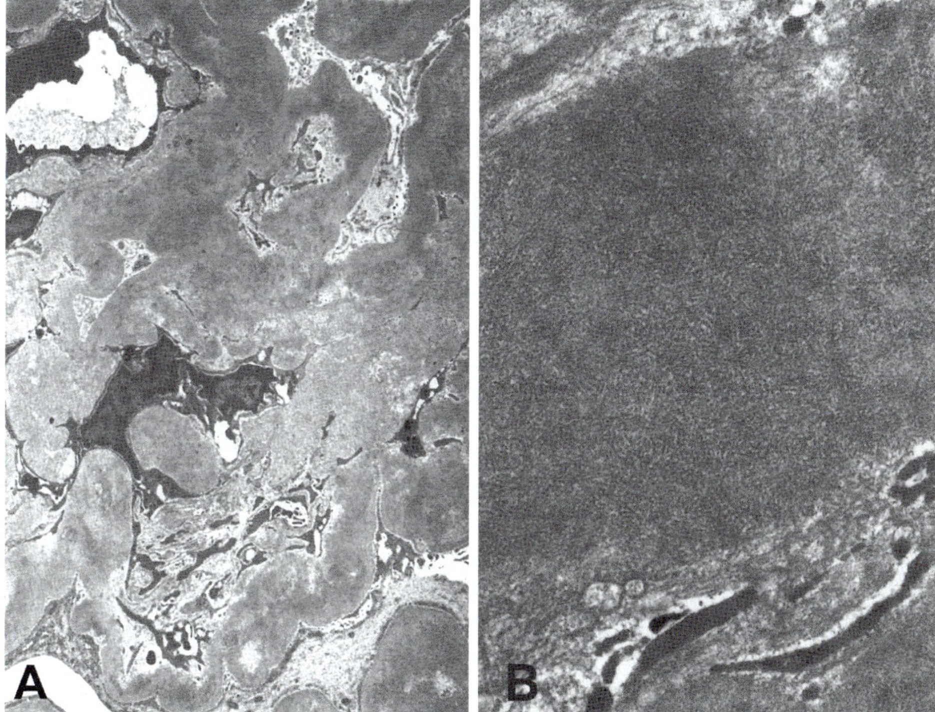

Fig. 5.20 (**a**, **b**) Transmission electron microscopy, uranyl acetate and lead citrate-AX8500, BX15000. Nodular glomerulosclerosis. Light chain deposition disease. Note mesangial nodule with increased matrix (**a**) and deposition of punctate electron dense material in mesangium best shown in (**b**)

arterioles with the typical immunofluorescence pattern and ultrastructural features, are sufficient to establish a solid diagnosis of diabetic nephropathy, nodular glomerulosclerosis.

The finding of nodular glomerulosclerosis should instigate a focused differential diagnosis. While diabetic nephropathy is by far the most common pathology responsible for the formation of mesangial nodules, these are not specific at all. The one important lesion to differentiate from nodular diabetic glomerulosclerosis is light/heavy chain deposition disease (Figs. 5.19 and 5.20) [45]. In this case detection of monotypical light or heavy chains in the glomerulus, interstitium, and or vasculature permits an accurate diagnosis.

However, there are situations where the deposition of the monoclonal proteins may be subtle or early and fluorescence and ultrastructural manifestations may be quite subtle. It is also a challenge to diagnose superimposed light or heavy chain deposition disease in a patient with diabetic nephropathy as the pathological glomerular findings overlap significantly and the glomerular diabetic milieu makes it difficult to detect the abnormal proteins in the glomerulus. It is often easier to look for the monoclonal protein in the tubular interstitial compartment generally along tubular basement membranes and confirm its presence by immunofluorescence and/or electron microscopy.

There is a subset of patients with so-called idiopathic nodular glomerulosclerosis. This entity was first described by Alpers [56] and Biava in 1989 and in 1999 [57]. Herzenberg et al. coined the term idiopathic nodular glomerulosclerosis to refer to this condition. These patients exhibit in their renal tissue findings identical to those observed in diabetic nephropathy by light, immunofluorescence and ultrastructural examination. This entity has been epidemiologically linked to hypertension and smoking. The incidence of this condition is low; it was found in 0.45 % of 5,073 renal biopsies examined at Columbia University in a 5-year period [58]. The authors of all idiopathic glomerulosclerosis publications carefully excluded cases with clinical or preclinical diabetes from their series. Idiopathic nodular glomerulosclerosis involves interplay of hypertension, smoking, increased glomerular extracellular matrix production, and angiogenesis [58]. Neovascularization in the affected glomeruli represents a rather constant finding in these cases. Secretion and activation of TGF-β is responsible in the same manner as it is in diabetic nephropathy, for the increased mesangial matrix and eventual mesangial nodularity.

Other entities in the differential diagnosis, though usually creating less of a dilemma in differentiation from diabetic nephropathy, include chronic thrombotic microangiopathy, membranoproliferative glomerulonephritis with "lobular" glomerular appearance, amyloidosis (Fig. 5.21), fibrillary and immunotactoid glomerulopathies which in some cases may mimic nodular glomerulosclerosis. The combination of light, special stains, immunofluorescence and electron microscopy suffices to make the correct diagnosis in the great majority of the cases [58].

Superimposed Pathology (Nondiabetic Lesions) That Can Alter Structural Alterations in Diabetic Nephropathy Cases

Diabetic patients with renal disease attributable to their disease are usually not biopsied unless the clinical course is not the usual one. There are a number of clinical situations that lead to a renal biopsy. Among these are progression to renal failure faster than expected, especially if other findings are detected such as the presence of circulating monoclonal proteins, positive serologies for collagen vascular disease, or ANCA (antineutrophilic cytoplasmic antibodies) in the serum, or nephrotic range proteinuria. One of the complicating factors in the understanding of structural changes that are part of diabetic nephropathy is that other conditions can coexist with diabetic nephropathy changing the characteristic structural alterations that are present. Virtually any immune complex-mediated process can be seen in a diabetic glomerulus. A renal biopsy is indicated if there is a clinical suspicion that this is the case. Immunofluorescence and electron microscopy will highlight the particular findings associated with these superimposed processes. The most common immune complex-mediated lesion found in diabetic patients superimposed on diabetic nephropathy is membranous nephropathy [19].

There are also tubular interstitial conditions such as acute tubular necrosis (Fig. 5.22) and acute tubular interstitial nephritis (Fig. 5.23) that may accelerate the pace of renal failure in patients with diabetic nephropathy. A renal biopsy will make the diagnosis.

The same is true of superimposed vascular diseases that may be uncovered in renal biopsies. Some of these include thrombotic microangiopathy and vasculitis.

The presence of monoclonal proteins in the renal biopsy detected by immunofluorescence, proliferative glomerular changes, glomerular necrosis/crescents, and immune complexes detectable by immunofluorescence/electron microscopy indicate a superimposed process in a diabetic patient with evidence of nephropathy.

A recent publication highlights nondiabetic conditions that can be seen in patients with diabetic nephropathy with focal segmental glomerulosclerosis being the most common followed by hypertensive nephrosclerosis and acute tubular necrosis [59].

Finding of concomitant diseases alerts the clinician to treat those with the hope to improve renal function. Frequently, the clinical response is slow and sometimes quite sluggish, as the damage in the renal parenchyma caused by the diabetic changes makes recuperation from these superimposed conditions much more difficult.

Conclusions

Diabetic nephropathy represents a well-characterized entity with structural abnormalities in the renal parenchyma that can generally be recognized with certainty in specimens submitted for pathological assessment.

The ideal biomarker for diabetic nephropathy does not exist. Despite the large number of biomarkers that have been discovered, none has been proven to be superior to albuminuria [60].

There are a number of experimental models that have provided crucial information regarding how lesions in this condition

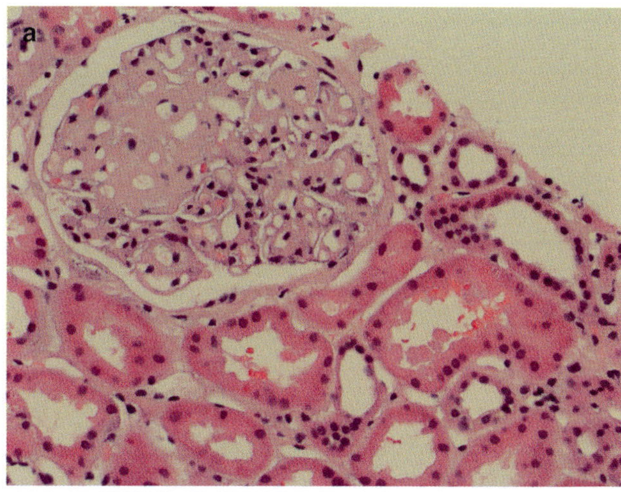

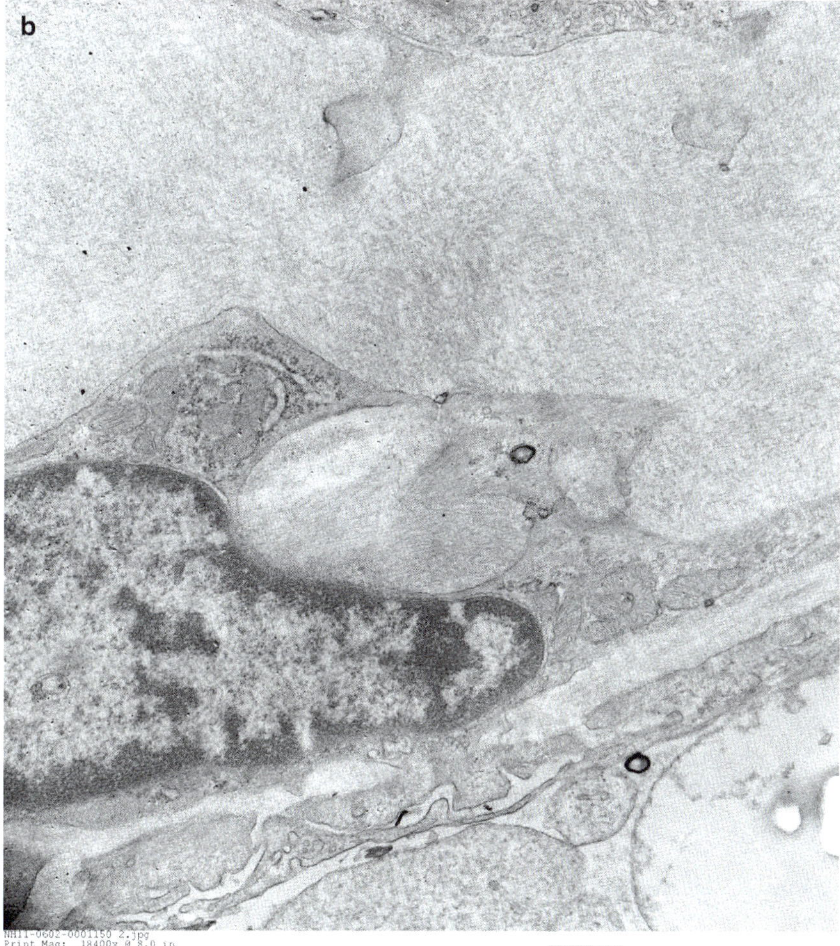

Fig. 5.21 (**a**) H&E; (**b**) Transmission electron microscopy, uranyl acetate and lead citrate-AX350; BX13500. AL-amyloidosis superimposed on diabetic nephropathy. Note amorphous, eosinophilic material in expanded mesangial area in (**a**). In (**b**) note randomly disposed, nonbranching fibrils indicative of amyloid

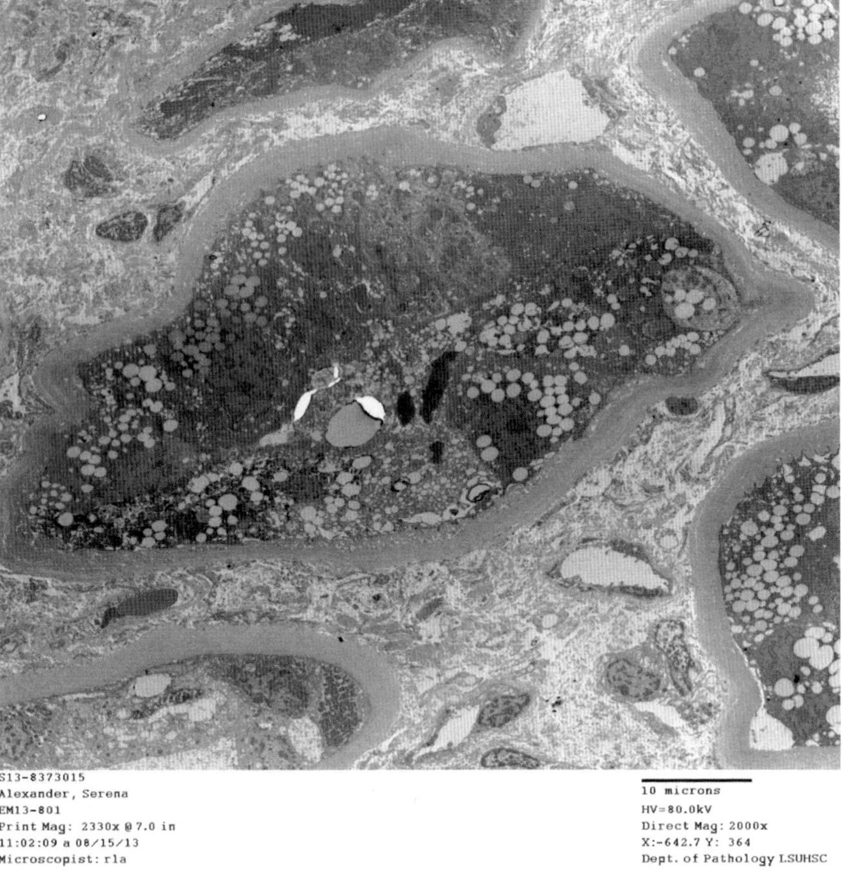

Fig. 5.22 X7500. Transmission electron microscopy, uranyl acetate and lead citrate. Acute tubular necrosis superimposed on diabetic nephropathy. Tubular injury in a background of interstitial edema and no inflammatory activity

develop and progress. The elucidation of mechanistic phenomena that lead to the morphological/structural changes provides a solid platform to device new therapeutic interventions to ameliorate or reduce the speed of progression to renal failure or to stop its progression altogether. The main problem is that there are many intertwined factors that are involved and teasing these becomes rather complicated. It is likely that a multiprong approach will remain necessary in the treatment of these patients in order to obtain positive results. Controlling blood sugar, blood pressure, and proteinuria are all beneficial and very much indicated for the management of these patients with diabetic nephropathy. These therapeutic interventions may be even considered milestones in the treatment of diabetic nephropathy. However, these maneuvers have not been proven to be enough to stop completely progression of the renal damage and eventual end-stage renal disease. The challenge for the future rests in a better understanding of the complex interactions between hyperglycemia, metabolic, hemodynamic, and intracellular factors together with the actions of growth factors and cytokines involved in the pathogenesis of diabetic nephropathy to design new therapeutic interventions with a broader range of action aimed directly at molecular mechanisms that play a role in progression to end-stage kidney disease. New approaches that have been proposed include those targeting oxygen biology, such as hypoxia, oxidative stress, and dyserythropoiesis, all of which have been implicated in diabetic nephropathy [61].

More recently used approaches such as transcriptome and proteome profiling and molecular genetics using cell lines, animal models, and human samples have increased our understanding of the mechanisms important in the progression of diabetic nephropathy. As a result, new biomarkers have been discovered which could lead to therapeutic maneuvers that can contribute to the amelioration of the diabetic nephropathy and decrease mortality and morbidity in chronic kidney disease patients that progress to end-stage renal disease. Target genes can also be modulated using data mining to identify those that are of relevance for the diagnosis and therapy of diabetic nephropathy [54].

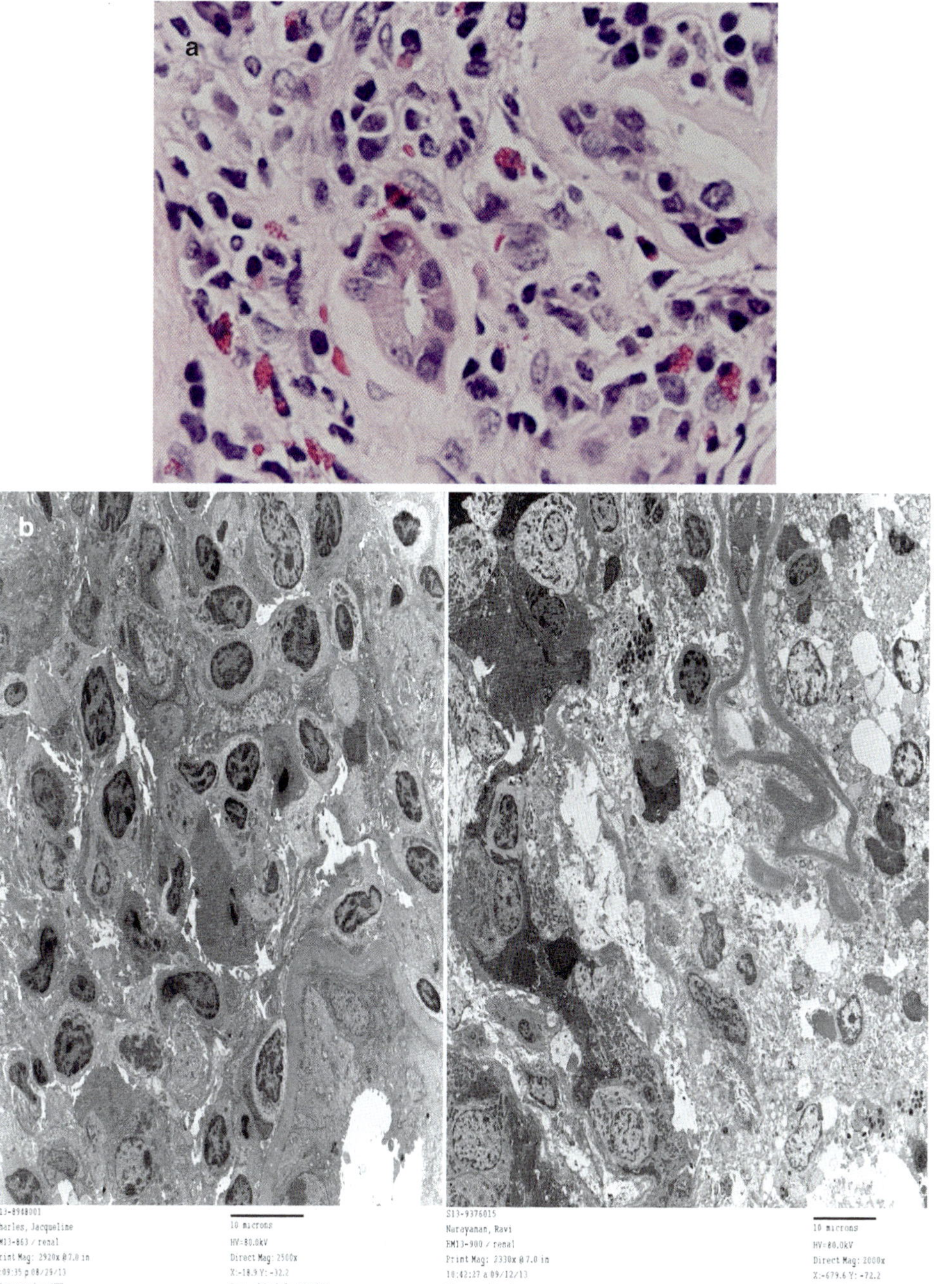

Fig. 5.23 (**a**) H&E stain; (**b**, **c**) transmission electron microscopy, uranyl acetate and lead citrate. AX500, BX7500, CX8500. In (**a**) note interstitial inflammatory process with eosinophils associated with focal tubulitis and tubular damage. (**b**, **c**) Illustrate corresponding ultrastructural findings with a dense interstitial inflammatory infiltrate associated with focal tubular damage and tubulitis

References

1. Kimmelstiel P, Wilson C. Intercapillary lesions in the glomeruli of the kidney. Am J Pathol. 1936;12:83–98.7.
2. Murakami R. Beitrag zur Kenntnis der Veränderung des Nierenkörperchens beim Diabetes mellitus. Trans Jpn Pathol Soc. 1936;26:657–64.
3. Gellman DD, Pirani CL, Soothill JF, Muehrcke RC, Kark RM. Diabetic nephropathy: a clinical and pathologic study based on renal biopsies. Medicine (Baltimore). 1959;38:321–67.
4. Dalla Vestra M, Saller A, Mauer M, Fioretto P. Role of mesangial expansion in the pathogenesis of diabetic nephropathy. J Nephrol. 2001;14 Suppl 4:S51–7.
5. Mogensen CE, Andersen MJ. Increased kidney size and glomerular filtration rate in early juvenile diabetes. Diabetes. 1973;22:706–12.
6. Drummond K, Mauer M. The early natural history of nephropathy in type 1 diabetes: II. Early renal structural changes in type 1 diabetes. Diabetes. 2002;51:1580–7.
7. Dalla Vestra M, Saller A, Bortoloso E, Mauer M, Fioretto P. Structural involvement in type 1 and type 2 diabetic nephropathy. Diabetes Metab. 2000;26 Suppl 4:8–14.

8. Mauer SM, Steffes MW, Ellis EN, Sutherland DE, Brown DM, Goetz FC. Structural-functional relationships in diabetic nephropathy. J Clin Invest. 1984;74:1143–55.
9. Ritz E, Zeng XX, Rychlik I. Clinical manifestation and natural history of diabetic nephropathy. Contrib Nephrol. 2011;170:19–27.
10. Ritz E. Diabetic nephropathy. Saudi J Kidney Dis Transpl. 2006;17:481–90.
11. Ellis EN, Warady BA, Wood EG, et al. Renal structural-functional relationships in early diabetes mellitus. Pediatr Nephrol. 1997;11:584–91.
12. Jeansson M, Granqvist AB, Nystrom JS, Haraldsson B. Functional and molecular alterations of the glomerular barrier in long-term diabetes in mice. Diabetologia. 2006;49:2200–9.
13. Flyvbjerg A. Inhibition and reversibility of renal changes: lessons from diabetic kidney disease. Acta Paediatr Suppl. 2006;95:83–92.
14. Qian Y, Feldman E, Pennathur S, Kretzler M, Brosius 3rd FC. From fibrosis to sclerosis: mechanisms of glomerulosclerosis in diabetic nephropathy. Diabetes. 2008;57:1439–45.
15. Osterby R, Gall MA, Schmitz A, Nielsen FS, Nyberg G, Parving HH. Glomerular structure and function in proteinuric type 2 (non-insulin-dependent) diabetic patients. Diabetologia. 1993;36:1064–70.
16. Dische FE. Measurement of glomerular basement membrane thickness and its application to the diagnosis of thin-membrane nephropathy. Arch Pathol Lab Med. 1992;116:43–9.
17. Haas M. Alport syndrome and thin glomerular basement membrane nephropathy: a practical approach to diagnosis. Arch Pathol Lab Med. 2009;133:224–32.
18. Nasr SH, Markowitz GS, Valeri AM, Yu Z, Chen L, D'Agati VD. Thin basement membrane nephropathy cannot be diagnosed reliably in deparaffinized, formalin-fixed tissue. Nephrol Dial Transplant. 2007;22:1228–32.
19. Najafian B, Alpers CE, Fogo AB. Pathology of human diabetic nephropathy. Contrib Nephrol. 2011;170:36–47.
20. Ziyadeh FN, Wolf G. Pathogenesis of the podocytopathy and proteinuria in diabetic glomerulopathy. Curr Diabetes Rev. 2008; 4:39–45.
21. Stout LC, Kumar S, Whorton EB. Focal mesangiolysis and the pathogenesis of the Kimmelstiel-Wilson nodule. Hum Pathol. 1993;24:77–89.
22. Wada T, Shimizu M, Yokoyama H, et al. Nodular lesions and mesangiolysis in diabetic nephropathy. Clin Exp Nephrol. 2013;17:3–9.
23. Tervaert TW, Mooyaart AL, Amann K, et al. Pathologic classification of diabetic nephropathy. J Am Soc Nephrol. 2010;21:556–63.
24. Matsusaka T, Xin J, Niwa S, et al. Genetic engineering of glomerular sclerosis in the mouse via control of onset and severity of podocyte-specific injury. J Am Soc Nephrol. 2005;16:1013–23.
25. Stout LC, Kumar S, Whorton EB. Insudative lesions—their pathogenesis and association with glomerular obsolescence in diabetes: a dynamic hypothesis based on single views of advancing human diabetic nephropathy. Hum Pathol. 1994;25:1213–27.
26. Alsaad KO, Herzenberg AM. Distinguishing diabetic nephropathy from other causes of glomerulosclerosis: an update. J Clin Pathol. 2007;60:18–26.
27. Bader R, Bader H, Grund KE, Mackensen-Haen S, Christ H, Bohle A. Structure and function of the kidney in diabetic glomerulosclerosis. Correlations between morphological and functional parameters. Pathol Res Pract. 1980;167:204–16.
28. Mauer SM, Sutherland DE, Steffes MW. Relationship of systemic blood pressure to nephropathology in insulin-dependent diabetes mellitus. Kidney Int. 1992;41:736–40.
29. Fioretto P, Steffes MW, Sutherland DE, Mauer M. Sequential renal biopsies in insulin-dependent diabetic patients: structural factors associated with clinical progression. Kidney Int. 1995;48:1929–35.
30. Caramori ML, Kim Y, Huang C, et al. Cellular basis of diabetic nephropathy: 1. Study design and renal structural-functional relationships in patients with long-standing type 1 diabetes. Diabetes. 2002;51:506–13.
31. Perrin NE, Torbjornsdotter TB, Jaremko GA, Berg UB. The course of diabetic glomerulopathy in patients with type I diabetes: a 6-year follow-up with serial biopsies. Kidney Int. 2006;69:699–705.
32. Caramori ML, Parks A, Mauer M. Renal lesions predict progression of diabetic nephropathy in type 1 diabetes. J Am Soc Nephrol. 2013;24:1175–81.
33. Teiken JM, Audettey JL, Laturnus DI, Zheng S, Epstein PN, Carlson EC. Podocyte loss in aging OVE26 diabetic mice. Anat Rec (Hoboken). 2008;291:114–21.
34. Bohle A, Wehrmann M, Bogenschutz O, Batz C, Muller CA, Muller GA. The pathogenesis of chronic renal failure in diabetic nephropathy. Investigation of 488 cases of diabetic glomerulosclerosis. Pathol Res Pract. 1991;187:251–9.
35. Mason RM, Wahab NA. Extracellular matrix metabolism in diabetic nephropathy. J Am Soc Nephrol. 2003;14:1358–73.
36. Pichaiwong W, Hudkins KL, Wietecha T, et al. Reversibility of structural and functional damage in a model of advanced diabetic nephropathy. J Am Soc Nephrol. 2013;24:1088–102.
37. Berg UB, Torbjornsdotter TB, Jaremko G, Thalme B. Kidney morphological changes in relation to long-term renal function and metabolic control in adolescents with IDDM. Diabetologia. 1998;41:1047–56.
38. Tamsma JT, van den Born J, Bruijn JA, et al. Expression of glomerular extracellular matrix components in human diabetic nephropathy: decrease of heparan sulphate in the glomerular basement membrane. Diabetologia. 1994;37:313–20.
39. Rossi M, Morita H, Sormunen R, et al. Heparan sulfate chains of perlecan are indispensable in the lens capsule but not in the kidney. EMBO J. 2003;22:236–45.
40. van den Born J, Pisa B, Bakker MA, et al. No change in glomerular heparan sulfate structure in early human and experimental diabetic nephropathy. J Biol Chem. 2006;281:29606–13.
41. Nerlich A, Schleicher E. Immunohistochemical localization of extracellular matrix components in human diabetic glomerular lesions. Am J Pathol. 1991;139:889–99.
42. Adler SG, Feld S, Striker L, et al. Glomerular type IV collagen in patients with diabetic nephropathy with and without additional glomerular disease. Kidney Int. 2000;57:2084–92.
43. Truong LD, Pindur J, Barrios R, et al. Tenascin is an important component of the glomerular extracellular matrix in normal and pathologic conditions. Kidney Int. 1994;45:201–10.
44. Tsilibary EC. Microvascular basement membranes in diabetes mellitus. J Pathol. 2003;200:537–46.
45. Turbat-Herrera EA. Overview of models for the study of renal disease. In: Herrera GA, editor. Experimental models of renal diseases: pathogenesis and diagnosis, Contributions to nephrology series, vol. 169. Basel: S Karger AG; 2011. p. 1–5.
46. Loy A, Lurie KG, Ghosh A, Wilson JM, MacGregor LC, Matschinsky FM. Diabetes and the myo-inositol paradox. Diabetes. 1990;39:1305–12.
47. Alpers CE, Hudkins KL. Mouse models of diabetic nephropathy. Curr Opin Nephrol Hypertens. 2011;20:278–84.
48. Breyer MD, Bottinger E, Brosius III FC, et al. Mouse models of diabetic nephropathy. J Am Soc Nephrol. 2005;16:27–45.
49. Chevalier J, Masurier C, Lavaud S, Michel O, Bariety J. Approach of cellular mechanisms of glomerulosclerosis in a model of accelerated aging the obese Zucker rat. C R Seances Soc Biol Fil. 1995;189:987–1007.
50. Dalla Vestra M, Masiero A, Roiter AM, Saller A, Crepaldi G, Fioretto P. Is podocyte injury relevant in diabetic nephropathy? Studies in patients with type 2 diabetes. Diabetes. 2003;52: 1031–5.
51. Regoli M, Bendayan M. Alterations in the expression of the alpha 3 beta 1 integrin in certain membrane domains of the glomerular epithelial cells (podocytes) in diabetes mellitus. Diabetologia. 1997;40:15–22.

52. Phillips A, Janssen U, Floege J. Progression of diabetic nephropathy. Insights from cell culture studies and animal models. Kidney Blood Press Res. 1999;22:81–97.
53. Gassler N, Elger M, Kranzlin B, et al. Podocyte injury underlies the progression of focal segmental glomerulosclerosis in the fa/fa Zucker rat. Kidney Int. 2001;60:106–16.
54. Wada J, Sun L, Kanwar YS. Discovery of genes related to diabetic nephropathy in various animal models by current techniques. In: Herrera GA, editor. Experimental models of renal diseases: pathogenesis and diagnosis, Contributions to nephrology series, vol. 159. Basel: S Karger AG; 2011. p. 161–74.
55. Anjaneyulu M, Chopra K. Nordihydroguairetic acid, a lignin, prevents oxidative stress and the development of diabetic nephropathy in rats. Pharmacology. 2004;72:42–50.
56. Alpers CE, Biava CG. Idiopathic lobular glomerulonephritis (nodular mesangial sclerosis): a distinct diagnostic entity. Clin Nephrol. 1989;32:68–74.
57. Herzenberg AM, Holden JK, Singh S, Magil AB. Idiopathic nodular glomerulosclerosis. Am J Kidney Dis. 1999;34:560–4.
58. Markowitz GS, Lin J, Valeri AM, Avila C, Nasr SH, D'Agati VD. Idiopathic nodular glomerulosclerosis is a distinct clinicopathologic entity linked to hypertension and smoking. Hum Pathol. 2002;33:826–35.
59. Sharma SG, Bomback AS, Radhakrishnan J, Herlitz LC, Stokes MB, Markowitz GS, D'Agati VD. The modern spectrum of renal biopsy findings in patients with diabetes. Clin J Am Soc Nephrol. 2013;8:1718–24.
60. Jim B, Santos J, Spath F, Cijiang He J. Biomarkers of diabetic nephropathy, the present and the future. Curr Diabetes Rev. 2012;8:317–28.
61. Miyata T, Suzuki N, de Strihou VY. Diabetic nephropathy: are there new and potentially promising therapies targeting oxygen biology? Kidney Int. 2013;84:693–702.

6 Diabetes in Children and Adolescents

Ihor V. Yosypiv

Introduction

Diabetes mellitus (DM) is a disease of the metabolic homeostasis characterized by chronic hyperglycemia resulting from defects in insulin secretion, insulin action, or both. There are two types of DM: type 1 and type 2 [1]. Type 1 DM (T1DM) is caused by an absolute insulin deficiency resulting from a loss of the insulin-producing β-cells of the pancreas. Type 2 DM (T2DM) is caused by the relative insulin deficiency where insulin resistance is compensated for initially by an increased insulin secretion followed by insufficient insulin secretion to match the increased requirements imposed by the insulin-resistant state.

Epidemiology of DM

In 2007, the total child population of the world (0–14 years) was estimated to be 1.8 billion, of whom 0.02 % have diabetes. This means that approximately 440,000 children around the world have diabetes with 70,000 new cases diagnosed each year [2]. In most industrialized countries, T1DM accounts for over 90 % of DM in children and adolescents [2]. Mean annual incidence rates for T1DM in 0–14 years of age group in different countries vary between 0.1 and 57.6 per 100,000. It is lowest in Asia (China—0.1 per 100,000, Japan—2.4 per 100,000) and highest in Finland (57.6 per 100,000). In the United States, it is highest in white (27 per 100,000), followed by African American (18 per 100,000) and Hispanic (15 per 100,000) children [2]. A rise in the incidence was reported in many countries with most cases presenting in cooler months of the year. T1DM is two to three times more common in the offspring of diabetic men (3.6–8.5 %) compared with diabetic women (1.3–3.6 %) [2]. When both parents are affected, the risk increases to 30 %. The age of clinical presentation of T1DM has a bimodal distribution with one peak at 4–6 years of age and a second at 10–14 years of age [3]. T2DM is becoming increasingly more common and accounts for up to 45 % of new-onset cases among adolescents in certain at-risk populations [4]. In the United States, T2DM accounted for 12 % of all new cases of pediatric diabetes in 1990, whereas by 2000, almost 50 % of patients diagnosed with diabetes had T2DM [5]. T2DM accounted for 26 % of prevalent black case subjects and 10 % of non-Hispanic white case subjects 0–19 years of age. Among black female subjects 10–19 years of age, 46 % of new cases of diabetes were classified as T2DM [6]. At mean age of 14 years in patients with T2DM, 41.1 % were Hispanic, 31.5 % black and 27.4 % white, 89.4 % had a family history of DM, and 64.9 % were female [7]. T2DM is diagnosed at a mean age of 13.5 years.

Etiology of DM

Etiological classification of DM is presented in Table 6.1 [1]. Major causes of non-monogenic DM include (1) a common polygenic predisposing pattern, (2) epigenetic mechanisms, at least partially linked to nutritional disturbances during gestation influencing fetal programming, and (3) detrimental societal environment promoting the development of obesity by (a) giving free access to excess food rich in calories, sucrose, and lipids, (b) limiting physical activity, or (c) exposing to pollutants or infectious agents that could exert a toxic effect on the β-cell. Although the exact prevalence of monogenic DM in children is unknown, the majority of patients with genetically proven monogenic DM are initially incorrectly diagnosed as T1DM or T2DM [8]. In children, almost all monogenic DM results from mutations in genes that regulate β-cell function with few cases resulting from insulin resistance [9].

I.V. Yosypiv, M.D. (✉)
Division of Pediatric Nephrology, Department of Pediatrics SL37, Tulane Hospital for Children, 1430 Tulane Avenue, New Orleans, LA 70112, USA
e-mail: iiosipi@tulane.edu

E.V. Lerma and V. Batuman (eds.), *Diabetes and Kidney Disease*,
DOI 10.1007/978-1-4939-0793-9_6, © Springer Science+Business Media New York 2014

Table 6.1 Etiological classification of DM

Type 1
(a) Immune mediated
(b) Idiopathic
Type 2
Genetic defects of β-cell function
HNF1α (MODY3)
HNF4α (MODY1)
HNF1β (MODY5)
Glucokinase (MODY2)
IPF1 (MODY4)
NeuroD1 (MODY6)
KCNJ11
Mitochondrial DNA mutation
Genetic defects of insulin action
Type A insulin resistance
Leprechaunism
Rabson–Mendenhall syndrome
Lipoatrophic diabetes
Diseases of exocrine pancreas
Pancreatitis
Pancreatic trauma or neoplasia
Cystic fibrosis
Hemochromatosis
Endocrinopathies
Acromegaly
Cushing's syndrome
Glucagonoma
Pheochromocytoma
Hyperthyroidism
Somatostatinoma
Aldosteroma
Drug- or chemical-induced
Glucocorticoids
Thyroid hormone
Diazoxide
β-adrenergic agonists
Thiazides
Dilantin
A-interferon
Infections
Congenital rubella
Cytomegalovirus
Uncommon forms of immune-mediated diabetes
Other genetic syndromes sometimes associated with diabetes
Down
Klinefelter
Turner
Wolfram
Friedreich's ataxia
Huntington's chorea
Laurence–Moon–Biedl
Myotonic dystrophy
Porphyria
Prader–Willi

HNF hepatocyte nuclear factor, *MODY* maturity-onset diabetes of the young

Pathophysiology of DM

Most cases of T1DM are due to T-cell mediated destruction of pancreatic β-cells. T1DM becomes clinically symptomatic when approximately 90 % of pancreatic β-cells are destroyed [10]. Susceptibility to autoimmune T1DM is determined by multiple genes with HLA genes having the strongest known association [11]. The environmental triggers (chemical or viral), except possible association with enterovirus infection, which initiate destruction of pancreatic β-cells remain largely unknown [12, 13]. In a recent study, 17.8 % of children with diabetic ketoacidosis (DKA) had viral and 12.9 % had bacterial infection [14]. Once the autoimmune process is triggered by infection, effector mechanisms like antibody-dependent cellular cytotoxicity, delayed hypersensitivity, complement activation, and cytotoxic concentrations of cytokines like interferon-γ and interleukin-1 could result in destruction of β-cells [13]. The pathophysiology of T2DM most likely represents autoimmune T1DM in overweight or obese individuals with underlying insulin resistance. This possibility is supported, in part, by the findings that 15–40 % of children and young adults with T2DM have T1DM-associated autoantibodies [15].

Development of the Pancreas

The mature pancreas is a glandular organ that carries out two major functions: exocrine and endocrine. The exocrine pancreas, constituting almost 99 % of the total mass of the organ, comprises a ramifying tubular tree of ductal branches, which drain the digestive enzymes secreted by acinar cells to the duodenum [16]. The endocrine pancreas comprises the islets of Langerhans, clusters of 100–1,000 hormone-secreting cells scattered throughout the exocrine tissue and interconnected via blood vessels. The primary function of islets is to maintain metabolic homeostasis through the production of hormones that regulate blood glucose levels. Five primary endocrine cell types, each responsible for secreting a particular hormone, are found in islets: α-cells (glucagon); β-cells (insulin); δ-cells (somatostatin); ε-cells (ghrelin); and PP-cells (pancreatic polypeptide) [16, 17].

Understanding how the pancreas develops is vital to finding new treatments for a range of pancreatic diseases, including DM. In the developing embryo, appropriate patterning of the endoderm destined to become pancreas requires the spatial and temporal coordination of transcription and soluble growth factors secreted by the surrounding tissues. Once pancreatic progenitor cells are specified in the developing epithelial endoderm, epithelial–mesenchymal interactions, as well as a networks of transcription factors, delineate three distinct lineages, including endocrine, exocrine, and ductal

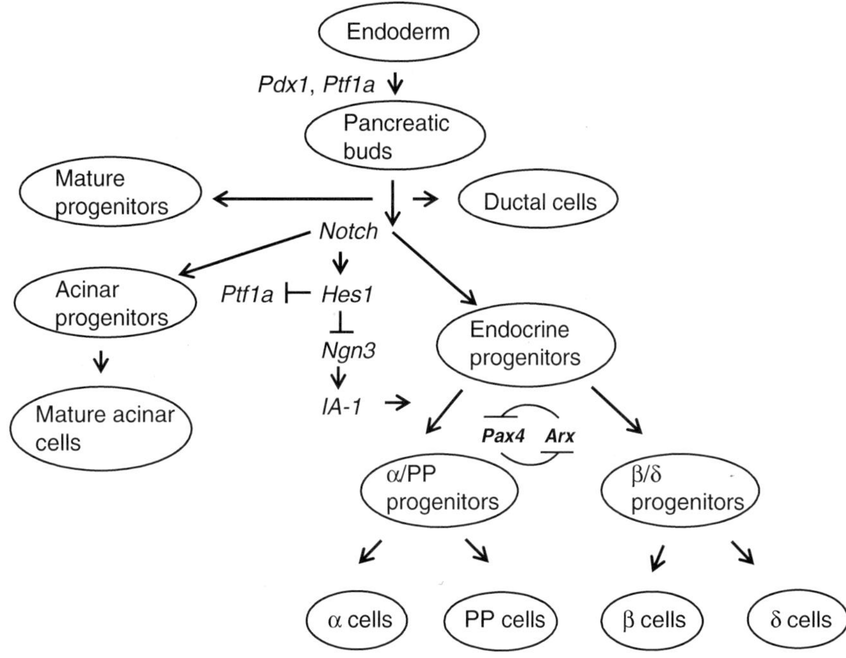

Fig. 6.1 Schematic diagram of key steps of development and differentiation of pancreatic cell types. Please see text for details

cells (Fig. 6.1). Both endocrine and exocrine lineages arise from embryonic endodermal epithelium (Fig. 6.1), which expresses the proteins pancreatic and duodenal homeobox 1 (Pdx1) and pancreas-specific transcription factor 1 (Ptf1a) [16, 18]. During development of the pancreatic epithelium, endocrine cells emerge in two waves of differentiation as they exit the tubular epithelium, differentiate, migrate, coalesce to form islets, and proliferate. In the mouse, endocrine differentiation begins on embryonic day 9.5 (E9.5) [18]. Following early differentiation, the epithelium undergoes a second wave of expansion and differentiation called the "secondary transition," starting around E12.5 in the mouse and the sixth week of embryonic development in humans [18, 19]. Scattered cells located within the "trunk" domain of the ductal epithelium individually take on an endocrine fate marked by transient expression of neurogenin 3 (Ngn3) and its downstream target gene, zinc finger transcription factor insulinoma-associated protein 1 (IA-1), delaminate, and form endocrine cell clusters, while acinar cells at branch tips actively proliferate and increase in size as they accumulate digestive enzyme. Lateral interactions between epithelial cells, mediated via Notch/Hes1 signaling, are central to the control of endocrine/exocrine specification [20, 21]. Downstream of the Ngn3-positive pan-endocrine progenitor cell population, α/PP and β/δ lineages are specified by the opposing actions of transcription factors aristaless-related homeobox gene (Arx) and paired box 4 (Pax4), respectively (Fig. 6.1). Secondary wave endocrine cells primarily differentiate into β-cells, along with other endocrine lineages, delaminate from the epithelium, and coalesce into small islet-like clusters that progressively form larger islet aggregates during postnatal development. In adults, the formation of new β-cells gradually ceases, but can be induced under conditions of increased metabolic demand, such as insulin resistance. Most available evidence suggests that duplication of preexisting differentiated β-cells, rather than differentiation of stem or progenitor cells, is the predominant mechanism [22]. Unraveling the cell intrinsic vs. extrinsic mechanisms that drive β-cell generation, either during development, homeostasis, or disease, remains a major and immediate challenge of the field [23].

Developmental Programming of DM

A growing body of evidence supports the concept that changes in the intrauterine milieu during "sensitive" periods of embryonic development or in infant diet after birth affect the developing individual, resulting in general health alterations later in life. This phenomenon is referred to as "developmental programming" or "developmental origins of health and disease." The risk of developing T2DM is increased in infants born prematurely at <37 weeks of gestation or in low birth weight (LBW) infants weighing <2,500 g at birth [24, 25]. Recent epidemiologic studies demonstrate a relationship between T2DM with both LBW and high birth weight (>4 kg) [26]. In addition, LBW neonates undergoing catch-up growth have impaired glucose tolerance at 7 years of age [27, 28]. Thus, accelerated postnatal growth during early postnatal life is an independent risk factor for adverse metabolic outcomes. In mono- and di-zygotic twins discordant for T2DM, LBW twins had higher rates of T2DM compared to their co-twin, indicating that nongenetic intrauterine factors are important in determining the risk of T2DM [29]. Developmental programming due to intrauterine growth retardation (IUGR) resulting from maternal undernutrition or gestational DM increases the risk of insulin resistance and T2DM [30, 31]. In gestational DM, intrauterine exposure to hyperglycemia and hyperinsulinemia may affect development of pancreatic β-cells and adipose tissue resulting in obesity and altered glucose metabolism in later life. Experimental animal studies demonstrate that exposure to intrauterine DM may be associated with impaired renal function and hypertension in an offspring. In this regard, maternal streptozotocin-induced DM in the rat results in glomerular hypertrophy, reduced GFR, and an elevated blood pressure in the offspring without change in total nephron number as early as at 1 month after birth [32]. Changes in vascular reactivity could be contributing to the hypertension observed in these offsprings of diabetic mothers [33].

Epigenetic modifications provide one potential mechanism for how environmental influences in early life cause long-term changes in chronic disease susceptibility. The major players in epigenetic mechanisms of gene expression regulation are DNA or chromatin protein methylation, acetylation, and chromatin remodeling. Posttranslational modifications of histones such as histone acetylation and methylation of cytosine bases adjacent to guanines (CpG dinucleotides) may affect chromatin function and alter gene expression in the absence of changes in DNA sequence [34, 35]. It has been shown that a maternal low protein diet or tobacco use is associated with reduced global methylation in the liver of the offspring in the rat or in the human placenta, a metabolic and endocrine organ that may be considered an "imprint" of fetal exposure in utero [36, 37]. In the rat model of IUGR, reduced expression of pancreatic and duodenal homeobox 1 (*Pdx1*), a key transcription factor that directs pancreatic progenitor cell development, was associated with changes in histone acetylation and methylation at this locus in an offspring [38]. Epigenetic modifications of the hepatocyte nuclear factor 4α (*HNF4α*), a key transcription factor that regulates differentiation of pancreatic β-cells, have been reported in an offspring of mothers subjected to dietary protein restriction during gestation [39]. In addition, histone modifications of *GLUT4*, an insulin-responsive glucose transporter gene in skeletal muscle, are observed in the rat IUGR offspring [40]. Together, these findings support a role for both pancreatic and peripheral epigenetic modifications in metabolic disease pathogenesis and represent a plausible mechanism by which early life environment may alter gene expression to influence an individual's susceptibility to metabolic disease in later life.

Environmental influences during an individual's early life are not the sole cause of long-term changes in chronic disease susceptibility. Emerging data suggest that integration of signals from an individual's mother's lifetime nutritional or health experience contributes to intergenerational transfer of environmental information. For example, offsprings of LBW or preterm mothers are more likely to be born LBW or preterm, indicating transgenerational effect for LBW or preterm birth [41]. Epigenetic imprinting, alteration of gene expression based on their methylation status, is likely to play a role in transmitting epigenetic information from previous generations [42].

Clinical Manifestations of DM

The classic symptoms of DM are polydipsia, polyuria, and weight loss. Reemergence of bedwetting, nocturia, daytime urine incontinence, and a need to leave classes in school to use the restroom suggest polyuria. In younger children who are not toilet trained, increased frequency of wet diapers and diapers that are more heavy (wet) may be noted by caregivers. In girls, perineal candidiasis may be observed [43]. Initially, appetite is increased, but over time, children may become anorexic, contributing to weight loss. Weight loss results from hypovolemia (from polyuria) and increased catabolism (from impaired glucose utilization in skeletal muscle and increased fat and muscle breakdown). In the absence of the classic symptoms, DM can be suspected in the presence of elevated plasma glucose levels or glucosuria. T2DM is also strongly associated with acanthosis nigricans, polycystic ovary syndrome (PCO), and metabolic syndrome [44–46].

Acute Complications of DM

DKA and hyperosmolar hyperglycemic state (HHS, also known as nonketotic hyperglycemia) are two of the most serious acute complications of DM. DKA results from absolute or relative insulin deficiency and the combined effects of increased levels of the counterregulatory hormones: catecholamines, glucagon, cortisol, and growth hormone [47]. The combination of low serum insulin and high levels of counterregulatory hormones results in an accelerated catabolic state with increased glucose production by the liver and kidney (via glycogenolysis and gluconeogenesis), impaired peripheral glucose utilization, resulting in hyperglycemia and hyperosmolality, increased lipolysis and ketogenesis, causing ketonemia and metabolic acidosis. DKA occurs in 15–70 % of children with DM at the time of diagnosis [48–50]. In the presence of DKA, tachypnea, deep respirations, a fruity breath secondary to exhaled acetone, neurologic findings ranging from drowsiness, lethargy, and obtundation to coma may be observed. Clinical signs of cerebral edema include fluctuating level of consciousness, sustained heart rate deceleration (decline more than 20 beats per minute) not attributable to improved intravascular volume or sleep state, age-inappropriate incontinence, vomiting, headache, lethargy or difficulty to be aroused from sleep, and diastolic blood pressure >90 mmHg [51]. The mortality rate from DKA in children is 0.15–0.30 % with cerebral edema accounting for 60–90 % of all DAK-related deaths [52, 53].

HHS may occur in children with T1DM, but is more common in T2DM [48]. In the United States, population rates for HHS hospitalization rose 52.4 % from 2.1 to 3.2 per one million children from 1997 to 2009 [54]. Symptoms of HHS develop more insidiously, as compared to DKA. The earliest symptoms of marked hyperglycemia are polyuria, polydipsia, and weight loss. As the degree or duration of hyperglycemia progresses, neurologic symptoms including lethargy, focal signs, and obtundation can be seen. Neurological symptoms are most common in HHS, while hyperventilation and abdominal pain are primarily limited to patients with DKA. The criteria for HHS include plasma glucose concentration >600 mg/dL (>33.3 mmol/L), serum osmolality >320 mOsm/kg, small ketonuria, absent to mild ketonemia, arterial pH>7.30, serum bicarbonate >15 mmol/L, stupor, or coma.

Diagnosis

It is important to diagnose DM promptly and differentiate T1DM from T2DM or monogenic DM. The diagnostic criteria for DM are based upon the guidelines of the American Diabetes Association (ADA) and are the same as those used in adults: fasting plasma glucose (FPG) >126 mg/dL (7 mmol/L), symptoms of hyperglycemia and a random venous plasma glucose >200 mg/dL (11.1 mmol/L), abnormal OGTT defined as plasma glucose >200 mg/dL (11.1 mmol/L) measured 2 h after a glucose load of 1.75 g/kg (maximum dose of 75 g), and hemoglobin A1C>6.5 % [55]. Patients who manifest impaired fasting glucose (100–125 mg/dL or 5.6–6.9 mmol/L) or glucose tolerance (140–199 mg/dL or 7.8–11.0 mmol/L) are considered to have prediabetes. The following findings generally suggest the presence of T2DM: BMI>85th percentile, presentation after the onset of puberty, presence of acanthosis nigricans, hypertension, dyslipidemia, PCO syndrome, and ethnicity (Hispanic, African, Native, and Asian American). In T1DM, the presence of pancreatic islet cell autoantibodies, reduced insulin and C-peptide levels, and no evidence of insulin resistance with fasting C-petide levels within the normal range (0–20 %) are usually observed. Patients with T1DM and T2DM can have a family history of DM and present with ketoacidosis. The following findings may suggest the presence of monogenic DM: diagnosis of DM before 6 months of age, family history of DM with a parent affected, non-obese patient, pancreatic islet autoantibodies are absent, and evidence of endogenous insulin production outside the "honeymoon" period (after 3 years of diabetes) with detectable C-peptide (>200 nmol/L) when glucose >8 mmol/L or presence of specific gene mutations known to be associated with DM (Table 6.1) [11, 56]. Overall, 70 % of patients fell into T1DM (55 %) or T2DM (16 %). An additional 20 % exhibit both autoimmunity and insulin resistance, a pattern typical for obese patients with T1DM. The final 10 % of patients are insulin sensitive in the absence of β-cell autoimmunity, suggesting that these patients need additional evaluation for the possibility of monogenic DM [57]. In addition, DM may result from other diseases of pancreatic exocrine system, endocrine anomalies in glucose regulation, and use of medications or viruses (Table 6.1).

Monogenic DM

Genetic Defects of β-Cell Function

DM associated with monogenetic defects in β-cell function is characterized by onset of hyperglycemia at an early age (generally before age 25 years). This spectrum of DM is referred to as maturity-onset diabetes of the young (MODY) and is characterized by impaired insulin secretion with minimal or no defects in insulin action. MODY is the most common form of monogenic DM, accounting for 2–5% of diabetes [58]. It is inherited in an autosomal dominant pattern. Abnormalities at six genetic loci on different chromosomes have been identified to date (Table 6.1). The most common form is associated with mutations in a hepatic transcription factor (HNF)-1α [59]. A second form is associated with mutations in the glucokinase gene resulting in a defective glucokinase, an enzyme that converts glucose to glucose-6-phosphate. Because of defects in the glucokinase gene, increased plasma levels of glucose are necessary to elicit normal levels of insulin secretion [60]. The less common forms of MODY result from mutations in other transcription factors, including HNF-4α, HNF-1β, insulin promoter factor (IPF)-1, and neurogenic differentiation factor-1 (NeuroD1). *IPF1* gene mutations can lead to MODY4 by reduced binding of the protein to the insulin gene promoter [61]. Mutations in the *HNF-1β* gene cause MODY5. In addition to early onset DM, affected patients can develop pancreatic atrophy, congenital anomalies of the kidney and urinary tract (CAKUT) (renal dysplasia, renal cysts, glomerulocystic disease, oligomeganephronia), chronic kidney disease (CKD), and genital abnormalities (epididymal cysts, atresia of vas deferens, and bicornuate uterus) [62]. Some patients may have a phenotype consistent with familial juvenile hyperuricemic nephropathy or autosomal recessive form of polycystic kidney disease [63, 64]. NeuroD1 normally functions as a regulatory switch for endocrine pancreatic development. *NeuroD1* mutations cause MODY6 [65].

Other Causes of Familial DM

Transient (TNDM) or permanent (PNDM) neonatal DM is usually diagnosed in the first 3 months of life. TNDM will resolve at a median age of 3 months, but can relapse in up to 50 % of cases [66]. Most patients with TNDM have abnormal imprinting of the *ZAC* and *HYMAI* genes on chromosome 6q. The most common known cause of PNDM is mutation in the KCNJ11 gene which encodes the Kir6.2 subunit of the β-cell K_{ATP} channel [67]. X-linked (IPEX) syndrome can also lead to neonatal DM. IPEX syndrome is a rare monogenic primary immunodeficiency due to mutations of *FOXP3*, a key transcription factor for regulatory T cells [68]. The initial presenting symptoms are severe enteritis and/or type-1 diabetes mellitus, alone or in combination with eczema and elevated serum IgE. Most patients with this disorder die within the first year of life regardless of the type and site of the mutation. Point mutations in mitochondrial DNA have been found to be associated with diabetes and deafness. The most common mutation occurs at position 3,243 in the tRNA gene [69]. Patients have a defect in insulin secretion and sensorineural hearing loss. The mean age of onset of diabetes and hearing loss is between the ages of 30 and 40.

Other types of monogenic DM result from a dominantly inherited missense mutation in the sulfonylurea 1 receptor subunit (Sur1) characterized by hyperinsulinemia in childhood and diabetes in adulthood, inability to convert proinsulin to insulin, production of mutant insulin molecules, or insulin resistance [70–73]. For example, Leprechaunism and the Rabson–Mendenhall syndrome are due to mutations in the insulin receptor gene with subsequent alterations in insulin receptor function and extreme insulin resistance [9]. Leprechaunism is usually fatal in infancy and is characterized by small body size, elfin facies, and enlarged clitoris and breasts. Rabson–Mendenhall syndrome is a rare, autosomal recessive disorder characterized by growth retardation, coarse and senile-looking faces, mental precocity, early dentition, and pineal hyperplasia. Particular forms of PCO syndrome with severe hyperandrogenism, acanthosis nigricans, and marked insulin resistance define the type A insulin resistance syndrome. Familial partial lipodystrophy (FPLD) is a monogenic form of dominantly inherited DM caused by a mutation in the *LMNA* gene and associated with the loss of subcutaneous fat from the limbs and trunk, with excess fat deposited around the face and neck [74]. Wolfram syndrome (diabetes insipidus, diabetes mellitus, optic atrophy, and deafness) is a rare autosomal recessive disorder with incomplete penetrance [75, 76]. Patients with Wolfram syndrome develop insulin-requiring DM and optic atrophy in early childhood. Later in adolescence, they develop diabetes insipidus, hydronephrosis, progressive sensorineural deafness, and neurologic dysfunction [77]. Wolcott–Rallison syndrome is another rare autosomal recessive disorder associated with mutations in *EIF2AK3* and characterized by onset of DM in the first 3 years of life, epiphyseal dysplasia, CKD, acute hepatic failure, and developmental restriction [78].

It is important to distinguish MODY from T1DM or T2DM because the optimal treatment and risk for diabetes complications varies with the underlying genetic defect. For example, patients with MODY due to HNF1α or HNF4 α mutations are frequently misdiagnosed as having insulin requiring T1DM because they present at an early age and are not obese. However, many of these patients can be successfully managed with sulfonylureas monotherapy. In addition, diagnosing monogenic DM allows earlier identification of family members at risk. In a patient with presumed T1DM, measurement of serum autoantibodies (islet-cell antibodies (ICA), glutamic acid decarboxylase (GAD65), insulin, tyrosine phosphatases, IA-2 and IA-2β) should be performed prior to consideration of genetic testing for MODY. The presence of autoantibodies makes MODY very unlikely. Unfortunately, there are currently no biochemical tests that reliably differentiate between the MODY and T2DM diseases. The diagnosis of MODY is made by performing diagnostic genetic testing by direct sequencing of the gene. A list of laboratories is available on at www.ncbi.nlm.nih.gov/sites/GeneTests or www.athenadiagnostics.com. Genetic testing should only be performed after informed consent and genetic counseling.

Treatment of DM

Therapy of DM by a multidisciplinary team involves training the caregivers and the patient to provide appropriate care, education and lifestyle modifications, specifically diet, exercise and weight loss, progressive increase in independence and self-care by the growing child, strict glycemic control, avoidance of severe hypoglycemia, control of comorbidities, including hypertension, dyslipidemia, nephropathy and hepatic steatosis, and maintenance of normal growth and development. Specific guidelines on how and when to administer insulin and other medications, how to rotate injection sites, test for and record blood glucose test results, timing and carbohydrate content of meals and snacks, how to adjust insulin dose based on blood glucose concentrations and carbohydrate intake, test urine for ketones at times of illness, or if two consecutive blood glucose readings are greater than 250 mg/dL (13.9 mmol/L), intervene with dietary measures and/or glucagon if blood glucose level is too low [55]. Adolescent drivers with DM should test blood glucose levels before driving and carry carbohydrate snacks with them at all times. Adolescents should be counseled on risky behaviors such as alcohol or drug use, eating disorders, cigarette smoking, and unprotected sexual intercourse. A system to ensure gradual transition into adult care should be in place.

Treatment of T1DM

Insulin

All insulin is now manufactured by recombinant DNA technology and is based on the amino acid sequence of human insulin. Three rapid-acting insulin analogues are available: lispro (Humalog), aspart (NovoLog), and glulisine (Apidra). These insulins start to act in 0.15–0.35 h and last for 3–5 h. Rapid acting analogues are used as prandial or snack boluses and in insulin pumps. Regular insulin is short-acting and is used in intravenous infusion to treat DKA. Neutral protamine Hagedorn (NPH) is intermediate in peak and duration of action (onset: 2–4, peak: 4–12, duration: 12–24 h). Basal long-acting analogues include detemir (Levemir) and glargine (Lantus) (onset: 1–4, peak: 6–12, duration: 20–24 h).

Insulin Regimens

During the honeymoon period, single daily injection of insulin may be sufficient. Ultimately, however, most patients will require at least two injections of insulin per day (at breakfast and dinner) with mixing short/rapid-acting (1/3 of a dose) and NPH (2/3 of a dose) insulin. Children on this regimen often require more (~2/3) of the total insulin dose in the morning and less (~1/3) in the evening. Basal-bolus regimens aim to achieve more physiologic insulin concentrations. The basal insulin provides fasting insulin needs and the bolus provides insulin to cover food requirements and to correct hyperglycemia. Of the total daily insulin requirements, 40–60 % should be basal insulin and the rest preprandial rapid-acting or regular insulin. Insulin dosage depends of such factors as age, weight, stage of puberty, duration and phase of DM, nutritional intake, exercise, results of blood glucose monitoring, and intercurrent illness. During the partial remission, the total daily insulin dose is <0.5 IU/kg/day. Outside the partial remission phase, prepubertal children usually require 0.7–1.0 IU/kg/day while pubertal children require 1–2 IU/kg/day of insulin [79].

Monitoring

Blood glucose is monitored before meals or snacks, at bedtime, when ill, and with sports. Reasonable goals for fasting and preprandial blood glucose levels are preschool age: 100–180 mg/dL (5.6–10.0 mmol/L), school age: 90–180 mg/dL (5.0–10.0 mmol/L), and teenagers: 90–130 mg/dL (5.0–7.2 mmol/L). The goals for HbA1C (reflecting average blood glucose concentration over the 2 previous months) are <6 year old: 7.5–8.5 %, 6–12 years: <8 %, 13–19 years: <7.5 %. Urine or blood ketones should be monitored when blood glucose values are >250 mg/dL (13.9 mmol/L) or when children are not feeling well to abort episodes of DKA.

Treatment of T2DM

Pharmacologic therapy should be started from metformin which has an advantage over sulfonylureas of similar reductions in HbA1C without the risk of hypoglycemia. Failure of monotherapy with metformin over 3 months indicates the need to add glitazone, sulfonylurea, or insulin alone or in combination with meglitidine, amylin, or DPP-IV inhibitor [80]. Only metformin and insulin are approved for use in children in most countries. Lifestyle changes in diet and exercise should be continued in addition to pharmacologic therapy. Patients at risk for pregnancy should be counseled on the effects of DM and oral agents on conception and fetal development. Bariatric surgery may be recommended in adolescents with T2DM with BMI > 35 [81]. Studies demonstrate resolution of T2DM in 91 % of adolescent patients who underwent gastric bypass surgery [82].

Treatment of DKA and HHS

The biochemical criteria for the diagnosis of DKA are hyperglycemia [>200 mg/dL (>11 mmol/L)], venous pH < 7.3, or bicarbonate <15 mmol/L, ketonemia or ketonuria. The severity of DKA is categorized by the degree of acidosis. Mild: venous pH < 7.3 or bicarbonate <15 mmol/L; moderate: pH < 7.2, bicarbonate < 10 mmol/L; severe: pH < 7.1, bicarbonate <5 mmol/L. Goals of therapy are correct dehydration, acidosis, reverse ketosis, restore blood glucose to near normal, and avoid complications of therapy. In severe volume depletion or shock, isotonic saline (or Ringer's lactate) in 20 mL/kg boluses should be given to restore circulatory volume. Insulin therapy is essential to normalize blood glucose and suppress lipolysis and ketogenesis. Insulin at 0.1 unit/kg/h should be administered after initial fluid replacement and continued until resolution of DKA (pH > 7.30, bicarbonate >15 mmol/L). Five percent glucose should be added to IV fluid when plasma glucose falls to 250–300 mg/dL (14–17 mmol/L) to prevent hypoglycemia. If the patient is hypokalemic, potassium replacement (40 mmol/L) should be initiated at the time of initial volume expansion. Otherwise, potassium should be given after initial volume expansion and concurrent with starting insulin therapy. If patient is hyperkalemic, potassium administration should be deferred until urine output is documented. Bicarbonate or phosphorus administration is not recommended unless the acidosis is profound. Transition from IV to subcutaneous insulin should be initiated when oral intake is tolerated before a mealtime 15–30 min (rapid insulin) or 1–2 h (regular insulin) before stopping insulin infusion [48]. Treatment of cerebral edema involves elevation of the head of the bed, reduction of fluid administration by one-third, and giving mannitol (0.5–1.0 g/kg IV over 20 min) or 3 % saline [83]. After treatment for cerebral edema has been started, a cranial CT scan should be obtained to rule out other possible intracranial causes of neurologic deterioration (e.g., thrombosis or hemorrhage). Intubation may be necessary for impending respiratory failure.

Treatment of Monogenic DM

TNDM or PNDM usually requires treatment with insulin [56]. These patients may be also treated with sulphonylureas which are used in higher doses compared to doses used in adults [84]. Patients with MODY3 (*HNF-1α* mutations) or MODY1 (*HNF-4α* mutations) can be treated with diet, insulin, and low doses of sulphonylureas (Gliclazide) [85]. Patients with MODY5 (*HNF-1β* mutations), mitochondrial DM, and Wolfram or Roger's syndrome are treated with insulin [86]. Treatment of insulin resistance syndromes (type A insulin resistance, lipodystrophy, leprechaunism, and Rabson–Mendenhall syndrome) includes the use of insulin sensitizers (metformin and glitazones) and insulin [9]. In patients with pancreatic aplasia exocrine pancreatic supplements are required. The only known effective cure for IPEX syndrome is hematopoietic stem cell transplantation [68]. Table 6.2 lists useful resources on DM for patients, parents, and caregivers.

Chronic Complications and Comorbidities of DM

Children and adolescents with DM are at risk for a number of comorbid conditions. Associated autoimmune diseases (e.g., thyroid dysfunction, celiac disease) occur more frequently in children with T1DM [87]. Linear growth is affected negatively by DM. Patients with DM are at increased risk for dyslipidemia, a major risk factor for cardiovascular disease. Dyslipidemia is observed in 33 % of children with T2DM [88]. Obesity and T2DM are also associated with nonalcoholic fatty liver disease (NAFLD) [89]. Microvascular complications of diabetes include retinopathy, nephropathy, and neuropathy [89]. Screening for retinopathy is recommended when the child has had DM for 3–5 years. DM-associated nephropathy is a progressive disorder of the microvasculature of the kidney, occurring in 14–22 % of children with T2DM at presentation [89]. The prevalence and risk of progression of neuropathy has not been systematically studied among children with DM. Macrovascular complications (coronary artery, peripheral, and cerebral vascular disease) are frequent in adolescents with T2DM. Observational studies of children report essential hypertension in 5.9 % and in 17–32 % of patients at presentation in T1DM and T2DM, respectively [90]. Left ventricular hypertrophy is observed in 22–47 % of children with T2DM [89]. Increased arterial stiffness is reported in adolescents with T2DM compared to obese and healthy-weight controls, indicating premature aging of the cardiovascular system [91]. Blunted nocturnal dipping of blood pressure is associated with nephropathy in children with T1DM and T2DM, and may be an early marker for impaired renal function [92, 93]. Clearly, the increasing prevalence of T2DM in children and adolescents, particularly among specific minority groups, requires additional large-scale studies to prospectively study hypertension as an important risk factor for cardiovascular disease. Psychological complications in adolescents with T2DM include an increased risk for depression and binge eating, observed in 15–26 % of patients [94, 95]. Notably, both men and woman with T1DM have a smaller number of live births than matched controls, indicating that T1DM has an effect on fertility and family size in humans [96].

Table 6.2 Useful resources on DM for patients, parents, and caregivers

http://www.childrenwithdiabetes.com
http://www.ndep.nih.gov
http://www.diabetes.org
http://www.childrensdiabetesfdn.org/publications.html
http://www.uchsc.edu/misc/diabetes/udform.html
http://www.designersink.com
http://www.henhousepress.com/index.html

Diabetic Nephropathy

Diabetic nephropathy is one of the most severe complications in patients with T1DM, leading to ESRD and the need for renal replacement therapy. The earliest sign of diabetic nephropathy is microalbuminuria (persistent albumin excretion between 30 and 300 mg/day or 20–200 μg/min).

Recent studies suggest that novel biomarkers for diabetic nephropathy in children may include profibrotic growth factors such as TGF-β1. In this regard, children with T1DM have increased levels of TGF-β1 in the urine at disease onset with reduction after metabolic control with insulin [97]. Microalbuminuria, if not treated successfully, may progress to overt proteinuria, defined as persistent albumin excretion >300 mg/day (>200 μg/min) [98]. In a large population-based study, the cumulative prevalence of microalbuminuria was 26 % after 10 years of diabetes and 51 % after 19 years of diabetes [99]. The prevalence of ESRD in pediatric DM differs between countries and ethnic groups. Studies from Canada demonstrate that children with T2DM have a 23-fold increased risk of ESRD and a 39-fold increased risk of dialysis compared with control subjects [100]. In this study, children with T2DM had a fourfold increased risk of renal failure compared to youth with T1DM. Presence of albuminuria was a risk factor associated with ESRD in adolescence [101]. During a 20-year follow-up of 11,681 young patients with T1DM in nationwide population-based study in Sweden, only 127 patients had developed ESRD due to diabetic nephropathy, a presumed reflection of better glycemic control [101]. The cumulative incidence at 30 years of T1DM duration was low, with a male predominance (4.1 % [95 % CI 3.1–5.3] vs. 2.5 % [1.7–3.5]). In addition, a reduced risk, or a delay, in development of ESRD in patients diagnosed with T1DM before the age 5 and 10 years was found [101, 102]. Strict control of the serum glucose concentration, adequate control of elevated blood pressure and dyslipidemia, and use of angiotensin converting enzyme (ACE) inhibitor can slow the rate of progression of microalbuminuria or even reduce proteinuria and progressive nephropathy in children with DM [103, 104]. A 5-year, double-blind, placebo-controlled study of candesartan in nonalbuminuric and normotensive young adults with T1DM reported a reduction in mesangial matrix volume and decline in blood pressure with the use of candesartan, suggesting that changes in renal morphology can be prevented or arrested by early intervention [105]. The strongest risk markers for the development of microalbuminuria and hypertension in young adults with T1DM were poor metabolic control after puberty, high daytime systolic blood pressure and increased glomerular basement membrane thickness at 10 years [106]. Antihypertensive therapy should be targeted to decrease blood pressure values below the 90th percentile for age, gender, and height. Preemptive living donor transplantation before initiation of dialysis is preferred in non-monogenic DM [107]. Screening for mutations associated with monogenic DM should be performed in potential living-related donors for children with known monogenic DM. Family history of T2DM, use of tacrolimus, and hyperglycemia in the first 2 weeks after kidney transplantation are the risk factors for posttransplant DM in children [108].

Screening and Prevention of DM

Screening for T2DM should begin in high-risk children (BMI>85th percentile for age and sex, family history of T2DM in a first- or second-degree relative, presence of acanthosis nigricans, PCO syndrome, hypertension dyslipidemia, maternal history of DM or gestational DM, American Indian, Asian/Pacific Islander, African American, or Latino ethnic background) at age of 10 years or at the onset of puberty [1]. The most commonly used screening tests for T2DM include measurement of FPG, 2-h plasma glucose during a 2-h OGTT, and A1C. A recent randomized controlled trial conducted in overweight or obese children in the United States demonstrated a reduction in the risk of T2DM as estimated by insulin area under the curve from an oral GTT after 13 weeks of 20 or 40 min/day of aerobic training regardless of sex or race [109].

For T1DM, screening for potential complications of the disease (microalbuminuria, retinopathy, dyslipidemia, and neuropathy) is recommended. Annual screening for microalbuminuria should be initiated when the child is 10 years old and has had T1DM for 5 years [110]. The preferred screening strategy for microalbuminuria is measurement of the urine albumin-to-creatinine ratio in an untimed urinary sample. All children who have had T1DM for 3–5 years or more should have an annual ophthalmologic evaluation starting at 10 years of age [55]. A fasting lipid profile should be obtained in prepubertal children (2–10 years), if there is a family history of hypercholesterolemia (defined as total cholesterol >240 mg/dL, [6.2 mmol/L]), a cardiovascular event before 55 years of age, or if the family history is unknown or the child is overweight or obese. Adolescents (puberty or >10 years of age) should be screened at the time of diagnosis. Testing for vibration (using a tuning fork) and pressure sensation (using a 10 g monofilament) is recommended at least annually in children older than 10 years of age.

Although no successful strategy for the prevention of T1DM has yet been identified, children who are at high risk for T1DM can be identified using a combination of immune, genetic, and metabolic markers. Genetic markers (e.g., major susceptibility genes for T1DM located in the HLA region on chromosome 6p) may be helpful in assessing the risk of T1DM in close relatives of a patient with T1DM [111]. Measurement of autoantibodies (GAD, IAA, and IA2/ICA512) was reported to prospectively identify all children without familial DM who developed diabetes within 8 years [112]. However, a large proportion of individuals with positive screening test results is found not to have DM upon further diagnostic testing [113]. Determination of the acute (or "first phase") insulin response to glucose (FPIR) during an intravenous glucose tolerance test (IVGTT) and 2-h glucose during OGTT can be used for prediction of DM.

In the FPIR test, the rise in serum insulin above baseline is measured during the first 10 min after an intravenous glucose challenge [114]. The response correlates with the functioning *β*-cell mass. Abnormalities of FPIR and 2-h glucose during OGTT have similar sensitivities for diabetes prediction within 6 months of diagnosis (76 % for OGTT [95 % CI 60–83 %] and 73 % for FPIR [95 % CI 60–83 %]) [115]. Considering the high prevalence of DM with strong evidence for a genetic predisposition, more efforts are needed to promote awareness around familial clustering and primary prevention [116]. Although such parameters as IGF-1, IGFBP3, fasting insulin, glucose, and lipid levels can be measured in LBW or small for gestational age infants to screen for DM, the predictive capacity of these factors as biological markers for later DM or obesity may not be of clinical use [117, 118].

Transition of Adolescents with DM to Adult Health Care Service

Due to advances in medical care, nearly all children with DM will survive into adult life. Adolescents leave behind their childhood taking new responsibilities and striving to become an independent adult. This coincides with their move from the children's into the adult health care service. This transition has a potential to cause instability in the adolescent's already vulnerable state [119, 120]. Therefore, an important role for the health care team is to ensure that the transition process will build up and develop a person empowered to become an independent individual. While children's health care service may be perceived as family centered, socially oriented, informal, and relaxed, adult service may be perceived as person centered, disease oriented, formal, and direct. Principles of a successful transition should be explained beforehand, allowing the adolescent and family sufficient time to familiarize themselves with the idea that care will be delivered in a different setting and by a different team at some point in the future. The most appropriate time to introduce this concept is debatable, but it is clear that its introduction at an early stage allows adequate time for preparation such as health education and promotion of independence. The timing of the transfer should take into account adolescent's physical development and emotional maturity, occur at a time of relative stability in their health, and be coordinated with other life transitions [121].

References

1. American Diabetes Association. Diagnosis and classification of diabetes mellitus. Diabetes Care. 2011;34 Suppl 1:S62–9.
2. Craig ME, Hattersley A, Donaghue KC. Definition, epidemiology and classification of diabetes in children and adolescents. Pediatr Diabetes. 2009;10 Suppl 12:3–12.
3. Felner EI, Klitz W, Ham M, Lazaro AM, Stastny P, Dupont B, White PC. Genetic interaction among three genomic regions creates distinct contributions to early- and late-onset type 1 diabetes mellitus. Pediatr Diabetes. 2005;6(4):213–20.
4. Pinhas-Hamiel O, Zeitler P. The global spread of type 2 diabetes mellitus in children and adolescents. J Pediatr. 2005;146(5):693–700.
5. Grinstein G, Muzumdar R, Aponte L, Vuguin P, Saenger P, DiMartino-Nardi J. Presentation and 5-year follow-up of type 2 diabetes mellitus in African-American and Caribbean-Hispanic adolescents. Horm Res. 2003;60(3):21–126.
6. Oeltmann JE, Liese AD, Heinze HJ, Addy CL, Mayer-Davis EJ. Prevalence of diagnosed diabetes among African-American and non-Hispanic white youth. Diabetes Care. 2003;26:2531–5.
7. Copeland KC, Zeitler P, Geffner M, Guandalini C, Higgins J, Hirst K, Kaufman FR, Linder B, Marcovina S, McGuigan P, Pyle L, Tamborlane W, Willi S, TODAY Study Group. Characteristics of adolescents and youth with recent-onset type 2 diabetes: the TODAY cohort at baseline. J Clin Endocrinol Metab. 2011;96(1):159–67.
8. Møller AM, Dalgaard LT, Pociot F, Nerup J, Hansen T, Pedersen O. Mutations in the hepatocyte nuclear factor-1alpha gene in Caucasian families originally classified as having Type I diabetes. Diabetologia. 1998;41(12):1528–31.
9. Musso C, Cochran E, Moran SA, Skarulis MC, Oral EA, Taylor S, Gorden P. Clinical course of genetic diseases of the insulin receptor (type A and Rabson-Mendenhall syndromes): a 30-year prospective. Medicine (Baltimore). 2004;83(4):209–22.
10. Gepts W. Pathologic anatomy of the pancreas in juvenile diabetes mellitus. Diabetes. 1965;14(10):619–33.
11. Lambert AP, Gillespie KM, Thomson G, Cordell HJ, Todd JA, Gale EA, Bingley PJ. Absolute risk of childhood-onset type 1 diabetes defined by human leukocyte antigen class II genotype: a population-based study in the United Kingdom. J Clin Endocrinol Metab. 2004;89(8):4037–43.
12. Lönnrot M, Korpela K, Knip M, Ilonen J, Simell O, Korhonen S, Savola K, Muona P, Simell T, Koskela P, Hyöty H. Enterovirus infection as a risk factor for beta-cell autoimmunity in a prospectively observed birth cohort: the Finnish Diabetes Prediction and Prevention Study. Diabetes. 2000;49(8):1314–8.
13. Atkinson MA, Mclaren NK. The pathogenesis of insulin dependent diabetes mellitus. N Engl J Med. 1994;331(21):1428–36.
14. Flood RG, Chiang VW. Rate and prediction of infection in children with diabetic ketoacidosis. Am J Emerg Med. 2001;19:270–3.
15. Umpaichitra V, Banerji MA, Castells S. Autoantibodies in children with type 2 diabetes mellitus. J Pediatr Endocrinol Metab. 2002;15 Suppl 1:525–30.
16. Bonal C, Herrera PL. Genes controlling pancreas ontogeny. Int J Dev Biol. 2008;52(7):823–35.
17. Oliver-Krasinski JM, Stoffers DA. On the origin of the beta cell. Genes Dev. 2008;22(15):1998–2021.
18. Jørgensen MC, Ahnfelt-Rønne J, Hald J, Madsen OD, Serup P, Hecksher-Sørensen J. An illustrated review of early pancreas development in the mouse. Endocr Rev. 2007;28(6):685–705.
19. Polak M, Bouchareb-Banaei L, Scharfmann R, Czernichow P. Early pattern of differentiation in the human pancreas. Diabetes. 2000;49(2):225–32.
20. Pearl EJ, Horb ME. Promoting ectopic pancreatic fates: pancreas development and future diabetes therapies. Clin Genet. 2008;74(4):316–24.
21. Mastracci TL, Sussel L. The Endocrine Pancreas: insights into development, differentiation and diabetes. Wiley Interdiscip Rev Membr Transp Signal. 2012;1(5):609–28.
22. Solar M, Cardalda C, Houbracken I, Martín M, Maestro MA, De Medts N, Xu X, Grau V, Heimberg H, Bouwens L, Ferrer J. Pancreatic exocrine duct cells give rise to insulin-producing

beta cells during embryogenesis but not after birth. Dev Cell. 2009;17(6):849–60.
23. Carolan PJ, Melton DA. New findings in pancreatic and intestinal endocrine development to advance regenerative medicine. Curr Opin Endocrinol Diabetes Obes. 2013;20(1):1–7.
24. Pilgaard K, Færch K, Carstensen B, Poulsen P, Pisinger C, Pedersen O, Witte DR, Hansen T, Jørgensen T, Vaag A. Low birthweight and premature birth are both associated with type 2 diabetes in a random sample of middle-aged Danes. Diabetologia. 2010;53(12):2526–30.
25. Barker DJ, Hales CN, Fall CH, Osmond C, Phipps K, Clark PM. Type 2 (non-insulin-dependent) diabetes mellitus, hypertension and hyperlipidaemia (syndrome X): relation to reduced fetal growth. Diabetologia. 1993;36(1):62–7.
26. Wei JN, Sung FC, Li CY, Chang CH, Lin RS, Lin CC, Chiang CC, Chuang LM. Low birth weight and high birth weight infants are both at an increased risk to have type 2 diabetes among schoolchildren in Taiwan. Diabetes Care. 2003;26(2):343–8.
27. Crowther NJ, Cameron N, Trusler J, Gray IP. Association between poor glucose tolerance and rapid post natal weight gain in seven-year-old children. Diabetologia. 1998;41(10):1163–7.
28. Crowther NJ, Cameron N, Trusler J, Toman M, Norris SA, Gray IP. Influence of catch-up growth on glucose tolerance and beta-cell function in 7-year-old children: results from the birth to twenty study. Pediatrics. 2008;121(6):e1715–22.
29. Poulsen P, Vaag AA, Kyvik KO, Møller Jensen D, Beck-Nielsen H. Low birth weight is associated with NIDDM in discordant monozygotic and dizygotic twin pairs. Diabetologia. 1997;40(4):439–46.
30. Forsén T, Eriksson J, Tuomilehto J, Reunanen A, Osmond C, Barker D. The fetal and childhood growth of persons who develop type 2 diabetes. Ann Intern Med. 2000;133(3):176–81.
31. Silverman BL, Rizzo TA, Cho NH, Metzger BE. Long-term effects of the intrauterine environment. The Northwestern University Diabetes in Pregnancy Center. Diabetes Care. 1998;21 Suppl 2:B142–8.
32. Magaton A, Gil FZ, Casarini DE, Cavanal Mde F, Gomes GN. Maternal diabetes mellitus—early consequences for the offspring. Pediatr Nephrol. 2007;22(1):37–43.
33. Rocha SO, Gomes GN, Forti AL, do Carmo Pinho Franco M, Fortes ZB, de Fátima Cavanal M, Gil FZ. Long-term effects of maternal diabetes on vascular reactivity and renal function in rat male offspring. Pediatr Res. 2005;58(6):1274–9.
34. Nottke A, Colaiácovo MP, Shi Y. Developmental roles of the histone lysine demethylases. Development. 2009;136(6):879–89.
35. Smith CL. A shifting paradigm: histone deacetylases and transcriptional activation. Bioessays. 2008;30(1):15–24.
36. Rees WD, Hay SM, Brown DS, Antipatis C, Palmer RM. Maternal protein deficiency causes hypermethylation of DNA in the livers of rat fetuses. J Nutr. 2000;130(7):1821–6.
37. Suter M, Ma J, Harris A, Patterson L, Brown KA, Shope C, Showalter L, Abramovici A, Aagaard-Tillery KM. Maternal tobacco use modestly alters correlated epigenome-wide placental DNA methylation and gene expression. Epigenetics. 2011;6(11):1284–94.
38. Park JH, Stoffers DA, Nicholls RD, Simmons RA. Development of type 2 diabetes following intrauterine growth retardation in rats is associated with progressive epigenetic silencing of Pdx1. J Clin Invest. 2008;118(6):2316–24.
39. Sandovici I, Smith NH, Nitert MD, Ackers-Johnson M, Uribe-Lewis S, Ito Y, Jones RH, Marquez VE, Cairns W, Tadayyon M, O'Neill LP, Murrell A, Ling C, Constância M, Ozanne SE. Maternal diet and aging alter the epigenetic control of a promoter-enhancer interaction at the Hnf4a gene in rat pancreatic islets. Proc Natl Acad Sci U S A. 2011;108(13):5449–54.
40. Raychaudhuri N, Raychaudhuri S, Thamotharan M, Devaskar SU. Histone code modifications repress glucose transporter 4 expression in the intrauterine growth-restricted offspring. J Biol Chem. 2008;283(20):13611–26.
41. Vélez MP, Santos IS, Matijasevich A, Gigante D, Gonçalves H, Barros FC, Victora CG. Maternal low birth weight and adverse perinatal outcomes: the 1982 Pelotas Birth Cohort Study, Brazil. Rev Panam Salud Publica. 2009;26(2):112–9.
42. Gluckman PD, Hanson MA, Cooper C, Thornburg KL. Effect of in utero and early-life conditions on adult health and disease. N Engl J Med. 2008;359(1):61–73.
43. Quinn M, Fleischman A, Rosner B, Nigrin DJ, Wolfsdorf JI. Characteristics at diagnosis of type 1 diabetes in children younger than 6 years. J Pediatr. 2006;148(3):366–71.
44. Kong AS, Williams RL, Rhyne R, Urias-Sandoval V, Cardinali G, Weller NF, Skipper B, Volk R, Daniels E, Parnes B, McPherson L. Acanthosis Nigricans: high prevalence and association with diabetes in a practice-based research network consortium—a PRImary care Multi-Ethnic network (PRIME Net) study. J Am Board Fam Med. 2010;23(4):476–81.
45. Lipton RB, Drum ML, Danielson KK, Greeley SA, Bell GI, Hagopian WA. Onset features and subsequent clinical evolution of childhood diabetes over several years. Pediatr Diabetes. 2011;12(4 Pt 1):326–34.
46. Chen F, Wang Y, Shan X, Cheng H, Hou D, Zhao X, Wang T, Zhao D, Mi J. Association between childhood obesity and metabolic syndrome: evidence from a large sample of Chinese children and adolescents. PLoS One. 2012;7(10):e47380.
47. Foster DW, McGarry JD. The metabolic derangements and treatment of diabetic ketoacidosis. N Engl J Med. 1983;309(3):159–69.
48. Wolfsdorf J, Craig ME, Daneman D, Dunger D, Edge J, Lee W, Rosenbloom A, Sperling M, Hanas R. Diabetic ketoacidosis in children and adolescents with diabetes. Pediatr Diabetes. 2009;10 Suppl 12:118–33.
49. Lévy-Marchal C, Papoz L, de Beaufort C, Doutreix J, Froment V, Voirin J, Czernichow P. Clinical and laboratory features of type 1 diabetic children at the time of diagnosis. Diabet Med. 1992;9(3):279–84.
50. Muir AB, Quisling RG, Yang MC, Rosenbloom AL. Cerebral edema in childhood diabetic ketoacidosis: natural history, radiographic findings, and early identification. Diabetes Care. 2004;27(7):1541–6.
51. Glaser N, Barnett P, McCaslin I, Nelso ND, Trainor J, Louie J, Kaufman F, Quayle K, Roback M, Malley R, Kuppermann N, Pediatric Emergency Medicine Collaborative Research Committee of the American Academy of Pediatrics. Risk factors for cerebral edema in children with diabetic ketoacidosis. The Pediatric Emergency Medicine Collaborative Research Committee of the American Academy of Pediatrics. N Engl J Med. 2001;344(4):264–9.
52. Curtis JR, To T, Muirhead S, Cummings E, Daneman D. Recent trends in hospitalization for diabetic ketoacidosis in Ontario children. Diabetes Care. 2002;25(9):1591–6.
53. Bagdure D, Rewers A, Campagna E, Sills MR. Epidemiology of hyperglycemic hyperosmolar syndrome in children hospitalized in USA. Pediatr Diabetes. 2013;14(1):18–24.
54. Rodacki M, Pereira JR, Nabuco de Oliveira AM, Barone B, Mac Dowell R, Perricelli P, Bravo MT, de Oliveira MM, Brum JD, Belem LC, de Ornellas PG, Berardo RS, Luescher J, Campos L, Vangelotti Ade M, Kupfer R, Zajdenverg L, Milech A, Paulo de Oliveira JE. Ethnicity and young age influence the frequency of diabetic ketoacidosis at the onset of type 1 diabetes. Diabetes Res Clin Pract. 2007;78(2):259–62.
55. American Diabetes Association. Standards of medical care in diabetes. Diabetes Care. 2011;34 Suppl 1:S11–21.
56. Hattersley A, Bruining J, Shield J, Njolstad P, Donaghue KC. The diagnosis and management of monogenic diabetes in children and adolescents. Pediatr Diabetes. 2009;10 Suppl 12:33–42.

57. Dabelea D, Pihoker C, Talton JW, D'Agostino Jr RB, Fujimoto W, Klingensmith GJ, Lawrence JM, Linder B, Marcovina SM, Mayer-Davis EJ, Imperatore G, Dolan LM, SEARCH for Diabetes in Youth Study. Etiological approach to characterization of diabetes type: the SEARCH for Diabetes in Youth Study. Diabetes Care. 2011;34(7):1628–34.
58. Gat-Yablonski G, Shalitin S, Phillip M. Maturity onset diabetes of the young. Pediatr Endocrinol Rev. 2006;3 Suppl 3:514–9.
59. Yamagata K, Furuta H, Oda N, Kaisaki PJ, Menzel S, Cox NJ, Fajans SS, Signorini S, Stoffel M, Bell GI. Mutations in the hepatocyte nuclear factor-4alpha gene in maturity-onset diabetes of the young (MODY1). Nature. 1996;384(6608):458–64.
60. Froguel P, Zouali H, Vionnet N, Velho G, Vaxillaire M, Sun F, Lesage S, Stoffel M, Takeda J, Passa P. Familial hyperglycemia due to mutations in glucokinase. Definition of a subtype of diabetes mellitus. N Engl J Med. 1993;328(10):697–702.
61. Macfarlane WM, Frayling TM, Ellard S, Evans JC, Allen LI, Bulman MP, Ayres S, Shepherd M, Clark P, Millward A, Demaine A, Wilkin T, Docherty K, Hattersley AT. Missense mutations in the insulin promoter factor-1 gene predispose to type 2 diabetes. J Clin Invest. 1999;104(9):R33–8.
62. Bellanné-Chantelot C, Chauveau D, Gautier JF, Dubois-Laforgue D, Clauin S, Beaufils S, Wilhelm JM, Boitard C, Noël LH, Velho G, Timsit J. Clinical spectrum associated with hepatocyte nuclear factor-1beta mutations. Ann Intern Med. 2004;140(7):510–4.
63. Bingham C, Ellard S, van't Hoff WG, Simmonds HA, Marinaki AM, Badman MK, Winocour PH, Stride A, Lockwood CR, Nicholls AJ, Owen KR, Spyer G, Pearson ER, Hattersley AT. Atypical familial juvenile hyperuricemic nephropathy associated with a hepatocyte nuclear factor-1beta gene mutation. Kidney Int. 2003;63(5):1645–9.
64. Hiesberger T, Bai Y, Shao X, McNally BT, Sinclair AM, Tian X, Somlo S, Igarashi P. Mutation of hepatocyte nuclear factor-1beta inhibits Pkhd1 gene expression and produces renal cysts in mice. J Clin Invest. 2004;113(6):814–9.
65. Kristinsson SY, Thorolfsdottir ET, Talseth B, Steingrimsson E, Thorsson AV, Helgason T, Hreidarsson AB, Arngrimsson R. MODY in Iceland is associated with mutations in HNF-1alpha and a novel mutation in NeuroD1. Diabetologia. 2001;44(11):2098–102.
66. Gardner RJ, Mackay DJ, Mungall AJ, Polychronakos C, Siebert R, Shield JP, Temple IK, Robinson DO. An imprinted locus associated with transient neonatal diabetes mellitus. Hum Mol Genet. 2000;9(4):589–96.
67. Gloyn AL, Pearson ER, Antcliff JF, Proks P, Bruining GJ, Slingerland AS, Howard N, Srinivasan S, Silva JM, Molnes J, Edghill EL, Frayling TM, Temple IK, Mackay D, Shield JP, Sumnik Z, van Rhijn A, Wales JK, Clark P, Gorman S, Aisenberg J, Ellard S, Njølstad PR, Ashcroft FM, Hattersley AT. Activating mutations in the gene encoding the ATP-sensitive potassium-channel subunit Kir6.2 and permanent neonatal diabetes. N Engl J Med. 2004;350(18):1838–49.
68. Bae KW, Kim BE, Choi JH, Lee JH, Park YS, Kim GH, Yoo HW, Seo JJ. A novel mutation and unusual clinical features in a patient with immune dysregulation, polyendocrinopathy, enteropathy, X-linked (IPEX) syndrome. Eur J Pediatr. 2011;170(12):1611–5.
69. Donovan LE, Severin NE. Maternally inherited diabetes and deafness in a North American kindred: tips for making the diagnosis and review of unique management issues. J Clin Endocrinol Metab. 2006;91(12):4737–41.
70. Huopio H, Reimann F, Ashfield R, Komulainen J, Lenko HL, Rahier J, Vauhkonen I, Kere J, Laakso M, Ashcroft F, Otonkoski T. Dominantly inherited hyperinsulinism caused by a mutation in the sulfonylurea receptor type 1. J Clin Invest. 2000;106(7):897–902.
71. Robbins DC, Shoelson SE, Rubenstein AH, Tager HS. Familial hyperproinsulinemia. Two cohorts secreting indistinguishable type II intermediates of proinsulin conversion. J Clin Invest. 1984;73(3):714–9.
72. Tager H, Given B, Baldwin D, Mako M, Markese J, Rubenstein A, Olefsky J, Kobayashi M, Kolterman O, Poucher R. A structurally abnormal insulin causing human diabetes. Nature. 1979;281(5727):122–7.
73. Moller DE, Flier JS. Insulin resistance—mechanisms, syndromes, and implications. N Engl J Med. 1991;325(13):938–44.
74. Owen KR, Donohoe M, Ellard S, Hattersley AT. Response to treatment with rosiglitazone in familial partial lipodystrophy due to a mutation in the LMNA gene. Diabet Med. 2003;20(10):823–7.
75. Cremers CW, Wijdeveld PG, Pinckers AJ. Juvenile diabetes mellitus, optic atrophy, hearing loss, diabetes insipidus, atonia of the urinary tract and bladder, and other abnormalities (Wolfram syndrome). A review of 88 cases from the literature with personal observations on 3 new patients. Acta Paediatr Scand Suppl. 1977;264:1–16.
76. Inoue H, Tanizawa Y, Wasson J, Behn P, Kalidas K, Bernal-Mizrachi E, Mueckler M, Marshall H, Donis-Keller H, Crock P, Rogers D, Mikuni M, Kumashiro H, Higashi K, Sobue G, Oka Y, Permutt MA. A gene encoding a transmembrane protein is mutated in patients with diabetes mellitus and optic atrophy (Wolfram syndrome). Nat Genet. 1998;20(2):143–7.
77. Chaussenot A, Bannwarth S, Rouzier C, Vialettes B, Mkadem SA, Chabrol B, Cano A, Labauge P, Paquis-Flucklinger V. Neurologic features and genotype-phenotype correlation in Wolfram syndrome. Ann Neurol. 2011;69(3):501–8.
78. Iyer S, Korada M, Rainbow L, Kirk J, Brown RM, Shaw N, Barrett TG. Wolcott-Rallison syndrome: a clinical and genetic study of three children, novel mutation in EIF2AK3 and a review of the literature. Acta Paediatr. 2004;93(9):1195–201.
79. Bangstad HJ, Danne T, Deeb LC, Jarosz-Chobot P, Urakami T, Hanas R. International Society for Pediatric and Adolescent Diabetes. SPAD Clinical Practice Consensus Guidelines 2006–2007. Insulin treatment in children and adolescents with diabetes. Pediatr Diabetes. 2007;8(2):88–102.
80. Rosenbloom AL, Silverstein JH, Amemiya S, Zeitler P, Klingensmith GJ, International Society for Pediatric and Adolescent Diabetes. ISPAD Clinical Practice Consensus Guidelines 2006–2007. Type 2 diabetes mellitus in the child and adolescent. Pediatr Diabetes. 2008;9(5):512–26.
81. Hsia DS, Fallon SC, Brandt ML. Adolescent bariatric surgery. Arch Pediatr Adolesc Med. 2012;166(8):757–66.
82. Inge TH, Miyano G, Bean J, Helmrath M, Courcoulas A, Harmon CM, Chen MK, Wilson K, Daniels SR, Garcia VF, Brandt ML, Dolan LM. Reversal of type 2 diabetes mellitus and improvements in cardiovascular risk factors after surgical weight loss in adolescents. Pediatrics. 2009;123(1):214–22.
83. Roberts MD, Slover RH, Chase HP. Diabetic ketoacidosis with intracerebral complications. Pediatr Diabetes. 2001;2(3):109–14.
84. Zung A, Glaser B, Nimri R, Zadik Z. Glibenclamide treatment in permanent neonatal diabetes mellitus due to an activating mutation in Kir6.2. J Clin Endocrinol Metab. 2004;89(11):5504–7.
85. Pearson ER, Starkey BJ, Powell RJ, Gribble FM, Clark PM, Hattersley AT. Genetic cause of hyperglycaemia and response to treatment in diabetes. Lancet. 2003;362(9392):1275–81.
86. Ozdemir MA, Akcakus M, Kurtoglu S, Gunes T, Torun YA. TRMA syndrome (thiamine-responsive megaloblastic anemia): a case report and review of the literature. Pediatr Diabetes. 2002;3(4):205–9.
87. Cooke DW, Plotnick L. Type 1 diabetes mellitus in pediatrics. Pediatr Rev. 2008;29(11):374–84.
88. Kershnar AK, Daniels SR, Imperatore G, Palla SL, Petitti DB, Pettitt DJ, Marcovina S, Dolan LM, Hamman RF, Liese AD, Pihoker C, Rodriguez BL. Lipid abnormalities are prevalent in youth with type 1 and type 2 diabetes: the SEARCH for Diabetes in Youth Study. J Pediatr. 2006;149(3):314–9.
89. Pinhas-Hamiel O, Zeitler P. Acute and chronic complications of type 2 diabetes mellitus in children and adolescents. Lancet. 2007;369(9575):1823–7.

90. Rodriguez BL, Dabelea D, Liese AD, Fujimoto W, Waitzfelder B, Liu L, Bell R, Talton J, Snively BM, Kershnar A, Urbina E, Daniels S, Imperatore G. Prevalence and correlates of elevated blood pressure in youth with diabetes mellitus: the SEARCH for diabetes in youth study. J Pediatr. 2010;157(2):245–51.
91. Gungor N, Thompson T, Sutton-Tyrrell K, Janosky J, Arslanian S. Early signs of cardiovascular disease in youth with obesity and type 2 diabetes. Diabetes Care. 2005;28(5):1219–21.
92. Ettinger LM, Freeman K, DiMartino-Nardi JR, Flynn JT. Microalbuminuria and abnormal ambulatory blood pressure in adolescents with type 2 diabetes mellitus. J Pediatr. 2005;147(1):67–73.
93. Lurbe E, Redon J, Kesani A, Pascual JM, Tacons J, Alvarez V, Batlle D. Increase in nocturnal blood pressure and progression to microalbuminuria in type 1 diabetes. N Engl J Med. 2002;347(11):797–805.
94. Wilfley D, Berkowitz R, Goebel-Fabbri A, Hirst K, Ievers-Landis C, Lipman TH, Marcus M, Ng D, Pham T, Saletsky R, Schanuel J, Van Buren D. Binge eating, mood, and quality of life in youth with type 2 diabetes: baseline data from the today study. Diabetes Care. 2011;34(4):858–62.
95. Stewart SM, Rao U, White P. Depression and diabetes in children and adolescents. Curr Opin Pediatr. 2005;17(5):626–31.
96. Sjöberg L, Pitkäniemi J, Haapala L, Kaaja R, Tuomilehto J. Fertility in people with childhood-onset type 1 diabetes. Diabetologia. 2013;56(1):78–81.
97. Holmquist P, Torffvit O. Urinary transforming growth factor-beta(1), collagen IV and the effect of insulin in children at diagnosis of diabetes mellitus. Scand J Urol Nephrol. 2009;43(2):142–7.
98. Rademacher ER, Sinaiko AR. Albuminuria in children. Curr Opin Nephrol Hypertens. 2009;18(3):246–51.
99. Amin R, Widmer B, Prevost AT, Schwarze P, Cooper J, Edge J, Marcovecchio L, Neil A, Dalton RN, Dunger DB. Risk of microalbuminuria and progression to macroalbuminuria in a cohort with childhood onset type 1 diabetes: prospective observational study. BMJ. 2008;336(7646):697–703.
100. Dart AB, Sellers EA, Martens PJ, Rigatto C, Brownell MD, Dean HJ. High burden of kidney disease in youth-onset type 2 diabetes. Diabetes Care. 2012;35(6):1265–71.
101. Möllsten A, Svensson M, Waernbaum I, Berhan Y, Schön S, Nyström L, Arnqvist HJ, Dahlquist G, Swedish Childhood Diabetes Study Group. Cumulative risk, age at onset, and sex-specific differences for developing end-stage renal disease in young patients with type 1 diabetes: a nationwide population-based cohort study. Diabetes. 2010;59(7):1803–8.
102. Nordwall M, Bojestig M, Arnqvist HJ, Ludvigsson J. Declining incidence of severe retinopathy and persisting decrease of nephropathy in an unselected population of type 1 diabetes-the Linkoping Diabetes Complications Study. Diabetologia. 2004;47:1266–72.
103. Basevi V, Di Mario S, Morciano C, Nonino F, Magrini N. Standards of medical care in diabetes-2011. Diabetes Care. May;34 Suppl 1:S11–61.
104. Hilgers KF, Dötsch J, Rascher W, Mann JF. Treatment strategies in patients with chronic renal disease: ACE inhibitors, angiotensin receptor antagonists, or both? Pediatr Nephrol. 2004;19(9):956–61.
105. Perrin NE, Jaremko GA, Berg UB. The effects of candesartan on diabetes glomerulopathy: a double-blind, placebo-controlled trial. Pediatr Nephrol. 2008;23(6):947–54.
106. Perrin NE, Torbjörnsdotter T, Jaremko GA, Berg UB. Risk markers of future microalbuminuria and hypertension based on clinical and morphological parameters in young type 1 diabetes patients. Pediatr Diabetes. 2010;11(5):305–13.
107. Becker BN, Rush SH, Dykstra DM, Becker YT, Port FK. Preemptive transplantation for patients with diabetes-related kidney disease. Arch Intern Med. 2006;166(1):44–8.
108. Greenspan LC, Gitelman SE, Leung MA, Glidden DV, Mathias RS. Increased incidence in post-transplant diabetes mellitus in children: a case-control analysis. Pediatr Nephrol. 2002;17(1):1–5.
109. Davis CL, Pollock NK, Waller JL, Allison JD, Dennis BA, Bassali R, Meléndez A, Boyle CA, Gower BA. Exercise dose and diabetes risk in overweight and obese children: a randomized controlled trial. JAMA. 2012;308(11):1103–12.
110. Silverstein J, Klingensmith G, Copeland K, Plotnick L, Kaufman F, Laffel L, Deeb L, Grey M, Anderson B, Holzmeister LA, Clark N, American Diabetes Association. Care of children and adolescents with type 1 diabetes: a statement of the American Diabetes Association. Diabetes Care. 2005;28(1):186–212.
111. Thomson G, Robinson WP, Kuhner MK, Joe S, MacDonald MJ, Gottschall JL, Barbosa J, Rich SS, Bertrams J, Baur MP. Genetic heterogeneity, modes of inheritance, and risk estimates for a joint study of Caucasians with insulin-dependent diabetes mellitus. Am J Hum Genet. 1988;43(6):799–816.
112. LaGasse JM, Brantley MS, Leech NJ, Rowe RE, Monks S, Palmer JP, Nepom GT, McCulloch DK, Hagopian WA, Washington State Diabetes Prediction Study. Successful prospective prediction of type 1 diabetes in schoolchildren through multiple defined autoantibodies: an 8-year follow-up of the Washington State Diabetes Prediction Study. Diabetes Care. 2002;25(3):505–11.
113. Ongagna JC, Levy-Marchal C. Sensitivity at diagnosis of combined beta-cell autoantibodies in insulin-dependent diabetic children. French Registry of IDDM in Children Study Group. Diabetes Metab. 1997;23(2):155–60.
114. Bingley PJ. Interactions of age, islet cell antibodies, insulin autoantibodies, and first-phase insulin response in predicting risk of progression to IDDM in ICA+ relatives: the ICARUS data set. Islet Cell Antibody Register Users Study. Diabetes. 1996;45(12):1720–8.
115. Barker JM, McFann K, Harrison LC, Fourlanos S, Krischer J, Cuthbertson D, Chase HP, Eisenbarth GS, DPT-1 Study Group. Pre-type 1 diabetes dysmetabolism: maximal sensitivity achieved with both oral and intravenous glucose tolerance testing. J Pediatr. 2007;150(1):31–6.
116. van Esch SC, Cornel MC, Snoek FJ. "I am pregnant and my husband has diabetes. Is there a risk for my child?" A qualitative study of questions asked by email about the role of genetic susceptibility to diabetes. BMC Public Health. 2010;10:688–92.
117. Lee PA, Chernausek SD, Hokken-Koelega AC, Czernichow P, International Small for Gestational Age Advisory Board. International Small for Gestational Age Advisory Board consensus development conference statement: management of short children born small for gestational age. Pediatrics. 2003;111(6 Pt 1):1253–61.
118. Leger J, Oury JF, Noel M, Baron S, Benali K, Blot P, Czernichow P. Growth factors and intrauterine growth retardation. I. Serum growth hormone, insulin-like growth factor (IGF)-I, IGF-II, and IGF binding protein 3 levels in normally grown and growth-retarded human fetuses during the second half of gestation. Pediatr Res. 1996;40(1):94–100.
119. Salamon KS, Brouwer AM, Fox MM, Olson KA, Yelich-Koth SL, Fleischman KM, Hains AA, Davies WH, Kichler JC. Experiencing type 2 diabetes mellitus: qualitative analysis of adolescents' concept of illness, adjustment, and motivation to engage in self-care behaviors. Diabetes Educ. 2012;38(4):543–51.
120. Pound N, Sturrock ND, Jeffcoate WJ. Age related changes in glycated haemoglobin in patients with insulin-dependent diabetes mellitus. Diabet Med. 1996;13(6):510–3.
121. Fleming E, Carter B, Gillibrand W. The transition of adolescents with diabetes from the children's health care service into the adult health care service: a review of the literature. J Clin Nurs. 2002;11(5):560–7.

Part II

Clinical Presentation and Associated Disorders

Screening, Early Diagnosis, Genetic Markers, and Predictors of Diabetic Nephropathy

7

Eric P. Cohen and Jean-Marie Krzesinski

Introduction

Kidney disease in diabetes greatly diminishes quality and quantity of life, and is very expensive. Focused attention to the early stages of diabetic nephropathy is urgently needed, to define better therapies that may slow it down or even stop its progression, thus reducing its heavy burden.

Current Screening and Early Diagnosis of Diabetic Nephropathy

The classical presentation of diabetic nephropathy is well known, as is its threat to life and limb. Sixty years ago, diabetics with proteinuria might only survive 3 years [1]. Today, that survival is much longer, but a great burden of morbidity persists. Chronic kidney disease (CKD) occurs in up to 40 % of all diabetics. Its feared complication of end-stage renal disease (ESRD) occurs in only a few percent of all diabetics [2] (Fig. 7.1), but it exacts a great toll in terms of expense, morbidity, and mortality. Earlier diagnosis is likely to lead to better treatment. The serum glucose and the glycohemoglobin levels correlate with outcome in diabetes, but are not markers of renal injury. The American Diabetes Association (ADA) recommends that urine albumin excretion be tested as an early marker of renal injury yearly in every patient with type 2 diabetes and yearly after 5 years of diabetes duration in every patient with type 1 diabetes [3]. Measurement of the serum creatinine should also be done yearly in all diabetics.

E.P. Cohen, M.D. (✉)
Department of Medicine, Zablocki VA Hospital,
5000 West National Avenue, Milwaukee, WI 53295, USA
e-mail: Eric.Cohen@va.gov

J.-M. Krzesinski, M.D., Ph.D.
Unité de Néphrologie, Centre Hospitalier Universitaire,
Université de Liège, Liège, Belgium
e-mail: jm.krzesinski@chu.ulg.ac.be

Methods and Approach

This chapter will address screening, early diagnosis, genetic markers, and predictors of diabetic nephropathy. The words "diabetic nephropathy" will be used throughout, rather than the separate term "diabetic kidney disease" for lesser degrees of injury. Type 1 diabetes will be distinguished from type 2, where possible. The literature on these topics was reviewed using multiple PubMed searches, with attention to publications of original data in the last 3 years. Studies in laboratory animals were excluded. Publications showing correlations with diagnosis and/or prognosis were sought, as were publications testing mechanism via therapies and their effects on one or more markers. It is possible that important publications were missed, which hopefully will be only a small imperfection.

Serum Creatinine and GFR

Established diabetic nephropathy will present as nephrotic syndrome with azotemia and hypertension. Those features are neither specific nor early. Their use is for diagnosis, not screening. But the serum creatinine and its derived estimated glomerular filtration rate (eGFR) can have a predictive value. In type 1 diabetics with proteinuria but an eGFR above 60 mL/min, the initial five estimates of the eGFR provided an accurate prediction of the risk of ESRD over long-term follow-up [4]. A fall in eGFR of more than 11 mL/min/year was associated with a 50 % risk of ESRD over 5 years, whereas a fall in eGFR of less than 7 mL/min/year was associated with a 5-year risk of ESRD of only 4 %. This prediction was better than use of baseline characteristics of glycohemoglobin, blood pressure, or urinary albumin. On modern electronic medical record systems, graphing functions can show this evolution of eGFR versus time, which enables predictions that may improve clinical care.

E.V. Lerma and V. Batuman (eds.), *Diabetes and Kidney Disease*,
DOI 10.1007/978-1-4939-0793-9_7, © Springer Science+Business Media New York 2014

Albuminuria

Proteinuria has been known as a sign of renal disease since the 1800s [5]. Kimmelstiel and Wilson documented its association with diabetic nephropathy in 1936 [6]. By 1980, the paradigm for diabetic nephropathy was that it started with an asymptomatic phase involving "microalbuminuria," or urinary albumin in amounts too low to be detected by usual methods for testing proteinuria [7]. These amounts of albumin are in the range of 30–300 mg/day. The "micro" prefix refers to smaller amounts of albumin, below the threshold of the dipstick test for proteinuria, not to smaller albumin molecules. This stage of microalbuminuria was felt to be an obligatory intermediate stage to the development of dipstick-positive proteinuria, then by a further increase in urinary protein to the nephrotic range with concurrent decline in GFR and subsequent evolution to renal failure. Microalbuminuria became a surrogate early marker for diabetic nephropathy. Its significance is underlined by its correlation with increased mortality, and the even higher mortality for higher amounts of proteinuria [8] (Fig. 7.2). Further, Gaede et al. showed that in type 2 diabetics with microalbuminuria, a multifactorial intervention not only reduced cardiovascular death but also reduced progression to ESRD [9]. This appears to justify the ADA guidelines as stated above.

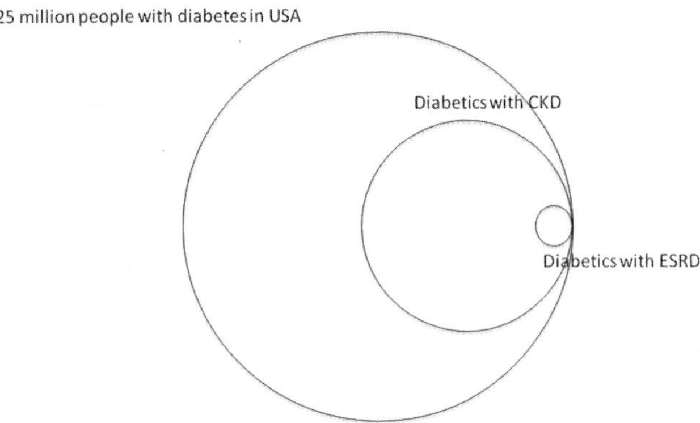

Fig. 7.1 Diagram of the epidemiology of diabetes and associated kidney disease. The area of the circles is proportional to the number of affected people. Estimate of the number of Americans with diabetes in 2013 is from the American Diabetes Association (www.diabetes.org), and the fraction of those with CKD is estimated as in Plantinga et al. [2]. The prevalence of diabetic ESRD now is ~300,000 in the USA, so the fraction of all current diabetics with ESRD is 300,000/25,000,000 = 0.01 or 1 %

But recent studies show that both type 1 and type 2 diabetics can develop CKD without albuminuria [10]. It is possible that part of this discrepancy results from measurement issues, i.e., that more sensitive measurement of urinary albumin might show positive results in subjects initially thought to have normoalbuminuria [11]. Nonetheless, only ~40 % of patients with microalbuminuria will develop proteinuria over a 10-year follow-up time [12]. This duality and unpredictability of microalbuminuria emphasize the need to search for and identify injury markers other than urinary albumin for identification of diabetics with impending kidney disease.

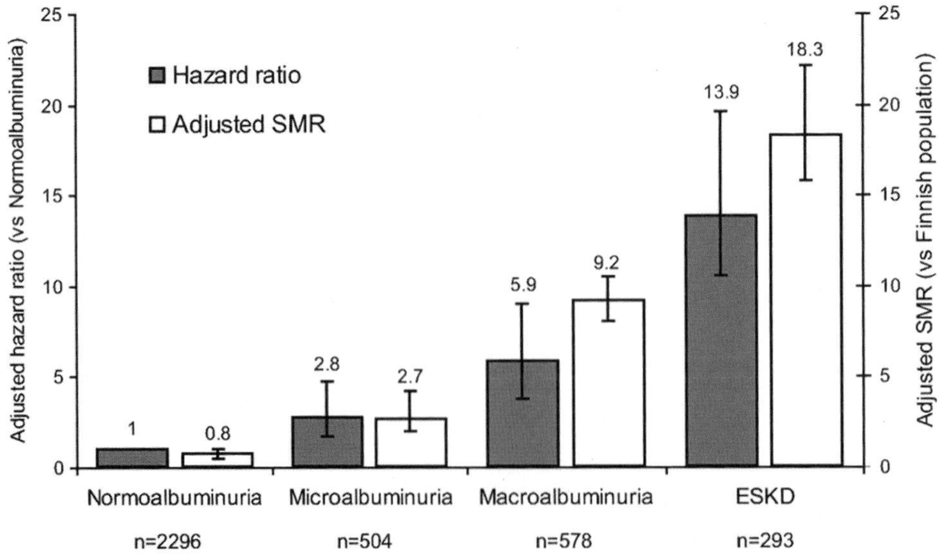

Fig. 7.2 Risk of mortality in individuals with type 1 diabetes from the FinnDiane study associated with each level of albuminuria and end-stage kidney disease (ESKD). The adjusted hazard ratios with 95 % c.i. are standardized against individuals with urinary albumin excretion in the normoalbuminuric range. Adjusted standardized mortality rates (SMRs) are shown, standardized for the Finnish population. Reprinted by permission from Groop et al. [8]. From Groop PH et al. The presence and severity of chronic kidney disease predicts all-cause mortality in type 1 diabetes. Diabetes 2009 Jul;58(7):1651–1658. Reprinted with permission from American Diabetes Association

Urinary Proteins

Increased urinary type IV collagen has been associated with loss of kidney function in subjects with type 2 diabetes [13]. This makes sense because type IV collagen is a substantial component of tubular and glomerular basement membranes, and its synthesis is stimulated by hyperglycemia [14]. An additional study showed that elevation in urinary collagen IV is associated with loss of kidney function in both type 1 and type 2 diabetes, without correlation to albuminuria [15]. Further study of urinary collagen is needed to confirm its utility as a marker for kidney disease in diabetics that have minimal or no elevations in urinary albumin.

The pro-fibrotic cytokine transforming growth factor beta-1 (TGFbeta) has been amply studied in experimental and human diabetic nephropathy [16]. Serum levels of TGFbeta appear to be increased in diabetics with albuminuria compared to those without it [17], and kidney biopsy studies of diabetic nephropathy have pointed to the mechanistic relevance of TGFbeta [18]. The renal expression of collagen IV and TGFbeta is reduced by ACE inhibitors. Urinary TGFbeta may be decreased by losartan [19] and may also be decreased by better control of the blood pressure in type 2 diabetics with proteinuria [20]. These data may confirm mechanisms but may not yet be useful for day-to-day patient care.

Inflammation could play a role in progressive diabetic nephropathy. Urinary interleukin-6, interleukin-8, monocyte chemoattractant protein-1, interferon gamma-inducible protein, and macrophage inflammatory protein-1 were significantly associated with declining renal function in a cohort of 145 type 1 diabetics [21]. The same group used a highly sensitive immunoassay to show elevations of urinary immunoglobulins in albuminuric and even normoalbuminuric diabetics; these were not found in healthy control subjects [22]. These observations require confirmation, especially in view of the emerging data on the serum marker of inflammation, tumor necrosis factor alpha, as discussed below.

Six recent publications report noninflammatory urinary protein markers of diabetic nephropathy. Merchant et al. evaluated the urinary peptidome in type 1 diabetics, and found decreased urinary alfa-1 (IV) and V collagens and tenascin-X, and increased FAT tumor suppressor 3, inositol pentakisphosphate kinase, and zona occludens-3 [23]. In renal biopsies of these patients, there was increased expression of the latter two proteins. Vaidya et al. showed elevations in urinary interleukin-6, CXCL 10/IP-10, *N*-acetyl glucosaminidase (NAG), and kidney injury molecule-1 (KIM-1), but progressive renal injury was only associated with urinary KIM-1 and NAG [24]. Nauta et al. tested six urinary biomarkers in subjects with diabetes and found that only heart fatty acid binding protein (H-FABP) was associated with kidney function independently of albuminuria [25]. Schlatzer et al. found four urinary protein biomarkers that predicted early renal injury in type 1 diabetics [26]. These were Tamm–Horsfall protein, progranulin, clusterin, and alpha-1 acid glycoprotein. But another large scale proteomic study found reduced urinary uromodulin (Tamm–Horsfall protein) as a marker of diabetic nephropathy [27]. Very recently, it was reported that urinary haptoglobin levels predicted early renal functional decline in patients with type 2 diabetes and microalbuminuria [28]. Each of these studies used albuminuria for comparison to the change in the urinary protein marker. Three included renal function decline as the comparison variable. Only one also included normoalbuminuric diabetics [27]. Thus, the markers reported in many studies may not accurately predict or correlate with normoalbuminuric diabetic nephropathy.

In the specific case of tubular markers, Nielsen et al. recently evaluated the urinary levels of neutrophil gelatinase-associated lipocalin (NGAL), KIM-1, and liver fatty acid binding protein (L-FABP) and found them to correlate with loss of kidney function in type 1 diabetics, but that correlation was lost when controlling for hypertension and albuminuria [29]. In type 2 diabetics, urinary NGAL and L-FABP did not add to albuminuria as a marker of injury in two recent studies [30, 31]. Nonetheless, another group reported correlations of urinary cystatin C and non-albumin protein with loss of renal function [32]. The variability of these results shows that further work is needed. Studies should move beyond testing for correlations with existing injury, such as albuminuria, and instead attempt to correlate markers with loss of kidney function, such as the slopes of eGFR versus time. Finally, defining the utility of tubular markers must include well-defined populations to enable robust conclusions.

Non-urinary Markers

Blood Pressure

In persons with type 1 diabetes, an increase in systolic blood pressure during sleep precedes the development of microalbuminuria [33]. Other data show that nocturnal dosing of antihypertensive medications reduces cardiovascular risk in subjects with CKD, including diabetics and nondiabetics [34]. A cross-sectional study has shown lesser renal injury, as proteinuria, in type 2 diabetics who ingest one or more of their antihypertensive medications at bedtime [35]. This tends to confirm nocturnal hypertension or non-dipping of blood pressure as a marker of risk in subjects with type 1 and type 2 diabetes. Prospective studies are needed in diabetics with kidney disease, to test whether nocturnal dosing of antihypertensives may prevent loss of kidney function.

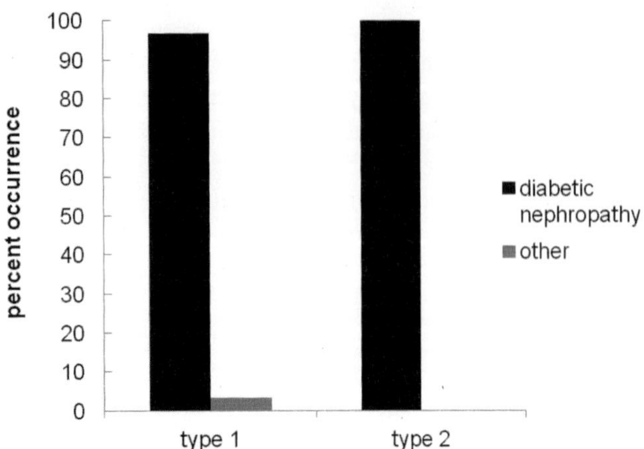

Fig. 7.3 The relationship of clinical neuropathy (numbness on exam) to the presence of diabetic nephropathy or nondiabetic kidney disease on kidney biopsy. Type 1 diabetics with clinical neuropathy had 90 % occurrence of diabetic nephropathy by kidney biopsy. No type 2 diabetic with neuropathy had nondiabetic kidney disease on biopsy. Adapted from Amoah et al. [40]

Funduscopic Exam

The coexistence of diabetic retinopathy (DR) and nephropathy has been known for many decades. Good control of glycemia in type 1 diabetics reduces the risk of retinopathy, as it does that of nephropathy [36], and a multifactorial approach in type 2 diabetics with microalbuminuria reduces the risk of retinopathy and nephropathy [9]. But diabetic retinopathy (DR) still occurs in up to 40 % of type 1 and type 2 diabetics [37]. Type 1 diabetics with diabetic nephropathy will almost always have DR, which will be present in 50 % of type 2 diabetics with diabetic nephropathy [38]. In a type 2 diabetic with kidney disease, the presence of proliferative DR strongly points to diabetic nephropathy [39]. The absence of DR is a useful feature in type 1 diabetics, less so in the type 2.

Neuropathy

In a series of 109 diabetics who underwent kidney biopsy, 18 had lesions other than diabetes [40]. Neuropathy by clinical exam was highly predictive of diabetic nephropathy on kidney biopsy (Fig. 7.3). Using neuropathy or retinopathy as associated features may thus be very useful for diagnosis. It is not known how these clinical features could be used for early identification of diabetic nephropathy.

Blood Testing

Good control of the blood glucose will reduce the risk of diabetic nephropathy [36]. But blood glucose and glycosylated hemoglobin levels are not good predictors of diabetic nephropathy. Indeed, in type 2 diabetics, while the average glycosylated hemoglobin level was not statistically associated with CKD, greater than 10 % variability in the glycosylated hemoglobin level was a significant predictor of CKD [41]. This observation may simply be the reflection of poor glucose control. Perhaps untoward swings of protein glycosylation have an independent and adverse effect.

Desai et al. showed that in diabetics with eGFR less than 40 mL/min, elevation in the cardiac marker troponin T to may be a significant predictor of ESRD, independent of proteinuria or eGFR [42]. These findings could simply be parallel markers of end-organ damage, rather than have mechanistic implications. But they do illustrate that useful biomarkers may be unexpected ones that are not typically associated with kidneys.

TNF Receptors

As discussed above, urinary markers for inflammation are found in diabetic nephropathy. The serum levels of tumor necrosis factor receptor 1 (TNFR1) have now been shown to predict risk for ESRD in type 2 diabetics even when adjusting for urinary albumin [43]. A similar risk for an early decline in GFR was found for elevated TNFRs in type 1 diabetics even before they developed proteinuria [44]. New therapies targeting inflammatory pathways are thus plausible. But enthusiasm for these data is tempered by the accompanying editorial that rightly points out that these observational studies may point to significant associations but not prove causality [45].

Uric Acid

Beyond its role in gout and nephrolithiasis, uric acid has received much attention as a correlate of cardiovascular disease [46]. It may be a marker and mechanism for CKD [47]. For baseline serum uric acid levels over 3 mg/dL, Ficociello et al. showed a direct dose–response relationship to the loss of GFR in type 1 diabetics with albuminuria [48]. Higher baseline serum uric acid levels predicted progression to albuminuria in another study of type 1 diabetics [49]. As shown (Fig. 7.4) these data are statistically significant but have limited clinical value because of the substantial overlap between the progressors and non-progressors. Nonetheless, treatment of the elevated uric acid levels could be beneficial and warrants testing.

Kidney Ultrasound

Hyperfiltration may occur in diabetes, perhaps mediated by tubular glucose and sodium reabsorption that leads to reduced distal nephron sodium delivery that causes an increase in GFR [50]. Renal hypertrophy may also occur, and lead to kidney enlargement. Type 1 diabetics with bigger kidneys may have a greater probability of developing microalbuminuria [51] (Fig. 7.5). The vascular resistive index as tested by Doppler ultrasound was found to be elevated in diabetic compared to nondiabetic children [52]. Thus, kidney ultrasound may serve as an early marker of diabetic nephropathy. Improving tissue-level resolution of ultrasound or other imaging technology may lead to even better imaging markers of diabetic nephropathy.

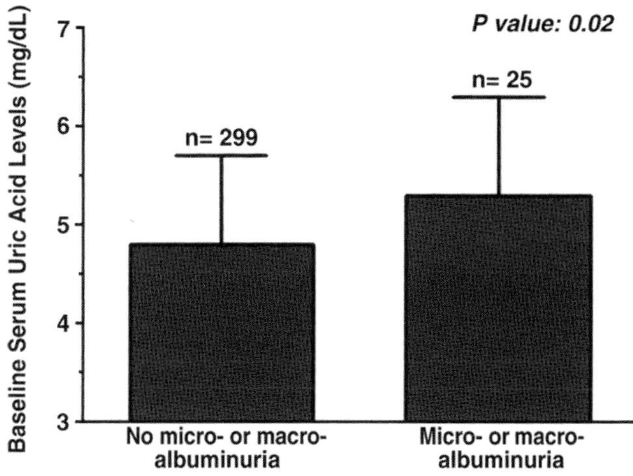

Fig. 7.4 Mean baseline serum uric acid levels according to albuminuria status at the 6-year follow-up visit in a cohort of type 1 diabetics. Elevated serum uric acid levels are a predictor of the development of albuminuria in patients with type 1 diabetes, but there is substantial overlap between the elevated and non-elevated serum uric acid levels. From Jalal et al. Serum uric acid levels predict the development of albuminuria over 6 years in patients with type 1 diabetes: findings from the Coronary Artery Calcification in Type 1 Diabetes study. *Nephrol Dial Transplant* 25:1865–1869, 2010. Reprinted with permission of Oxford University Press

Genetic Markers and Prediction of Diabetic Nephropathy

Beyond well-recognized diseases such as autosomal dominant polycystic kidney disease (ADPKD) or Alport syndrome, the familial predisposition to ESRD was clearly recognized 20 years ago [53]. The presence of a first-degree relative with ESRD increases an African American's risk for developing ESRD by ninefold and a white American's risk by fourfold. A gradient of risk is evident, whereby first-order relatives of a subject with ESRD have a higher risk of developing ESRD than do second-order relatives, who in turn have a higher risk than third-order relatives of a subject with ESRD. This points to genetic determinants of kidney disease. For nondiabetic kidney disease, identification of allelic variation at chromosome 22q12.3 has been extensively studied and risk variants of the APOL1 gene have been identified [54]. The odds ratios for the predisposition to nondiabetic kidney disease by the APOL1 risk alleles are between 7 and 10 [55]. Diabetic nephropathy has other genetic associations, of which some are shown in the table below (Table 7.1).

The odds ratios for the positively associated genes are well below the odds ratio of having the APOL1 risk allele. The low odds ratios show that testing for the genes of Table 7.1 cannot serve to screen for diabetic nephropathy. In addition, the genetic influences on diabetic nephropathy are likely to be multifactorial in their effect to predispose a particular diabetic patient to kidney disease. Confirmatory studies are needed for any genetic marker before it can be considered reliable or even useful for mechanistic studies.

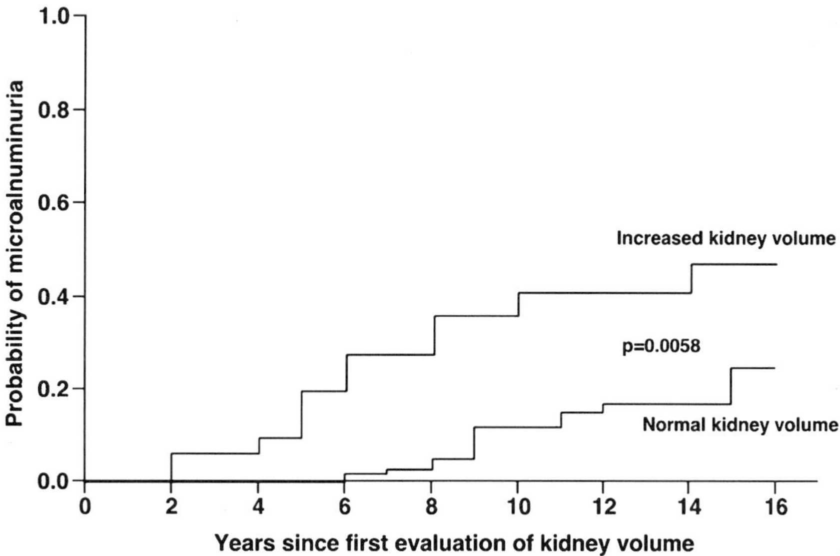

Fig. 7.5 The actuarial risk of developing microalbuminuria in type 1 diabetics, according to the baseline kidney volume as assessed by ultrasound. There is a significantly greater risk of developing microalbuminuria in subjects with enlarged kidneys at baseline. Reproduced by permission, from Zerbini et al. [51]. From Zerbini G, et al. Persistent renal hypertrophy and faster decline of glomerular filtration rate precede the development of microalbuminuria in type 1 diabetes. Diabetes 2006 Sep;55(9):2620–2625. Reprinted with permission from American Diabetes Association

Table 7.1 Genetic markers of diabetic nephropathy

Marker	Type 1 or type 2 diabetes	Odds ratio	Reference
PPAR gamma Ala (PPARG2 Ala12 allele)	Type 2	0.47	[56]
GLUT1 mutation (Xba-)	Type 2	0.6	[57]
ACE genotype (II versus D)	Both	0.78	[58]
ACE2, AII receptor	Type 1	Not significant (n.s.)	[59]
M235T AGT (angiotensinogen variant)	Type 1	n.s.	[60]
APOE (apolipoprotein E)	Both	Contradictory	[61]
ADIPOQ (adiponectin)	Type 1	1.46	[62]
Gremlin	Type 1	1.69	[63]
GLUT1 mutation (Xba-)	Type 2	1.9	[64]
CNDP1 (carnosinase)	Type 2	2.46	[65]
ELMO1 (engulfment and motility)	Type 2	2.67	[66]
ACE D allele	Type 1	5.0	[60]

The Role of MicroRNA

MicroRNAs (miRNAs) are single-stranded RNAs that regulate gene expression by blocking translation or by promoting breakdown of mRNAs. Many recent studies have pointed to the potential role of miRNA in diabetic nephropathy but these studies have been either in vitro or in rodent models [67]. A PubMed search yielded only one study that tested miRNA in humans, in which it was reported that urinary miR-15 was low in subjects with glomerulosclerosis [68]. Further human studies are eagerly awaited.

Glomerular Markers

Kidney biopsy studies of diabetic nephropathy have reported the mechanistic relevance of TGFbeta1 and nephrin [18, 69, 70]. The increased renal expression of TGFbeta is reduced by ACE inhibitors, and that of nephrin is restored [18, 70]. Urinary mRNA for podocyte markers nephrin, podocin, synaptopodin, and alpha-actinin-4 may be increased in subjects with diabetic nephropathy, but had no correlation with GFR decline in one study [71]. The same group showed in a subsequent report that ACE inhibition decreased urinary mRNA for synaptopodin [72]. Data such as this may clarify the mechanism of benefit of known therapies, but since podocyte injury occurs in many glomerular diseases, evidence for it cannot be considered as a discriminatory marker.

The glomerular and tubular basement membrane thickening, and the mesangial expansion of diabetic nephropathy are diagnostic, but they are invasive markers that cannot be applied to all patients. Nonetheless, kidney biopsy studies are of great value in defining diabetic nephropathy and can usefully be added to studies that aim to identify accurate noninvasive biomarkers.

Utility of Markers

The utility of any marker for present or future injuries can be shown by its predictive value for those injuries. The modification of the injury marker by known therapies provides additional insight. This has been reported for microalbuminuria. The Steno-2 study showed the benefit of intensive multifactorial intervention for type 2 diabetics with microalbuminuria, as a reduction in mortality and in occurrence of ESRD [9]. These optimistic data are tempered by the fact that type 2 diabetics may have quite variable histology upon kidney biopsy, unrelated to age, duration of diabetes, renal function, blood pressure, or urinary protein excretion [73]. The kidney biopsy may show classical diabetic nephropathy, or show more vascular than glomerular disease, or even nondiabetic disease superimposed on diabetic nephropathy. It is very likely that these different histopathologies will have different patterns of biomarkers and will respond differently to treatment.

"Unbiased" Insight to New Mechanisms

Many of the above-cited studies have tested markers and their correlates based on existing knowledge, i.e., have used a "likely candidate" approach. A two-species and unbiased approach using mice and humans was used by Hodgin et al., which identified hitherto unsuspected pathways in the pathogenesis of diabetic nephropathy [74]. These were the Janus kinase/signal transducer and activator of transcription (JAK/STAT) and vascular endothelial growth factor receptor (VEGFR) pathways. Phase II studies of JAK/STAT inhibitors have been started based on these data.

Urinary proteomic studies have been done, also in an unbiased approach. Otu et al. unfortunately provide no identification of the proteins identified in their report [75]. Alkhalaf et al. did identify collagen I and III fragments as promising urinary biomarkers [76]. Although collagens I and III are localized to interstitium in normal kidneys, they may participate in glomerular scarring [77], which links these observations to those of Araki, cited above.

Markers of Other Disease

Evaluation of a diabetic patient with proteinuria or azotemia must also test for other kidney diseases. Superimposed or nondiabetic kidney disease was reported in 10 of 122 kidney biopsies done for diagnosis in diabetics [78], and 30 % of biopsies of type 1 and type 2 diabetic patients showed nondiabetic kidney disease in a more recent report [79]. Urinalysis findings of microhematuria, i.e., more than ten red cells per high power field [80], are unusual for diabetic nephropathy and will suggest other kidney disease. As stated above, an absence of retinopathy is associated with nondiabetic kidney disease especially in type 1 diabetics. Markers of other kidney diseases, such as paraproteins, antineutrophil cytoplasmic antibodies, or antinuclear antibodies, will clearly point to disease other than or at least superimposed on diabetes. Reliable identification of diabetic nephropathy, rather than nondiabetic kidney disease, is important clinically. It is also important for clinical research in diabetic nephropathy, because the results of interventions will be distorted if some of the studied population does not have diabetic nephropathy.

Markers May Lead Us Astray

The benefits of using ACE inhibitors or angiotensin receptor blockers (ARBs) led to testing their combination [81], the rationale being that using ACE inhibitor plus ARB to suppress the RAS might be expected to yield more benefit than using one drug alone. This was found to lower albuminuria but was associated with adverse effects including worse renal function [82]. There has been a similar experience with the renin antagonist aliskiren. In combination with the ARB losartan, it reduces proteinuria in patients with diabetic nephropathy [83], but aliskiren in combination therapy does not improve renal outcomes and increases the risk of adverse effects, including hyperkalemia [84, 85]. Similarly, knowledge of the role of hypertension as marker and mechanism of renal injury led to study of intensive blood pressure control in diabetics. Data from the Reduction of Endpoints in NIDDM with the Angiotensin II Antagonist Losartan (RENAAL) study shows a progressive rise in risk of death or ESRD for systolic blood pressure (BP) above 140 systolic [86]. But the Action to Control Cardiovascular Risk in Diabetes (ACCORD) trial showed that diabetics reaching an average systolic BP of 120 mmHg had more serious adverse events and no overall cardiovascular endpoint improvement when compared to those with an average systolic BP of 134 mmHg [87]. In diabetics with albuminuria or frank proteinuria, no trial appears to show a benefit of lowering the systolic BP to less than 130 mmHg. Because cardiovascular morbidity and mortality are the major problem in diabetics, our interest in biomarkers for renal injury must not distract us. A large Danish study reports 45 times more cardiovascular than ESRD deaths in subjects with type 2 diabetes [88]. In this regard, one trial showed that a single ARB, olmesartan, could delay the occurrence of microalbuminuria in type 2 diabetics, but at the price of increased fatal cardiovascular events [89]. In this trial, the average achieved systolic BP was 126 mmHg in the olmesartan-treated patients. Achieving a reduction in the albuminuria biomarker will be counterproductive if it leads to greater mortality. One is faced with similar problems if markers other than urinary albumin become the target for mitigation or treatment of diabetic nephropathy.

Statistical Issues

The use of microalbuminuria is now a standard for care of diabetic patients. As noted above, decline in GFR can occur without an increase in albuminuria, so that this marker has an incomplete sensitivity for kidney disease in diabetics. It is also not specific, because elevations in urine albumin may occur in many kidney diseases. A similar analysis must be done for any biomarker that is proposed as mechanistically important in diabetic nephropathy. The proposed marker must survive a stringent statistical validation before it could be used for clinical care.

Cost–Benefit and Deficiencies in Current Studies

As of April 2013, PubMed reports over 500 publications since 2010 for the search term "biomarkers diabetic nephropathy." This is a lot of data and a lot of publication, and is nearly impossible for one person to know, let alone implement in practice. Indeed, most of the current data are at the discovery and correlation phase. We found only a few recent studies that addressed cost–benefit of testing proteinuria as a biomarker [90–92]. None of the newer markers have undergone cost–benefit analysis. "Newer" molecules such as miRNAs appear to be more popular than "older" ones, such as uric acid, without regard to cost.

Table 7.2 Biomarkers of diabetic nephropathy: current use and future needs

Diabetic nephropathy KDOQI stages	Goal	Markers	Markers needed
I	Diagnosis	Albuminuria, retinopathy, kidney hypertrophy, uric acid	Distinguish nondiabetic kidney disease
II	Predict progression	Serial eGFR, blood pressure	
III	Identify effect of therapy	Albuminuria, blood pressure	For normoalbuminuric disease
IV	Identify progression	Serial eGFR	Irreversibility
V	Identify irreversibility	Troponin	Irreversibility

Many studies correlate one or more biomarkers to categories of disease, such as micro- or macroalbuminuric subjects. Not enough studies test the relation of the biomarker to progressive loss of kidney function. Few studies have the certainty of diagnosis by kidney biopsy, which may show unsuspected nondiabetic kidney disease in 10–30 % of cases. No studies have careful phenotypic case definition, including funduscopic exam and assessment of neuropathy. Only one study has identified a marker that defines subjects who have irreversible disease that will progress to ESRD. Reliable markers of irreversibility are needed, because reliable identification of patients with irreversible disease will compel the planning for renal replacement therapy, i.e., dialysis and/or kidney transplantation.

Use of Markers at Different Stages of Disease

It is useful to consider the stage of kidney disease and current use of biomarkers for diabetic nephropathy. Table 7.2 shows our interpretation of current knowledge. One should also add the information that one gets from the history and physical examination. A patient who has kidney disease but with a less than 5-year duration of diabetes, a normal funduscopic exam, and no evidence of neuropathy is unlikely to have diabetic nephropathy. Conversely, one needs no special biomarker to make the diagnosis of diabetic nephropathy for a patient who has had diabetes for more than 10 years, dot hemorrhages on funduscopic exam, and a symptomatic sensorimotor neuropathy. There are many patients between these extremes, for whom new markers may be needed.

Recommendations

Going forward, we recommend the performance of comprehensive and cost-sensitive biomarker studies in diabetic nephropathy. These studies will include cases that are clearly diabetic nephropathy, and for which the phenotype is extensively documented, including the essential variables of blood pressure and albuminuria. The population will include diabetics with macro-, micro-, and normoalbuminuria. Suitable normal controls and also subjects with nondiabetic kidney disease will be included. Use of a few well-studied cohorts in which there is testing of multiple markers may be preferable to many cohorts that each test a separate biomarker.

The ideal biomarker will be noninvasive, easily and cheaply measured, and will closely correlate with loss of kidney function. It will improve on the diagnostic and predictive value of the clinical evaluation that includes history, physical exam, funduscopic exam, and urinalysis. The best biomarkers will be cost-effective, sensitive, and specific, and their measurement will relieve illness and prolong life.

References

1. Fishberg AM. Hypertension and nephritis. Philadelphia: Lea and Febiger; 1954.
2. Plantinga LC, Crews DC, Coresh J, Miller 3rd ER, Saran R, Yee J, et al. Prevalence of chronic kidney disease in US adults with undiagnosed diabetes or prediabetes. Clin J Am Soc Nephrol. 2010; 5(4):673–82.
3. American Diabetes Association. Standards of medical care in diabetes—2013. Diabetes Care. 2013;36 Suppl 1:S11–66.
4. Skupien J, Warram JH, Smiles AM, Niewczas MA, Gohda T, Pezzolesi MG, et al. The early decline in renal function in patients with type 1 diabetes and proteinuria predicts the risk of end-stage renal disease. Kidney Int. 2012;82(5):589–97.
5. Bright R. Cases and observations illustrative of renal disease accompanied with the secretion of albumenous urine. Guys Hosp Rep. 1836;1:338–79.
6. Kimmelstiel P, Wilson C. Intercapillary lesions in the glomeruli of the kidney. Am J Pathol. 1936;12:83–97.
7. Mogensen CE, Christensen CK, Vittinghus E. The stages in diabetic renal disease. With emphasis on the stage of incipient diabetic nephropathy. Diabetes. 1983;32 Suppl 2:64–78.
8. Groop PH, Thomas MC, Moran JL, Waden J, Thorn LM, Makinen VP, et al. The presence and severity of chronic kidney disease predicts all-cause mortality in type 1 diabetes. Diabetes. 2009;58(7): 1651–8.
9. Gaede P, Lund-Andersen H, Parving HH, Pedersen O. Effect of a multifactorial intervention on mortality in type 2 diabetes. N Engl J Med. 2008;358(6):580–91.
10. Macisaac RJ, Jerums G. Diabetic kidney disease with and without albuminuria. Curr Opin Nephrol Hypertens. 2011;20(3):246–57.
11. Magliano DJ, Polkinghorne KR, Barr EL, Su Q, Chadban SJ, Zimmet PZ, et al. HPLC-detected albuminuria predicts mortality. J Am Soc Nephrol. 2007;18(12):3171–6.
12. Caramori ML, Fioretto P, Mauer M. The need for early predictors of diabetic nephropathy risk: is albumin excretion rate sufficient? Diabetes. 2000;49(9):1399–408.

13. Araki S, Haneda M, Koya D, Isshiki K, Kume S, Sugimoto T, et al. Association between urinary type IV collagen level and deterioration of renal function in type 2 diabetic patients without overt proteinuria. Diabetes Care. 2010;33(8):1805–10.
14. Ziyadeh FN. Renal tubular basement membrane and collagen type IV in diabetes mellitus. Kidney Int. 1993;43(1):114–20.
15. Cohen MP, Lautenslager GT, Shearman CW. Increased collagen IV excretion in diabetes. A marker of compromised filtration function. Diabetes Care. 2001;24(5):914–8.
16. Yamamoto T, Nakamura T, Noble NA, Ruoslahti E, Border WA. Expression of transforming growth factor beta is elevated in human and experimental diabetic nephropathy. Proc Natl Acad Sci U S A. 1993;90(5):1814–8.
17. Shaker OG, Sadik NA. Transforming growth factor beta 1 and monocyte chemoattractant protein-1 as prognostic markers of diabetic nephropathy. Hum Exp Toxicol. 2013;32(10):1089–96.
18. Langham RG, Kelly DJ, Gow RM, Zhang Y, Cordonnier DJ, Pinel N, et al. Transforming growth factor-beta in human diabetic nephropathy: effects of ACE inhibition. Diabetes Care. 2006; 29(12):2670–5.
19. Houlihan CA, Akdeniz A, Tsalamandris C, Cooper ME, Jerums G, Gilbert RE. Urinary transforming growth factor-beta excretion in patients with hypertension, type 2 diabetes, and elevated albumin excretion rate: effects of angiotensin receptor blockade and sodium restriction. Diabetes Care. 2002;25(6):1072–7.
20. Bertoluci MC, Uebel D, Schmidt A, Thomazelli FC, Oliveira FR, Schmid H. Urinary TGF-beta1 reduction related to a decrease of systolic blood pressure in patients with type 2 diabetes and clinical diabetic nephropathy. Diabetes Res Clin Pract. 2006;72(3): 258–64.
21. Wolkow PP, Niewczas MA, Perkins B, Ficociello LH, Lipinski B, Warram JH, et al. Association of urinary inflammatory markers and renal decline in microalbuminuric type 1 diabetics. J Am Soc Nephrol. 2008;19(4):789–97.
22. Gohda T, Walker WH, Wolkow P, Lee JE, Warram JH, Krolewski AS, et al. Elevated urinary excretion of immunoglobulins in nonproteinuric patients with type 1 diabetes. Am J Physiol Renal Physiol. 2012;303(1):F157–62.
23. Merchant ML, Perkins BA, Boratyn GM, Ficociello LH, Wilkey DW, Barati MT, et al. Urinary peptidome may predict renal function decline in type 1 diabetes and microalbuminuria. J Am Soc Nephrol. 2009;20(9):2065–74.
24. Vaidya VS, Niewczas MA, Ficociello LH, Johnson AC, Collings FB, Warram JH, et al. Regression of microalbuminuria in type 1 diabetes is associated with lower levels of urinary tubular injury biomarkers, kidney injury molecule-1, and *N*-acetyl-beta-D-glucosaminidase. Kidney Int. 2011;79(4):464–70.
25. Nauta FL, Boertien WE, Bakker SJ, van Goor H, van Oeveren W, de Jong PE, et al. Glomerular and tubular damage markers are elevated in patients with diabetes. Diabetes Care. 2011;34(4): 975–81.
26. Schlatzer D, Maahs DM, Chance MR, Dazard JE, Li X, Hazlett F, et al. Novel urinary protein biomarkers predicting the development of microalbuminuria and renal function decline in type 1 diabetes. Diabetes Care. 2012;35(3):549–55.
27. Rossing K, Mischak H, Dakna M, Zurbig P, Novak J, Julian BA, et al. Urinary proteomics in diabetes and CKD. J Am Soc Nephrol. 2008;19(7):1283–90.
28. Bhensdadia NM, Hunt KJ, Lopes-Virella MF, Michael Tucker J, Mataria MR, Alge JL, et al. Urine haptoglobin levels predict early renal functional decline in patients with type 2 diabetes. Kidney Int. 2013;83(6):1136–43.
29. Nielsen SE, Andersen S, Zdunek D, Hess G, Parving HH, Rossing P. Tubular markers do not predict the decline in glomerular filtration rate in type 1 diabetic patients with overt nephropathy. Kidney Int. 2011;79(10):1113–8.
30. Chou KM, Lee CC, Chen CH, Sun CY. Clinical value of NGAL, L-FABP and albuminuria in predicting GFR decline in type 2 diabetes mellitus patients. PLoS One. 2013;8(1):e54863.
31. Conway BR, Manoharan D, Manoharan D, Jenks S, Dear JW, McLachlan S, et al. Measuring urinary tubular biomarkers in type 2 diabetes does not add prognostic value beyond established risk factors. Kidney Int. 2012;82(7):812–8.
32. Kim SS, Song SH, Kim IJ, Jeon YK, Kim BH, Kwak IS, et al. Urinary cystatin C and tubular proteinuria predict progression of diabetic nephropathy. Diabetes Care. 2013;36(3):656–61.
33. Lurbe E, Redon J, Kesani A, Pascual JM, Tacons J, Alvarez V, et al. Increase in nocturnal blood pressure and progression to microalbuminuria in type 1 diabetes. N Engl J Med. 2002;347(11):797–805.
34. Hermida RC, Ayala DE, Mojon A, Fernandez JR. Bedtime dosing of antihypertensive medications reduces cardiovascular risk in CKD. J Am Soc Nephrol. 2011;22(12):2313–21.
35. Moya A, Crespo JJ, Ayala DE, Rios MT, Pousa L, Callejas PA, et al. Effects of time-of-day of hypertension treatment on ambulatory blood pressure and clinical characteristics of patients with type 2 diabetes. Chronobiol Int. 2013;30(1–2):116–31.
36. Diabetes Control and Complications Trial/Epidemiology of Diabetes Interventions and Complications (DCCT/EDIC) Research Group, Nathan DM, Zinman B, Cleary PA, Backlund JY, Genuth S, et al. Modern-day clinical course of type 1 diabetes mellitus after 30 years' duration: the diabetes control and complications trial/epidemiology of diabetes interventions and complications and Pittsburgh epidemiology of diabetes complications experience (1983–2005). Arch Intern Med. 2009;169(14):1307–16.
37. Cheung N, Mitchell P, Wong TY. Diabetic retinopathy. Lancet. 2010;376(9735):124–36.
38. El-Asrar AM, Al-Rubeaan KA, Al-Amro SA, Moharram OA, Kangave D. Retinopathy as a predictor of other diabetic complications. Int Ophthalmol. 2001;24(1):1–11.
39. He F, Xia X, Wu XF, Yu XQ, Huang FX. Diabetic retinopathy in predicting diabetic nephropathy in patients with type 2 diabetes and renal disease: a meta-analysis. Diabetologia. 2013;56(3):457–66.
40. Amoah E, Glickman JL, Malchoff CD, Sturgill BC, Kaiser DL, Bolton WK. Clinical identification of nondiabetic renal disease in diabetic patients with type I and type II disease presenting with renal dysfunction. Am J Nephrol. 1988;8(3):204–11.
41. Penno G, Solini A, Bonora E, Fondelli C, Orsi E, Zerbini G, et al. HbA1c variability as an independent correlate of nephropathy, but not retinopathy, in patients with type 2 diabetes: The Renal Insufficiency And Cardiovascular Events (RIACE) Italian multicenter study. Diabetes Care. 2013;36(8):2301–10.
42. Desai AS, Toto R, Jarolim P, Uno H, Eckardt KU, Kewalramani R, et al. Association between cardiac biomarkers and the development of ESRD in patients with type 2 diabetes mellitus, anemia, and CKD. Am J Kidney Dis. 2011;58(5):717–28.
43. Niewczas MA, Gohda T, Skupien J, Smiles AM, Walker WH, Rosetti F, et al. Circulating TNF receptors 1 and 2 predict ESRD in type 2 diabetes. J Am Soc Nephrol. 2012;23(3):507–15.
44. Gohda T, Niewczas MA, Ficociello LH, Walker WH, Skupien J, Rosetti F, et al. Circulating TNF receptors 1 and 2 predict stage 3 CKD in type 1 diabetes. J Am Soc Nephrol. 2012;23(3):516–24.
45. Brosius FC, Saran R. Do we now have a prognostic biomarker for progressive diabetic nephropathy? J Am Soc Nephrol. 2012; 23(3):376–7.
46. Kanbay M, Segal M, Afsar B, Kang DH, Rodriguez-Iturbe B, Johnson RJ. The role of uric acid in the pathogenesis of human cardiovascular disease. Heart. 2013;99(11):759–66.
47. Johnson RJ, Nakagawa T, Jalal D, Sanchez-Lozada LG, Kang DH, Ritz E. Uric acid and chronic kidney disease: which is chasing which? Nephrol Dial Transplant. 2013;28(9):2221–8.
48. Ficociello LH, Rosolowsky ET, Niewczas MA, Maselli NJ, Weinberg JM, Aschengrau A, et al. High-normal serum uric acid

increases risk of early progressive renal function loss in type 1 diabetes: results of a 6-year follow-up. Diabetes Care. 2010;33(6):1337–43.
49. Jalal DI, Rivard CJ, Johnson RJ, Maahs DM, McFann K, Rewers M, et al. Serum uric acid levels predict the development of albuminuria over 6 years in patients with type 1 diabetes: findings from the Coronary Artery Calcification in Type 1 Diabetes study. Nephrol Dial Transplant. 2010;25(6):1865–9.
50. Thomson SC, Vallon V, Blantz RC. Kidney function in early diabetes: the tubular hypothesis of glomerular filtration. Am J Physiol Renal Physiol. 2004;286(1):F8–15.
51. Zerbini G, Bonfanti R, Meschi F, Bognetti E, Paesano PL, Gianolli L, et al. Persistent renal hypertrophy and faster decline of glomerular filtration rate precede the development of microalbuminuria in type 1 diabetes. Diabetes. 2006;55(9):2620–5.
52. Youssef DM, Fawzy FM. Value of renal resistive index as an early marker of diabetic nephropathy in children with type-1 diabetes mellitus. Saudi J Kidney Dis Transpl. 2012;23(5):985–92.
53. Freedman BI, Spray BJ, Tuttle AB, Buckalew Jr VM. The familial risk of end-stage renal disease in African Americans. Am J Kidney Dis. 1993;21(4):387–93.
54. Wasser WG, Tzur S, Wolday D, Adu D, Baumstein D, Rosset S, et al. Population genetics of chronic kidney disease: the evolving story of APOL1. J Nephrol. 2012;25(5):603–18.
55. Freedman BI, Kopp JB, Langefeld CD, Genovese G, Friedman DJ, Nelson GW, et al. The apolipoprotein L1 (APOL1) gene and nondiabetic nephropathy in African Americans. J Am Soc Nephrol. 2010;21(9):1422–6.
56. Caramori ML, Canani LH, Costa LA, Gross JL. The human peroxisome proliferator-activated receptor gamma2 (PPARgamma2) Pro12Ala polymorphism is associated with decreased risk of diabetic nephropathy in patients with type 2 diabetes. Diabetes. 2003; 52(12):3010–3.
57. Grzeszczak W, Moczulski DK, Zychma M, Zukowska-Szczechowska E, Trautsolt W, Szydlowska I. Role of GLUT1 gene in susceptibility to diabetic nephropathy in type 2 diabetes. Kidney Int. 2001;59(2):631–6.
58. Ng DP, Tai BC, Koh D, Tan KW, Chia KS. Angiotensin-I converting enzyme insertion/deletion polymorphism and its association with diabetic nephropathy: a meta-analysis of studies reported between 1994 and 2004 and comprising 14,727 subjects. Diabetologia. 2005;48(5):1008–16.
59. Currie D, McKnight AJ, Patterson CC, Sadlier DM, Maxwell AP, UK Warren 3/GoKinD Study Group. Investigation of ACE, ACE2 and AGTR1 genes for association with nephropathy in type 1 diabetes mellitus. Diabet Med. 2010;27(10):1188–94.
60. Hadjadj S, Belloum R, Bouhanick B, Gallois Y, Guilloteau G, Chatellier G, et al. Prognostic value of angiotensin-I converting enzyme I/D polymorphism for nephropathy in type 1 diabetes mellitus: a prospective study. J Am Soc Nephrol. 2001;12(3):541–9.
61. Freedman BI, Bostrom M, Daeihagh P, Bowden DW. Genetic factors in diabetic nephropathy. Clin J Am Soc Nephrol. 2007;2(6):1306–16.
62. Vionnet N, Tregouet D, Kazeem G, Gut I, Groop PH, Tarnow L, et al. Analysis of 14 candidate genes for diabetic nephropathy on chromosome 3q in European populations: strongest evidence for association with a variant in the promoter region of the adiponectin gene. Diabetes. 2006;55(11):3166–74.
63. McKnight AJ, Patterson CC, Pettigrew KA, Savage DA, Kilner J, Murphy M, et al. A GREM1 gene variant associates with diabetic nephropathy. J Am Soc Nephrol. 2010;21(5):773–81.
64. Liu ZH, Guan TJ, Chen ZH, Li LS. Glucose transporter (GLUT1) allele (XbaI-) associated with nephropathy in non-insulin-dependent diabetes mellitus. Kidney Int. 1999;55(5):1843–8.
65. Janssen B, Hohenadel D, Brinkkoetter P, Peters V, Rind N, Fischer C, et al. Carnosine as a protective factor in diabetic nephropathy: association with a leucine repeat of the carnosinase gene CNDP1. Diabetes. 2005;54(8):2320–7.
66. Shimazaki A, Kawamura Y, Kanazawa A, Sekine A, Saito S, Tsunoda T, et al. Genetic variations in the gene encoding ELMO1 are associated with susceptibility to diabetic nephropathy. Diabetes. 2005;54(4):1171–8.
67. Alvarez ML, DiStefano JK. Towards microRNA-based therapeutics for diabetic nephropathy. Diabetologia. 2013;56(3):444–56.
68. Szeto CC, Ching-Ha KB, Ka-Bik L, Mac-Moune LF, Cheung-Lung CP, Gang W, et al. Micro-RNA expression in the urinary sediment of patients with chronic kidney diseases. Dis Markers. 2012; 33(3):137–44.
69. Langham RG, Kelly DJ, Cox AJ, Thomson NM, Holthofer H, Zaoui P, et al. Proteinuria and the expression of the podocyte slit diaphragm protein, nephrin, in diabetic nephropathy: effects of angiotensin converting enzyme inhibition. Diabetologia. 2002; 45(11):1572–6.
70. Jim B, Ghanta M, Qipo A, Fan Y, Chuang PY, Cohen HW, et al. Dysregulated nephrin in diabetic nephropathy of type 2 diabetes: a cross sectional study. PLoS One. 2012;7(5):e36041.
71. Wang G, Lai FM, Lai KB, Chow KM, Li KT, Szeto CC. Messenger RNA expression of podocyte-associated molecules in the urinary sediment of patients with diabetic nephropathy. Nephron Clin Pract. 2007;106(4):c169–79.
72. Wang G, Lai FM, Lai KB, Chow KM, Kwan BC, Li PK, et al. Urinary messenger RNA expression of podocyte-associated molecules in patients with diabetic nephropathy treated by angiotensin-converting enzyme inhibitor and angiotensin receptor blocker. Eur J Endocrinol. 2008;158(3):317–22.
73. Gambara V, Mecca G, Remuzzi G, Bertani T. Heterogeneous nature of renal lesions in type II diabetes. J Am Soc Nephrol. 1993; 3(8):1458–66.
74. Hodgin JB, Nair V, Zhang H, Randolph A, Harris RC, Nelson RG, et al. Identification of cross-species shared transcriptional networks of diabetic nephropathy in human and mouse glomeruli. Diabetes. 2013;62(1):299–308.
75. Otu HH, Can H, Spentzos D, Nelson RG, Hanson RL, Looker HC, et al. Prediction of diabetic nephropathy using urine proteomic profiling 10 years prior to development of nephropathy. Diabetes Care. 2007;30(3):638–43.
76. Alkhalaf A, Zurbig P, Bakker SJ, Bilo HJ, Cerna M, Fischer C, et al. Multicentric validation of proteomic biomarkers in urine specific for diabetic nephropathy. PLoS One. 2010;5(10):e13421.
77. Yoshioka K, Tohda M, Takemura T, Akano N, Matsubara K, Ooshima A, et al. Distribution of type I collagen in human kidney diseases in comparison with type III collagen. J Pathol. 1990; 162(2):141–8.
78. Kasinath BS, Mujais SK, Spargo BH, Katz AI. Nondiabetic renal disease in patients with diabetes mellitus. Am J Med. 1983; 75(4):613–7.
79. Haider DG, Peric S, Friedl A, Fuhrmann V, Wolzt M, Horl WH, et al. Kidney biopsy in patients with diabetes mellitus. Clin Nephrol. 2011;76(3):180–5.
80. Akimoto T, Ito C, Saito O, Takahashi H, Takeda S, Ando Y, et al. Microscopic hematuria and diabetic glomerulosclerosis—clinicopathological analysis of type 2 diabetic patients associated with overt proteinuria. Nephron Clin Pract. 2008;109(3):c119–26.
81. Mann JF, Anderson C, Gao P, Gerstein HC, Boehm M, Ryden L, et al. Dual inhibition of the renin-angiotensin system in high-risk diabetes and risk for stroke and other outcomes: results of the ONTARGET trial. J Hypertens. 2013;31(2):414–21.
82. Mann JF, Schmieder RE, McQueen M, Dyal L, Schumacher H, Pogue J, et al. Renal outcomes with telmisartan, ramipril, or both, in people at high vascular risk (the ONTARGET study): a multicentre, randomised, double-blind, controlled trial. Lancet. 2008; 372(9638):547–53.

83. Parving HH, Persson F, Lewis JB, Lewis EJ, Hollenberg NK, Avoid Study Investigators. Aliskiren combined with losartan in type 2 diabetes and nephropathy. N Engl J Med. 2008;358(23): 2433–46.
84. Parving HH, Brenner BM, McMurray JJ, de Zeeuw D, Haffner SM, Solomon SD, et al. Cardiorenal end points in a trial of aliskiren for type 2 diabetes. N Engl J Med. 2012;367(23):2204–13.
85. de Leeuw PW. Aliskiren increased adverse events in patients with diabetes and kidney disease who were receiving ACE inhibitors or ARBs. Ann Intern Med. 2013;158(6):JC7.
86. Bakris GL, Weir MR, Shanifar S, Zhang Z, Douglas J, van Dijk DJ, et al. Effects of blood pressure level on progression of diabetic nephropathy: results from the RENAAL study. Arch Intern Med. 2003;163(13):1555–65.
87. ACCORD Study Group, Cushman WC, Evans GW, Byington RP, Goff Jr DC, Grimm Jr RH, et al. Effects of intensive blood-pressure control in type 2 diabetes mellitus. N Engl J Med. 2010; 362(17):1575–85.
88. Hansen MB, Jensen ML, Carstensen B. Causes of death among diabetic patients in Denmark. Diabetologia. 2012;55(2):294–302.
89. Haller H, Ito S, Izzo Jr JL, Januszewicz A, Katayama S, Menne J, et al. Olmesartan for the delay or prevention of microalbuminuria in type 2 diabetes. N Engl J Med. 2011;364(10):907–17.
90. Palmer AJ, Chen R, Valentine WJ, Roze S, Bregman B, Mehin N, et al. Cost-consequence analysis in a French setting of screening and optimal treatment of nephropathy in hypertensive patients with type 2 diabetes. Diabetes Metab. 2006;32(1): 69–76.
91. Howard K, White S, Salkeld G, McDonald S, Craig JC, Chadban S, et al. Cost-effectiveness of screening and optimal management for diabetes, hypertension, and chronic kidney disease: a modeled analysis. Value Health. 2010;13(2):196–208.
92. Kessler R, Keusch G, Szucs TD, Wittenborn JS, Hoerger TJ, Brugger U, et al. Health economic modelling of the cost-effectiveness of microalbuminuria screening in Switzerland. Swiss Med Wkly. 2012;142:w13508.

8 Atypical Presentations of Diabetic Nephropathy and Novel Therapies

Louis J. Imbriano, John K. Maesaka, Joseph Mattana, Shayan Shirazian, and George Jerums

Overview of Traditional and Nontraditional Concepts in Diabetic Nephropathy

Diabetic nephropathy is the leading cause of end stage renal disease (ESRD) and can develop in 20–25 % of patients with type 1 or type 2 diabetes (T1DM or T2DM). The "typical" classic definition of diabetic nephropathy has previously included persistent macroalbuminuria (>300 mg/24 h or >200 µg/min), the presence of diabetic retinopathy, and the absence of nondiabetic renal diseases. Albuminuria has been thought to be the hallmark of glomerular disease for decades and was presumed to increase proportionately with the damage to the glomerular basement membrane (GBM). However, the association of diabetes and albuminuria has now been questioned because of the increasing recognition of "atypical" cases of diabetic nephropathy with normoalbuminuria.

Because the onset of T1DM can be ascertained with greater certainty, the development of diabetic nephropathy has been more accurately monitored and defined over time for T1DM compared to T2DM. The natural history of the "typical" T1DM patient has been classically described in stepwise stages, during which pathophysiologic and clinical changes develop over an extended period of time. The first 5–10 years after the onset of diabetes are associated with "silent" changes in renal structure and function, which include glomerular hypertrophy, hyperplasia, and hyperfiltration (HF) with increased glomerular filtration rate (GFR), and increased kidney size. The "typical" pathologic changes include mesangial cell hypertrophy, hyperplasia, increased mesangial matrix, thickening of the GBM, and tubular basement membrane (TBM), as well as varying degrees of tubulointerstitial injury and fibrosis. Microalbuminuria, defined as 30–300 mg/24 h [20–200 µg/min] if it occurs, is considered a strong predictor of the development of nephropathy. After 10 years of T1DM, about 40–50 % of patients with microalbuminuria begin to excrete increasing amounts of albumin into the range of macroalbuminuria (>300 mg/24 h or >200 µg/min). This is associated with progressive decline of the GFR, from supernormal HF rates to "normal" and eventually to reduced levels. Albuminuria is ostensibly attributed to thickening and distortion of the GBM and is an independent agent of injury to the tubules and interstitium. About 50 % of patients with T1DM and macroalbuminuria reach ESRD after 15–20 year, and the diagnosis of diabetic nephropathy is rare in T1DM before 10 years duration (Tables 8.1 and 8.2).

The progression of diabetic nephropathy in T2DM has not been clearly delineated because of prolonged periods of asymptomatic, undiagnosed disease. About 3 % of "newly diagnosed" T2DM patients have overt nephropathy and macroalbuminuria, reflecting the delay in diagnosis. It is, however, estimated that the time to albuminuria from the onset of diabetes and the time to ESRD from the onset of albuminuria is similar in T1DM and T2DM [1]. Overall, diabetic nephropathy develops in 30–50 % of patients with T1DM within 5–10 years after the onset of diabetes, and in 20–30 % of patients with T2DM, often after a considerable duration of undiagnosed diabetes.

Many "atypical" features of T1DM and T2DM have become apparent over the last two decades. The prevalence of normoalbuminuria in subjects with T2DM and GFR <60 mL/min/1.73 m^2 was reported to be 39 % [2]. After accounting for the use of renin-angiotensin system inhibitors (RAS), the prevalence of normoalbuminuria in subjects with GFR <60 mL/min/1.73 m^2 was 23 %. Another study reported

L.J. Imbriano, M.D. (✉) • S. Shirazian, M.D.
Department of Medicine, Winthrop-University Hospital, 200 Old Country Road, Suite 135, Mineola, NY 11501, USA
e-mail: limbriano@winthrop.org; sshirazian@winthrop.org

J.K. Maesaka, M.D. • J. Mattana, M.D.
Department of Medicine, Division of Nephrology and Hypertension, 200 Old Country Road, Suite 135, Mineola, NY 11501, USA
e-mail: JMaesaka@winthrop.org; jmattana@winthrop.org

G. Jerums, M.D.
Austin Health, Endocrine Centre of Excellence, Heidelberg Repatriation Hospital, Heidelberg West, VIC 3081, Australia
e-mail: ah-endo@unimelb.edu.au

E.V. Lerma and V. Batuman (eds.), *Diabetes and Kidney Disease*,
DOI 10.1007/978-1-4939-0793-9_8, © Springer Science+Business Media New York 2014

a relatively high prevalence of discordance between impaired renal function and urinary albumin excretion—approximately 22 % of participants in a population survey had an estimated GFR <60 mL/min/1.73 m^2 and in these subjects 17 % had normoalbuminuria [3]. For hyperglycemic subjects with GFR between 60 and 89 mL/min, the prevalence of normoalbuminuria was reported to be 51 % [4]. This is noteworthy because albuminuria was thought to be linked to diabetic nephropathy and progression of renal insufficiency. The dissociation of albuminuria from declining GFR and even from the renal pathologic changes suggests alternative mechanisms are responsible for renal injury and the use of albuminuria as a biomarker of diabetic renal disease may not be reliable. In the early stages of diabetic nephropathy, changes in albumin excretion rates (AERs) and GFR may occur independently. Despite the lack of association of albuminuria with GFR, Jerums et al. report that patients with increasing amounts of proteinuria have a more rapid decline of GFR. Urinary albumin has classically been attributed to permeability defects in the glomerular filter. Russo et al. has suggested that the "normal-appearing" glomerulus may filter large amounts of albumin and albuminuria may result from failure of the proximal convoluted tubule (PCT) to reabsorb it [5]. This theory may explain the discordance between glomerular ultrastructural changes and albuminuria, but remains controversial. Nonetheless, PCT aberrations may play an important role in the induction and progression of diabetic nephropathy [6]. We intend to discuss some common but atypical features of diabetic nephropathy that do not follow the traditional sequence of hyperfiltration, microalbuminuria, and macroalbuminuria with gradual loss of nephron function. The process, however, appears to begin with the putative role of hyperglycemia and its effect on PCT function and induction of hyperfiltration.

Table 8.1 Categories of albuminuria

Relationship among categories for albuminuria and proteinuria			
	Categories		
Measure	Normal to mildly increased (A1)	Moderately increased (A2)	Severely increased (A3)
AER (mg/24 h)	<30	30–300	>300
PER (mg/24 h)	<150	150–500	>500
ACR			
(mg/mmol)	<3	3–30	>30
(mg/g)	<30	30–300	>300
PCR			
(mg/mmol)	<15	15–50	>50
(mg/g)	<150	150–500	>500
Protein reagent strip	Negative to trace	Trace to +	+ or greater

From KDIGO 2012 Clinical Practice Guidelines for the Evaluation and Management of Chronic Kidney Disease. Kidney Int. Supplement (3), issue 1: 2013. Used with permission

ACR albumin-to-creatinine ratio, *AER* albumin excretion rate, *PCR* protein-to-creatinine ratio, *PER* protein excretion rate [159]

Hyperfiltration and Kidney Growth

At the onset of diabetes mellitus, and within days of hyperglycemia [7] a series of changes occur that include the induction of multiple growth factors that stimulate hyperplasia of PCT cells and soon thereafter hypertrophy and lengthening of the proximal tubule [8]. In addition to the enlarged PCT, there is glucose-dependent up-regulation of transporters such as SGLT2 in the early PCT and SGLT1 in more distal sites of the PCT, which increase sodium-dependent transport of glucose and other solutes such as amino acids and phosphate [9]. Consequently, relatively less of the filtered sodium

Table 8.2 Prognosis of CKD by GFR and albuminuria categories: KDIGO 2012

				Persistent albuminuria categories		
				Description and range		
				A1	A2	A3
				Normal to mildly increased	Moderately increased	Severely increased
				<30 mg/g	30–300 mg/g	>300 mg/g
				<3 mg/mmol	3–30 mg/mmol	>30 mg/mmol
GFR categories (mL/min/1.73 m^2) Description and range	G1	Normal or high	≥90	Low risk	Moderately increased risk	High risk
	G2	Mildly decreased	60–89	Low risk	Moderately increased risk	High risk
	G3a	Mildly to moderately decreased	45–59	Moderately increased risk	High Risk	Very high risk
	G3b	Moderately to severely decreased	30–44	High risk	Very high risk	Very high risk
	G4	Severely decreased	15–29	Very high risk	Very high risk	Very high risk
	G5	Kidney failure	<15	Very high risk	Very high risk	Very high risk

From KDIGO 2012 Clinical Practice Guidelines for the Evaluation and Management of Chronic Kidney Disease. Kidney Int. Supplement (3), issue 1: 2013. Used with permission [159]

load is delivered to distal sites such as the macula densa, which activates the tubuloglomerular feedback (TGF) mechanism to dilate the afferent arteriole (via nitric oxide-mediated inhibition of adenosine) and increase renal blood flow (RBF), and GFR, in an attempt to correct the perceived low filtered load of sodium. Dilatation of the afferent glomerular arteriole increases RBF and intra-glomerular pressure well before the onset of albuminuria [10]. These changes occur more frequently in patients with T1DM. The increased blood flow to the glomerulus via the dilated afferent arteriole increases intra-glomerular hydrostatic pressure, which stimulates growth factors such as platelet-derived growth factor to increase glomerular size and increase GFR to supernormal levels or HF [11]. The increased reabsorption of solute and filtrate in the hypertrophied PCT may lower the hydrostatic pressure in Bowman's capsule (BC), creating a favorable pressure gradient that might contribute to HF [12, 13]. Advanced glycation end products (AGEs) may also contribute to HF. Infusion of early glycation products in rats increases RBF, GFR, and intra-glomerular pressure—mimicking poorly controlled diabetes [14]. Also, increased tubular exposure to glucose can lead to overexpression of the enzyme ornithine decarboxylase (ODC), which has been shown to induce hyperplasia and hypertrophy of PCT, contributing to HF by increasing PCT sodium reabsorption [15]. The ODC-induced kidney growth and increase in PCT sodium reabsorption could be attenuated by difluoromethylornithine (DFMO), an inhibitor of ODC [16]. Thomson et al. proposed the "tubulo-centric" model of HF, in which HF results mainly from a "primary" increase in PCT sodium reabsorption, decreasing sodium delivery to the distal tubule and activating TGF which dilates the afferent arteriole [17]. The PCT in diabetic subjects may respond paradoxically to salt delivery and inappropriately induce vasodilation on low salt diet and vasoconstriction on a high salt diet—the so-called salt paradox [18, 19]. It appears that HF appears to reflect a fundamental defect in PCT function in diabetes mellitus. HF may then increase the risk of developing micro- or macroalbuminuria, a complication that could be ameliorated by strict blood pressure (BP) control or improved glycemic control [20]. BP lowering may reduce the shear stress injury on dilated, patulous afferent and glomerular capillaries. We can conclude that the cause of HF remains atypical and may be due to several different mechanisms.

Classical vs. Nonclassical Definitions of Diabetic Nephropathy Based on Proteinuria

Classical albuminuric diabetic nephropathy develops in four consecutive stages over time: (a) renal hypertrophy and HF which occur early, with increased GFR and normoalbuminuria; (b) renal hypertrophy and HF are followed by a phase of intermittent to persistent microalbuminuria in T1DM which may persist for many years and during which structural changes develop; (c) persistent microalbuminuria, likely with hypertension, converts to macroalbuminuria which is associated with normal GFR, but reduced from the previous stage of HF; and (d) increasing levels of macroalbuminuria are associated with reduced GFR, and progression to ESRD and a GFR <15 cc/min. However, the relationships between HF, albuminuria, and development of decreased GFR are not entirely clear. For example, one study estimated HF by using an equation based on the reciprocal of serum cystatin C levels and found no evidence that HF predisposed to the development of microalbuminuria in T1DM [21]. This disparate finding may be related to better control of glucose, blood pressure, and hyperlipidemia over many years, thus minimizing the role of HF as a predictor of microalbuminuria. Studies have shown a less predictive value of microalbuminuria and even spontaneous remissions of microalbuminuria in 25–40 % of patients [22]. Also, the GFR may progressively decrease even in normoalbuminuric patients with either T1DM or T2DM [23] contradicting the concept that albuminuria induces progressive renal insufficiency. Some patients with diabetes and albuminuria remain stable; some show regression of microalbuminuria, while others can develop renal insufficiency without albuminuria. Albuminuria is a presumed tubular toxin, but non-albuminuric T2DM can still develop ESRD, although their rate of decline in eGFR is reduced after reaching eGFR of 60 mL/min/1.73 m^2. In subjects with T2DM and GFR <60 cc/min the prevalence of normo-, micro-, and macroalbuminuria has been reported as 39 %, 35 %, and 26 %, respectively. After accounting for the use of angiotensin-converting enzyme (ACE)-inhibition, the prevalence of normoalbuminuria was 23 % [2]. The discordance between albuminuria and GFR argues against using the urinary AER as a marker for renal injury [24, 25] and has led to a search for a different biomarker of diabetic nephropathy. To further magnify the dilemma of albuminuria vs. normoalbuminuria, Russo et al. suggested that albumin filtration at the glomerulus may be much greater than previously thought and the discovery of albuminuria may be primarily due to failure of an albumin retrieval pathway in the PCT [5]. However, this proposal does not address the finding of normoalbuminuria in some T2DM patients with renal insufficiency. An animal model of T2DM with normoalbuminuria (the Cohen diabetic rat) has been shown to develop progressive renal insufficiency with typical diabetic glomerulosclerosis, but without proteinuria [26]. Similarly, typical changes of diabetic nephropathy have been reported in normoalbuminuric patients with T1DM who have reduced GFR. In the last 5 years, there has been much debate on the roles of the glomerular filtration barrier (podocyte, slit diaphragm, GBM) and the PCT cells in albuminuria [27]. Data suggest that the podocyte slit diaphragm has pores that are much larger than previously known, large enough to permit albumin filtration [28]. Several studies have indicated that PCT cells reclaim filtered proteins, including albumin, to minimize proteinuria [29–31]. Could this reclamation/retrieval system, if true, play a role in the non-proteinuric diabetic patient? Further studies in diabetic rats might clarify the postulated mechanisms for non-proteinuric diabetic nephropathy.

Non-albuminuric Diabetic Nephropathy

HF predisposes to the development of micro- and macroalbuminuria, with a hazard ratio of 2.3 when compared with a concurrent (normoalbuminuric) control group [32]. But there is no evidence as yet that HF predicts declining GFR [1]. Microalbuminuria (dipstick negative) has been classically associated with progression to macroalbuminuria (dipstick positivity) in the majority of T1DM and T2DM patients. Others report that only 30–45 % of patients with microalbuminuria progress to more advanced stages of kidney disease [33]. In the Joslin Clinic Study of 386 patients with microalbuminuria who were followed for 6 years, regression of microalbuminuria was reported in 58 % of the subjects—especially in younger patients, patients with microalbuminuria of short duration, HbA1c < 8 %, systolic BP < 115 mmHg, cholesterol <5.12 mmol/L (92 mg/dL), and triglycerides <1.64 mmol/L (29 mg/dL). Interestingly, the use of ACE inhibitors was not associated with regression of microalbuminuria [34]. In contrast, the Melbourne Diabetic Nephropathy Study Group investigation showed regression of microalbuminuria in 54 % of normotensive subjects with T1DM when treated with the ACE inhibitor, perindopril [35]. The reason for reversion to normoalbuminuria without ACE-inhibition (Joslin) or with ACE-inhibition (Melbourne) remains unexplained, but may be due to hemodynamic factors, reduced glucose toxicity, improved integrity of the microcirculation, or due to a separate phenotype of diabetes, which might explain the failure of therapies designed to attenuate increasing albumin excretion to salvage renal function [36]. A cohort of 79 T1DM patients who developed new onset microalbuminuria after 4 years of follow-up were tracked by estimating their GFR by the Modification of Diet in Renal Disease formula for an additional 12 years. There was no concordance between GFR and degree of microalbuminuria. In this study, 11 of 23 patients, who progressed to stages 3–5 chronic kidney disease (CKD), never developed overt proteinuria that was independent of ACE inhibition. Perkins et al. also dissociated declining renal function from proteinuria [37]. Yokoyama et al. studied a population of patients with T2DM, renal insufficiency (eGFR < 60 mL/min/m^2), and normoalbuminuria. This clinical presentation was more likely in older patients, female sex, with longer duration of diabetes, higher prevalence of hypertension, hyperlipidemia, diabetic neuropathy, and cardiovascular disease. They ascribed these findings to age-associated senescence, interstitial fibrosis, renal ischemia due to intra-renal arteriosclerosis, and/or cholesterol emboli [4, 38, 39]. In another study there were no differences in the duration of diabetes, BMI, prevalence of retinopathy, vascular disease, smoking history, HbA1c levels, diastolic BP, total cholesterol (LDL or triglycerides), or the use of RAS-blockers in the normoalbuminuric as compared to the microalbuminuric patients [40]. It was proposed that intravascular disease of the afferent arteriole may contribute to the normoalbuminuric model, but intra-renal vascular resistance on renal duplex Doppler scan was elevated to a similar degree in patients with and without proteinuria in a study of patients with T2DM and GFR < 60 cc/min suggesting that normoalbuminuria in CKD is not likely to be due to vascular disease. A similar non-proteinuric progression of CKD in younger T1DM patients with less likelihood for intra-renal vascular disease supports the notion that intra-renal vascular disease is not an important contributor to non-albuminuric CKD. There were no associations between renal Doppler-resistive index (RI) and AER, systolic BP, or levels of HbA1c or cholesterol (total, LDL, HDL, or triglyceride level). The RI is increased to the same extent in T2DM with CKD regardless of their albuminuric status, whether normo-, micro-, or macroalbuminuric and was independent of the use of RAS inhibitors. Thus, hemodynamic manipulation or microvascular disease does not appear to explain CKD in normoalbuminuric diabetics [40]. Yokoyama et al. studied the slope of eGFR based on serial measurements of serum creatinine in normoalbuminuric patients with and without diabetes and hypertension [38]. They found that the slope (%/year decline in eGFR) was significantly larger in subjects with diabetes and normoalbuminuria than in subjects without diabetes and normoalbuminuria. Also, the degree of hyperglycemia and HbA1c contributed to the induction of HF and accelerating the subsequent decline in GFR even in normoalbuminuric T2DM patients [41]. The authors concluded that the renal pathophysiologic mechanisms that explain the relationship between declining GFR and UAE in T2DM are not well characterized, as they were unable to demonstrate a relationship between a declining GFR and UAE in T2DM. In summary, many, but not all, patients with T2DM or even T1DM develop renal failure during their lifetime. The classical concept of worsening proteinuria as a cause of progressive renal dysfunction has been recast by increasing recognition of non-albuminuric diabetic nephropathy. Investigators are seeking other risk factors and biomarkers that may predict poor outcomes, so that strategies may be developed for early intervention.

Atypical Pathology in Diabetic Nephropathy

Chronic hyperglycemia is a major cause of diabetic nephropathy. A number of circulating factors (growth factors, angiotensin II, TGF-β (TGF-beta), endothelin (ET), AGE, and oxidants), as well as glomerular HF with increased glomerular capillary hydrostatic pressure eventually result in the structural changes of diabetic nephropathy that include—mesangial expansion with mesangial cell proliferation and increased deposition of extracellular matrix proteins, such as types IV and V collagen, laminin, and fibronectin. Mesangial expansion restricts the glomerular capillary lumen and reduces filtration surface. Mesangial cellularity later diminishes as homogeneous acellular collagen nodules develop into diabetic nodular glomerulosclerosis (DNG). DNG is characterized by acellular nodular accumulations of extracellular mesangial matrix (Kimmelstiel Wilson lesion), diffuse mesangial sclerosis, diffuse thickening of the GBM and TBM, chronic interstitial inflammation, tubulointerstitial fibrosis and scarring, moderate to severe intimal and medial sclerosis of arteries, and hyalinosis of the afferent and efferent arterioles of the glomerulus. However, there is much heterogeneity of renal biopsy findings. Renal biopsies in 34 T2DM patients with eGFR>90 mL/min/1.73 m^2, microalbuminuria and preserved GFR revealed near normal findings, disproportionately severe tubular-interstitial lesions, advanced glomerular arteriolar hyalinosis, or global glomerulosclerosis—with less than one third having typical diabetic nephropathy [41]. It is important to consider that these biopsy findings in early T2DM may be due to the effects of aging, hypertension, and atherosclerosis, compared to younger patients with T1DM. Also, microalbuminuria is not specific for diabetic nephropathy and may be a manifestation of microvascular and endothelial injury in nondiabetic nephropathies. Furthermore it is estimated that 10–30 % of patients with T2DM and macroalbuminuria may have non-diabetic renal morphologic changes, while the majority of T2DM patients with eGFR<60 mL/min/1.73 m^2 and micro- or macroalbuminuria demonstrate the typical diabetic nephropathy (DN) pattern on renal biopsy. Patients with early diabetes and microalbuminuria exhibited moderate increases in glomerular and mesangial volume on kidney biopsy and could not be distinguished from subjects who remained normoalbuminuric after an equal duration of diabetes. The exact relationship between proteinuria, regression to non-albuminuria, renal morphologic change, and progressive loss of GFR in T2DM remains unclear, since the various patterns of glomerular change do not always correlate with the rate of decline in GFR [42]. Data suggest that progressively declining GFR and albuminuria are separate and independent events in the diabetic kidney. This break in the traditional concept of diabetic nephropathy has led to consideration of other factors that can alter the filtration and/or excretion of albumin including the possibilities of alterations of the slit diaphragm proteins [43, 44], or change in the reabsorptive capacity of the PCT cells.

Genetics of Diabetic Nephropathy

The genetic variations that affect the development of T2DM are generally unknown. Genome-wide association studies have identified gene targets that predispose individuals to diabetic nephropathy. In Japanese patients with T2DM, Maeda and colleagues demonstrated a role for transcription factor 7-like 2 (TCF7L2), which mediates part of the Wnt-signaling pathway and maps onto chromosome 10q250 [45]. They also identified polymorphisms in SLC12A3 (which encodes a renal thiazide-sensitive sodium-chloride co-transporter) in Caucasian patients with T2DM [46]. They also demonstrated that overexpression of the engulfment and cell motility-1 gene (ELMO1) is associated with development of diabetic nephropathy in white patients with T1DM. Increased expression of ELMO1 might enhance the expression of extracellular matrix proteins [47]. Pezzolesi reported an association between susceptibility to diabetic nephropathy and two loci; FRMD3 (chromosome 9q21-22) and CARS (chromosome 11p15.5) in the GoKinD cross-sectional cohort. FRMD3 contains genes that maintain red blood cell (RBC) shape and mechanical properties of membranes in several cell types, while CARS codes for the attachment of amino acids to their cognate transfer (t) 0052NA iso-accepting families [48]. Genetic susceptibility may also include the role of the ACE gene genotype. Patients with T2DM and the DD polymorphism are at increased risk for diabetic nephropathy, more severe proteinuria and ESRD [49]. Granhall demonstrated that several different loci in the Niddm1i region, a major glucose controlling region on chromosome 1, conferred various defects in insulin secretion in non-obese spontaneously diabetic Goto-Kakizaki (GK) rats [50]. The defects were not caused by a reduction in the pancreatic β-cell mass, but were due to alterations in glucose-stimulated calcium-dependent insulin release and to altered β-cell mitochondrial glucose handling, depending on the defective gene locus. Altered expression of exocytotic genes contributing to impaired insulin secretion was also reported by Andersson et al. [51]. Interestingly, the gene encoding for transcription factor TCF7L2 is located in the Niddm1i locus, and has recently been identified as a candidate gene for T2DM in humans [52]. Esguerra identified a perturbed miRNA network in the GK rat islets, which may contribute to decreased production of key proteins of the insulin exocytotic machinery [53]. miRNAs are short regulatory RNAs involved in many fundamental biological processes, which may increase or decrease expression of functional proteins such as silencing pancreatic duodenal homeobox 1 (PDX-1) in pancreatic islet cells. Yang et al. have shown that PDX-1 expression was decreased in pancreatic islets from patients with T2DM compared with nondiabetic human donors, due to increased DNA methylation of PDX-1 in the islet cells [54]. They also showed that hyperglycemia and elevated glycosylated hemoglobin (HbA1c) correlated negatively with mRNA expression and increased DNA methylation of PDX-1 in human islets. T2DM also includes insulin resistance at peripheral sites. Studies indicate that insulin resistance alone does not result in T2DM unless there is a β-cell inability to compensate for the insulin resistance with appropriate hyperinsulinemia [55]. Genetic susceptibility and the environment (obesity) may combine to impair insulin signaling, and lead to varying degrees of insulin resistance and T2DM. Increased levels of non-esterified fatty acid (NEFA) affect insulin signaling [56]. Adipose tissue normally secretes adipokines such as leptin and adiponectin, which enhance the sequestration of FFA as adipose triglyceride stores, reducing the deleterious effects of circulating FFAs and enhancing insulin sensitivity [57]. The polygenic nature of diabetes heredity, with many islet genes which may impair β-cell glucose metabolism, islet K+ channel function, expression of transcription factors, as well as a number of environmental factors have made for slow progress in the understanding of the genetic basis of diabetes and diabetic nephropathy. Aside from glucotoxicity and its effect on mesangial cells and podocytes, a congenital/genetic decrease in renal expression of nephrin and fewer slit diaphragms has been described [58]. Genetic susceptibility may also include the role of the ACE gene genotype. Patients with type 2 diabetes and the DD polymorphism are at increased risk for diabetic nephropathy, more severe proteinuria and ESRD [49]. Diabetic nephropathy represents only one target of the polymorphic genetic alteration resulting in diabetes. Whether this is due to an altered miRNA expression, adiponectin defects, or to one of the myriad proteins which are responsible for normal mesangial function, collagen assembly or protein handling remains to be determined.

The Toll of Inflammation and Oxidative Stress Induced by Glucotoxicity

Because normoalbuminuric diabetic patients can develop CKD with eGFR < 60 mL/min/1.73 m^2, consideration must be given that other mechanisms lead to CKD in these patients. Hyperglycemia has been shown to be associated with inflammation [59]. Hyperglycemia suppresses the monocyte membrane receptor (CD-33), which normally down-regulates cytokine production, resulting in increased production of inflammatory cytokines TNFα (TNF-alpha), IL-1β (IL-1-beta), and IL-8 [60]. Diabetes begets diabetes because TNFα inhibits pancreatic insulin production [61]. Hyperglycemia also leads to enhanced glycolysis and mitochondrial overproduction of superoxide (O_2^-) and other reactive oxygen species (ROS), which directly activate protein kinase-C (PKC) and nuclear factor-κ (kappa) B (NF-κB) [62, 63]. In turn, glucose-activated PKC increases the production of extracellular matrix, increases permeability and vascular cell proliferation, leading to renal and retinal anomalies. Niewczas found a strong correlation between the levels of inflammatory mediators (TNF-α and Fas) and reduced cystatin-C-estimated GFR (cC-GFR) in T1DM patients, independent of the degree of proteinuria [64]. TNF-α and Fas mediate inflammation and apoptosis, respectively. TNF-α mediates its signal via TNF-receptors 1 and 2 (TNFR-1, TNFR-2), which are membrane bound as well as circulating soluble receptors. Induction of the receptors releases a broad spectrum of inflammatory substances including IL-8 (CXCL-8), monocyte chemotactic protein-1 (MCP-1 or CCL-2), interferon gamma-inducible protein-10 (CXCL-10), intercellular adhesion molecule-1 (ICAM-1), and vascular cell adhesion molecule-1 (VCAM-1). TNF-α increases permeability (as does PKC) and reduces GFR in animal models [65, 66]. Exposure of kidney cells to TNF-α or sTNFR-1 increases mRNA expression of TNFRs in the tubulointerstitium, triggering cell death [67]. Circulating levels of TNFRs 1 and 2 (not free or total TNF-α) were strongly associated with the risk of ESRD in T2DM independently of all relevant clinical covariates, and regardless of whether urinary albumin excretion was in the normoalbuminuric or macroalbuminuric range [68]. The levels of TNF-α and TNFRs 1 and 2 did not appear to be due to reduced GFR since most patients in Niewczas' study had normal renal function, and even the renal function loss resulting from uninephrectomy (in animals) does not raise serum TNFR concentrations [69]. Thus, glucotoxicity appears to cause inflammation, tubulointerstitial changes, and reduced GFR even before the onset of proteinuria, and may explain why even mildly increased HbA1c levels correlate strongly with progressive CKD [70].

Contribution of Immunoglobulin Light Chains to Diabetic Nephropathy

There is evidence that immunoglobulin light chains may play a role in diabetic nephropathy as well. Free light chains (FLCs) fit into the proposal that endocytosis of albumin induces cytokine production by the PCT to promote tubulointerstitial nephritis [71]. The relevance of FLC in this cascade of inflammatory cytokine production becomes evident after reviewing studies which demonstrate FLC to be much more injurious to proximal tubule cell function than albumin. Immunoglobulin light chains are 22,000 Da polypeptides that are synthesized by plasma cells and assembled with heavy chains to form different classes of intact immunoglobulins, e.g., immunoglobulin G (IgG) and immunoglobulin A (IgA). Plasma cells normally produce a slight excess of light chains, which can be measured with the FLC radioimmunoassay. The circulating levels are fairly constant in the normal adult; normal levels of κ (kappa) 3.3–19.4 mg/L and of λ (lambda) 5.71–26.3 mg/L, yielding a κ (kappa)/λ (lambda) ratio of 0.25–1.65. Serum FLC may rise during chronic inflammatory states such as rheumatoid arthritis, multiple sclerosis, or when malignant B-cells or plasma cells produce a monoclonal FLC. κ (kappa)-FLC exist primarily as monomers (~22.5 kDa molecular mass) while λ (lambda)-FLC circulate as covalently linked dimers with a molecular mass of ~45 kDa. The smaller κ (kappa)-FLC has a higher renal clearance than the larger λ (lambda)-FLC to account for the higher κ (kappa)/λ (lambda) FLC ratio of 2.04–10.37 in normal urine. The kidney is the major site of metabolism of light chains. The FLC are endocytosed by the PCT cells via megalin/cubilin receptors and are eventually catabolized within lysosomes with only minute quantities appearing in normal urine [72].

Increased urine FLC may be due to increased production as in multiple myeloma or lymphoma or injury to the proximal tubule brush border receptors. Patients with paraproteinemic diseases produce monoclonal glomerulopathic light chains, which have altered molecular structure and misfold, resulting in light chain deposition disease or amyloidosis, or produce monoclonal tubulopathic light chains, which can induce cast nephropathy or the myeloma kidney.

Studies have shown that myeloma light chains become endocytosed by PCT cells, activate NF-κB and induce the production and release of interleukins IL-6 and IL-8, and monocyte chemoattractant protein-1 (MCP-1) [73]. There was variability among six different types of myeloma light chains, although the induction of inflammatory cytokines was >10-fold higher than equal doses of albumin [73]. A similar greater potency of myeloma light chains over that of albumin was also demonstrated in the induction of IL-6, and MCP-1 by activation of MAP kinases ERK1,2, JNK, and p38 in the PCT [74]. Light chains from patients with plasma cell dyscrasia can also induce production of hydrogen peroxide and MCP-1, effects which were inhibited by pyrrolidine dithiocarbamate, an inhibitor of NF-κB [75]. Human serum albumin had no effect on cytokine production. It would appear that light chains, when present, are a more potent contributor than albumin to the initiation and progression of tubulointerstitial inflammation and fibrosis, which is a superior marker of risk for progression of CKD than changes noted in glomeruli [76]. The contribution of FLC to diabetic nephropathy becomes compelling after noting their effects on PCT. Polyclonal FLCs in plasma of T2DM are increased before the onset of proteinuria or reduction in GFR [77]. This increase can have potentially profound effects on PCT because of the HF that accompanies it. As noted above, hyperglycemia sequentially induces PCT hyperplasia, hypertrophy, lengthening of the proximal tubule and glomerular HF. The combination of increased serum FLC and HF leads to increase in the filtered load of FLC, which can be endocytosed in larger quantities by an increase in megalin and cubilin receptors resulting from a lengthened proximal tubule. The endocytosed FLC would then activate NF-κB and MAP kinases to increase ROS, IL-6, IL-8, and MCP-1 in greater quantities than equidoses of albumin to increase interstitial inflammation, fibrosis, and apoptosis [73]. It is plausible that this process early in the course of diabetic nephropathy might contribute to the eventual decrease in GFR and risk for advancing CKD. The reduction in whole-kidney GFR would be expected to induce HF of the remaining glomeruli by afferent arteriolar vasodilatation resulting from vasodilators such as prostaglandin I_2, and possibly E_2, and D_2 [78]. As whole-kidney GFR decreases, the filtered load of polyclonal FLCs progressively increases to progressively higher levels through hyperfiltering nephrons as the patient progresses from stage 1 to stage 5 CKD. Moreover, FLCs have been shown to be prominently higher in CKD associated with diabetes than in other causes of CKD [77]. Mean serum and urine polyclonal κ (kappa) and λ (lambda) FLC were significantly higher in patients with diabetic nephropathy (mean eGFR 25 mL/min) when compared to the entire CKD subjects (mean eGFR 29.4 mL/min). Serum FLC levels progressively increased with each stage of CKD, being fivefold higher at a pre-dialysis stage of their disease. The fractional excretion of FLCs was also higher in the diabetic group, suggesting a defective proximal tubule function [6]. As in the early stages of diabetes, the combination of progressively increasing levels of FLC in plasma and maximally hyperfiltrating glomeruli significantly increases the filtered load of FLC per nephron. In this scenario, the FLC-induction of inflammatory cytokines would increase apoptosis and interstitial inflammation and fibrosis to a greater extent and contribute to and possibly accelerate progression of CKD. Based on the combination of increased and increasing serum levels of FLCs and HF in early and at each stage of CKD in diabetes, there are reasons to implicate FLC as a contributor to diabetic nephropathy, irrespective of whether or not there is albuminuria or decreased whole-kidney GFR. The contribution of the PCT to this process is also in keeping with the proposal that the PCT is a major site for the initiation and progression of kidney disease in diabetes. Despite the known nephrotoxicity of monoclonal FLC, the toxicity of polyclonal FLCs has not been thoroughly appreciated. Polyclonal FLCs may be toxic to renal tubule cells. Groop et al. showed that newly diagnosed T1DM, long standing T1DM, or T2DM had increased excretion of κ (kappa) light chains with normal serum concentration of κ (kappa) light chains, implying that the increased urinary κ (kappa) light chains were of renal origin, although it can be explained by a higher fractional excretion of κ (kappa) light chains, suggesting either increased κ (kappa) light chain production or decreased proximal tubule reabsorption possibly implicating early PCT dysfunction [79]. Urinary IgLCs can be higher in T2DM with albuminuria and normoalbuminuria than in normal controls before the onset of renal disease [80].

Antigenic stimulation of immunoglobulin light chains can induce plasma extravasation, cutaneous swelling, and mast cell degranulation whereas cross-linking of receptor-bound IgLC by an antigen leads to mast cell degranulation, release of pro-inflammatory IL-8, and the induction of a local inflammatory response [81, 82]. Immunoglobulin light chains and IgE could exert similar pro-inflammatory effects via polymorphonuclear cells (PMNs) by sharing a common functionality [82]. Non-clonal FLC do not appear to be merely spillover products, but are mediators of inflammation by targeting various cell lines that are capable of anti-angiogenic, proteolytic, and complement-activating activities. It is, therefore, possible that monoclonal and polyclonal FLC would have similar patterns of affecting cell function, which gives credence to the proposal that polyclonal FLC can induce and possibly accelerate progression of diabetic nephropathy. Future studies must examine this interesting possibility.

Type IV RTA

Hyporeninemic hypoaldosteronism or type IV renal tubular acidosis (RTA) is frequently encountered in patients with diabetic nephropathy. Type IV RTA is characterized by impaired secretion of both H+ and K+ due to a decrease in renin and/or aldosterone release, resulting in metabolic acidosis and hyperkalemia. Hyperkalemia compounds the degree of acidosis by impairing NH_4^+ production and excretion. The metabolic acidosis is usually mild with the plasma HCO_3^- concentration remaining above 15 mEq/L. The urine pH is usually below 5.3, unlike distal RTA (RTA-I) where urine pH is nearly always over 5.5. The metabolic anomaly is disproportionately severe while the GFR is only mild to moderately decreased. There are no recent estimates of its prevalence or associations. Potassium concentrations were studied in 1,764 consecutive diabetic patients at a hospital clinic, normal potassium defined as 3.5–5.0 mmol/L. They found potassium levels >5 mmol/L in 369 patients (21 %) as compared to 4 % with hypokalemia whereas 14 of 67 (20 %) had potassium >5.4 mmol/L due to potassium-sparing medications and 12 of 67 (18 %) had serum creatinine greater than 140 μmol/L or 1.58 mg/dL [82]. Hyperkalemia appears to be relatively common in unselected diabetic outpatients, and physicians must consider the dangers of prescribing medications that increase potassium [83]. The treatment of type IV RTA includes a low potassium diet, polystyrene sulfonate, fludrocortisone, sodium bicarbonate, and loop diuretics.

Diabetes and Renal Tumors

A population-based retrospective cohort study of Swedish inpatients discharged with a diagnosis of diabetes mellitus between 1965 and 1983, followed up until 1989, showed an increased incidence of renal cell cancer (267 cases vs. the 182.4 that had been expected using age-specific, sex-specific, and period-specific standardized incidence ratios, SIRs). Increased risks were observed in both women (SIR = 1.7, 95 % confidence interval, CI = 1.4–2.0) and men (SIR 1.3, 95 % CI = 1.1–1.6) throughout the 25-year observation period. A higher risk was observed for kidney cancer mortality (SMR = 1.9; 95 % CI = 1.7–2.2 for women and SMR 1.7; 95 % CI = 1.4–1.9 for men). Compared with the general population, patients with DM showed an increased risk of renal cancer [84]. The marked increase of solid tumors in patients with diabetes mellitus was investigated by Habib and others in a retrospective analysis of 473 patients who underwent nephrectomy for RCC in a South Texas population [85]. Of the 473 cases with RCC, 120 patients (25.4 %) had a history of DM, more common in women and in Hispanics compared to White and other ethnic backgrounds. The majority of patients were 50–59 years of age. Clear cell histology predominated in 90 % of the cases of RCC in these diabetic patients. In 98 % of these tumors, the clear cell subtype resulted from a somatic mutation within the VHL tumor-suppressor gene found on the short arm of chromosome 3 3p25 [86–88]. Mutation of VHL activate hypoxia-inducible factor-1 (HIF-1) which leads to increased expression of pro-angiogenic factors including PDGF and VEGF, factors that play a key role in renal cell tumor genesis. Renal tumor incidence in diabetic patients may also be related to prolonged exposure to pro-insulin produces with homology to IGF-1, other growth factors, increased endogenous estrogen levels or hypertension [84]. The authors showed that HbA1c values were significantly higher in patients with tumors 1–5 cm, compared to tumors >5–10 cm suggesting that HbA1c might be a useful marker for early detection of small, silent RCCs, before they become clinically manifest. Hispanics have a higher prevalence of obesity, type 2 diabetes and high fat diet, factors which may play a role in increased incidence of RCC. Evidence exists of an association between obesity and risk of RCC [89].

Diabetic Cystopathy

Diabetic cystopathy (DC) is a newer term for neurogenic bladder and refers to motor and sensory dysregulation of the bladder detrusor and the entire contractile apparatus. Poor emptying will progress to urgency, urge incontinence, and overflow incontinence. Bladder dysfunction was discovered in diabetic patients without retinopathy, and in patients without subjective urinary symptoms [90]. A 2011 study of 52 diabetic men with lower urinary tract symptoms (LUTS), with mean age of 61 years, and mean duration of diabetes of 11 years described their urodynamic profile. Impaired first sensation (>250 mL) was noted in 23 %, increased capacity (> 600 mL) in 25 %, detrusor underactivity in 79 %, detrusor overactivity in 38.5 %, high post-void residual volume (>1/3 capacity) in 65 %, and bladder outlet obstruction in 29 %. Both sensory and motor diabetic cystopathy correlated with abnormal motor and sensory nerve conduction velocity studies on these patients. Bansal et al. concluded that electrophysiological evidence of motor or sensory neuropathy can predict the presence of cystopathy in a large proportion of diabetic patients [91].

Papillary Necrosis

Renal papillary necrosis (RPN) is a coagulative necrosis of the renal medullary pyramid and its tip—the papilla. RPN may be caused by conditions, medications, or toxins that share the ability to induce local ischemia. Since the kidney has multiple mechanisms to maintain kidney oxygenation during renal ischemia papillary necrosis usually occurs when several conditions coexist in the same patient [91]. Patients with hemoglobinopathies or microvascular disease (vasculitides, diabetes mellitus) become increasingly susceptible to ischemia when hypovolemia, hypoxia, or shock coexists. Most cases of RPN occur during the fifth and sixth decade of life, and is very uncommon in patients under 40 years of age or in children, unless they have several coexisting conditions, for example, sickle cell disease or trait, combined with nonsteroidal use, and/or volume depletion. RPN may be acute or chronic. It is often bilateral. The clinical severity depends on the degree of ischemia [92], the number of papillae involved, concurrent hemodynamic status/medications, and the presence or absence of obstruction.

Diabetes and Contrast-Induced Nephropathy

Diabetics are at increased risk of contrast-induced nephropathy (CIN) when exposed to radiocontrast dye. CIN refers to acute kidney injury (AKI) which develops after radiocontrast infusion. Among patients with no risk factors the risk of CIN is <1 %, while patients with risk factors (DM, CHF, CKD, myeloma, or dehydration) have risk of 10–20 % [93]. The typical morphologic change associated with CIN is acute tubular necrosis (ATN). CIN is generally reversible within 3–6 days, unlike the recovery from other forms of ATN, which resolve slowly over 3–5 weeks. The mechanism of CIN-ATN is not clearly understood; the ATN may be caused by renal vasoconstriction (mediated by endothelin and adenosine) with resulting hypoxia/ischemia or the ATN is a direct result of the cytotoxic nature of radiocontrast agents, inducing the production of oxygen-free radicals and ROS. The quick recovery from CIN may be related to less destructive effects on the renal tubule cells. Protein excretion is absent or negligible. This is hard to determine if the urine is checked by dipstick within 24–36 h of contrast exposure because iodinated contrast agents induce a false positive result with the dipstick or the sulfosalicylic acid method is used to detect protein. It remains puzzling why CIN-ATN is associated with an FENa <1 % while most patients remain nonoliguric. Patients with DM are at increased risk of CIN, possibly related to impaired nitric oxide generation [94]. Diabetic patients with CKD (creatinine > 1.69 mg/dL) are at higher risk for CIN than nondiabetics with CKD and creatinine > 1.69 mg/dL. After having IV contrast for a CT scan, the incidence of CIN was 8.8 % in the diabetics with CKD, vs. 4.4 % in the nondiabetics with CKD [95]. Among diabetic patients with normal renal function, diabetes did not increase the risk of CIN [96]. It has been well established that glucotoxicity and hyperglycemia result in cellular imbalance favoring ROS over natural antioxidant defenses. Hyperglycemia causes gradual deterioration of glomerular mesangial cells (MCs). Wasaki et al. studied the response of rat mesangial cells (MCs) cultured in normal glucose and high-glucose medium when exposed to diatrizoate (a high-osmolar contrast agent) and to iohexol (a low osmolar contrast agent) [97]. Cytotoxic effects were monitored by neutral red uptake in the MCs. Both contrast media decreased the viability of the cells pre-cultured under basal-glucose conditions. MCs that were pre-cultured under high-glucose conditions showed increased cytotoxic effects with both contrast media, showing increased intracellular peroxide levels. Interestingly, pre-culture treatment with the antioxidant, D-alpha-tocopherol (Toc) prevented the increased cytotoxic effects of diatrizoate on the high-glucose cells. No protective effect was noted for the Toc-treated cells exposed to a different agent, iohexol. It appears that MCs exposed to high glucose are already experiencing oxidative stress, and demonstrate increased susceptibility to the cytotoxic effects of contrast media. Recent studies comparing short-term high loading dose of atorvastatin alone or combined with *N*-acetylcysteine showed a significant beneficial effect of atorvastatin in reducing the rate of contrast-induced AKI in low to medium risk patients [98–100]. Atorvastatin has been shown to have immediate antioxidant activity and antiplatelet effects via inhibition of Nox-2. Patients with hypercholesterolemia were assigned to either a low cholesterol diet or atorvastatin (40 mg/day). Oxidative stress (as assessed by serum Nox-2 and urinary isoprostanes), was reduced, as well as platelet aggregation (as assessed by platelet recruitment, platelet isoprostanes, Nox2, and PKC) in the atorvastatin group, while no change was noted in the low cholesterol group [101]. Many studies have focused on the use of oral *N*-acetylcysteine with or without i.v. isotonic saline or sodium bicarbonate infusion to reduce the risk of contrast nephropathy in at risk patients. Mueller et al. reported isotonic saline hydration was superior to half-isotonic hydration in the prevention of contrast media-associated nephropathy [102]. The efficacy of such treatments varies considerably by center, by specific contrast procedure, by type of contrast, and by dose of contrast [103–106]. In general, a variety of preventative measures may individually or in combination reduce the risk of contrast nephropathy; (a) alternative imaging studies, such as ultrasound, CT without contrast, MRI; (b) lower doses of contrast, preferably less than 30 mL; (c) low or iso-osmolal nonionic (iodixanol) contrast agents; (d) avoid repetitive contrast studies within 72 h; (e) avoid volume depletion; (f) avoid nonsteroidal anti-inflammatory medications; (g) administration of intravenous isotonic saline or sodium bicarbonate; (h) administration of antioxidants, *N*-acetylcysteine, atorvastatin.

Nondiabetic Renal Disease in the Diabetic Patient

Since the realization that albuminuria is not necessarily linked to renal function loss in patients with diabetes, it has become increasingly important to clarify the prevailing renal disorder when certain parameters indicate that the renal disorder is not related to diabetes. The major clues which can be used to justify renal biopsy in diabetic patients in search of nondiabetic glomerular disease are: (a) the onset of proteinuria less than 5 years from the onset of T1DM, since the latent period for overt macroalbuminuria is usually 10–15 years from diagnosis. To estimate the precise time of the onset of diabetes is often difficult in T2DM, but the latent period is likely similar; (b) the presence of active urine sediment such as RBC, RBC casts, or acanthocytes; (c) acute deterioration of renal function; diabetic nephropathy is a slowly progressive loss of GFR; (d) the absence of retinopathy or neuropathy in T1DM; in contrast, retinopathy is relatively less prevalent in T2DM with biopsy-proven diabetic nephropathy [107]; (e) signs and symptoms of another systemic disease; (f) reduction in GFR > 30 % within 2 months of start of angiotensin blockade [108]; (g) loss of GFR > 10 mL/min/year with increasing albuminuria, in the absence of retinopathy; (h) hypercalcemia.

Therapeutic Measures for Diabetic Nephropathy

In addition to the use of approved medications for the treatment of diabetes mellitus, several investigational agents have been studied, with mixed results.

Antihypertensive Therapy

RAS blockade has been shown to reduce proteinuria and slow the progression of diabetic renal disease. An extension of this concept, specifically dual inhibition of the RA System with ACE-inhibitor + ARB, or ACE-I or ARB + renin blocker [109] has not shown benefit for preservation of renal function or for stroke prevention [110, 111]. Dual blockade actually increased the risk of requiring dialysis, and in another study it increased cardiovascular risk.

Aldosterone Blockade

Aldosterone blockade confers the theoretical advantage of inhibiting mineralocorticoid receptors on podocytes [112, 113], possibly being more effective in reducing proteinuria than an ARB [114]. Elevation of serum potassium may limit the use of aldosterone receptor blockers whether they are used as a sole treatment or in combination with and ACE inhibitor or an ARB.

Endothelin Receptor Blockade

Avosentan lowers the albumin-to-creatinine ratio by nearly 45 % and lowers BP when added to ACE inhibitors, but was associated with increasing edema and heart failure, terminating the trial [115].

SGLT 2 Inhibitors

SGLT 2 inhibitors are a new class of oral drugs in phase II development for the treatment of type 2 DM [116]. Agents that block the sodium-glucose transporter-2 in the PCT allow excessively filtered glucose to be excreted in the urine—effectively lowering blood glucose levels, HbA1c, and possibly BP. The reduction in systemic hyperglycemia may be the renoprotective benefit. This is an insulin-independent method of lowering blood glucose. Glucose control is improved, and weight loss and BP reduction are associated with their use, with low risk of hypoglycemia. A mean reduction in HbA1c ranging from 0.58 to 0.89 % was observed in the dapagliflozin group compared with 0.23 % in the placebo group [117]. Mean systolic BP was reduced by 3–5 mm/Hg and diastolic BP by approx. 2 mm/Hg, which could potentially convey additional cardiovascular benefit. The use of SGLT-2 inhibitors may increase the frequency of UTIs [118]. Genital tract infections (vulvovaginitis/balanitis) were more frequent.

Inhibitors of Advanced Glycation End-Product Production and Action

The accumulation of advanced glycated proteins may play a role in the progression of microvascular and macro-vascular complications [119, 120]. Studies with nonspecific blockers of AGE formation were found to be unsafe [121, 122]. New agents, which block the receptor for AGE (RAGE) are being studied [123, 124].

Inhibition of Inflammation

Metabolic pathways linked to inflammation play significant roles in the development of diabetes. Insulin resistance has been found to be modulated by macrophages [125]. Adipose tissue macrophages may regulate a variety of cytokines that affect insulin resistance [126]. Adiponectin, an adipocyte-derived hormone activates an energy-sensing enzyme, AMPK, which suppresses inflammation, in part via inhibition of NF-κB activation and NADPH oxidase production [127, 128].

MCP-1 (chemokine CC motif ligand-2 [CCL-2]) recruits macrophages to experimental diabetic kidneys [129, 130]. Blockade of MCP-1 or its receptor CCR-2 may affect progression of diabetic kidney disease. Other inflammatory cytokines are unregulated in models of diabetic kidney disease, including TNF-α, IL-6, IL-1β, and IL-18. Mycophenolate mofetil and pentoxiphyline have been shown to reduce cytokine elevation in preclinical models [131].

Modification of m-Tor Pathway

Activation of AMPK by AMPK activators, AICAR, berberine [132–135], resveratrol [136, 137], calorie restriction, exercise, metformin, or rosiglitazone offer renoprotection and cardiovascular protection, the latter two reducing the rate of renal decline when compared to sulfonylurea agents [138]. Metformin activates AMPK (amp-activated protein kinase) and orchestrates the regulation of pathways that consume or generate ATP; the phosphorylation of AMPK is the mechanism whereby metformin suppresses hepatic gluconeogenesis, lowering blood glucose, and reducing kidney hypertrophy (independent of blood glucose) [133]. The mammalian target of rapamycin, mTOR, is downstream of AMPK, and plays an important role in diabetic kidney hypertrophy. Rapamycin inhibits renal hypertrophy in mouse and rat models [139–141]. mTOR, a serine/threonine protein kinase, controls cell growth and metabolism in response to energy (via AMPK). Rapamycin binding to the intracellular receptor, FK-506-binding protein FKBP12, inhibits growth via inhibition of mTORC1. Diabetes is associated with increased mTORC1 activity, and inhibiting mTORC1 may be protective against diabetes podocyte dysfunction [142]. Diabetic renal hypertrophy and the effects of hyperglycemia on mesangial cells has been closely linked to mTOR activity and its downstream effector proteins; mTORC1, mTORC2 and 4E-BP1 [143].

Inhibiting Fibrosis and Oxidative Stress

Bardoxolone, an anti-inflammatory and antioxidant, targets Nrf-2 signaling and mitochondrial oxidative stress, up-regulating a variety of antioxidant molecules (SOD, GPX, and catalase) [144, 145]. One clinical trial found that bardoxolone dosing resulted in reductions of serum creatinine and increased GFR in diabetic patients with CKD [146]. The effects may relate to the blockade of oxidative damage, a hemodynamic effect, or to the ability to stimulate AMPK binding mTOR [147, 148]. Unfortunately while bardoxolone increased GFR it also increased proteinuria [149]. Other side effects were related to low magnesium, phosphorus, and increased liver enzymes. Recently however the Beacon Study of bardoxolone revealed excess adverse reactions, excess mortality, and the study was halted; diminishing hopes that bardoxolone would benefit patients with diabetic nephropathy [150].

Pirfenidone

Another anti-inflammatory, antifibrotic agent, pirfenidone, has been found to be effective in animal models of kidney disease [151–153]. Anti-TGF-β-mediated antifibrotic approaches have been shown in mouse models of kidney disease [154, 155]. A multicenter phase-2 trial of an anti-TGF-β-1-specific antibody in patients with diabetic kidney disease is currently ongoing (clinicaltrials.gov # NCT 01113801).

microRNA Therapy

miRNA such as miR-192 is up-regulated in diabetes, possibly induced by hyperglycemia and/or TGF-β. miR-192 is the master regulator of other key renal miRNAs and downstream genes, which regulate TGF-β signaling for renal mesangial cell fibrosis [156]. RNA-based therapeutics for blocking disease associated genes and noncoding RNAs such as chemically modified oligonucleotide (oligo) small interfering RNAs (siRNAs) and anti-miRNAs have been used before [157]. Locked nucleic acid (LNA)-modified oligos have shown promise in the field of small interfering RNA and miRNA therapies. Treatment with LNA-anti-miRNA-192 down-regulated the mRNA expression of key extra-cellular matrix-associated pro-fibrotic genes such as collagen Iα2 (COLA42), COLA41, TGF-β, connective tissue growth factor and fibronectin. The cumulative effect of LNA-anti-miRNA-192 was a decrease in kidney injury and an improvement in proteinuria [156].

Allopurinol

Allopurinol treatment to lower serum uric acid levels in patients with CKD may slow the rate of renal function decline. Long term studies in T1DM patients with CKD and proteinuria are underway [158].

Summary and Conclusions

The pathogenesis of diabetic nephropathy may be casually perceived to be due to hyperglycemia, but interplay of many atypical mechanisms has been formulated. The earliest event is increased growth of the PCT and dilation of the glomerular afferent arteriole, leading to hyperfiltration. Several theories relate hyperfiltration to overexpression of ODC, a primary increase in sodium reabsorption, TGF, or to AGEs. The "classic" association of DN with albuminuria has been shown to be nondiagnostic, as many diabetic patients may progress to renal failure without albuminuria. Genetic alterations increase susceptibility to diabetes and DN. A dozen or more cytokines and hormones interact and create an inflammatory state. It is possible that this results in an increase in FLC production and filtration—with increased reabsorption of the FLC by the longer and larger PCT. It may be possible that the excessive light chain reabsorption injures the PCT cells resulting in renal pathological changes, as well as reduced reabsorption and increased excretion of the filtered FLC. The renal injury may be a tubulointerstitial injury, which could possibly explain the discrepancies in renal biopsy findings in diabetic patients, many of whom do not present the classical DNG. Hyperglycemia alone induces the production of several cytokines including TNF-α, IL-1β, IL-8, TGF-β, ROS, and VEGF. Hyperglycemia may also cause the rearrangement of nuclear proteins so that they code for increased matrix and fibrosis. The chronic inflammatory state may induce endothelial cell injury, with increasing levels of extracellular microparticles (EMPs), which may serve as a marker the progressive micro- and macro-vascular disease accompanying diabetes. We hope that this chapter provides clinical and experimental information which can be used to improve the diagnosis and treatment of diabetic patients. The increasing incidence of this systemic disease with pleiotropic and atypical manifestations warrants continued intense scrutiny to uncover the pathophysiologic mechanisms which lead to renal injury and death.

References

1. Ritz E, Orth SR. Nephropathy in patients with type 2 diabetes mellitus. N Engl J Med. 1999;341:1127.
2. MacIsaac RJ, Tsalamandris C, Panagiotopoulos S, Smith TS, McNeil KJ, Jerums G. Nonalbuminuric renal insufficiency in type 2 diabetes. Diabetes Care. 2004;27:195–200.
3. Parving HH, Lewis JB, Ravid M, Wajman A, Tadgell C, Remuzzi G, et al. Prevalence and risk factors for microalbuminuria in type 2 diabetic patients: a global perspective. Diabetologia. 2004;47 Suppl 1:A64.
4. Bakris G, McGill JB, Chen S, Li S, Collins A, Brown W. Microalbuminuria and hyperglycemia: the changing landscape of chronic kidney disease (CKD). Diabetes. 2005;54 Suppl 1:A54.
5. Russo LM, Sandoval RM, McKee M, Osicka TM, Collins AB, Brown D, Molitoris BA, Comper WD. The normal kidney filters nephrotic levels of albumin retrieved by proximal tubule cells; retrieval is disrupted in nephrotic states. Kidney Int. 2007;71: 505–13.
6. Vallon V. The proximal tubule in the pathophysiology of the diabetic kidney. Am J Physiol Regul Integr Comp Physiol. 2011; 300(5):R1009–22.
7. Brocco E, Firoetto P, Maurer M, et al. Renal structure and function in non-insulin dependent diabetic patients with microalbuminuria. Kidney Int Suppl. 1997;63:S40–4.
8. Rasch R, Dorup J. Quantitative morphology of the rat kidney during diabetes mellitus and insulin treatment. Diabetologia. 1997;40: 802–9.
9. Vallon V, Richter K, Blantz RC, Thomson S, Osswald H. Glomerular hyperfiltration in experimental diabetes mellitus: potential role of tubular reabsorption. J Am Soc Nephrol. 1999;10: 2569–76.
10. Jin Y, Moriya T, Tanaka K, Matsubara M, Fujita Y. Glomerular hyperfiltration in non-proteinuric and non-hypertensive Japanese type 2 diabetic patients. Diabetes Res Clin Pract. 2006;71(3): 264–71.
11. Jerums G, Premaratne E, Panagiotopoulos S, MacIsaac RJ. The clinical significance of hyperfiltration in diabetes. Diabetologia. 2010;53(10):2093–104.
12. Persson P, Hansell P, Palm F. Tubular reabsorption and diabetes-induced glomerular hyperfiltration. Acta Physiol (Oxf). 2010; 200(1):3–10.
13. Hannedouche TP, Delgado AG, Gnionsahe DA, et al. Renal hemodynamics and segmental tubular reabsorption in early type I diabetes. Kidney Int. 1990;37:1126.
14. Sabbatini M, Sansone G, Uccello F, et al. Early glycosylation products induce glomerular hyperfiltration in normal rats. Kidney Int. 1992;42:875.
15. Thomson SC, Deng A, Bao D, Satriano J, Blantz RC, Vallon V. Ornithine decarboxylase, kidney size, and the tubular hypothesis of glomerular hyperfiltration in experimental diabetes. J Clin Invest. 2001;107:217–24.
16. Pedersen SB, Flyvbjerg A, Richelsen B. Inhibition of renal ornithine decarboxylase activity prevents kidney hypertrophy in experimental diabetes. Am J Physiol. 1993;264:C433–56.
17. Vallon V, Blantz RC, Thomson S. Glomerular hyperfiltration and the salt paradox in early type 1 diabetes mellitus: a tubulo-centric view. J Am Soc Nephrol. 2003;14:530–7.
18. Vallon V, Wead LM, Blantz RC. Renal hemodynamics and plasma and kidney angiotensin II in established diabetes mellitus in rats: effect of sodium and salt restriction. J Am Soc Nephrol. 1995;5: 1761–7.
19. Miller JA. Renal responses to sodium restriction in patients with early diabetes mellitus. J Am Soc Nephrol. 1997;8:749–55.
20. Ruggenenti P, Porrini EL, Gaspari F, Motterlini N, Cannata A, et al. Glomerular hyperfiltration and renal disease progression in type II diabetes. Diabetes Care. 2012;35(10):2061–8. Epub 2012 Jul 6.
21. Ficociello LH, Perkins BA, Roshan B, et al. Renal hyperfiltration and the development of microalbuminuria in type 1 diabetes. Diabetes Care. 2009;32:889–93.
22. Yokoyama H, Kanno S, Takahashi S, Yamada D, Itoh H, Saito K, Sone H, Haneda M. Determinants of decline in glomerular filtration rate in non-proteinuric subjects with or without diabetes and hypertension. Clin J Am Soc Nephrol. 2009;4:1432–40.

23. Tsalamandris C, Allen TJ, Gilbert RE, Sinha A, Panagiotopoulos S, Cooper ME, Jerums G. Progressive decline in renal function in diabetic patients with and without albuminuria. Diabetes. 1994;43:649–55.
24. Molitch ME, Steffes M, Sun W, Rutledge B, Cleary P, De Boer IH, Zinman B, Lachin J. Development and progression of renal insufficiency with and without albuminuria in adults with type 1 diabetes in the Diabetes Control and Complications Trial (DCCT) and the Epidemiology of Diabetes Interventions and Complications Study (EDIC). Diabetes Care. 2010;33(7):1536–43.
25. Perkins BA, Ficociello LH, Ostrander BE, et al. Microalbuminuria and the risk for early progressive renal function decline in type 1 diabetes. J Am Soc Nephrol. 2007;18:1353–61.
26. Yagil C, Barak A, Ben-Dor D, Rosenmann E, Bernheim J, Rosner M, et al. Non-proteinuric diabetes-associated nephropathy in the Cohen rat model of type 2 diabetes. Diabetes. 2005;54:1487–96.
27. Remuzzi A, Sangalli F, Fassi A, Remuzzi G. Albumin concentration in the Bowman's capsule: multiphoton microscopy vs micropuncture technique. Kidney Int. 2007;72:1410–1.
28. Gagliardini E, Conti S, Benigni A, Remuzzi G, Remuzzi A. Imaging of the porous ultrastructure of the glomerular epithelial filtration slit. J Am Soc Nephrol. 2010;21:2081–9.
29. Amsellem S, Gburek J, Hamard G, Nielsen R, Willnow TE, Devuyst O, Nexo E, Verroust PJ, Christensen EI, Kozyraki R. Cubilin is essential for albumin reabsorption in the renal proximal tubule. J Am Soc Nephrol. 2010;21:1859–67.
30. Rangel-Filho A, Sharma M, Datta YH, Moreno C, Roman RJ, Iwamoto Y, Provoost AP, Lazar J, Jacob HJ. RF-2 gene modulates proteinuria and albuminuria independently of changes in glomerular permeability in the fawn-hooded hypertensive rat. J Am Soc Nephrol. 2005;16:852–6.
31. Sidaway JE, Davidson RG, McTaggart F, Orton TC, Scott RC, Smith GJ, Brunskill NJ. Inhibitors of 3-hydroxy-3methylglutaryl-CoA reductase reduce receptor-mediated endocytosis in opossum kidney cells. J Am Soc Nephrol. 2004;15:2258–65.
32. Magee GM, Bilous RW, Caldwell CR, et al. Is hyperfiltration associated with the future risk of developing diabetic nephropathy? A meta-analysis. Diabetologia. 2009;52:691–7.
33. Caramori ML, Fioretto P, Maurer M. The need for early predictors of diabetic nephropathy risk: is albumin excretion rate sufficient? Diabetes. 2000;49:1300–408.
34. Perkins BA, Ficociello LH, Silva KH, et al. Regression of microalbuminuria in type 1 diabetes. N Engl J Med. 2003;348:2285–93.
35. Jerums G, Allen TJ, Campbell DJ, Cooper ME, Gilbert RE, Hammond JJ, et al. Long term comparison between perindopril and nifedipine in normotensive patients with type 1 diabetes and microalbuminuria. Am J Kidney Dis. 2001;37:890–9.
36. Jerums G, Panagiotopoulos S, Premaratne E, Power DA, MacIsaac RJ. Lowering of proteinuria in response to antihypertensive therapy predicts improved renal function in late but not in early diabetic nephropathy: a pooled analysis. Am J Nephrol. 2008;28:614–27.
37. Perkins BA, Ficociello LH, Roshan B, Warram JH, Krolewski AS. In patients with type 1 diabetes and new onset microalbuminuria the development of advanced chronic kidney disease may not require progression to proteinuria. Kidney Int. 2010;77(1):57–64.
38. Yokoyama H, Hirohito S, Oishi M, Kawai K, Fukumoto Y, Kobayashi M. Prevalence of albuminuria and renal insufficiency and associated clinical factors in type 2 diabetes: the Japan Diabetes Clinical Data Management study (JDDM15). Nephrol Dial Transplant. 2009;24:1212–9.
39. Ritz E. Type 2 diabetes: absence of proteinuria does not preclude loss of renal function. J Am Soc Nephrol. 2004;16:284–5.
40. MacIsaac RJ, Panagiotopoulos S, McNeil KJ, et al. Is nonalbuminuric renal insufficiency in type 2 diabetes related to an increase in intra-renal vascular disease? Diabetes Care. 2006;29:1560.
41. Fioretto P, Maurer M, Brocco E, Velussi M, Frigato F, Muollo B, Sambataro M, Abaterusso C, Baggio B, Crepaldi G, Nosadini R. Patterns of renal injury in NIDDM patients with microalbuminuria. Diabetologia. 1996;39:1569–76.
42. Ruggenenti P, Gambara V, Perna A, Bertani T, Remuzzi G. The nephropathy of non-insulin dependent diabetes: predictors of outcome relative to diverse patterns of renal injury. J Am Soc Nephrol. 1998;9:2336–43.
43. Bonnet F, Cooper ME, Kawachi H, Allen TJ, Boner G, Cao Z. Irbesartan normalizes the deficiency in glomerular nephrin expression in a model of diabetes and hypertension. Diabetologia. 2001;44:874–7.
44. Langham RG, Kelly DJ, Cox AJ, Thomson NM, Holthofer H, Zaoui P, et al. Proteinuria and the expression of the podocyte slit diaphragm protein, nephrin, in diabetic nephropathy: effects of angiotensin converting enzyme inhibition. Diabetologia. 2002;45:1572–6.
45. Maeda S, Osawa N, Hayashi T, Tsukada S, Kobayashi M, Kikkawa R. Genetic variations associated with diabetic nephropathy and type II diabetes in a Japanese population. Kidney Int Suppl. 2007;106:S43–8.
46. Ng DP, Nurbaya S, Choo S, Koh D, Chia KS, Krolewski AS. Genetic variation at the SLC12A3 locus is unlikely to explain risk for advanced diabetic nephropathy in Caucasians with type II diabetes. Nephrol Dial Transplant. 2008;23:2260–4.
47. Shimazaki A, Tanaka Y, Shinosaki T, Ikeda M, Watada H, Hirose T, Kawamori R, Maeda S. ELMO-1 increases expression of extracellular matrix proteins and inhibits cell adhesion to ECMs. Kidney Int. 2006;70:1769–76.
48. Pezzolesi MG, Poznik GD, Mychaleckyj JC, Paterson AD, Barati MT, Klein JB, Ng DP, Placha G, Canani LH, Bochenski J, Waggott D, Merchant ML, Mirea L, Wanic K, Katavetin P, Kure M, Wolkow P, Dunn JS, Smiles A, Walker WH, Boright AP, Bull SB, DCCT/EDIC Research Group, Doria A, Rogus JJ, Rich SS, Warram JH, Krolewski AS. Genome-wide association scans for diabetic nephropathy susceptibility genes in type 1 diabetes. Diabetes. 2009;58:1403–10.
49. Jeffers BW, Estacio RO, Ranolds MV, Schrier RW. Angiotensin converting enzyme gene polymorphism in non-insulin dependent diabetes mellitus and its relationship with diabetic nephropathy. Kidney Int. 1997;52:473.
50. Granhall C, Park HB, Fakhrai-Rad H, Luthman H. High-resolution quantitative trait locus analysis reveals multiple diabetes susceptibility loci mapped to intervals<800 kb in the species-conserved Niddm1i of the GK rat. Genetics. 2006;174:1565–72.
51. Andersson SA, Olsson AH, Esguerra JL, Heimann E, Ladenvall C, Edlund A, Salehi A, Taneera J, Degerman E, Groop L, Ling C, Eliasson L. Reduced insulin secretion correlates with decreased expression of exocytotic genes in pancreatic islets from patients with type 2 diabetes. Mol Cell Endocrinol. 2012;364(1–2):36–45.
52. Grant SF, Thorleifsson G, Reynisdottir I, Benediktsson R, Manolescu A, Sainz J, Helgason A, Stefansson H, Emilsson V, Helgadottir A, Styrarsdottir U, Magnusson KP, Walters GB, et al. Variant of transcription factor 7-like 2 (TCF7L2) gene confers risk of type 2 diabetes. Nat Genet. 2006;38:320–3.
53. Esguerra JL, Bolmeson C, Cilio CM, Eliasson L. Differential glucose-regulation of micro-RNAs in pancreatic islets of non-obese type 2 diabetes model Goto-Kakizaki rat. PLoS One. 2011;6(4):e18613.
54. Yang BT, Dayeh TA, Volkov PA, Kirkpatrick CL, Malmgren S, Jing X, Renstrom E, Wollheim CB, Nitert MD, Ling C. Increased DNA methylation and decreased expression of PDX-1 in pancreatic islets from patients with type 2 diabetes. Mol Endocrinol. 2012;26(7):1203–12.
55. Lebovitz HE. Type 2 diabetes: an overview. Clin Chem. 1999;45:1339–45.

56. Kahn SE, Hull RL, Utzschneider KM. Mechanisms linking obesity to insulin resistance and type 2 diabetes. Nature. 2006;444:840–6.
57. Unger RH. Lipotoxic diseases. Annu Rev Med. 2002;53:319–26.
58. Benigni A, Gagliardini E, Tomasoni S, et al. Selective impairment of gene expression and assembly of nephrin in human diabetic nephropathy. Kidney Int. 2004;65:2193.
59. Esposito K, Nappo F, Marfella R, Giugliano G, Giugliano F, Ciotola M, Quagliaro L, Ceriello A, Giugliano D. Inflammatory cytokine concentrations are acutely increased by hyperglycemia in humans: role of oxidative stress. Circulation. 2002;106:2067–72.
60. Gonzalez Y, Herrera MT, Soldevila G, Garcia-Garcia L, Fabian G, Perez-Armendariz EM, Bobadilla K, Guzman-Beltran S, Sada E, Torres M. High glucose concentrations induce TNF-α production through the down-regulation of CD33 in primary human monocytes. BMC Immunol. 2012;13:19.
61. Pickup JC. Inflammation and activated innate immunity in the pathogenesis of type 2 diabetes. Diabetes Care. 2004;27:813–23.
62. Nishikawa T, Edelstein D, Du XL, Yamagishi S, Matsumura T, Kaneda Y, Yorek MA, Beebe D, Oates PJ, Hammes HP, et al. Normalizing mitochondrial superoxide production blocks three pathways of hyperglycaemic damage. Nature. 2000;404:787–90.
63. Orie NN, Zidek W, Tepel M. Increased intracellular generation of reactive oxygen species in mononuclear leukocytes from patients with diabetes type 2. Exp Clin Endocrinol Diabetes. 2000;108: 175–80.
64. Niewczas MA, Ficociello LH, Johnson AC, Walker W, Rosolowsky ET, Roshan B, Warram JH, Krolewski AS. Serum concentrations of markers of TNFα and Fas-mediated pathways and renal function in nonproteinuric patients with type 1 diabetes. Clin J Am Soc Nephrol. 2009;4(1):62–70.
65. Navarro JF, Mora-Fernandez C. The role of TNFα in diabetic nephropathy: pathogenic and therapeutic implications. Cytokine Growth Factor Rev. 2006;17:441–50 [PubMed17113815].
66. Ortiz A, Lorz C, Egido J. The Fas ligand/Fas system in renal injury. Nephrol Dial Transplant. 1999;14:1831–4 [PubMed 10462254].
67. Al Lamki RS, Wang J, Vandenabeele P, Bradley JA, Thiru S, Luo D, Min W, Pober JS, Bradley JR. TNFR1- and TNFR2-mediated signaling pathways in human kidney are cell type-specific and differentially contribute to renal injury. FASEB J. 2005;19:1637–45 [PubMed 16195372].
68. Niewczas MA, Gohda T, Skupien J, Smiles AM, Walker WH, Rosetti F, Cullere X, Mayadas TN, Warram JH, Krolewski AS. Circulating TNF receptors 1 and 2 predict ESRD in type 2 diabetes. J Am Soc Nephrol. 2012;23:507–15.
69. Bemelmans MH, Gouma DJ, Buurman WA. Tissue distribution and clearance of soluble murine TNF receptors in mice. Cytokine. 1994;6:608–15.
70. Bash LD, Selvin E, Steffes M, Coresh J, Astor BC. Poor glycemic control in diabetes and the risk of incident chronic kidney disease even in the absence of albuminuria and retinopathy: the atherosclerosis risk in communities (ARIC) study. Arch Intern Med. 2008;168(22):2440–7.
71. Abbate C, Corna M, Capitanio M, Bertani T, Remuzxi G. In progressive nephropathies, overload of tubular cells with filtered proteins translates glomerular permeability dysfunction into cellular signals of interstitial inflammation. J Am Soc Nephrol. 1998;9: 1213–24.
72. Li M, Balamuthusamy S, Simon EE, Batuman V. Silencing megalin and cubilin genes inhibits myeloma light chain endocytosis and ameliorates toxicity in human renal proximal tubule epithelial cells. Am J Physiol Renal Physiol. 2008;295(1):F82–90.
73. Sengul S, Zwizinski C, Simon EE, Kapasi A, Singhal PC, Batuman V. Endocytosis of light chains induces cytokines through activation of NF-κB in human proximal tubule cells. Kidney Int. 2002;62:1977–88.
74. Sengul S, Zwizinski C, Batuman V. Role of MAPK pathways in light chain-induced cytokine production in human proximal tubule cells. Am J Physiol Renal Physiol. 2003;284:F1245–54.
75. Wang PX, Sanders PW. Immunoglobulin light chains generate hydrogen peroxide. J Am Soc Nephrol. 2007;18(4):1239–45.
76. Gilbert RE, Cooper ME. The tubulo-interstitium in progressive diabetic kidney disease; more than an aftermath of glomerular injury? Kidney Int. 1999;56:1627–37.
77. Hutchison CA, Harding S, Hewins P, Mead GP, Townsend J, Bradwell AR, Cockwell P. Quantitative assessment of serum and urinary polyclonal free light chains in patients with chronic kidney disease. Clin J Am Soc Nephrol. 2008;3:1684–90.
78. Hostetter TH, Nath KA. Role of prostaglandins in experimental renal disease. Contrib Nephrol. 1989;75:13–8.
79. Groop L, Makipernaa A, Stenman S, DeFronzo RA, Teppo AM. Urinary excretion of kappa light chains in patients with diabetes mellitus. Kidney Int. 1990;37:1120–5.
80. Hassan SB, Hanna MOF. Urinary κ and λ immunoglobulin light chains in normoalbuminuric type 2 diabetes mellitus patients. J Clin Lab Anal. 2011;25:229–32.
81. Redegeld FA, van der Heijden MW, Kool M, Heijdra BM, Garssen J, Kraneveld AD, Van Loveren H, Roholl P, Saito T, Verbeek JS, Claassens J, Koster AS, Nijkamp FP. Immunoglobulin-free light chains elicit immediate hypersensitivity-like responses. Nat Med. 2002;8(7):694–701.
82. Rijnierse A, Kroese ABA, Redegeld FA, Blokhuis BRJ, van der Heijdan MW, Koster AS, Timmermans JP, Nijkamp FP, Kraneveld AD. Immunoglobulin-free light chains mediate antigen-specific responses of murine dorsal root ganglion neurons. J Neuroimmunol. 2009;208(1):80–6.
83. Jarman PR, Kehely AM, Mather HM. Hyperkalaemia in diabetes: prevalence and associations. Postgrad Med J. 1995;71:551–2.
84. Lindblad P, Chow WH, Chan J, Bergstrom A, Wolk A, Gridley G, McLaughlin JK, Nyren O, Adami HO. The role of diabetes mellitus in the aetiology of renal cell cancer. Diabetologia. 1999;42(1): 107–12.
85. Habib SL, Prihoda TJ, Luna M, Werner SA. Diabetes and risk of renal cell carcinoma. J Cancer. 2012;3:42–8.
86. Giovannucci E. Insulin, insulin like growth factors and colon cancer: a review of the evidence. J Nutr. 2001;131:3109S–20.
87. Bruce WR, Giacca A, Medline A. Possible mechanisms relating diet and risk of colon cancer. Cancer Epidemiol Biomarkers Prev. 2000;9:1271–9.
88. Lowrance WT, Thompson RH, Yee DS, Kaag M, Donat SM, Russo P. Obesity is associated with a higher risk of clear-cell renal carcinoma than with other histologies. BJU Int. 2009;105:16–20.
89. Hjartaker A, Langseth H, Weiderpass E. Obesity and diabetes epidemics: cancer repercussions. Adv Exp Med Biol. 2008;630: 72–93.
90. Ueda T, Yoshimura N, Yoshida O. Diabetic cystopathy: relationship to autonomic neuropathy detected by sympathetic skin responses. J Urol. 1997;157(2):580–4.
91. Bansal R, Agarwal MM, Modi M, Mandal AK, Singh SK. Urodynamic profile of diabetic patients with lower urinary tract symptoms: association of diabetic cystopathy with autonomic and peripheral neuropathy. Urology. 2011;77(3):699–705.
92. Evans R, Eppel GA, Michaels S, Burke SL, Nematbakhsh M, Head GA, Carroll JF, O'Connor PM. Multi-mechanisms act to maintain kidney oxygenation during renal ischemia in anesthetized rats. Am J Physiol Renal Physiol. 2010;298:F1235–43.
93. Aspelin P, Aubry P, Fransson SG, et al. Nephrotoxic effects in high-risk patients undergoing angiography. N Engl J Med. 2003;348:491.
94. Agmon Y, Peleg H, Greenfeld Z, et al. Regional alterations in renal haemodynamics and oxygenation: a role in contrast medium-induced nephropathy. Nephrol Dial Transplant. 2005;20 Suppl 1:i6.

95. Parfrey PS, Griffiths SM, Barrett BJ, et al. Contrast material-induced renal failure in patients with diabetes mellitus, renal insufficiency, or both. A prospective controlled study. N Engl J Med. 1989;320:143.
96. Rudnick MR, Goldfarb S, Wexler L, et al. Nephrotoxicity of ionic and nonionic contrast media in 1196 patients: a randomized trial. The Iohexol Cooperative Study. Kidney Int. 1995;47:254.
97. Wasaki M, Sugimoto J, Shirota K. Glucose alters the susceptibility of mesangial cells to contrast media. Invest Radiol. 2001;36(7): 355–62.
98. Patti G, Ricottini E, Nusca A, Colonna G, Pasceri V, D'Ambrosio A, Montinaro A, DiSciascio G. Short term high dose atorvastatin pre-treatment to prevent contrast-induced nephropathy in patients with acute coronary syndrome undergoing percutaneous coronary intervention (from ARMYDA-CIN—atorvastatin for reduction of myocardial damage during angioplasty—contrast induced nephropathy) trial. Am J Cardiol. 2011;108(1):1–7.
99. Ozhan H, Erden I, Ordu S, Aydin M, Caglar O, Basar C, Yalein S, Alemdar R. Efficacy of short-term high dose atorvastatin for prevention of contrast-induced nephropathy in patients undergoing coronary arteriography. Angiology. 2010;61(7):711–4.
100. Quintavalle C, Fiore D, DeMicco F, Visconti G, Focaccio A, Golia B, Ricciardelli B, Donnarumma E, Bianco A, Zabatta MA, Troncone G, Colomo A, Briguori C, Condorelli G. Impact of a high loading dose of atorvastatin on contrast-induced kidney injury. Circulation. 2012;126(25):3008–16.
101. Pignatelli P, Carnevale R, Pastori D, Napoleone L, et al. Immediate antioxidant and antiplatelet effect of atorvastatin via inhibition of Nox2. Circulation. 2012;126(1):92–103.
102. Mueller C, Buerkle G, Buettner HJ, Petersen J, Perruchoud AP, Eriksson U, Marsch S, Roskamm H. Prevention of contrast media-associated nephropathy. Arch Intern Med. 2002;162:329–36.
103. Leone AM, DeCaterina AR, Sciabasi A, Aurelio A, Basile E, Porto I, Trani C, Burzotta F, Niccoli G, Mongiardo R, Mazzari MA, Buffon A, Panocchia N, Romagnoli E, Lioy E, Rebuzzi AG, Crea F. Sodium bicarbonate plus N-acetylcysteine to prevent contrast-induced nephropathy in primary and rescue percutaneous coronary interventions: the BINARIO study. EuroIntervention. 2012;8(7):839–47.
104. Briguori C. Renalguard system in high-risk patients for contrast-induced acute kidney injury. Minerva Cardioangiol. 2012;60(3): 291–7.
105. Duong MH, MacKenzie TA, Malenka DJ. N-acetylcysteine prophylaxis significantly reduces the risk of radiocontrast-induced nephropathy: comprehensive meta-analysis. Catheter Cardiovasc Interv. 2005;64(4):471–9.
106. Momeni A, Mirhoseini M, Beigi FM, Esfahani MR, Kheiri S, Amiri M, Seidain Z. Effect of N-acetylcysteine in prevention of contrast nephropathy on patients under intravenous pyelography and contrast CT. Adv Biomed Res. 2012;1:28. Epub 2012 July 6.
107. Parving HH, Gall MA, Scott P, et al. Prevalence and causes of albuminuria in non-insulin dependent diabetic patients. Kidney Int. 1992;41:758.
108. KDOQI. KDOQI clinical practice guidelines and clinical practice recommendations for diabetes and chronic kidney disease. Am J Kidney Dis. 2007;49:S12.
109. Wood S. ALTITUDE halted: adverse events when aliskiren added to ACE, ARB therapy. Heart Wire. Available at: http://www.theheart.org/article/1331173.co. Accessed 3 July 2012.
110. Titan SM, Vieira J Jr M, Dominguez WV, Barros RT, Zatz R. ACEI and ARB combination therapy in patients with macro-albuminuric diabetic nephropathy and low socioeconomic level: a double-blind randomized clinical trial. Clin Nephrol. 2011;76:273–83.
111. Krairittichai U, Chaisuvannarat V. Effects of dual blockade of renin-angiotensin system in type Shibata S, Fujita T: mineralocorticoid receptors in the pathophysiology of chronic kidney diseases and the metabolic syndrome. Mol Cell Endocrinol 350: 273–280, 20122 diabetes patients with diabetic nephropathy. J Med Assoc Thai. 2009;92:611–7.
112. Shibata S, Fujita T. Mineralocorticoid receptors in the pathophysiology of chronic kidney diseases and the metabolic syndrome. Mol Cell Endocrinol. 2012;350:273–80.
113. Nagase M, Fugita T. Aldosterone and glomerular podocyte injury. Clin Exp Nephrol. 2008;12:233–42.
114. Medhi UF, Adams-Huet B, Raskin P, Vega GL, Toto RD. Addition of angiotensin receptor blockade or mineralocorticoid antagonism to maximal angiotensin-converting enzyme inhibition in diabetic nephropathy. J Am Soc Nephrol. 2009;20:2641–50.
115. Mann JF, Green D, Jamerson K, Ruilope LM, Kuranoff SJ, Littke T, Viberti G, ASCEND Study Group. Avosentan for overt diabetic nephropathy. J Am Soc Nephrol. 2010;21(3):527–35.
116. MacEwen A, McKay GA, Fisher M. Drugs for diabetes: part 8, SGLT2 inhibitors. Br J Cardiol. 2012;19:26–9.
117. Ferannini E, Ramos SJ, Salsali A, Tang W, List JF. Dapagliflozin monotherapy in type 2 diabetes patients with inadequate glycaemic control by diet and exercise: a randomized, double-blind, placebo-controlled phase III trial. Diabetes Care. 2010;3:217–24.
118. Abdul-Ghani MA, Norton L, DeFronzo RA. Efficacy and safety of SGLT-2 inhibitors in the treatment of type 2 diabetes mellitus. Curr Diab Rep. 2012;12(3):230–8. Review.
119. Brownlee M, Cerami A, Vlassara H. Advanced glycosylation end products in tissue and the biochemical basis of diabetic complications. N Engl J Med. 1988;318:1315–21.
120. Makita Z, Radoff S, Rayfield EJ, Yang Z, Skolnik E, Delaney V, Friedman EA, Cerami A, Vlassara H. Advanced glycosylation end products in patients with diabetic nephropathy. N Engl J Med. 1991;325:836–42.
121. He C, Sabol J, Mitsuhashi T, Vlassara H. Dietary glycotoxins: inhibition of reactive products by aminoguanidine facilitates renal clearance and reduces tissue sequestration. Diabetes. 1999;48: 1308–15.
122. Freedman BI, Wuerth JP, Cartwright K, Bain RP, Dippe S, Hershon K, Mooradian AD, Spinowitz BS. Design and baseline characteristics for the aminoguanidine Clinical Trial in Overt Type 2 Diabetic Nephropathy (ACTION II). Control Clin Trials. 1999;20:493–510.
123. Ramasamy R, Yan SF, Schmidt AM. Advanced glycation end-products: from precursors to RAGE: round and round we go. Amino Acids. 2012;42:1151–61.
124. D'Agati V, Yan SF, Ramasamy R, Schmidt AM. RAGE, glomerulosclerosis and proteinuria. roles in podocytes and endothelial cells. Trends Endocrinol Metab. 2010;21:50–6.
125. Olefsky JM, Glass CK. Macrophages, inflammation and insulin resistance. Annu Rev Physiol. 2010;72:219–46.
126. Fan W, Morinaga H, Kim JJ, Bae E, Spann NJ, Heinz S, Glass CK, Olefsky JM. Fox01 regulates Tlr- 4 inflammatory pathway signaling in macrophages. EMBO J. 2010;29:4223–36.
127. Sharma K, Ramachandrarao S, Qiu G, Usui HK, Zhu Y, Dunn SR, Ouedraogo R, Hough K, McCue P, Chan L, Falkner B, Goldstein BJ. Adiponectin regulates albuminuria and podocyte function in mice. J Clin Invest. 2008;118:1645–56.
128. Shirwany NA, Zou MH. AMPK in cardiovascular health and disease. Acta Pharmacol Sin. 2010;31:1075–84.
129. Darisipudi MN, Kulkami OP, Sayyed SG, Ryu M, Migliorini A, Sagrinati C, Parente E, Vater A, Eulberg D, Klussmann S, Romagnani P, Anders HJ. Dual blockade of the homeostatic chemokine CXCLl2 and the pro-inflammatory chemokine CCL2 has additive protective effects on diabetic kidney disease. Am J Pathol. 2011;179:116–24.
130. Giunti S, Barutta F, Perin PC, Gruden G. Targeting the MCP-1/CCR2 system in diabetic kidney disease. Curr Vasc Pharmacol. 2010;8:849–60.

131. Ortiz-Munoz G, Lopez-Parra V, Lopez-Franco O, Fernandez-Vizarra P, Mallavia B, Flores C, Sanz A, Blanco J, Mezzano S, Ortiz A, Egido J, Gomez-Guerrero C. Suppressors of cytokine signaling abrogate diabetic nephropathy. J Am Soc Nephrol. 2010;21:763–72.
132. Wang Q, Zhang M, Liang B, Shirwany N, Zhu Y, Zou MH. Activation of AMP-activated protein kinase is required for berberine-induced reduction of atherosclerosis in mice: the role of uncoupling protein 2. PLoS One. 2011;6:e25436.
133. Lee MJ, Feliers D, Mariappan MM, Sataranatarajan K, Mahimainathan L, Musi N, Foretz M, Viollet B, Weinberg JM, Choudhury GG, Kasinath BS. A role for AMP-activated protein kinase in diabetes-induced renal hypertrophy. Am J Physiol Renal Physiol. 2007;292:F617–27.
134. Eid AA, Ford BM, Block K, Kasinath BS, Gorin Y, Ghosh-Choudhury G, Barnes JL, Abboud HE. AMP-activated protein kinase (AMPK) negatively regulates Nox4-dependent activation of p53 and epithelial cell apoptosis in diabetes. J Biol Chem. 2010;285:37503–12.
135. Decleves AI, Mathew AV, Cunard R, Sharma K. AMPK medicates the initiation of kidney disease induced by a high fat diet. J Am Soc Nephrol. 2011;22:1846–55.
136. Lee MJ, Feliers D, Sataranatarajan K, Mariappan MM, Li M, Barnes JL, Choudhury GG, Kasinath BS. Resveratrol ameliorates high glucose-induced protein synthesis in glomerular epithelial cells. Cell Signal. 2010;22:65–70.
137. Pearson KJ, Baur JA, Lewis KN, Peshkin L, Price NL, Labinskyy N, Swindell WR, Kamara D, Minor RK, Perez E, Jamieson HA, Zhang Y, Dunn SR, Sharma K, Pleshko N, Woollett LA, Csiszar A, Ikeno Y, Le Couteur D, Elliott PJ, Becker KG, Navas P, Ingram DK, Wolf NS, Ungvari Z, Sinclair DA, de Cabo R. Resveratrol delays age-related deterioration and mimics transcriptional aspects of dietary restriction without extending life span. Cell Metab. 2008;8:157–68.
138. Hung AM, Roumie CL, Greevy RA, Liu X, Grijalva CG, Murff HJ, Ikizler TA, Griffin MR. Comparative effectiveness of incident oral anti-diabetic drugs on kidney function. Kidney Int. 2012; 81:698–706.
139. Sakaguchi M, Isono M, Isshiki K, Sugimoto T, Koya D, Kashiwagi A. Inhibition of mTOR signaling with rapamycin attenuates renal hypertrophy in the early diabetic mice. Biochem Biophys Res Commun. 2006;340:296–301.
140. Chen JK, Chen J, Thomas G, Kozma SC, Harris RC. S6 kinase 1 knockout inhibits uni-nephrectomy- or diabetes-induced renal hypertrophy. Am J Physiol Renal Physiol. 2009;297:F585–93.
141. Lloberas N, Cruzado JM, Franquesa M, Herrero-Fresneda I, Torras J, Alperovich G, Rama I, Vidal A, Grinyo JM. Mammalian target of rapamycin pathway blockade slows progression of diabetic kidney disease in rats. J Am Soc Nephrol. 2006;17:1395–404.
142. Godel M, Hartleben B, Herbach N, Liu S, Zschiedrich S, Lu S, Debreczeni-Mór A, Lindenmeyer MT, Rastaldi MP, Hartleben G, Wiech T, Fornoni A, Nelson RG, Kretzler M, Wanke R, Pavenstadt H, Kerjaschki D, Cohen CD, Hall MN, Ruegg MA, Inoki K, Walz G, Huber TB. Role of mTOR in podocyte function and diabetic nephropathy in humans and mice. J Clin Invest. 2011;121:2197–209.
143. Kasinath BS, Mariappan MM, Sataranatarajan K, Lee MJ, Ghosh-Choudhury G, Feliers D. Novel mechanisms of protein synthesis in diabetic nephropathy-role of mRNA translation. Rev Endocr Metab Disord. 2008;9:255–66.
144. Wu QQ, Wang Y, Senitko M, Meyer C, Wigley WC, Ferguson DA, Grossman E, Chen J, Zhou XL, Hartono J, Winterberg P, Chen B, Agarwal A, Lu CY. Bardoxolone methyl (BARD) ameliorates ischemic AKI and increases expression of protective genes Nrf2, PPARγ, and HO-1. Am J Physiol Renal Physiol. 2011;300:F1180–92.
145. Pareek TK, Belkadi A, Kesavapany S, Zaremba A, Loh SL, Bai L, Cohen ML, Meyer C, Liby KT, Miller RH, Sporn MB, Letterio JJ. Triterpenoid modulation of IL-17 and Nrf-2 expression ameliorates neuro-inflammation and promotes re-myelination in autoimmune encephalomyelitis. Sci Rep. 2011;1:201.
146. Pergola PE, Raskin P, Toto RD, Meyer CJ, Huff JW, Grossman EB, Krauth M, Ruiz S, Audhya P, Christ-Schmidt H, Wittes J, Wamock DG. BEAM Study Investigators: bardoxolone methyl and kidney function in CKD with type 2 diabetes. N Engl J Med. 2011;365:327–36.
147. Saha PK, Reddy VT, Konopleva M, Andreeff M, Chan L. The triterpenoid 2-cyano-3, 12-dioxooleana-1,9-dien-28-oic-acid methyl ester has potent anti-diabetic effects in diet-induced diabetic mice and Lepr(db/db) mice. J Biol Chem. 2010;285:40581–92.
148. Yore MM, Kettenbach AN, Sporn MB, Gerber SA, Liby KT. Proteomic analysis shows synthetic oleanane triterpenoid binds to mTOR. PLoS One. 2011;6:e22862.
149. Tayek JA, Kalantar-Zadeh K. The extinguished BEACON of bardoxolone: not a Monday quarterback story. Am J Nephrol. 2013;37(3):208–11.
150. Reata Pharmaceuticals press release, October 18, 2012: Reata halts its phase 3 trial of bardoxolone secondary to mortality in the treatment arm.
151. Al-Bayati MA, Xie Y, Mohr FC, Margolin SB, Giri SN. Effect of pirfenidone against vanadate induced kidney fibrosis in rats. Biochem Pharmacol. 2002;64:517–25.
152. Shimizu T, Fukagawa M, Kuroda T, Hata S, Iwasaki Y, Nemoto M, Shirai K, Yamanchi S, Margolin SB, Shimizu F, Kurokawa K. Pirfenidone prevents collagen accumulation in the remnant kidney in rats with partial nephrectomy. Kidney Int Suppl. 1997;63:S239–43.
153. Sharma K, Ix JH, Mathew AV, Cho M, Pflueger A, Dunn SR, Francos B, Sharma S, Falkner B, McGowan TA, Donohue M, Ramachandrarao S, Xu R, Fervenza FC, Kopp JB. Pirfenidone for diabetic nephropathy. J Am Soc Nephrol. 2011;22:1144–51.
154. Sharma K, Jin Y, Guo J, Ziyadeh FN. Neutralization of TGF-beta by anti-TGF-beta antibody attenuates kidney hypertrophy and the enhanced extracellular matrix gene expression in STZ-induced diabetic mice. Diabetes. 1996;45:522–30.
155. Ziyadeh FN, Hoffman BB, Han DC, Iglesias-De La Cruz MC, Hong SW, Isono M, Chen S, McGowan TA, Sharma K. Long-term prevention of renal insufficiency, excess matrix gene expression, and glomerular mesangial matrix expansion by treatment with monoclonal anti-transforming growth factor-beta antibody in db/db diabetic mice. Proc Natl Acad Sci U S A. 2000;97:8015–20.
156. Putta S, Lanting L, Sun G, Lawson G, Kato M, Natarajan R. Inhibiting MicroRNA-192 ameliorates renal fibrosis in diabetic nephropathy. J Am Soc Nephrol. 2012;23:458–69.
157. Krutzfeldt J, Rajewsky N, Braich R, Rajeef KG, Tuschl T, Manoharan M, Stoffel M. Silencing of microRNAs in vivo with "antagomirs". Nature. 2005;438:685–9.
158. Goicoechea M, de Vinuesa SG, Verdalles U, Ruiz-Caro C, Ampuero J, Rincon A, Arroyo D, Luno J. Effect of allopurinol in chronic kidney disease progression and cardiovascular risk. Clin J Am Soc Nephrol. 2010;5:1388–93.
159. KDIGO Board Members; Eknoyan G, Lameire N, Eckardt KU, Kasiske B, Wheeler DC, Abboud OI, Adler S, Agarwal R, Andreoli SP, Becker GJ, Brown F, Cattran DC, Collins AJ, Coppo R, Coresh J, Correa-Rotter R, Covic A, Craig JC, de Francisco Angel LM, de Jong PE, Figueiredo A, Gharbi MB, Guyatt G, Harris D, Hooi LS, Imai E, Inker LA, Jadoul M, Jenkins S, Kim S, Kuhlmann MK, Levin NW, Li PKT, Liu ZH, Massari P, McCullough PA, Moosa R, Riella MC, Rizvi AH, Rodriguez-Iturbe B, Schrier R, Silver J, Tonelli M, Tsukamoto Y, Vogels T, Wang A Yee-Moon, Wanner C, Zakharova E. KDIGO 2012 clinical practice guidelines for the evaluation and management of chronic kidney disease. Kidney Int Suppl. 2013;3(1):1–50.

Albuminuria–Proteinuria in Diabetes Mellitus

9

Surya V. Seshan and Alluru S. Reddi

Healthy subjects excrete <150 mg of protein in a 24-h period. Of this protein, only 10–20 % is albumin, and the remaining portion is composed of immunoglobulins, enzymes, low molecular weight proteins and peptides as well as Tamm–Horsfall proteins. Thus, normal albumin excretion is extremely small. Routinely used dipsticks measure albumin only, but its detection is not evident until the concentration of albumin exceeds 300 mg. Therefore routine testing for urinary albumin requires either a chemical method or a dipstick that recognizes only albumin at very low concentrations.

In recent years, the leading cause of proteinuria (albuminuria) in the United States and Europe is the diabetic kidney disease or diabetic nephropathy (DN) rather than primary glomerular diseases [1, 2]. Proteinuria of glomerular origin represents the most important, singular sign of kidney disease and heralds the onset of clinical DN. *Not proteinuria but albuminuria is more specific and is commonly used to define the earliest stages of DN.* In particular, raised urinary albumin levels between 30 and 300 mg/day are considered pathognomonic of diabetic kidney disease in both type 1 and in newly diagnosed type 2 diabetic subjects. Albuminuria <30 mg/day is considered normal, and its prognostic significance in the progression of diabetic kidney disease is less clear. It should be noted that proteinuria may be an early manifestation of an isolated nondiabetic renal disease or nondiabetic renal disease superimposed on typical DN, in nearly 35–50 % of patients with type 2 and less commonly with type 1 diabetes [3, 4].

S.V. Seshan, M.D.
Department of Pathology and Laboratory Medicine, Weill Cornell Medical College, 525 East 68th Street, New York, NY, USA
e-mail: SVS2002@med.cornell.edu

A.S. Reddi, M.D. (✉)
Department of Medicine, Division of Nephrology & Hypertension, Rutgers New Jersey Medical School, 185 South Orange Avenue, Newark, NJ 07103, USA
e-mail: reddias@njms.rutgers.edu

Definitions of Proteinuric States in Diabetic Nephropathy

The preferred measure of proteinuria in diabetic patients is urine albumin excretion or albuminuria in the diagnosis of DN [5]. Effective potential therapeutic interventions at the earlier stages of albuminuria are available with complete, partial, or no reversal/resolution in DN. The latter usually correlates with nondiabetic renal diseases, particularly in the absence of diabetic retinopathy. Early studies have shown that diabetic patients, particularly type 1 diabetics, demonstrate various levels of albuminuria–proteinuria during the evolution of DN. This evolutionary course has been divided into various stages for proper management of DN [6, 7].

Stages 1 and 2 develop within the first 5 years and refer to normoalbuminuric state defined as albumin excretion rate in urine up to 30 mg/24-h.

Stage 3, also known as incipient diabetic nephropathy, generally occurs in 35–40 % of patients after 6–15 years of the onset of diabetes. This stage is characterized by albumin excretion 30–300 mg/24-h (20–200 μg/min), which is defined as microalbuminuria. Microalbuminuria represents the earliest clinical sign of DN and is significant in predicting further deterioration of renal function and development of hypertension without adequate metabolic and blood pressure control. This transition from normo- to microalbuminuria is a crucial step in the evolution of DN, as 35–44 % of diabetic patients may progress to renal failure between 15 and 25 years.

The stage 4 is overt DN, which occurs between 15 and 25 years and is qualified by proteinuria of >500 mg/24 h or albuminuria >300 mg/24 h, detectable by routine urinalysis by dipstick along with hypertension and decline in estimated glomerular filtration rate (eGFR).

The magnitude of proteinuria may increase with progression of renal disease to nephrotic range (3–3.5 g/day) or nephrotic

E.V. Lerma and V. Batuman (eds.), *Diabetes and Kidney Disease*,
DOI 10.1007/978-1-4939-0793-9_9, © Springer Science+Business Media New York 2014

range albuminuria (2.2 g/day), within the next 5–10 years, leading to end stage renal disease (ESRD) in a fraction of cases in type 1 diabetes. However, several studies have shown that regression of microalbuminuria is more common than progression to overt (clinical) proteinuria or ESRD in some type 1 diabetic patients [8]. In type 2 diabetic patients, the progression to ESRD is faster but varied depending on ethnicity, age, male gender, presence of retinopathy, and increased baseline albumin excretion [8].

It should be noted that renal impairment can occur in both type 1 and type 2 diabetic patients without albuminuria, or without progression from microalbuminuria to overt proteinuria [9].

Should We Use the Terms "Microalbuminuria and Overt Proteinuria"?

Some investigators [10, 11] and a consensus panel [12] propose that the use of terms microalbuminuria and overt proteinuria should be discontinued and replaced by such terms as albuminuria or albuminuria–proteinuria. Their proposal is based on the observations from several studies that reported an associated high risk of cardiovascular events even in the presence of extremely low urinary albumin excretion rate [10–14]. Also, albuminuria is a continuous variable that should be regarded as a significant marker of endothelial dysfunction, causing systemic complications. Some investigators believe that microalbuminuria is a misnomer and implies "small size" albumin molecule rather than small quantity of albumin in the urine and has restricted or limited usage.

The use of the term "albuminuria–proteinuria" appears to be the more meaningful terminology than microalbuminuria [11], as most of the clinicians routinely measure proteinuria than albuminuria in their management of nondiabetic kidney disease. The clinicians, however, order the urine albumin measurement only in diabetics, but they follow protein to creatinine ratio in nondiabetic patients. Therefore, the use of the term "albuminuria–proteinuria" is justified.

It should be noted that almost all therapeutic trials in diabetic patients were conducted either with normoalbuminuria, microalbuminuria, or overt proteinuria. Also, this type of classification is important, as the disease progression is dependent on the extent of albuminuria, particularly in type 1 diabetic patients. Until further studies are available that confirm the safety lower limits of albuminuria, we will retain this terminology of microalbuminuria in this chapter in order to discuss the prognosis and treatment of albuminuria in diabetic subjects.

Measurement of Urinary Albumin

Urine Collection

Most of the studies suggest that the first morning void urine specimen, if analyzed immediately, provides the best results of albuminuria with little variability. If the first voided sample is not available, second morning void sample can be used.

Urine Storage

Determination of albumin is preferred in a fresh sample. However, it is not possible in clinical studies with large number of samples. It is suggested that the urine samples can be kept at 4 °C for at least 1–2 weeks before analysis, or at −80 °C for prolonged period of time. Albumin seems to be stable at these temperatures.

Current Methods for Albumin Determination

There are several methods to determine small amounts of albumin in the urine. In the laboratory, a large number of samples can be analyzed in a few hours, which is cost-effective. The most commonly used techniques are radioimmunoassay, immunoturbidimetry, laser immunonephelometry, enzyme-linked immunosorbent assay, and single radial immunodiffusion assay. High performance liquid chromatography (HPLC) method seems to measure both the fragments and the entire albumin molecule and is the suggested methodology for urine albumin determination. Therefore, urine albumin concentrations by HPLC method are higher than with other routine immunoassay methods, resulting in much higher incidence rates of albuminuria in diabetic patients.

In the office setting, a number of dipsticks were developed to test for albumin. These dipsticks take only few minutes for analysis, but they are expensive. Several dipsticks have been developed over the years to detect low grade albuminuria and are useful in the primary care setting and diabetes clinics. Table 9.1 shows various in-office albumin tests.

Reporting Urinary Albumin

Historically, urinary albumin is expressed as mg/24-h. Since collection of urine for 24 h is not feasible in all patients, it has become a common practice to express as the ratio of urinary

Table 9.1 Albumin tests in the office and clinics

Name	Test description
Micral test strips	Color match strips with results in 1 min
Clinitek microalbumin 2 reagent strips	Provides albumin, creatinine, and albumin–creatinine results in 1 min
ImmunoDip microalbumin strips	Color match strips with results in 3 min
HemoCue Albumin 201	Urine sample is drawn into the cuvette and read in an analyzer with the result in 90 s

Table 9.2 Definitions of albuminuria

Category	24-h collection (mg/24-h)	Timed collection (μg/min)	Spot collection ACR: mg/mg (μg/mg)
Normoalbuminuria	<30	<20	<0.02 (<30)
Microalbuminuria	30–300	20–200	0.02–0.2 (30–300)
Overt or clinical proteinuria or macroalbuminuria	>300	>200	>0.2 (≥300)

ACR albumin:creatinine ratio

albumin to urinary creatinine (ACR) in a spot urine sample. However, confusion arises from reporting results in units of "mg albumin/mmol creatinine," "mg albumin/g creatinine," "μg albumin/mg creatinine," "g albumin/mol creatinine," or "mg albumin/mg creatinine" [12]. Since there are no uniform guidelines, the clinician should follow the individual laboratory reporting system. The following Table 9.2 is one of the representations of defining albuminuria.

Significance of Albuminuria in Type 1 Diabetic Patients

Several prospective studies from various laboratories have demonstrated that an elevation in albumin excretion rate without clinical proteinuria predicts the risk of developing clinical diabetic nephropathy later in life [15–19]. From Table 9.3, it is evident that higher percentage of microalbuminuric patients progress to clinical proteinuria than patients with normoalbuminuria.

Significance of Albuminuria in Type 2 Diabetic Patients

The renal prognostic value of microalbuminuria in type 2 diabetes is not as clear as in type 1 diabetes. This is probably related to several factors, including the onset of diabetes, coexisting hypertension, obesity, and hyperinsulinemia. It is

Table 9.3 Predictive value of microalbuminuria for the development of diabetic nephropathy in type 1 diabetic patients with normo- or microalbuminuria

Study [Ref.]	Patients (no.)	Follow-up period (years)	Cut-off UAE (μg/min)	Patients progressed to clinical proteinuria (%)
Viberti et al. [15]	63	14	>30 <30	87 4
Parving et al. [16]	23	6	>28 <28	75 13
Mogensen and Christensen [17]	43	10	>15 <15	86 0
Mathiesen et al. [18]	71	6	>70 <70	100 5
Almdal et al. [19]	118	5	>20 <20	19 2

Table 9.4 Progression of microalbuminuria to nephropathy in patients with type 2 diabetes (adapted from [20])

Author [Ref.]	No.	Observation period (year)	Patients developing clinical proteinuria (%/year)
Mogensen [21]	59	9	2.4
Nelson et al. [22]	50	4	9.3
Ravid et al. [23]	49	5	8.4
Ahmad et al. [24]	51	5	4.8
Gæde et al. [25]	80	4	5.8
Estacio et al. [26]	150	5	4.0
HOPE Study Group [27]	1,140	4.5	4.5
Parving et al. [28]	201	2	7.5
Parving et al. [29]	86	5	7.0

generally accepted that type 2 diabetics demonstrate either micro- or macroalbuminuria at the time of diagnosis. Also, the majority of the patients are either hypertensive, obese, or hyperinsulinemic at the onset of diagnosis. In addition, some of the so-called type 2 diabetics may have a nondiabetic renal disease causing heavy proteinuria. Despite the above limitations, several studies have shown that microalbuminuria can predict the later development of overt proteinuria in type 2 diabetic patients (Table 9.4).

A recent study confirmed the observations shown in Table 9.4. Berhane et al. [30] evaluated the predictive value of albuminuria and eGFR for ESRD in 2,420 Pima Indians with type 2 diabetes. Based on ACR, the patients were classified into normoalbuminuric (ACR <30 mg/g), microalbuminuric (ACR 30–300 mg/g), and macroalbuminuric (≥300 mg/g) groups. During a mean follow-up of 10.2 years, 287 patients developed ESRD. The incidence of ESRD increased with increasing albuminuria, and the highest incidence was associated with macroalbuminuria.

Also, low GFR was associated with the highest incidence of ESRD. Combined albuminuria and eGFR had an additive effect on the development of ESRD. A recent meta-analysis also confirmed that both albuminuria and estimated GFR predicted an additive risk for ESRD [31]. Thus, albuminuria can predict the development of ESRD.

Mechanisms of Albuminuria-Proteinuria in Diabetes

The mechanisms responsible for albuminuria–proteinuria in diabetes have been thoroughly studied. Hemodynamic alterations, hyperglycemia, hormones, size and charge-selective properties of the glomerular capillary wall, alterations in the glomerular basement membrane (GBM) composition, reactive oxygen species, glycation of proteins, and altered podocyte biology have been implicated. Mesangial cell pathophysiology has long been considered central to the development of albuminuria and glomerulosclerosis in diabetes. In recent years, however, the participation of podocytes in proteinuria and glomerulosclerosis has been extensively studied at the molecular level [32–38]. We, therefore, focus our discussion on podocyte biology in albuminuria–proteinuria of diabetes.

Podocyte Biology

In order to reach the Bowman space, the ultrafiltrate passes through the fenestrae of the endothelium, the GBM, and the slit pore or slit diaphragm of the podocytes. These podocytes are highly specialized cells with primary, secondary, and complex tertiary cellular processes, the latter being the foot processes which interdigitate with adjacent epithelial foot processes and anchor firmly on the basement membranes. Since they are terminally differentiated, they are incapable of being replaced by compensatory proliferation of the adjacent epithelial cells.

The slit diaphragms lie between two foot processes of the podocyte and form the final barrier to filtration of water and solutes. Although low molecular weight proteins may pass through these barriers easily, proteins such as albumin are not easily filtered.

Studies have shown that the slit diaphragms contain a number of proteins that restrict the passage of albumin into the Bowman space. The first protein to be identified was nephrin. Mutations in the gene-encoding nephrin (NPHS1) causes congenital nephrotic syndrome of the Finnish type. The other slit diaphragm proteins include P-cadherin, Neph1 and 2, FAT1 (fatty acid transporter tumor suppressor homolog-1), and FAT2. The foot processes are not static, but they contain a contractile cytoskeleton. This cytoskeleton contains actin, α-actinin-4, synaptopodin, myosin-II, talin, and vinculin. The cytoskeleton of the foot processes connects to both the GBM and the slit diaphragm. The slit diaphragm proteins are connected to the cytoskeleton by various proteins, including podocin, CD2AP (CD2-associated protein), ZO-1 (zonula occludens-1), and densin. Podocin seems to play a key role in nephrin signaling and also in activating TRPC6 (transient receptor potential cation channel subfamily C, member 6). The foot processes are attached to the GBM via $\alpha_3\beta_1$ integrin and dystroglycan. The integrin dimers specifically interconnect TVP (talin, paxillin, vinculin) complex to laminin 11 of the GBM.

In addition to several proteins, the podocytes express receptors for angiotensin II and many other cytokines and growth factors. Therefore, drugs aimed at blocking these receptors may prevent proteinuria and glomerulosclerosis.

In diabetes, abnormalities in podocyte-specific proteins have been reported. For example, nephrin, P-cadherin, and ZO-1 expressions are reduced in diabetic glomeruli and podocytes [39–42]. Decreased synthesis or loss of these proteins has been shown to cause proteinuria. Combined structural and functional changes have been observed in these podocytes, as a result of injury, even in the earlier stages of DN. The structural changes are best visualized by electron microscopy demonstrating decreased podocyte number and/or density, via apoptosis or varying degrees of podocyte detachment and broadening of the foot processes, leading to diminished width of the slit diaphragm as well as reduced nephrin protein and significant loss of negative charge [39–42]. Podocyte or foot process denudation from the GBM has been attributed to suppression of anchor protein integrin α_3 and overexpression of β_1 integrin in response to high glucose levels and angiotensin II. Furthermore, other actin-binding proteins in the podocytes, such as α-actinin-4, synaptopodin, and surface anionic protein podocalyxin were all down-regulated, contributing towards podocyte damage and dysfunction. These structural and molecular changes of the podocytes have been shown to promote albuminuria–proteinuria in both experimental and human studies [39–42]. Concurrent activation of the growth factors and cytokine systems by hyperglycemia, glycated proteins, hypertension-induced mechanical stress and high renal angiotensin II induce transforming growth factor-beta 1 (TGB-β1) and increased vascular endothelial growth factor A (VEGF-A), a permeability and angiogenic factor by the podocytes. TGF-β1 causes podocyte apoptosis and increased extracellular matrix deposition [43]. Podocyte loss also causes decreased VEGF-A messenger RNA expression in DN [44]. Thus, podocytes play an important role in the development of albuminuria and glomerulosclerosis in diabetes.

Extrarenal Manifestations of Albuminuria

There are several associated extrarenal abnormalities in patients with albuminuria or microalbuminuria. The microalbuminuric patients are at a higher risk not only for cardiovascular and other microvascular diseases such as retinopathy and neuropathy than normoalbuminuric diabetic patients as well. The mechanisms responsible for increased cardiovascular mortality in microalbuminuric patients are poorly understood. However, microalbuminuria seems to be a marker for widespread endothelial dysfunction, and a number of cardiovascular risk factors are present in microalbuminuric patients. Table 9.5 summarizes some of the abnormalities (associations) that are found in microalbuminuric patients, which predispose them to increased early morbidity and mortality from cardiovascular disease (CVD).

Table 9.5 Extrarenal manifestations of microalbuminuria in both types of diabetic patients (adapted from [45])

Functional parameter	Change
Hemodynamic	
Blood pressure	↑
Left ventricular function	↓
Left ventricular mass	↑
End-diastolic volume	↓
Maximal oxygen uptake	↓
Cardiovascular risk factors	
Total cholesterol	↑
VLDL cholesterol	↑
LDL cholesterol	↑
Apolipoprotein B	↑
HDL cholesterol	↓
Plasma fibrinogen	↑
Endothelial cell function	
von Willebrand factor	↑
PAI	↑
Adhesion molecules	↑
Function of nitric oxide	↓
$TER_{albumin}$	↑
$TER_{fibrinogen}$	↑
ACE level	↑
Homocystine level	↑
Microvascular disease	
Proliferative retinopathy	↑
Peripheral neuropathy	↑

↑ Increase, ↓ decrease, *PAI* plasminogen activator inhibitor, *TER* transcapillary escape, *ACE* angiotensin-converting enzyme

Albuminuria and Cardiovascular Disease

Albuminuria is a risk factor for CVD [46]. Even normal albumin excretion rates, i.e., below 30 mg/24-h are associated with CVD complications. It is imperative that microalbuminuria carries even more CVD complications [14]. In earlier studies, it has been shown that the relative mortality from CVD is increased 40-fold in type 1 diabetic patients with proteinuria as compared with the general population [47]. Subsequently, follow-up studies in type 1 diabetic patients for 10, 18, or 23 years suggested that microalbuminuria is a strong risk factor for early death, particularly CV death (reviewed in [45]). In another cross-sectional study [48], 476 type 1 adult diabetic patients were followed for a 5-year period. During this follow-up, 19 patients died and 30 developed CV or renal disease, such as myocardial infarction ($N=8$), stroke ($N=3$), amputation ($N=6$), and renal insufficiency ($N=13$). Urinary albumin concentration in a single early morning urine sample was found to be a strong prognostic marker for the development of CVD or death.

The relationship between the degree of albuminuria and CV risk was examined by the investigators of the Heart Outcomes Prevention Evaluation (HOPE) study [49]. This was a cohort study conducted between 1994 and 1999 with a median follow-up of 4.5 years. The prevalence of microalbuminuria in diabetic patients was 32.6 % as compared with 14.8 % in patients without diabetes. The results suggest that any degree of albuminuria is a risk factor for CV events, such as myocardial infarction, stroke or CV death, or hospitalization for congestive heart failure. The risk of CVD increases with an increase in ACR, starting well below the microalbuminuria cut-off. This study is thus consistent with many other previous studies [45].

Dinneeen and Gerstein [50] critically analyzed the literature linking microalbuminuria with total and cardiovascular morbidity and mortality in type 2 diabetic patients. A total of 11 cohort studies were selected from 264 citations for analysis. These 11 studies included a total of 2,138 patients with a mean follow-up of 6.4 years. The duration of diabetes ranged from newly diagnosed to 13 years. The prevalence of microalbuminuria ranged from 20 to 36 % in the eight cohorts that excluded patients with clinical proteinuria. All studies reported significant association between microalbuminuria and total mortality or cardiovascular morbidity and mortality. The authors concluded that microalbuminuria is a strong predictor of total and cardiovascular morbidity and mortality in patients with type 2 diabetes. The observations that a reduction in albuminuria parallels an improvement in CVD prognosis supports the concept that microalbuminuria is a strong risk factor for CVD.

Albuminuria and Hypertension

As shown in Table 9.5, one of the concomitant abnormalities in microalbuminuric patients is elevated blood pressure. Studies have shown that microalbuminuria precedes the increase in systemic blood pressure during the development of diabetic nephropathy in type 1 patients. Also, a significant correlation was found between arterial blood pressure and albumin excretion rate in microalbuminuric patients [51]. The prevalence of hypertension was greater than 80 % in both male and female patients with overt proteinuria.

The association between ambulatory blood pressure monitoring (ABPM) and microalbuminuria has been studied in normotensive type 1 diabetic patients by several investigators, in order to define the variability in blood pressure and albumin excretion rate (reviewed in [45]). These studies have shown that 24-h blood pressure is significantly higher in micro- than in normoalbuminuric patients. Furthermore, the physiological nocturnal fall in systolic blood pressure was blunted. Some of these studies found a correlation between microalbuminuria and ABPM and not with casual or office blood pressure readings. The conclusion from all these studies is that 24-h blood pressure recording is a useful technique in detecting abnormalities in blood pressure that are not apparent in casual blood pressure measurement in normotensive type 1 diabetic patients.

Table 9.6 summarizes ABPM in normotensive adult type 1 diabetic patients with normo- and microalbuminuria. Also, the ambulatory blood pressure recordings were compared with office or clinic blood pressures in these diabetics and matched healthy controls.

Determinants of Albuminuria

Several factors can influence albuminuria or microalbuminuria. The most important determinants are hyperglycemia and blood pressure. Determinants such as familial predisposition to proteinuria, duration of diabetes, age, endothelial cell dysfunction, lipid abnormalities, and probably smoking may be involved in the development and progression of microalbuminuria.

Table 9.6 Ambulatory blood pressure (mmHg) recordings in normotensive type 1 diabetic patients with or without microalbuminuria (adapted from [45])

	Daytime		Nighttime		24-h		Office	
Subjects	SBP	DBP	SBP	DBP	SBP	DBP	SBP	DBP
Controls	122	72	114	60	118	68	116	68
Normoalbuminuria	122	75	112	63	118	70	118	71
Microalbuminuria	128	79	121	70	126	75	122	74

SBP systolic blood pressure, *DBP* diastolic blood pressure

Screening for Albuminuria

A routine urinalysis should be performed in all patients before screening for microalbuminuria. If the dipstick is positive for proteinuria, there is no need to screen for microalbuminuria because the patient already has overt proteinuria. If the dipstick is negative, then screening for microalbuminuria is indicated. The consensus is that the screening should begin from puberty and 5 years after the diagnosis of type 1 diabetes. Urine samples can be collected over a 24-h period, early morning specimen or a random spot collection, whichever is convenient to the patient, and follow the criteria shown in Table 9.1 to define albuminuria.

Before albuminuria is established in any patient, it is essential to rule out other causes that increase or decrease albumin excretion (Table 9.7). Also, two of three collections done in a 3–6 month period should show elevated albumin levels before the diagnosis of microalbuminuria is entertained. A suggested schema for screening type 1 or type 2 patients for microalbuminuria is shown in Fig. 9.1.

Proteinuria of Nondiabetic Origin

Occasionally, patients with established diabetes present with dipstick positive or heavy proteinuria that is not expected for the duration or control of hyperglycemia. Also, unexpected deterioration in renal function is seen. Such atypical presentation is more common in type 2 diabetic than type 1 diabetic patients. These patients require a thorough clinical work-up of proteinuria. Such patients usually undergo a renal biopsy to establish DN and its various stages, but also to document existence of a nondiabetic renal disease alone or superimposed on DN. In addition to a definitive diagnosis, the histopathologic findings provide pertinent prognostic information

Table 9.7 Clinical conditions associated with increased or decreased albumin excretion

Increase	Decrease
Urinary tract infection	Nonsteroidal antiinflammatory drugs
Blood in urine	ACE-inhibitors or angiotensin receptor-blockers
Fever	Malnutrition
Exercise within 24-h	Low protein diets
Uncontrolled hyperglycemia	Inadequate 24-h urine collection
Uncontrolled hypertension	Overnight urine collection
Congestive heart failure	
High protein intake	
Excessive diuresis	
Upright posture	
Menstrual and vaginal bleeding	

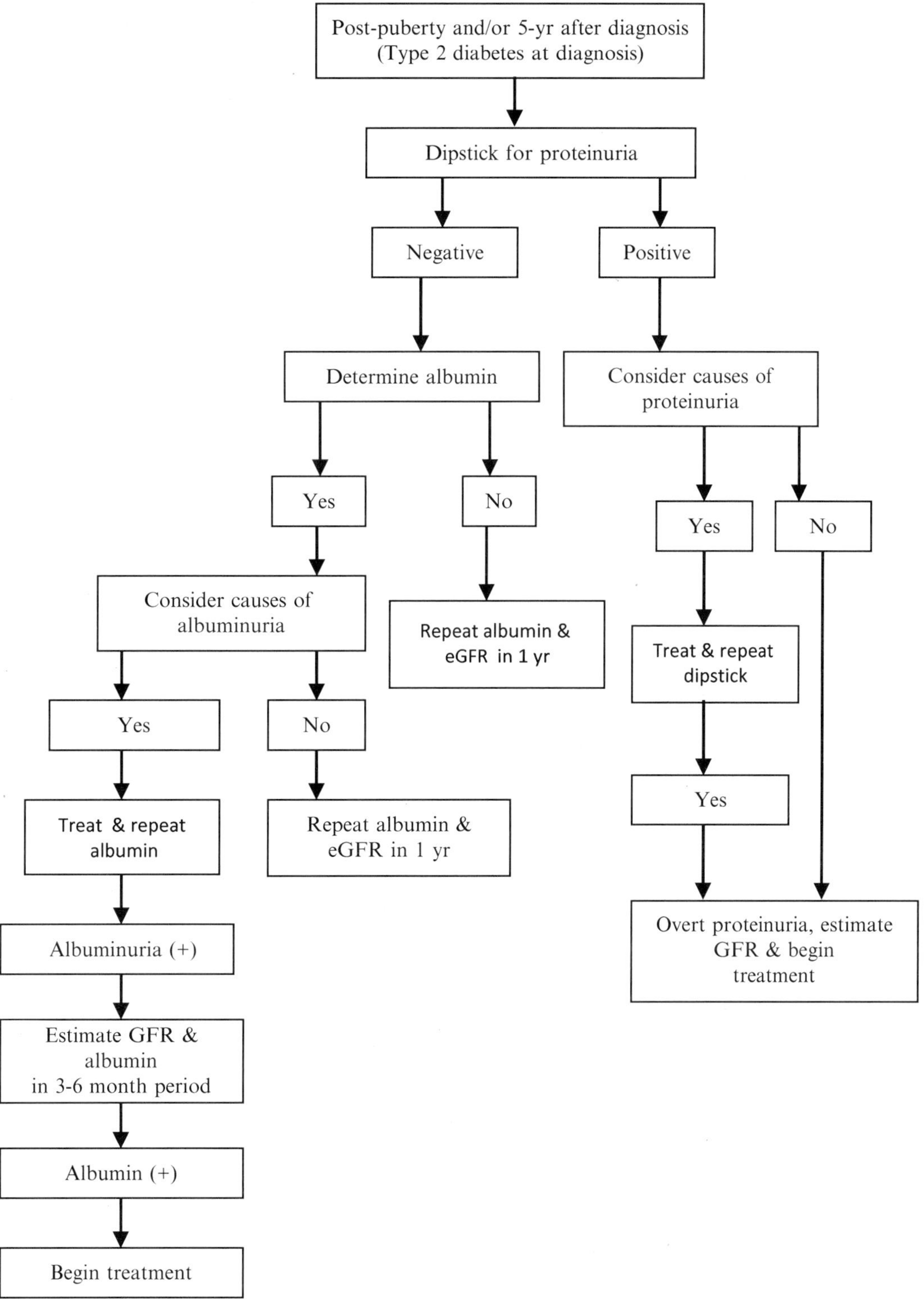

Fig. 9.1 Screening for albuminuria and estimated GFR (eGFR) in type 1 and type 2 diabetic patients

as well as a direction for appropriate therapy and management. The indications for renal biopsy are shown in Table 9.8.

When renal biopsies were performed in patients with atypical presentation, as shown in Table 9.8, a variety of nondiabetic renal diseases were observed. Such renal lesions were present either alone or superimposed on DN, making management more difficult. The following glomerular lesions have been documented.

Table 9.8 Indications for kidney biopsy in diabetic patients with renal disease

1. Proteinuria or nephrotic syndrome of sudden onset, appearing less than 5–10 years of type 1 DM
2. Proteinuria and/or impaired renal function in the absence of retinopathy in type 1 DM[a]
3. Proteinuria associated with a nephritic syndrome characterized by micro- or macrohematuria, renal insufficiency with RBC casts in types 1 and 2 DM
4. Unexplained renal failure with or without proteinuria
5. Presence of a systemic disease with abnormal serologic findings and clinical renal disease
6. Abnormal imaging studies such as ultrasonography and Doppler studies, after excluding renovascular disease
7. Absence of urologic disease or infection

[a]Prevalence of retinopathy less predictable for DN in type 2 DM

Table 9.9 Differential diagnosis of diabetic and nondiabetic renal diseases

Diagnosis	Proteinuria	Hematuria	Creatinine	S Alb	Serology	BP	Systemic symptoms
Diabetic nephropathy	Variable	Cr 30 %	Gradual increase	Nl or low	Negative	Variable	Long duration >10 year, nonspecific
Minimal change disease	NRP	None	Normal	Low	Negative	–	–
Focal segmental sclerosis	NRP	None	Normal	Low	Negative	–	–
Membranous GN, primary	NRP	<20 %	Normal	Low	PLA2R abs	–	
Membranous GN, secondary	NRP	None-1+	Normal	Low	Depending on systemic disease	–	Disease specific
Post-infectious GN	Mild to moderate	1–3+	Elevated	Nl or low	+ or neg blood cultures	Variable	Evidence of infection
IgAN	Mild	1–3+	Variable	Nl or low	Negative	Variable	Some cases with MRSA infection
Crescentic GN	Mild	3+	Elevated	Nl	ANCA, antiGBM	–	Rash, lung symptoms
Lupus nephritis	Variable to NRP	1–3+	Variable	Nl or low	ANA+	Variable	SLE symptoms
HCV/HBV infection	Variable to NRP	1–3+	Variable	Low	HBV+, HCV+	–	Extrarenal or hepatic disease
Fibrillary GN	Mild to NRP	1+	Variable	Low	Negative	–	–
Monoclonal protein disease	Mild to NRP	1–3+	Variable	Nl or low	M-spike	–	Depending on type of disease

NRP nephrotic range proteinuria >3 g/24 h, *Nl* normal, *Neg* negative, variable: creatinine levels may depend on active/proliferative GN or chronic sclerosing changes

Minimal change nephrotic syndrome/focal segmental glomerulosclerosis
Membranous glomerulonephritis
Crescentic glomerulonephritis
Postinfectious glomerulonephritis
IgA nephropathy-primary/secondary
Lupus nephritis
HCV-associated glomerulonephritis
Fibrillary glomerulonephritis
Monoclonal immunoglobulin-mediated diseases
Collapsing glomerulopathy

It is, therefore, suggested that the nephrologist should include nondiabetic renal lesions in the differential diagnosis of abnormal proteinuria. Table 9.9 shows clinical features of various glomerular diseases with proteinuria that may be helpful for appropriate management.

Treatment of Albuminuria–Proteinuria

A detailed review of treatment of albuminuria is beyond the scope of this chapter. Only generalizations are presented here. Almost all studies recommend an angiotensin-converting enzyme inhibitor (ACE-I), or an angiotensin receptor-blocker (ARB) as an initial drug of choice for albuminuria. In addition, control of glucose to achieve HbA1c ≤7 % has an independent positive effect in reducing albuminuria. Lowering blood pressure and controlling glucose have an additive effect in preventing the progression of albuminuria and renal dysfunction.

ACE-Is provide a selective benefit over other antihypertensive agents in both delaying the progression of albuminuria and decline in GFR in patients with high levels of albuminuria.

Table 9.10 Medical management of diabetic kidney disease

Proven benefit	Probable benefit	Benefit to be proven[a]
Blood glucose control	Control of hyperlipidemia	Aldose reductase inhibitors
Blood pressure control	Smoking cessation	Inhibitors of AGE
Low protein diet	Low salt diet	Antiplatelet and related therapy
		Antioxidants
		PKC inhibitors
		Sulodexide
		Growth factor inhibitors
		Gene therapy

AGE advanced glycation end products, *PKC* protein kinase C, *GAG* glycosaminoglycans
[a]Need large human studies

Also, the use of ACE-Is has been shown to reduce major CV events, such as stroke, myocardial infarction, or death, in diabetic patients. In normoalbuminuric type 2 diabetic patients, ACE-Is have been shown to delay the onset of microalbuminuria. ARBs seem to have minimal effect in preventing the onset of albuminuria in normotensive type 1 and type 2 diabetic subjects. However, ARBs have been shown to reduce the progression from micro- to macroalbuminuria as well as the development of ESRD in type 2 diabetic patients. Furthermore, the CV events were prevented by ARBs in type 2 diabetics.

A combination of an ACE-I and an ARB is not suggested at this time, although such a combination has been shown to have an additive effect in reducing proteinuria in both types of diabetics in the past. Also, addition of renin inhibitor is not suggested at this time. An additive benefit in terms of proteinuria can be achieved with a combination of an ACE-I or an ARB and an aldosterone blocker in patients with eGFR >60 mL/mL. Even in these patients, serum potassium levels may be slightly elevated. Therefore, close monitoring of serum potassium is warranted with this combination therapy.

Other antihypertensive drugs such as calcium channel blockers, diuretics, or β-blockers have been shown to lower proteinuria and can be used as additional drugs to lower blood pressure who are on either ACE-Is or ARBs. These drugs can be used as first-line therapy in selected individuals who cannot tolerate either ACE-Is or ARBs. Serum electrolytes, creatinine, and lipid panel should be obtained periodically in patients on diuretics.

Low protein diet (0.8 g/kg/day) can be used in selected diabetic patients whose proteinuria is progressing despite good glucose and blood pressure control and on adequate dosage of an ACE-I or ARB.

Several other therapies have been applied to improve both proteinuria and eGFR. Table 9.10 summarizes therapies that have been tried with variable success.

Table 9.11 Potential therapies for treatment of diabetic kidney disease

Therapeutic agent	Proposed mechanism
Pirfenidone	Inhibition of TGF-β1, TNF-α, collagen synthesis
Tranilast	Inhibition of TGF-β1
Doxycycline	Inhibition of matrix metalloproteinase activity
Pentoxifyline	Inhibition of proinflammatory cytokines
Connective tissue growth factor (CTGF) antagonist	Inhibition of matrix production and TGF-β1
Anti-TGF-β1	Inhibition of matrix formation
Bardoxolone	Decrease in oxidative stress
Bosentan	Endothelin (ET)-a and b antagonist
Atrasentan	ET-a selective receptor antagonist
Avosentan	ET-a antagonist
Pericalcitol	Inhibition of pro-fibrotic cytokines
Allopurinol	Inhibition of xanthine oxidase
B vitamin (folic acid, B_6, B_{12})	Decrease in oxidative stress and glycation
Adiponectin	Activation of an energy-sensing enzyme, AMPK
Rapamycin	Inhibition of mTOR (mammalian target of rapamycin)

Table 9.12 Podocyte-specific drugs

Vehicle	Target	Result
PKCα-inhibitor	Prevents nephrin loss	↓Proteinuria
Low molecular weight heparin	Binding to RAGE and inactivates its actions	↓Albuminuria
RAGE-antibody	Inactivation of RAGE	↓Albuminuria
BMP7	Podocyte overexpression	↓Albuminuria
BMP7 injection	Podocyte preservation of BMP7	↓Albuminuria
CTGF-AS-ODN	Counteracts CTGF action	↓Albuminuria
sFlt-1	Podocyte overexpression	↓Albuminuria
Handle region peptide (a decoy peptide)	Inhibits binding of prorenin to its receptor	↓Proteinuria

BMP bone morphogenetic protein 7, *CTGF-AS-ODN* connective tissue growth factor antisense oligodeoxynucleotide, *PKC* protein kinase C, *RAGE* receptor for advanced glycation end product, *(Flt-1* soluble fms-like tyrosine kinase 1, or soluble vascular endothelial growth receptor-1)

In recent years, a number of new therapeutic drugs have been tried in animals and humans for diabetic kidney disease. These therapeutic drugs are summarized in Table 9.11 [52–56].

Podocyte-Specific Drugs

As discussed under "Mechanisms of Albuminuria-Proteinuria," either decreased synthesis or mutations in genes that encode the podocyte proteins cause albuminuria. Therefore, development of podocyte-specific drugs is clearly indicated. In diabetic animal models, a number of pharmaceutical strategies have been tried with success. These studies are summarized in Table 9.12 [57, 58].

Conclusions

The presence of albuminuria–proteinuria in diabetic patients is an indication of early renal disease and signifies systemic endothelial dysfunction. Even a small amount of albuminuria (<30 mg/day) carries a risk for CVD. Abnormalities in podocyte-specific proteins seem to be the underlying mechanisms for albuminuria–proteinuria. Whenever a diabetic patient presents with heavy albuminuria–proteinuria, the nephrologist should consider the coexistence of nondiabetic primary glomerular diseases. Renal biopsy in such a patient is clearly warranted (Table 9.8).

The screening for albuminuria should begin from puberty and 5 years after the diagnosis of diabetes in type 1 patients. Urine samples can be collected over a 24-h period, early morning specimen or a random spot collection, whichever is convenient to the patient. ACR in a morning voided specimen is usually the standard way of expressing the excretion of albuminuria in the outpatient setting. Reagent strips for documenting the minute quantities of albuminuria are available in the office setting and diabetes clinics. Screening for albuminuria should begin during the first visit in type 2 diabetic patients.

ACE-Is or ARBs are the drugs of choice for the treatment of albuminuria. Prevention of albuminuria delays the progression of kidney disease as well as CVD. Combination of an ACE-I and an ARB is not recommended; however, a combination of either one of these drugs and an aldosterone antagonist seems to have an added benefit in the prevention of renal and CV diseases. Many new drugs targeting podocytes are being evaluated in animals and humans to prevent albuminuria–proteinuria in diabetic and nondiabetic patients. It is hoped that their introduction into the clinical practice is expected to decrease the morbidity and mortality in patients with albuminuria–proteinuria.

References

1. Vassalotti JA, Stevens LA, Levey AS. Testing for chronic kidney disease: a position statement from the National Kidney Foundation. Am J Kidney Dis. 2007;50:169–80.
2. Stoycheff N, Stevens LA, Schmid CH, et al. Nephrotic syndrome in diabetic kidney disease: an evaluation and update of the definition. Am J Kidney Dis. 2009;54:840–9.
3. Ruggenenti P, Gambara V, Perna A, et al. The nephropathy of non-insulin-dependent diabetes: predictors of outcome relative to diverse patterns of renal injury. J Am Soc Nephrol. 1998;9:2336–43.
4. Pham TT, Sim JJ, Kujubu DA, et al. Prevalence of nondiabetic renal disease in diabetic patients. Am J Nephrol. 2007;27:322–8.
5. KDOQI. KDOQI clinical practice guidelines and clinical practice recommendations for diabetes and chronic kidney disease. Am J Kidney Dis. 2007;49(2 Suppl 2):S12–54.
6. Mogensen CE, Christensen CK, Vittinghus E. The stages in diabetic renal disease. With emphasis on the stage of incipient diabetic nephropathy. Diabetes. 1983;32 Suppl 2:64–78.
7. Reddi AS. Diabetic nephropathy: theory & practice. East Hanover: College Book Publishers; 2004. Chapter 2, Natural history and clinical course of diabetic nephropathy. p. 5–26.
8. Reutens AT. Epidemiology of diabetic kidney disease. Med Clin North Am. 2013;97:1–18.
9. Dwyer JP, Lewis JB. Nonproteinuric diabetic nephropathy. Med Clin North Am. 2013;97:53–8.
10. Forman JP, Brenner BM. 'Hypertension' and 'microalbuminuria': the bell tolls for thee. Kidney Int. 2006;69:22–9.
11. Ruggenenti P, Remuzzi G. Time to abandon microalbuminuria. Kidney Int. 2006;70:1214–22.
12. Miller WG, Bruns DE, Hortin GL, Sandberg S, Aakre KM, McQueen MJ, et al. Current issues in measurement and reporting of urinary albumin excretion. Clin Chem. 2009;55:24–38.
13. Danziger J. Importance of low-grade albuminuria. Mayo Clin Proc. 2008;83:806–12.
14. Matshushita K, van de Velde M, Astor BC, et al. Association of estimated glomerular filtration rate and albuminuria with all-cause and cardiovascular mortality in general population cohorts: a collaborative meta-analysis. Lancet. 2010;375:2073–81.
15. Viberti GC, Jarrett RJ, Mahmud U, et al. Microalbuminuria as a predictor of clinical nephropathy in insulin-dependent diabetes mellitus. Lancet. 1982;I:1430–32.
16. Parving H-H, Oxenboll B, Svendson PA, et al. Early detection of patients at risk of developing diabetic nephropathy. A longitudinal study of urinary albumin excretion. Acta Endocrinol. 1982;100: 550–5.
17. Mogensen CE, Christensen CK. Predicting diabetic nephropathy in insulin-dependent patients. N Engl J Med. 1984;311:89–93.
18. Mathiesen ER, Oxenboll B, Johansen K, et al. Incipient nephropathy in type 1 (insulin-dependent) diabetes. Diabetologia. 1984;26: 406–10.
19. Almdal T, Norgaard K, Feldt-Rasmussen B, et al. The predictive value of microalbuminuria in IDDM. A five-year follow-up study. Diabetes Care. 1994;1(7):120–5.
20. Parving H-H, Chaturvedi N, Viberti GC, et al. Does microalbuminuria predict diabetic nephropathy? Diabetes Care. 2002;25:406–7.
21. Mogensen CE. Microalbuminuria predicts clinical proteinuria and early mortality in maturity-onset diabetes. N Engl J Med. 1984;310:356–60.
22. Nelson RG, Bennett PH, Beck GJ, et al. Development and progression of renal disease in Pima Indians with non-insulin-dependent diabetes mellitus. N Engl J Med. 1996;335:1636–42.
23. Ravid M, Lang R, Rachmani R, et al. Long-term renoprotective effect of angiotensin-converting enzyme inhibition in non-insulin-dependent diabetes mellitus. Arch Intern Med. 1996;156:286–9.
24. Ahmad J, Siddiqui MA, Ahmad H. Effect of postponement of diabetic nephropathy with enalapril in normotensive type 2 diabetic patients with microalbuminuria. Diabetes Care. 1997;20:1576–81.
25. Gæde P, Vedel P, Parving H-H, et al. Intensified multifactorial intervention in patients with type 2 diabetes mellitus and microalbuminuria: the Steno type 2 randomised study. Lancet. 1999;353:617–22.
26. Estacio RO, Jeffers BW, Gifford N, et al. Effect of blood pressure control on diabetic microvascular complications in patients with hypertension and type 2 diabetes. Diabetes Care. 2000;23:B54–64.
27. Heart Outcomes Prevention Evaluation Study Investigators. Effects of ramipril on cardiovascular and microvascular outcomes in people with diabetes mellitus: results of the HOPE study and MICRO-HOPE substudy. Lancet. 2000;355:253–9.
28. Parving H-H, Lehnert H, Bröchner-Mortensen J, et al. The effect of irbesartan on the development of diabetic nephropathy in patients with type 2 diabetes. N Engl J Med. 2001;345:870–8.
29. Parving H-H. Diabetic nephropathy: prevention and treatment. Kidney Int. 2001;60:2041–55.
30. Berhane AM, Weil EJ, Knowler WC, et al. Albuminuria and estimated glomerular filtration rate as predictors of diabetic end-stage renal disease and death. Clin J Am Soc Nephrol. 2011;6:2444–51.

31. Gansevoort RT, Matsushita K, van der Velde M, et al. Chronic kidney disease prognosis consortium: lower estimated GFR and higher albuminuria are associated with adverse kidney outcomes. A collaborative meta-analysis of general and high-risk population cohorts. Kidney Int. 2011;80:93–104.
32. Mundel P, Shankland SJ. Podocyte biology and response to injury. J Am Soc Nephrol. 2002;13:3005–13.
33. Pavenstädt H, Kriz W, Kretzler M. Cell biology of the glomerular podocyte. Phys Rev. 2003;83:253–307.
34. Tryggvason K, Patrakka J, Wartiovaara J. Hereditary proteinuria syndromes and mechanisms. N Engl J Med. 2006;354:1387–401.
35. Asanuma K, Yanagida-Asanuma E, Takagi M, et al. The role of podocytes in proteinuria. Nephrology. 2007;12:S15–20.
36. Mundel P, Reiser J. Proteinuria: an enzymatic disease of the podocyte? Kidney Int. 2010;77:571–80.
37. Garg P, Rabelink T. Glomerular proteinuria: a complex interplay between unique players. Adv Chronic Kidney Dis. 2011;18:233–42.
38. Reiser J, Sever S. Podocyte biology and pathogenesis of kidney disease. Annu Rev Med. 2013;64:357–66.
39. Li JJ, Kwak SJ, Jung DS, et al. Podocyte biology in diabetic nephropathy. Kidney Int. 2007;72:S36–42.
40. Jefferson JA, Shankland SJ, Pichler RH. Proteinuria in diabetic kidney disease: a mechanistic viewpoint. Kidney Int. 2008;74:22–36.
41. Ziyadeh FN, Wolf G. Pathogenesis of the podocytopathy and proteinuria in diabetic glomerulopathy. Curr Diabetes Rev. 2008;4:39–45.
42. Weil EJ, Lemley K, Mason CC, et al. Podocyte detachment and reduced glomerular capillary endothelial fenestration promote kidney disease in type 2 diabetic nephropathy. Kidney Int. 2012;82:1010–7.
43. Edelstein MH, Weinstein T, Grafter U. TGFβ1-dependent podocyte dysfunction. Curr Opin Nephrol Hypertens. 2013;22:93–9.
44. Baelde HJ, Eikmans M, Lappin DWP, et al. Reduction of VEGF-A and CTGF expression in diabetic nephropathy is associated with podocyte loss. Kidney Int. 2007;71:637–45.
45. Reddi AS. Diabetic nephropathy: theory & practice. East Hanover: College Book Publishers; 2004. Chapter 4, Microalbuminuria in type 1 diabetes. p. 55–88.
46. Weir MR. Microalbuminuria and cardiovascular disease. Clin J Am Soc Nephrol. 2007;2:581–90.
47. Borch-Johnsen K, Kreiner S. Proteinuria: value as predictor of cardiovascular mortality in insulin-dependent diabetes mellitus. Br Med J. 1987;294:1651–4.
48. Tarffvit O, Agardh C-D. The predictive value of albuminuria for cardiovascular and renal disease. A 5-year follow-up study of 476 patients with type 1 diabetes mellitus. J Diabetes Complications. 1993;7:49–56.
49. Gerstein HC, Mann JFE, Yi Q, et al. Albuminuria and risk of cardiovascular events, death, and heart failure in diabetic and nondiabetic individuals. JAMA. 2001;286:421–6.
50. Dinneeen SF, Gerstein HC. The association of microalbuminuria and mortality in non-insulin-dependent diabetes mellitus. A systematic overview of the literature. Arch Intern Med. 1997;157:1413–8.
51. Wiseman M, Viberti G, Mackintosh D, et al. Glycaemia, arterial pressure and micro-albuminuria in type 1 (insulin-dependent) diabetes mellitus. Diabetologia. 1984;26:401–5.
52. Turgut F, Bolton WK. Potential new therapeutic agents for diabetic kidney disease. Am J Kidney Dis. 2010;55:928–40.
53. Mathew A, Cunard R, Sharma K. Antifibrotic treatment and other new strategies for improving renal outcomes. Contrib Nephrol. 2011;170:217–27.
54. Ruggennent P, Cravedi P, Remuzzi G. Mechanisms and treatment of CKD. J Am Soc Nephrol. 2012;23:1917–28.
55. Shepler B, Nash C, Smith C, et al. Update on potential drugs for the treatment of diabetic kidney disease. Clin Ther. 2012;34:1237–46.
56. Kania DS, Smith CT, Nash CL, et al. Potential new treatments for diabetic kidney disease. Med Clin North Am. 2013;97:115–34.
57. Leeuwis JW, Nguyen TQ, Dendooven A, et al. Targeting podocyte-associated diseases. Adv Drug Deliv Rev. 2010;62:1325–36.
58. Reiser J, Gupta V, Kistler AD. Toward the development of podocyte-specific drugs. Kidney Int. 2010;77:662–8.

Hypertension in Diabetes Mellitus

10

William J. Elliott

Introduction

Hypertension (typically diagnosed if two office blood pressures are ≥140/90 mmHg) is currently the most common chronic condition for which Americans obtain medical care [1]. Across the USA, the age-adjusted prevalence of hypertension has remained relatively stable from 1994 to 2010 at around 30 %, but because of aging and obesity, it is expected to increase by a further 7.2 % by the year 2030 [1]. Diabetes mellitus (traditionally diagnosed after two fasting blood glucose measurements are >125 mg/dL, but more recently if A1c is >6.5 % [2]), especially the more common type 2, also has a prevalence that is strongly influenced by age and obesity; multiple datasets suggest there has been a near doubling of the incidence of diabetes in the last three decades in the USA. The age- and gender-dependence of the prevalence of hypertension and diabetes in the USA (derived primarily from the most recent National Health and Nutritional Examination Surveys, NHANES [1, 3]) is shown in Figs. 10.1 and 10.2.

The burden of hypertension, diabetes, and their combination is substantial. For example, in 2009–2010 data from the National Center for Health Statistics and National Health Interview Survey, 57 % of American women and 54 % of American men had been diagnosed with hypertension; the corresponding proportions for diabetes were 18 % for women and 24 % for men. These figures are likely to be underestimates, because undiagnosed hypertension was found in 6 % of the US adults in the NHANES of 2007–2010, and undiagnosed diabetes was estimated at 2.3 % of Americans ≥20 years of age in extrapolations of the 2007–2008 NHANES data to 2010 [4]. In 2010, diagnosed or undiagnosed hypertension affected an estimated 77.9 million Americans ≥20 years of age, compared to 25.8 million with diagnosed or undiagnosed diabetes [1, 3].

Hypertension and diabetes are just two of the all-too-commonly clustered cardiovascular risk factors in many Americans, which also include obesity and dyslipidemia (especially elevated serum levels of triglycerides and, perhaps more importantly, low-density lipoprotein cholesterol). A summary of the estimated prevalence of these interrelated risk factors, based on recent national survey data, extrapolated from the entire US adult population [1–3] (and for their overlap in a 60-year-old person, the closest age of the average American with diabetes, from the Framingham Heart Study in 2000–2005 [4]), is shown in Fig. 10.3. One of the more important features of this figure is the 67–90 % overlap of diabetes with hypertension (depending on age, body-mass index, and kidney function), which provides a very strong impetus for population-based strategies to improve outcomes in diabetics (see below).

Across the globe, both diabetes and hypertension contribute strongly to disability and death. Worldwide, high blood pressure was identified as the largest (and most important) risk factor for the Global Burden of Disease in 2010, accounting for 7 % of the global disability-adjusted life-years, edging out tobacco smoking (6.3 %) and household air pollution from solid fuels (4.3 %) [6]. This was a huge change from 1990, when childhood infectious diseases were more often fatal, and reflects the increasing incidence of cardiovascular disease (and its risk factors) across the earth. Using existing epidemiological data through 2002, another group estimated that 26.4 % (or about 972 million) of the world's population had hypertension in 2000, with 29.2 % (or 1.56 billion) projected to have the condition by 2025. Most of the growth was expected to occur in developing nations [7]. The International Diabetes Federation estimates that 366 million people had diabetes in 2011, which will increase to 552 million by 2030, because the prevalence of type 2 diabetes is increasing in every country surveyed. Perhaps because 80 % of people

The writing of this manuscript was not supported by any specific entity. For a list of the author's "Real or Potential Conflicts of Interest," see the attached "Standard Financial Disclosure Form."

W.J. Elliott, M.D., Ph.D. (✉)
Division of Pharmacology, Pacific Northwest University of Health Sciences, 200 University Parkway, Yakima, WA 98901, USA
e-mail: wj.elliott@yahoo.com

E.V. Lerma and V. Batuman (eds.), *Diabetes and Kidney Disease*,
DOI 10.1007/978-1-4939-0793-9_10, © Springer Science+Business Media New York 2014

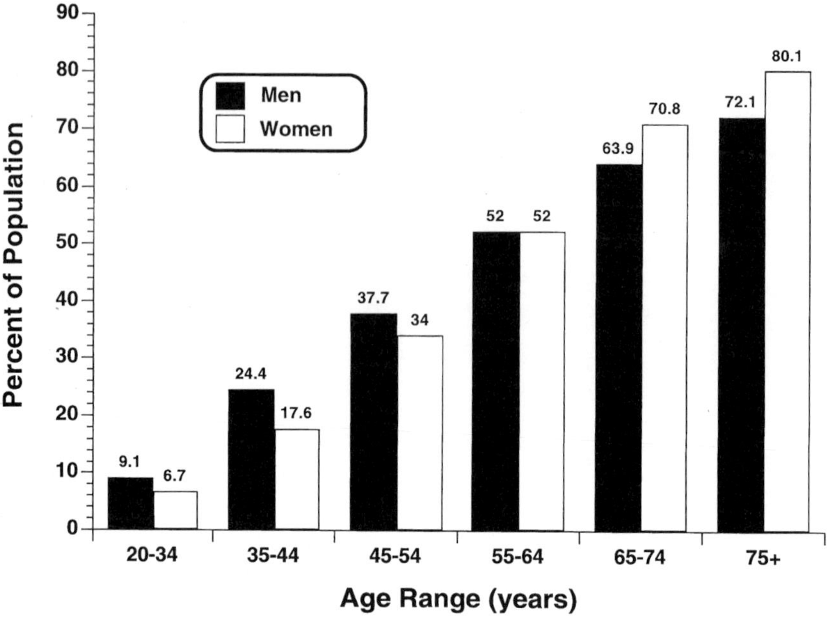

Fig. 10.1 Age- and gender-specific prevalence of hypertension in the USA, according to the National Health and Nutrition Examination Surveys 2007–2010 (Adapted from reference [1]). Note that men have a higher prevalence of hypertension than women until about age 60, after which the reverse is true. Whether this can be attributed to a survivorship effect is not clear

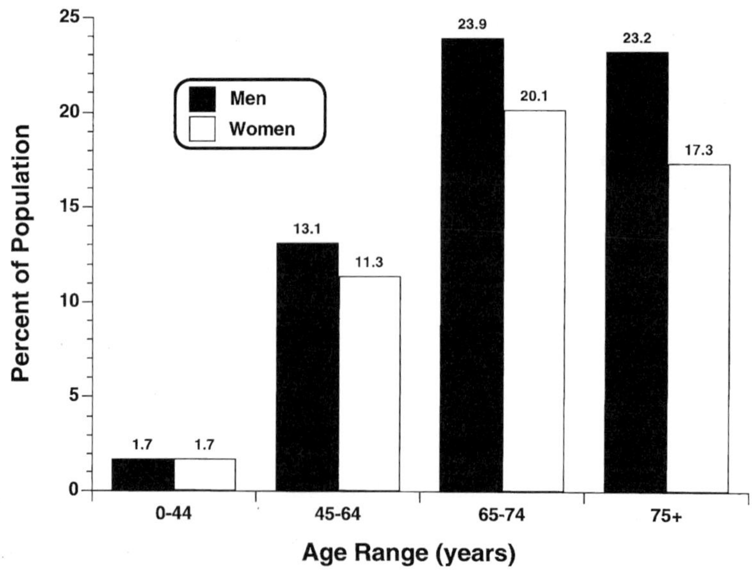

Fig. 10.2 Age- and gender-specific prevalence of diabetes mellitus in the USA in 2010, according to the US Centers for Disease Control and Prevention's National Center for Chronic Disease Prevention and Health Promotion, Division of Diabetes Translation (data from reference [2])

with diabetes live in low- and middle-income countries, about half of those with diabetes have not yet been diagnosed. Reflecting its importance as a risk factor for mortality (with 4.6 million deaths in 2011), the prevalence of diabetes is greatest worldwide between the ages of 40 and 59 years [8].

Pathophysiology of Hypertension in Diabetics

Although perhaps something of an oversimplification, one of the most important factors in the co-development of hypertension and diabetes is insulin resistance. This problem can be most directly studied using insulin-clamp techniques that are most appropriate in a research setting, but surrogates have been developed, including fasting and postprandial serum insulin levels that lend themselves to large studies, including clinical trials. The results of such studies suggest that nearly 50 % of Americans with primary hypertension have insulin resistance. Genetics have also been implicated, because first-degree relatives of patients with hypertension also have an increased risk of insulin resistance and dyslipidemia, even if they are normotensive. Probably more important for most Americans are environmental factors, like high-fat and high-calorie diets and sedentary lifestyles that lead to central adiposity and ectopic lipid deposition. These factors probably combine with the increased risk of insulin resistance to cause inflammatory and oxidative stress, which has many negative

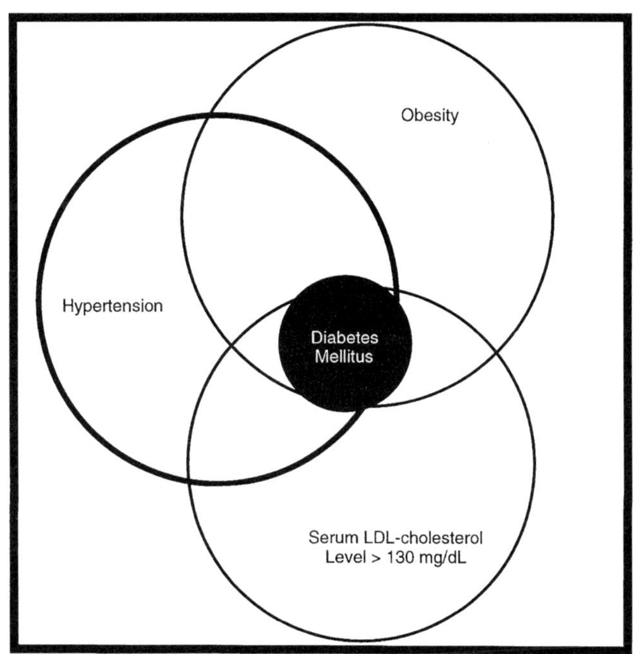

Fig. 10.3 Venn diagram representing the prevalence (and strong overlap) of hypertension (33 %), diabetes (11.8 %), obesity (34.6 %), and elevated serum low-density lipoprotein cholesterol level (>130 mg/dL, 31.1 %) in the civilian, non-institutionalized US adult population (represented by the area within the *square box*) in recent National Surveys that included the year 2010 [1–4]. The overlap proportions are taken from either national survey data (when available) or reference [5]

effects. In addition to enhancing the activity of the renin–angiotensin–aldosterone and sympathetic nervous systems, and causing sodium/water retention, many maladaptive derangements occur in blood vessels. These include an increase in vascular smooth muscle cell proliferation, arterial stiffness, and vascular tone, and endothelial dysfunction, a decreased ability to vasodilate in response to appropriate stimuli (e.g., nitric oxide) [9]. Some of these effects (especially closely linked to hyperinsulinemia) appear to be mediated by an elevation in intracellular calcium concentrations within vascular smooth muscle cells, which has, in turn, been recently linked to abnormal vitamin D levels and metabolism. Some believe that better understanding of these pathophysiological links between hypertension and diabetes has implications for better treatment of either condition, as antihypertensive drug classes may have differential effects on incident diabetes, and some hypoglycemic drugs may increase blood pressure (see below).

Hypertension and Type 1 Diabetes Mellitus

Type 1 diabetes (characterized by a complete lack of insulin) constitutes only about 6-8% of Americans with diabetes, as the other 92-94% have type 2 diabetes (characterized by peripheral insulin insensitivity). Most affected patients are children or adolescents, who, because of their young ages, are at low risk for hypertension. They are therefore also at low risk for competing causes of death (compared to their type 2 diabetic counterparts, discussed below), so a larger proportion of type 1 diabetics develop chronic kidney disease (compared to type 2 diabetics). Most type 1 diabetic patients develop microalbuminuria, proteinuria, and subsequently renal disease before hypertension (see Chaps. 3 and 7 of this book for more details). However, elevated blood pressure accelerates the disease processes in these young individuals, and greatly increases their risk of both macrovascular and microvascular manifestations of diabetes. For this reason, *early*, intensive antihypertensive therapy is often recommended, particularly with an inhibitor of the renin–angiotensin system (for which there are clinical trial data using macroalbuminuria as the endpoint) [2]. Typically, beta-blockers are best avoided as antihypertensive therapy for type 1 diabetics, as such patients are more prone to hypoglycemia, signs and symptoms of which can be diminished and even masked by beta-blockade [2]. Otherwise considerations about blood pressure management in type 1 diabetics are quite similar to those for the much more common type 2 diabetics, which have been more extensively studied (see below).

Hypertension and Type 2 Diabetes

We have far more data, and thus much stronger evidence (even including some from randomized clinical trials, see below), for the role of blood pressure as a major contributor to the risk of both cardiovascular and renal disease in type 2 diabetics. Nearly all epidemiological studies, starting with the Framingham Heart Study, have consistently identified hypertension as an independent risk factor for heart disease, stroke, cardiovascular death, and end-stage renal disease, whether the subject was initially diabetic or not. Perhaps the most revealing of the recent literature on the prognostic importance of hypertension in diabetics comes from a roughly 4-year follow-up study of 1,145 Framingham participants after the new diagnosis of diabetes, of whom 125 died and 204 experienced a cardiovascular event [10]. After appropriate adjustments for demographic and other clinical variables, hypertension was associated with a highly significant 72 % increase in the risk of mortality, and a similarly significant 57 % increase in the risk of cardiovascular event in individuals with newly diagnosed diabetes. Hypertension carried a far greater population-attributable risk than diabetes for both death (30 % vs. 7 %) and cardiovascular event (25 % vs. 9 %) in these subjects. Some would argue that conclusions drawn from observational studies are inherently weaker than observations made about primary analyses of clinical trials. Fortunately, we have abundant data from clinical trials in both diabetic subjects treated with antihypertensive drug therapy (compared to those who did not receive such therapy) and hypertensive subjects who were or were not diabetic (at baseline) that consistently show significant benefits of lowering blood pressure to prevent major cardiovascular and/or renal endpoints.

Cardiovascular Outcomes in Hypertensive Diabetics vs. Hypertensive Nondiabetics

The Blood Pressure Lowering Treatment Trialists' Collaboration most recently published data comparing outcomes in clinical trials of antihypertensive drug therapy in diabetics vs. nondiabetics in 2005 [11]. Although their original intent was not to directly compare risks among diabetics and nondiabetics, but instead to identify the benefits of similar blood pressure-lowering treatments in these groups, their data about fatal or nonfatal myocardial infarctions ("Coronary Heart Disease") can be rearranged as in Fig. 10.4. Random-effects meta-analysis of these data shows that diabetics consistently have a higher risk of coronary heart disease events than nondiabetics, even when treated with similar, if not identical, antihypertensive regimens. On average, diabetics in these trials (who were well treated with all appropriate other therapies at the times the trials were executed) experienced an 88 % (95 % confidence interval, CI: 83–99 %) increased risk of fatal or nonfatal myocardial infarction ($P \ll 0.0001$), compared to nondiabetics. Similar calculations indicate that the risk of fatal or nonfatal stroke in clinical trials of antihypertensive agents is highly significantly increased by 43 % (95 % CI: 38–52 %) in diabetics, compared to nondiabetics. Similarly, cardiovascular death was significantly increased by 90 % (95 % CI: 84–101 %) for diabetics compared to nondiabetics. These estimates are in substantial agreement with many other datasets, including those from large epidemiological studies, indicating that diabetes usually doubles long-term cardiovascular risk, in both hypertensive and non-hypertensive individuals.

Renal Outcomes in Hypertensive Diabetics

Although there are fewer data from randomized clinical trials for renal vs. cardiovascular endpoints, many lines of evidence strongly implicate hypertension as a major risk factor for end-stage renal disease and progressive renal disease in diabetics. Perhaps most tragic are the data collected for each patient who starts renal replacement therapy in the USA on the "Intake Form," which are summarized annually by the United States Renal Data Systems [12]. According to the 2012 report, 50,305 of the 114,032 (or 44.1 %) individuals who were diagnosed with end-stage renal disease in 2010 had diabetes as the primary reason for their fate; a further

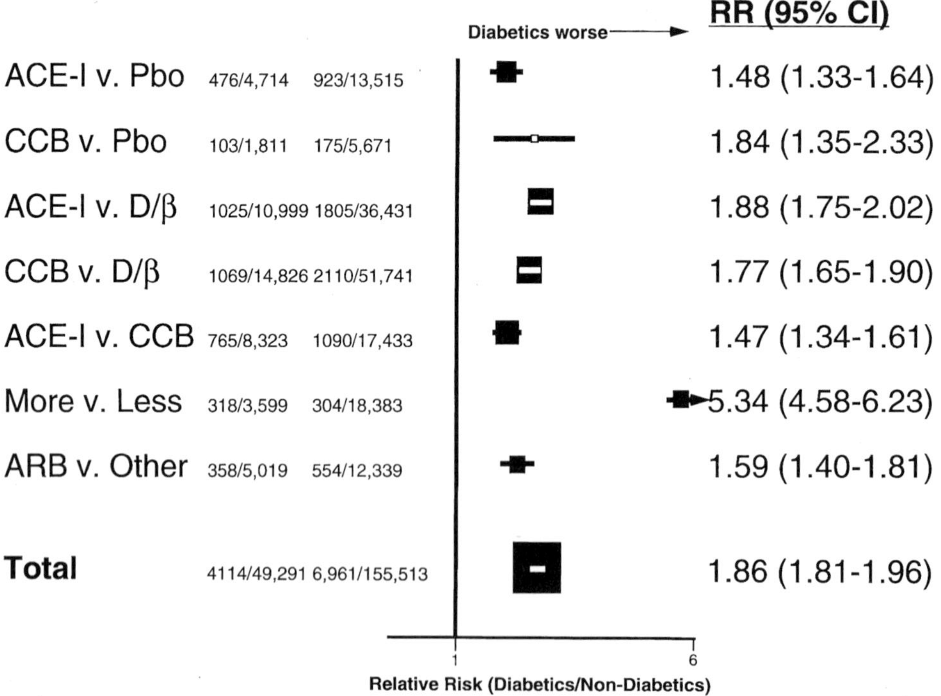

Fig. 10.4 Meta-analysis of coronary heart disease (fatal or nonfatal myocardial infarction) in randomized clinical trials comparing antihypertensive drug regimens in hypertensive diabetics vs. hypertensive nondiabetics. Data from reference [11]. The summary odds ratio for coronary heart disease across 186,620 subjects was 1.88 (95 % CI: 1.83–1.99) for diabetic compared to nondiabetic hypertensives

28.5 % had hypertension as the primary cause of kidney failure. However, these data are likely biased, because the Intake Form allows only a single answer to a typically complex question, and the options are given alphabetically (putting "Diabetes" ahead of "Hypertension" in the list). The Intake Form was modified once, in 2001, to allow identification of more than one condition that resulted in renal replacement therapy. In that year, 15 % of those reaching end-stage renal disease had diabetes alone as the cause, 33 % had hypertension alone, and 39 % had both hypertension and diabetes checked on the Intake Form. These data, which have not been replicated, suggest that, even (or perhaps especially) among diabetics, hypertension is a major contributor to the risk of end-stage renal disease.

In addition to these population-based epidemiological data about the risk of end-stage renal disease being significantly higher in hypertensive diabetics, many longitudinal databases also show a highly significant increase in the risk for several renal endpoints in hypertensive (compared to normotensive) diabetics. Interestingly, the Framingham Heart Study has not contributed extensively to this literature, primarily because they originally enrolled only 5,209 subjects in their study, and it is far more likely that these individuals died of cardiovascular causes before they developed end-stage renal disease. However, large databases from the Multiple Risk Factor Intervention Trial [13], the Department of Veterans Affairs Medical Centers [14], and the Kaiser Permanente of Northern California Health Plan [15] have consistently shown that hypertension is a major, significant contributor to both chronic kidney disease and end-stage renal disease, even (or perhaps especially) among diabetics. Similar conclusions have been reached in long-term follow-up of populations from Finland [16], China [17], and Norway [18].

Perhaps even more compelling than epidemiological data about the importance of elevated blood pressures in diabetics in preventing kidney disease are the large number of successful clinical trials, summarized in detail below, that have shown major benefits in retarding the progression of kidney disease, and sometimes even preventing or delaying the onset of end-stage renal disease.

Hypertension Treatment Strategies in Diabetics

Lifestyle Modifications

Few would argue that intensive non-pharmacological intervention, typically starting with diet and exercise, should not be highly recommended for diabetics with elevated blood pressures [2]. Recent clinical trial data supporting these interventions in hypertensive diabetics, however, are scarce, as it is probably unethical now to randomize diabetic hypertensive patients to a strategy that does not include diet and exercise. A summary of the effects of dietary modifications (typically to lower both calories and sodium) on blood pressure can be found in two excellent, recent reviews [19, 20]. Many other lifestyle modifications have a salutary effect on blood pressure, but those highlighted in a recent American Heart Association Scientific Statement [21] included increased physical activity (typically aerobic exercise) and device-guided breathing. The benefits of aerobic exercise in hypertensive diabetics probably derive from both weight loss (with or without a diet plan) and improved insulin sensitivity. The best data on this point come from a large epidemiological study in Finland [22], and the Finnish Diabetes Prevention Study [23], which showed that overweight subjects with impaired glucose tolerance experienced a 58 % reduction in the risk of diabetes over an average of 3.2 years after being randomized to individualized counseling about reducing weight, total and saturated fat, and increasing dietary fiber and physical activity; the benefits were directly related to successful achievement of these goals.

A beneficial lifestyle modification that should not really require much discussion is tobacco avoidance [2]. Cigarettes and other forms of tobacco use increase the risk of atherosclerotic cardiovascular disease, independently of blood pressure and diabetes. Although the "evidence-base" for tobacco avoidance in diabetics, hypertensives, or the combination is lacking (primarily because it would be unethical to recommend that smokers with these problems continue using tobacco), all current guidelines recommend cessation of tobacco use, which has been shown in long-term epidemiological studies to significantly decrease the risk of most of the chronic complications of hypertension and diabetes (including cardiovascular death, myocardial infarction, stroke, and amputation).

Effects of Antihypertensive Drugs on Incident Diabetes

Although lowering elevated blood pressure is highly beneficial in preventing both cardiovascular and renal endpoints in individuals with hypertension, different classes of antihypertensive agents have disparate effects on glucose tolerance (and incident diabetes). It has been known since the late 1950s that thiazide diuretics may increase insulin requirements in diabetics, or increase the risk of incident diabetes in those who are not yet diabetic. Data on this point are confounded by the fact that hypertension itself increases these risks, presumably due to both the higher risk of overweight/obesity and increased insulin resistance. Some beta-blockers have been noted to increase both these risks, perhaps by limiting exercise tolerance and decreasing peripheral arterial flow (and glucose uptake by large skeletal muscles).

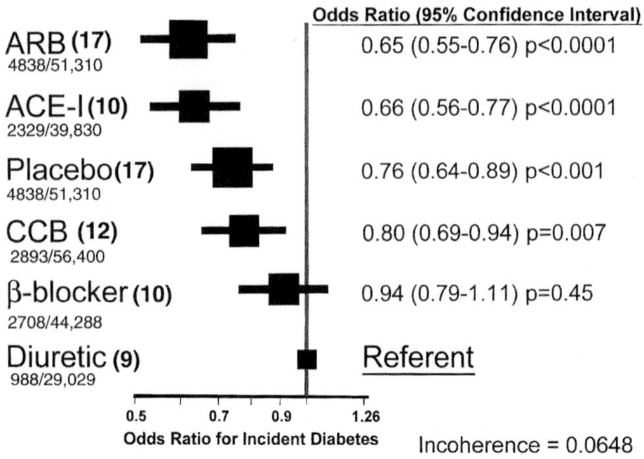

Fig. 10.5 Results of network meta-analysis of incident diabetes in 34 clinical trials involving antihypertensive drugs (and placebo/no treatment). The numbers in *parentheses* after each class of drug are the frequency of use in clinical trials; the numbers separated by the *slash* below the drug class correspond to the number of incident diabetics/number of subjects at risk. Data from reference [25]

On the other hand, both angiotensin-converting enzyme (ACE) inhibitors and angiotensin receptor blockers (ARBs) have been shown in randomized clinical trials to improve insulin sensitivity and reduce the risk of incident diabetes. Network meta-analyses have been used to compare the risks of incident diabetes across all antihypertensive drug classes (including placebo/no treatment) in long-term randomized clinical trials in hypertensive individuals [24]. The most recent of these is summarized in Fig. 10.5 [25].

The clinical implications of these data are controversial [24, 26]. The Multiple Risk Factor Intervention Trial [27], the population-based Finnish Monitoring of Trends and Determinants in Cardiovascular Disease Experience [28], the Antihypertensive and Lipid-Lowering treatment to prevent Heart Attack Trial (ALLHAT) [29], and the long-term follow-up of the Systolic Hypertension in the Elderly Trial [30] all showed no significant increase in cardiovascular risk among individuals who were not diabetic at baseline, but who developed it during the time of observation, compared to those who maintained euglycemia during follow-up. This conclusion can be easily faulted, however, because the duration of follow-up, particularly in clinical trials, was relatively short (e.g., in ALLHAT, the protocol called for initial testing for incident diabetes at 2 years of follow-up, and therefore limited the time for development of subsequent cardiovascular disease to 2.9 years, on average). A population-based observational study from Italy suggested (based on 11 outcome events in the new diabetic population) that new-onset diabetes was associated with a significantly higher risk of cardiovascular events (compared to nondiabetics), which did not differ from cardiovascular event rates over 13 years in those who were diabetic at baseline [31]. A population-based study from Gothenburg, Sweden, concluded that it took 9 years for the cardiovascular risk of new-onset diabetes to achieve statistical significance [32]. The Framingham Heart Study also concluded that the cardiovascular risk associated with incident diabetes was time-dependent, and became significant after more than a decade of type 2 diabetes for coronary heart disease, but only ~7 years for coronary heart disease death [33]. This experience was similar to that seen in the Valsartan Long-term Use Evaluation (VALUE) trial, in which the 1,298 patients who developed diabetes during follow-up had a cardiac morbidity that was intermediate (hazard ratio 1.43, 95 % CI: 1.16–1.77) between those who were diabetic at randomization (hazard ratio 2.20, 95 % CI: 1.95–2.49), compared to the referent group who remained euglycemic throughout [34].

There is little doubt that, in large populations, the increased risk of incident diabetes associated with diuretics or beta-blockers (even though statistically significant) is vastly outweighed by the overwhelmingly beneficial effects of blood pressure lowering. Even if the cardiovascular and/or renal risk of incident diabetes does not increase significantly for a decade, the short-term incremental costs involved in routine medical care for diabetics will be substantial: monitoring blood glucose (and A1c twice yearly), lowering serum lipids to a lower threshold, monitoring renal function (albuminuria and serum creatinine), and ophthalmological and podiatric screening [2]. These types of considerations have led to the common recommendation to begin antihypertensive drug therapy for most diabetics with either an ACE-inhibitor or an ARB, as they are least likely to increase plasma glucose levels or insulin requirements [2].

Pharmacological Treatment of Hypertension in Diabetes

Overview

Essentially all authorities agree that controlling blood pressure is beneficial for diabetics [2], but disagreement has recently emerged regarding which class of antihypertensive agent should be preferred as first-line drug therapy, and what the target blood pressure should be. The American Diabetes Association still recommends either an ACE-inhibitor or an ARB, although it has softened its wording about initial therapy, and now recommends only that the antihypertensive regimen include one of these agents [2]. In 2005, the Blood Pressure Lowering Treatment Trialists' Collaboration found "comparable" differences across four initial types of antihypertensive drugs (ACE-inhibitor, ARB, calcium antagonist, diuretic/beta-blocker) vs. placebo for preventing total major cardiovascular events in diabetics, and "limited evidence" that lower blood pressure goals produced larger reductions in total major cardiovascular events in diabetics [11]. This last conclusion was soundly rejected by the results of the Action to Control Cardiovascular Risk in Diabetes (ACCORD)-Blood

Table 10.1 Major cardiovascular events observed (or estimated*) in outcome-based clinical trials of antihypertensive drugs in diabetics

Trial acronym	Drug class	Events/at risk	Drug class	Events/at risk	Drug class	Events/at risk
SHEP*	Diuretic	39/283	Placebo	58/300		
ABCD	CCB	47/235	ACE	29/235		
FACET	CCB	23/191	ACE	14/189		
UKPDS	ACE	94/400	Beta-blocker	72/358		
NORDIL	CCB	44/351	Beta-blocker[a]	44/376		
Syst-Eur*	CCB	13/252	Placebo	31/240		
MICRO-HOPE	ACE	277/1,808	Placebo	351/1,769		
Syst-China*	CCB	5/51	Placebo	10/47		
INSIGHT*	CCB	46/649	Diuretic	49/653		
PROGRESS	ACE	82/394	Placebo	91/368		
IDNT	ARB	138/579	Placebo	144/569	CCB	128/567
RENAAL	ARB	124/751	Placebo	118/762		
IRMA-2*	ARB	11/194	Placebo	18/201		
LIFE	ARB	103/586	Beta-blocker	139/609		
ALLHAT	Diuretic	906/5,393	CCB	555/3,214	ACE	521/3129
CONVINCE	CCB	101/1,616	Beta-blocker	116/1,623		
INVEST*	CCB	463/3,169	Beta-blocker	450/3,231		
SCOPE	ARB	46/313	Placebo	51/284		
PERSUADE	ACE	103/721	Placebo	130/781		
DIAB-HYCAR	ACE	282/2,443	Placebo	276/2,469		
DETAIL	ACE	12/130	ARB	150/120		
ASCOT	CCB	246/2,565	Beta-blocker	257/2,572		
ADVANCE	ACE	480/5,569	Placebo	520/5,571		
CASE-J	ARB	68/1,011	CCB	70/1,007		
ONTARGET	ARB	568/3,246	ACE	558/3,146		
ACCOMPLISH	CCB	170/3,347	Diuretic	203/3,468		
PRoFESS	ARB	498/2,840	Placebo	511/2,903		
TRANSCEND	ARB	211/1,059	Placebo	211/1,059		

SHEP Systolic Hypertension in the Elderly Program [64]; *ABCD* Appropriate Blood pressure Control in Diabetes (N Engl J Med. 2000;343:1969); *FACET* Fosinopril Amlodipine Cardiovascular Events Trial (Diabetes Care. 1998;21:1779–1780); *UKPDS* United Kingdom Prospective Diabetes Study #39 [63]; *NORDIL* Nordic DILtiazem study (Lancet. 2000;356:359–365); *Syst-Eur* Systolic hypertension in Europe trial (N Engl J Med. 1999;340:677–684); *MICRO-HOPE* MIcroalbuminuria, Cardiovascular and Renal Outcomes-Heart Outcomes Prevention Evaluation [52]; *Syst-China* Systolic Hypertension in China study (Arch Intern Med. 2000;160:211–220); *INSIGHT* International Nifedipine GITS Study: Intervention as a Goal in Hypertension Treatment (Hypertension. 2003;41:431–6); *PROGRESS* Perindopril pROtection aGainst Recurrent Stroke Study (Blood Press. 2004;13:7–13); *IDNT* Irbesartan Diabetic Nephropathy Trial [41]; *RENAAL* Reduction of Endpoints in Non-Insulin Dependent Diabetes Mellitus with the Angiotensin II Antagonist Losartan [42]; *IRMA-2* IRbesartan in patients with type 2 diabetes and Microalbuminuria study #2 [44]; *LIFE* Losartan Intervention For Endpoint reduction trial [36]; *ALLHAT* Antihypertensive and Lipid-Lowering to prevent Heart Attack Trial [53]; *CONVINCE* Controlled ONset Verapamil INvestigation of Cardiovascular Endpoints (JAMA. 2003;289:2073–2082); *INVEST* International Verapamil-trandolapril STudy (Hypertension. 2004;44:637–642); *SCOPE* Study on Cognition and Prognosis in the Elderly (Blood Press. 2005;14:31–37); *PERSUADE* PERindopril SUbstudy in coronary Artery disease and DiabetEs (Eur Heart J. 2005;26:1369–1378); *DIAB-HYCAR* DIABetes, Hypertension, microalbuminuria or proteinuria, Cardiovascular events And Ramipril study (BMJ. 2004;328:495, erratum 686); *DETAIL* Diabetics Exposed to Telmisartan And enalaprIL Study[50]; *ASCOT* Anglo-Scandinavian Cardiac Outcomes Trial [61]; *ADVANCE* Action in Diabetes and Vascular disease: preterAx® and diamicroN-mr® Controlled Evaluation (Lancet. 2007;370:829–840); *CASE-J* Candesartan Antihypertensive Survival Evaluation in Japan (Hypertens Res. 2010;33:600–606); *ONTARGET* ONgoing Telmisartan Alone or in combination with Ramipril Global Endpoint Trial [56]; *ACCOMPLISH* Avoiding Cardiovascular events through COMbination therapy in Patients LIving with Systolic Hypertension [62]; *PRoFESS* Prevention Regimen for Effectively Avoiding Second Strokes (N Engl J Med. 2008:359:1225–1237); *TRANSCEND* Telmisartan Randomized AssessmeNt Study in angiotensin Converting Enzyme-inhibitor iNtolerant subjects with cardiovascular Disease (Lancet. 2008;371:1174–1183)

Pressure trial [35], which caused a revision of the decade-old recommendation for diabetics to achieve a blood pressure <130/80 mmHg [2], discussed in detail below. Some have suggested that the argument about initial antihypertensive therapy in diabetics is (or should be) moot, as nearly all diabetics (in clinical trials, as well as in general clinical practice) have required two or more blood pressure-lowering agents to achieve even the currently recommended blood pressure target of <140/90 mmHg [2].

The numbers of diabetics with major cardiovascular events (composite of cardiovascular death, stroke, or myocardial infarction) observed (or estimated) in 28 randomized clinical trials of antihypertensive drugs involving 78,754 subjects are summarized in Table 10.1.

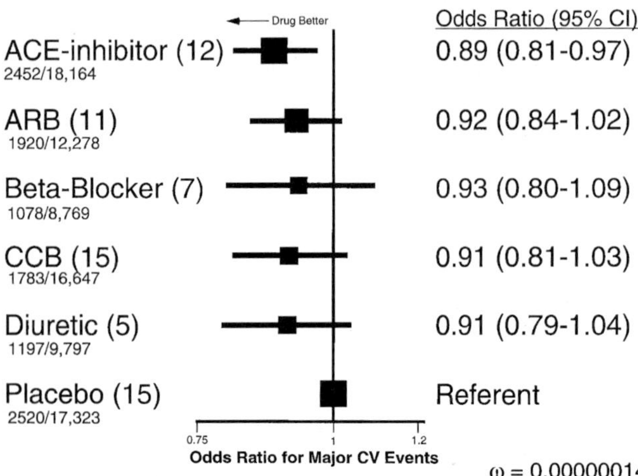

Fig. 10.6 Results of a network meta-analysis comparing the risk of major cardiovascular events (cardiovascular death, myocardial infarction, or stroke) in 78,754 diabetic subjects across all randomized drug classes (placebo, diuretic, beta-blocker, calcium antagonist, ACE-inhibitor, angiotensin II receptor blocker) in 28 clinical trials of antihypertensive drugs (excluding the combination arms of ONTARGET). Numbers in *parentheses* are the number of trials using this randomized drug class. *Horizontal bars* indicate the 95 % confidence limits; the *boxes* represent the odds ratios (drawn with area proportional to available statistical information). *CI* confidence interval, *ACE-inhibitor* angiotensin-converting enzyme inhibitor, *ARB* angiotensin receptor blocker, *CCB* calcium channel blocker, *CV* cardiovascular. Numbers separated by the *slash* below the drug class represent the numbers of diabetics with major cardiovascular events/numbers randomized across all trials

The results from a new network meta-analysis of these data are shown in Fig. 10.6. These data support (and extend) the 2005 analyses of the Blood Pressure Lowering Treatment Trialists' Collaboration, which suggested that there were few important outcome differences across randomized agents. These data are confounded by the fact that most placebo-treated patients in these studies received other antihypertensive agents, in addition to the randomized therapy, which dilutes the protective effect of the active agent. Most authorities now hold that most truly significant differences (when they exist) in these analyses are more likely due to lack of statistical power, study design issues, and other technical factors, rather than a clear superiority of one drug class over another.

Angiotensin Receptor Blockers

Angiotensin II receptor blockers offer many advantages for the treatment of hypertension in type 2 diabetics. They are generally effective in lowering blood pressure (particularly when combined with a diuretic or calcium antagonist), are well tolerated (even better than placebo in several comparative trials in nondiabetics), reduce proteinuria and albuminuria (both acutely and chronically), prevent major cardiovascular and renal events, and are contraindicated only in patients immediately before or during pregnancy, with known renovascular hypertension, or prior allergy to the specific agent. Several ARBs are now generically available, although none are currently on most $4/month lists.

Probably the best clinical trial evidence for an ARB to prevent major cardiovascular events comes from the type 2 diabetic subgroup enrolled in the Losartan Intervention For Endpoint (LIFE) reduction trial [36]. Critics will argue that this study enrolled only patients with very strict criteria for left ventricular hypertrophy, and therefore its results should not be generalizable to other patients without such abnormalities. Two years after its publication, the first author of this very report pointed out that atenolol, the initial comparator agent in LIFE, is a suboptimal once-daily antihypertensive agent [37]. Despite these objections, however, the 1,195 subjects in LIFE all had hypertension, type 2 diabetes, and electrocardiographic evidence for left ventricular hypertrophy, and were randomized to initial antihypertensive therapy with either losartan or atenolol, followed by hydrochlorothiazide, and other antihypertensive drugs, as needed. Blood pressures fell from an average of 177/96 mmHg at randomization to 146/79 mmHg in the losartan group, compared to 148/79 mmHg in the atenolol group. The primary composite endpoint was cardiovascular death, stroke, or myocardial infarction, which was significantly reduced in the group randomized to losartan (relative risk: 0.76, 95 % CI: 0.58–0.98, $P=0.031$), even after statistical adjustment for both baseline Framingham risk score and the degree of left ventricular hypertrophy. This unusual, post hoc, step was pre-specified in the LIFE data analysis protocol, to reduce the probability of a Type II statistical error, which was felt to most likely arise from an unbalanced randomization process. Both all-cause and cardiovascular mortality were also significantly reduced in the losartan group (by 39 % and 37 %, respectively). These data were consistent with a suggestion, popular from 1995 to 2005, that how one lowered blood pressure might be an important determinant of outcomes [38]; today, most authorities agree that lowering blood pressure is more important than which agent is selected to start the process [39, 40].

Two classic, placebo-controlled, multicenter, prospective, randomized clinical trials have made type 2 diabetic nephropathy a "compelling indication" for an ARB, resulting in two FDA-approvals for this condition. Many are not aware that in both the Irbesartan Diabetic Nephropathy Trial (IDNT) [41] and the Reduction of Endpoints in Non-Insulin Dependent Diabetes Mellitus with the Angiotensin II Antagonist Losartan (RENAAL) Trial [42], potentially eligible type 2 diabetics had their blood pressures treated with diuretics, beta-blockers, and/or other antihypertensive drugs, *before* randomization to an ARB or placebo or amlodipine (in IDNT). The entry criteria for the two studies were only slightly different: IDNT required type 2 diabetics between 30 and 70 years of age, a blood pressure >135/85 mmHg, >900 mg/day of proteinuria, and a serum creatinine between 1 and 3 mg/dL in women or 1.2–3.0 mg/dL in men.

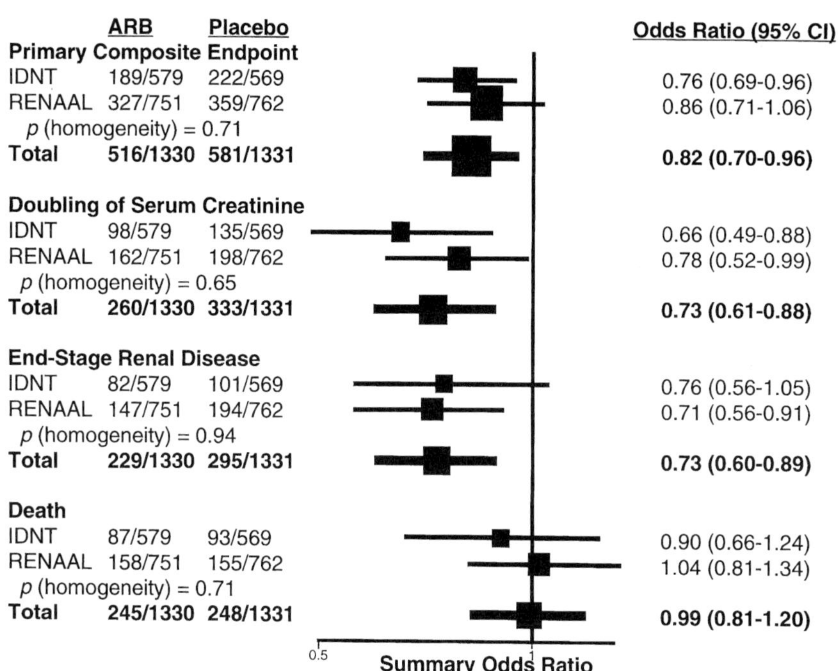

Fig. 10.7 Results of traditional Mantel–Haenzsel meta-analyses of comparisons of an angiotensin receptor blocker (irbesartan or losartan) vs. placebo in two landmark trials of type 2 diabetic nephropathy. Data from references [41, 42]. Horizontal bars correspond to the 95 % confidence limits for each comparison; *solid boxes* are drawn in proportion to the number of subjects experiencing each endpoint (compared to the referent primary composite endpoint). *ARB* angiotensin receptor blocker, *95 % CI* 95 % confidence interval, *IDNT* Irbesartan Diabetic Nephropathy Trial, *RENAAL* Reduction of Endpoints in Non-Insulin Dependent Diabetes Mellitus with the Angiotensin II Antagonist Losartan. Note that these analyses ignore otherwise valid data from the amlodipine arm of IDNT

For RENAAL, type 2 diabetics had to be 30–70 years old, with urinary albumin/creatinine ratios of >300 mg/g, and serum creatinine levels between 1.3 and 3.0 mg/dL. The results, published back-to-back in the *New England Journal of Medicine*, were astonishingly similar. Blood pressure was reduced in IDNT from 159/87 mmHg at randomization, to 140/77 mm in the group randomized to irbesartan, 141/77 mmHg in the group randomized to amlodipine, and 144/80 mmHg in the group randomized to placebo. In RENAAL, blood pressures were reduced from 152/82 mmHg at randomization, to 140/74 mmHg in the losartan group, and 142/74 mmHg in the placebo group (at the end of the study). Not only was the primary composite endpoint for both trials identical (doubling of serum creatinine, end-stage renal disease, or death), but also the final *P*-value comparing the incidence of the primary endpoint across the ARB and placebo was exactly 0.02 for each trial! The results of traditional meta-analyses summarizing these two landmark trials are shown in Fig. 10.7. It is probably not surprising that there was no overall effect on mortality, as the average age of the diabetic subjects was nearly 60 years, and nearly two-thirds had retinopathy at randomization. However, the overall highly significant delay of the primary endpoint, and the significant reduction in the number of people requiring renal replacement therapy were impressive. Pharmacoeconomic analyses of these and similar outcomes studies indicate that ARBs (even at pre-generic prices!) are cost-saving within 2 years of institution of therapy in patients with either early or late diabetic nephropathy [43].

Although not recognized by the US FDA as a valid surrogate endpoint, albuminuria and/or proteinuria have been extensively studied in both type 1 and type 2 diabetics. In nearly all trials, ARBs are quite effective in both reducing albuminuria in the short term and preventing its development in the longer term (typically 2–4 years). Perhaps the most famous trial of this type was the Irbesartan Microalbuminuria trial [44], published simultaneously with IDNT and RENAAL. In this prospective trial, 610 type 2 hypertensive diabetics with microalbuminuria (20–200 μg/min) were randomized to placebo or low or high dose irbesartan for 2 years, and followed for the development of frank proteinuria (≥288 mg/day, and an increase from baseline of ≥15 %). Blood pressures were barely different across the groups (145/84 mmHg with placebo, 143/84 mmHg with 150 mg/day, and 142/84 mmHg with 300 mg/day of irbesartan), and there were fewer adverse effects and discontinuations in the drug-treated groups. After 2 years, only the group receiving irbesartan at 300 mg/day showed a significant (70 %) reduction in the incidence of proteinuria; the lower dose had only a trend at 39 %. A recent meta-analysis suggested that renin–angiotensin–aldosterone system inhibitors significantly reduced albuminuria in both type 1 and type 2 diabetics, with a larger effect on those with higher levels of baseline albuminuria [45].

Several of the many objections to albuminuria as a valid or useful surrogate endpoint in kidney disease in diabetics can be summarized by the conclusions of important studies. In type 1 diabetes especially, the degree of albuminuria varies considerably, depending on recent blood pressure control, volume status, dietary sodium intake, and other factors. One prospective study of 75 normotensive type 1 diabetics without albuminuria at baseline suggested that patients with an increase in blood pressure during sleep predicted the development of microalbuminuria [46]. This issue can presumably be overcome by requiring two successive determinations above threshold (e.g., as in the Irbesartan Microalbuminuria trial [44]). Secondly, a 3.2-year clinical trial that enrolled 4,447 type 2 diabetics without albuminuria, comparing 40 mg of olmesartan vs. placebo, showed a slightly lower office blood pressure (by 3.1/1.9 mmHg), a slowing of the rate of onset of microalbuminuria (by 23 %, 95 % CI: 6 %–37 %, $P=0.01$), no difference in nonfatal cardiovascular events ($P=0.37$), but an increase in cardiovascular death (15 vs. 3, $P=0.01$) in the olmesartan group [47]. Although the excess death rate has been attributed to chance, an imbalance in the numbers of patients with known coronary heart disease, and other factors, many would argue that it takes far longer than 3.2 years for the disease process in hypertensive diabetics to progress from microalbuminuria to clinical cardiovascular events, suggesting that this study was underpowered to detect a significant difference in the "hard endpoints" of stroke, myocardial infarction, or cardiovascular death. The role of albuminuria as an outcomes effect modifier in chronic kidney disease is likely to remain controversial for some years to come [48].

ACE-Inhibitors

ACE-inhibitors share many of the advantages of ARBs for the treatment of diabetics with hypertension, but carry the added risk of chronic, nonproductive cough (~13 %) and angioedema (0.7 %). Perhaps because they were the first available agents that directly inhibited the renin–angiotensin system, they have been well tested in clinical trials that included diabetics. Perhaps the most illustrative is the Captopril Collaborative Study Group's comparison of captopril vs. placebo in type 1 diabetics with nephropathy [49]. This trial enrolled 409 type 1 diabetics with urinary protein excretion >500 mg/day and serum creatinine <2.5 mg/dL, and used doubling of serum creatinine as the primary endpoint. After a 3-year median follow-up period, blood pressure differences between the groups were <2/4 mmHg; significantly fewer patients in the captopril-treated group experienced doubling of serum creatinine (25 vs. 43, $P=0.007$), or the secondary composite (but clinically important) endpoint of death, dialysis, or transplantation (23 vs. 42, $P=0.006$).

This landmark study made it difficult to justify doing similar placebo-controlled renal outcome trials in type 2 diabetics, as it was widely assumed that similar benefits should accrue. One head-to-head comparison of an ARB with an ACE-inhibitor has been done in type 2 diabetics, but it used the surrogate endpoint of decline in glomerular filtration rate (measured by iohexol clearance) as its primary outcome measure, and was successful in establishing statistical "non-inferiority" of telmisartan with enalapril in a 5-year study of 250 type 2 diabetics [50]. Many feel that this endpoint was not as robust as those used in previous renal studies, and may have been unduly influenced by lack of a final measurement in 14 % of the telmisartan- and 13 % of the enalapril-treated subjects. Many other trials have established ACE-inhibitors as being particularly valuable for reducing proteinuria and delaying the progression of chronic kidney disease in patients without diabetes [51].

ACE-inhibitors have also been studied extensively to prevent cardiovascular disease events in diabetics. Perhaps the most optimistic effects were seen with ramipril in the 3,677 diabetics randomized in the Heart Outcomes Prevention Evaluation (HOPE) [52]. Although stopped 6 months earlier than planned, the diabetics randomized to ramipril enjoyed a highly significant 25 % relative risk reduction for the primary composite endpoint of cardiovascular death, myocardial infarction, or stroke, as well as significant reductions in each of its components, as well as a 24 % reduction in all-cause mortality and development of >300 mg/day of proteinuria. Later trials enrolling large numbers of diabetics and nondiabetics, which compared placebo with either perindopril or trandolapril, were not nearly as positive, probably because of more extensive and appropriate treatment of other risk factors in both randomized groups (including antiplatelet agents, beta-blockers in subjects with a history of myocardial infarction, and lipid-lowering agents). The overwhelmingly positive results of HOPE and its diabetic substudy might be attributed to the reluctance of the Data Safety and Monitoring Board to halt the trial, which would be far more likely today (for many reasons) than in 1999.

It is important to balance the perhaps uniquely positive results of HOPE and its diabetic substudy by contrasting it with the results of the clinical trial that enrolled the largest number of type 2 diabetics ever, the Antihypertensive and Lipid-Lowering to prevent Heart Attack Trial (ALLHAT) [53], discussed further below. In their enrolled cohort of 13,101 diabetics, lisinopril was not superior to chlorthalidone in preventing any type of cardiovascular event, and may have been significantly worse in preventing stroke in black subjects (diabetic or not).

Many small studies in diabetes, heart failure, chronic kidney disease, and other conditions suggested that combining an ACE-inhibitor and an ARB might be beneficial. This seemed especially promising for reduction of albuminuria in diabetics [54], or prevention of death or rehospitalization in patients with systolic heart failure [55]. However, when the large trial (with 25,620 randomized subjects) was undertaken combining full doses of telmisartan+ramipril, there was a slightly lower blood pressure in the group given the combination, but no improvement in cardiovascular events, significantly more hyperkalemia and renal dysfunction [56], and a significantly greater risk of the composite of doubling of serum creatinine, end-stage renal disease, or death [57]. Among the 9,612 enrolled diabetics, similar (nonsignificant) trends were observed for these important endpoints. These data suggested that there were few differences between full doses of an ACE-inhibitor and an ARB, and that the combination might be harmful to the kidney. More recently, losartan (100 mg/day) was given to 1,448 type 2 diabetics with an albumin/creatinine ratio of >300 mg/g and a baseline estimated glomerular filtration rate (*e*GFR) between 30 and 89.9 mL/min/1.73 m^2, to which was added either placebo or lisinopril (10–40 mg/day). Although originally intended to compare regimens with regard to a "hard renal endpoint" (a composite of the first occurrence of decline in *e*GFR ≥30 mL/min/1.73 m^2 if baseline *e*GFR was ≥60 mL/min/1.73 m^2, decline in *e*GFR of ≥50 %, end-stage renal disease, or death), the trial was terminated early (despite a nonsignificant 12 % reduction in the primary composite endpoint) because of excess hyperkalemia (6.3 vs. 2.6 events per 1,000 person-years in the combination vs. monotherapy arms) and acute kidney injury (12.2 vs. 6.7 events per 1,000 person-years) [58]. These data confirmed the potential harms of combining an ACE-inhibitor + ARB in type 2 diabetics, which increased the risk of shared toxicities (e.g., hyperkalemia, increase in serum creatinine), with no major benefit on cardiovascular or renal outcomes.

Renin Inhibitor(s)

The newest method of interfering with the renin–angiotensin system attacks the rate limiting step: hydrolysis of angiotensinogen to angiotensin I, by directly inhibiting renin. Aliskiren, the original renin inhibitor, was launched in 2007, and seemed to have many of the advantages of an ARB: dose-dependent blood pressure reductions, excellent tolerability profile, and contraindications only for pregnancy and renal artery disease. The initial trial in hypertensive type 2 diabetics with an early morning albumin/creatinine ratio between 300 and 3,499 mg/g compared losartan 100 mg/day, with or without aliskiren force-titrated from 150 mg/day for 3 months, to 300 mg/day, for another 3 months [59]. The results were quite promising: only a little (and nonsignificant) lowering of blood pressure, quite similar adverse effects, and a 20 % overall reduction in albumin/creatinine ratio, with aliskiren + losartan, compared to losartan alone. This led to high expectations about the "hard outcomes study" that compared adding aliskiren (300 mg/day) to either an ACE-inhibitor or an ARB in 8,561 diabetics with chronic kidney disease, cardiovascular disease, or both. Although blood pressure and albuminuria were slightly lower in the group given aliskiren, the study was stopped prematurely because of significantly higher risk of hyperkalemia, hypotension, or adverse effects requiring discontinuation of drug therapy in the aliskiren group [60]. After the announcement of the trial's early termination, other trials of aliskiren in diabetics and marketing efforts for all dose forms of the aliskiren + valsartan combination were halted, and the FDA-approved product information for aliskiren was updated to include a contraindication for combining aliskiren with either an ARB or ACE-inhibitor in diabetics, and a warning against using aliskiren in patients with an *e*GFR <60 mL/min/1.73 m^2, if the patient is already taking an ACE-inhibitor or ARB.

A recent post hoc analysis of the trial comparing the combination of telmisartan + ramipril to monotherapy with either in type 2 diabetics also showed a higher risk of hypotension, hyperkalemia, and the need for acute dialysis in those receiving dual inhibitors of the renin–angiotensin system [61]; excess risk was also observed in the losartan + lisinopril-treated group of the more recent trial funded by the Department of Veterans Affairs [58]. Taken together, these data indicate that monotherapy should be more advantageous than combining two drugs that interfere at different sites of the renin–angiotensin–aldosterone cascade.

Calcium Antagonists

Both dihydropyridine and non-dihydropyridine calcium antagonists have been used to lower blood pressure in many diabetic patients, based on a number of clinical trials. Early studies of non-dihydropyridine calcium antagonists showed mild-to-moderate reductions in proteinuria, which are often additive to those of renin–angiotensin system inhibitors, whereas "naked" dihydropyridine calcium antagonists tend to increase proteinuria, and were significantly inferior to an ARB in IDNT in preventing its renal endpoints [41]. As a result, most physicians now use calcium antagonists in combination with a renin–angiotensin-system inhibitor, as was commonly the case in RENAAL [42]. Calcium antagonists have no major adverse effect on glucose or cholesterol metabolism, are reasonably well tolerated, and have plentiful outcomes data from randomized clinical trials in both diabetic and nondiabetic hypertensives.

Two trials are especially illustrative of the potential benefits of calcium antagonists in diabetics: the Anglo-Scandinavian Cardiac Outcomes Trial (ASCOT) and the Avoiding Cardiovascular events through COMbination therapy in Patients LIving with Systolic Hypertension (ACCOMPLISH). The former compared amlodipine (with perindopril, as needed) and atenolol (with bendroflumethiazide, as needed), with fatal or nonfatal myocardial infarction as the primary endpoint. Concomitantly, eligible subjects were randomized to atorvastatin or placebo, which was so successful in reducing the incidence of the primary endpoint that it was stopped early, leaving the blood pressure-lowering arm of the trial with lower-than-expected statistical power. This was thought to justify a change in the primary outcome measure to total cardiovascular events and procedures for all pre-specified subgroup analyses, including that for the 5,137 diabetics [62]. Although the study protocol recommended a target of <130/80 mmHg for diabetics, their blood pressure was reduced, at 1 year, to 143/81 and 148/84 mmHg, in the amlodipine and atenolol groups, respectively, and to 137/76 and 136/75 mmHg at the end of the study. During follow-up, the Kaplan–Meier curves for total cardiovascular events and procedures in diabetics were superimposable for the first 3 years, but diverged thereafter, resulting in an overall significant advantage for the amlodipine-treated group ($P=0.0261$). This difference was presumably driven by putatively significant differences ($P<0.05$, uncorrected for multiple comparisons) in fatal and nonfatal stroke, chronic stable angina, nonfatal stroke, peripheral arterial disease, and other revascularization procedures, all favoring amlodipine. The original primary outcome measure was not significant ($P=0.46$), although the trend favored amlodipine. Overall, these results in diabetics paralleled those seen in the entire ASCOT study cohort, and have been criticized by those who believe that secondary outcomes can be properly evaluated only if the primary outcome is significant.

The ACCOMPLISH trial enrolled 11,505 high-risk hypertensive subjects (including 6,946 with diabetes), and randomized them to initial therapy with benazepril and either amlodipine or hydrochlorothiazide [63]. The primary outcome measure was a composite of cardiovascular death, myocardial infarction, stroke, hospitalization for angina, resuscitated cardiac arrest, or coronary revascularization. The protocol recommended a target blood pressure of <130/80 mmHg for all diabetics, but the average office blood pressures were 132/73 and 133/74 mmHg in the amlodipine- and hydrochlorothiazide-treated groups during follow-up. Despite its early termination due to superiority of amlodipine over hydrochlorothiazide, diabetics randomized to the former therapy enjoyed a significant 23 % reduction in the primary endpoint ($P=0.003$), with significantly lower rates of coronary events (revascularization and the composite of myocardial infarction, unstable angina pectoris, or sudden cardiac death). In addition, the post hoc renal endpoint (increase in serum creatinine by >50 % and above the reference range) was significantly reduced in incidence by 47 % (95 % CI: 36–55 %, $P<0.001$) in diabetics, and even more in nondiabetics (62 %). These data have caused some guideline committees to favor a calcium antagonist over hydrochlorothiazide as second-line antihypertensive therapy for diabetics, but most ALLHAT investigators believe that chlorthalidone may have produced different results, if it had been used instead of the much shorter-acting and less potent hydrochlorothiazide.

Beta-Blockers

As discussed above, most authorities currently recommend a beta-blocker for diabetics only if there is a compelling indication (e.g., post-MI, heart failure with preserved left ventricular function), because of their propensity to mask hypoglycemic signs and symptoms, potential hyperglycemia, and reduction of exercise tolerance (which may promote weight gain). Before concerns about atenolol were raised [36, 37, 62], the United Kingdom Prospective Diabetes Study (UKPDS) 39 randomized 1,158 newly diagnosed type 2 diabetics with hypertension to twice-daily captopril or once-daily atenolol, with a second randomization (discussed below) to different target office blood pressure levels. During 9 years of follow-up, significantly more subjects abandoned atenolol than captopril, but there were no significant differences across treatment arms for any of the several prespecified endpoints (although they all favored atenolol) [64].

Diuretics

Diuretics have long been used to lower blood pressure in diabetics; for many such patients, attainment of blood pressure goals is difficult to impossible without a diuretic. These agents decrease the intravascular volume that is common in many type 2 diabetics, prevent heart failure, and counter the hyperkalemic effects of renin–angiotensin system inhibitors. Their adverse effects sometimes include erectile dysfunction, hypokalemia, and an increased risk of worsening glycemic control.

There is nonetheless a solid base of clinical trial evidence supporting the use of diuretics for hypertensive diabetics. In the Systolic Hypertension in the Elderly Program (SHEP) trial, chlorthalidone-based therapy was significantly better than placebo in reducing major cardiovascular disease events, with the same 34 % relative risk reduction, but a two-fold higher absolute risk reduction [65]. A meta-analysis from the Individual Data Analysis of Antihypertensive Drug Interventions project that included the Hypertension Detection and Follow-up Program, European Working Party on Hypertension in the Elderly, Swedish Trial of Older Patients with Hypertension, and SHEP showed a significant reduction in stroke (36 %) and major cardiovascular events (20 %) with an initial diuretic, compared to control intervention [66]. Lastly, and perhaps most importantly, as briefly mentioned above, the ALLHAT trial enrolled more diabetics than any other trial, and concluded that the diuretic they chose, chlorthalidone, was superior to all other classes of initial antihypertensive drugs for preventing one or more forms of cardiovascular disease among all hypertensives, as well as diabetics [53]. This conclusion, based largely on the inclusion of heart failure as an independent endpoint, rather than part of a composite (as originally planned), was originally quite controversial. Since then, the controversy has shifted to how large the differences are between chlorthalidone and the much more popular hydrochlorothiazide. Using very selective criteria that included data from only 9 trials, investigators from Connecticut concluded that chlorthalidone was clearly superior to hydrochlorothiazide in preventing cardiovascular events [67]; other investigators did not find a significant difference in outcomes between the two drugs in two other network meta-analyses that included data from 5 and 83 clinical trials [68, 69], although outcomes data (particularly in preventing heart failure) are far more plentiful with chlorthalidone [70].

Other Drug Classes

Most authorities agree that an alpha-1 adrenergic antagonist was inferior to low-dose chlorthalidone in preventing heart failure and combined cardiovascular disease events in ALLHAT diabetics [71]. There are many possible explanations for this disparity, including the use of seated (rather than standing) blood pressures, but it reinforces the importance of hard endpoints in clinical decision-making. Many previous studies had shown putatively beneficial effects of alpha-1 blockers on blood pressure and glucose and lipid metabolism, which were also seen in ALLHAT, but eventually found to be less important for preventing cardiovascular disease outcomes. Centrally acting alpha-2 agonists are sometimes needed to control blood pressure, and have few adverse metabolic effects, but sedation, dry mouth, and other common adverse effects make them less popular for routine therapy of hypertension. Aldosterone antagonists are also occasionally useful, but hyperkalemia and worsened renal impairment are common adverse effects.

Blood Pressure Treatment Targets for All Diabetics?

Controversy currently exists regarding the wisdom of a lower-than-usual blood pressure target for all diabetics. This had been a basic tenet in the diabetes and hypertension communities for many years, but has recently been challenged by the ACCORD trial.

Evidence supporting a lower-than-usual blood pressure target came from at least three clinical trials: the UKPDS, the Hypertension Optimal Treatment Study, and a small multiple-intervention trial in Denmark. Back in 1985, 1,148 newly diagnosed type 2 diabetics in the United Kingdom were randomized to a "lower blood pressure target" (≤150/85 mmHg) or "less tight control" (≤180/100 mmHg), and followed for 8.4 years [72]. The group randomized to the lower target achieved a mean blood pressure of 144/84 mmHg, compared to 154/87 mmHg for the other group, and suffered significantly fewer diabetes-related endpoints (the primary outcome measure, by 24 %), deaths (32 %), strokes (44 %), and microvascular endpoints (37 %). Formal cost-effectiveness analyses, based on then-current British health-care costs, indicated that lowering blood pressure to the lower target saved both discounted disease-free life-years *and* money (£1,049 per endpoint-free year of life saved) [73]. Note that the incremental blood pressure reduction between the two randomized groups seen in UKPDS (10/5 mmHg) was *exactly* that recommended a year earlier (for diabetics compared to nondiabetics) by the 1997 US hypertension guidelines committee, which was also supported by a pharmacoeconomic analysis showing overall cost-savings for the lower target [74]. The second trial that showed a significant benefit of a lower-than-usual blood pressure target for diabetics randomized 1,501 diabetics (among the enrolled total of 18,790 subjects) to diastolic blood pressures of ≤80, ≤85, or ≤90 mmHg [75]. Over a median of 3.8 years of follow-up, diabetics randomized to the lowest diastolic BP had a significant, 51 % lower risk of major cardiovascular events, compared to those randomized to ≤90 mmHg. The results of this trial were therefore used to support lowering the diastolic blood pressure target for diabetics to <80 mmHg in many national and international guidelines written between 1998 and 2012. This target was seemingly supported by a small trial of 180 type 2 diabetics in Denmark, which showed a significant 55 % reduction in the risk of cardiovascular complications in those who received "intensive therapy," which included a lower-than-usual blood pressure target [76]. Extended follow-up for another 5.5 years demonstrated a significant 45 % reduction in overall mortality in the "intensive therapy" group [77].

The largest and most direct test of the lower blood pressure target for diabetics was the ACCORD trial, which enrolled 10,251 subjects, and randomized them to a systolic blood pressure of <140 or <120 mmHg [35]. Although some argue that the <120 mmHg is too low, the average achieved systolic blood pressure in this group was 119 mmHg, proving that it was possible to meet such a low goal. However, the overall cardiovascular event rates were not significantly different ($P=0.20$), although the 12 % relative risk reduction favored the lower goal; only the secondary endpoint of fatal or nonfatal stroke was reduced significantly (by 41 %, $P=0.01$). Because of its large size, the ACCORD results overwhelm those of earlier trials, and have influenced many recent guideline committees to revise or reject previous recommendations for a lower-than-usual blood pressure treatment target for all diabetics.

There does seem to be some support, however, for a lower-than-usual blood pressure treatment target for diabetics with nephropathy, based on post hoc analyses of both IDNT and RENAAL. This makes perfect sense from the precepts of preventive medicine, as the recommended treatments are nearly always more intensive (and more beneficial) for high-risk, compared to low-risk, groups. This principle is supported by analyses of stroke prevention with antihypertensive drugs, previously recommended targets for LDL-cholesterol reduction across the cardiovascular risk continuum, and former post-exposure prophylaxis for needlesticks that might transmit the human immunodeficiency virus. So several very recent guidelines have recommended a lower-than-usual blood pressure for diabetics [2] (and nondiabetics) [48] if microalbuminuria (albumin/creatinine ratio >30 mg/g) is present. While one might argue that this recommendation is not completely evidence based, it fits with the more intensive treatment of predictors of outcomes that is common in other disease states.

To summarize, the optimal treatment of hypertension in diabetics is still quite controversial, but probably includes lifestyle modifications whenever feasible, one inhibitor of the renin–angiotensin system, and sufficient other antihypertensive medications to keep the blood pressure at a level inversely proportional to the absolute risk of cardiovascular and renal disease in the individual patient, based on assessment of all other risk factors, including albuminuria.

References

1. Go AS, Mozaffarian D, Roger VL, Benjamin EJ, Berry JD, Borden WB, Bravata DM, Dia S, Ford ES, Fox CS, Franco S, Fullerton HJ, Gillespie C, Hailpern SM, Heit JA, Howard VJ, Huffman MD, Kissela BM, Kittner SJ, Lackland DT, Lichtman JH, Lisabeth LD, Magid D, Marcus GM, Maraelli A, Matchar DB, McGuire DK, Mohler ER, Moy CS, Mussolino ME, Nichol G, Paynter NP, Schreiner PJ, Sorlie PD, Stein J, Turan TN, Virani SS, Wong ND, Woo D, Turner MB, on behalf of the American Heart Association Statistics Committee and Stroke Statistics Subcommittee. Heart disease and stroke statistics—2013 update: a report from the American Heart Association. Circulation. 2013;127:e6–245.
2. American Diabetes Association. Executive summary: standards of medical care in diabetes—2013. Diabetes Care. 2013;36 Suppl 1: S11–66.
3. US Centers for Disease Control and Prevention's National Center for Chronic Disease Prevention and Health Promotion, Division of Diabetes Translation. Detailed data for diagnosed diabetes. www.cdc.gov/diabetes/statistics/prev/national/tprevmage.htm, and www.cdc.gov/diabetes/statistics/prev/national/tprevfemage.htm. Accessed 20 May 13.
4. Centers for Disease Control and Prevention. National diabetes fact sheet: national estimates and general information on diabetes and prediabetes in the United States, 2011. Atlanta, GA: US Department of Health and Human Services, Centers for Disease Control and Prevention; 2011. http://www.cdc.gov/diabetes/pubs/pdf/ndfs_2011.pdf. Accessed 11 May 13.
5. Preis SR, Pencina MJ, Hwang S-J, D'Agostino Sr RB, Savage PJ, Levy D, Fox CS. Trends in cardiovascular risk factors in individuals with and without diabetes in the Framingham Heart Study. Circulation. 2009;120:212–20.
6. Lim SS, Vos T, Flaxman AD, Danael G, Shibuya K, Adair-Rohani H, et al. A comparative risk assessment of burden of disease and injury attributable to 67 risk factors and risk factor clusters in 21 regions, 1990-2010: a systematic analysis for the Global Burden of Disease Study 2010. Lancet. 2012;380:2224–60.
7. Kearney PM, Whelton M, Reynolds K, Muntner P, Whelton PK, He J. Global burden of hypertension: analysis of worldwide data. Lancet. 2005;365:217–23.
8. International Diabetes Federation. Diabetes atlas: The global burden. Available at www.idf.org/diabetesatlas/5e/the-global-burden, Accessed 21 May 13.
9. Matheus AS, Tannus LR, Cobas RA, Palma CC, Negrato CA, Gomes Mde B. Impact of diabetes on cardiovascular disease: an update. Int J Hypertens. 2013;2013:653789. doi: 10.1155/2013/653789. Epub 2013 Mar 4.
10. Chen G, McAlister FA, Walker RL, Hemmelgarn BR, Campbell NRC. Cardiovascular outcomes in Framingham participants with diabetes: the importance of blood pressure. Hypertension. 2011;57: 891–7.
11. Turnbull F, Neal B, Algert C, Chalmers J, Chapman N, Cutler J, Woodward M, MacMahon S; Blood Pressure Lowering Treatment Trialists' Collaboration. Effects of different blood pressure-lowering regimens on major cardiovascular events in individuals with and without diabetes mellitus: results of prospectively designed overviews of randomized trials. Arch Intern Med. 2005;165:1410–9.
12. US Renal Data System. USRDS 2012 annual data report. Atlas of chronic kidney disease and end-stage renal disease in the United States. Bethesda, MD: National Institutes of Health, National Institute of Diabetes and Digestive and Kidney Diseases; 2012. http://www.usrds.org/2012/pdf/v1_ch1_12.pdf. Accessed 11 May 13.
13. Ishani A, Grandits GA, Grimm Jr RH, Svendsen KH, Collins AJ, Prineas RJ, Neaton JD. Association of single-measurements of dipstick proteinuria, estimated glomerular filtration rate, and hematocrit with 25-year incidence of end-stage renal disease in the Multiple Risk Factor Intervention Trial. J Am Soc Nephrol. 2006;17:2444–52.
14. Perry Jr HM, Miller JP, Fornoff JR, Baty JD, Sambhi MP, Rutan G, Moskowitz DW, Carmody SE. Early predictors of 15-year end-stage renal disease in hypertensive patients. Hypertension. 1995;25:587–94.
15. Hsu C, Iribarren C, McCulloch CE, Darbinian J, Go AS. Risk factors for end-stage renal disease: 25-year follow-up. Arch Intern Med. 2009;169:342–50.
16. Kastarinen M, Juutilainen A, Kastarinen H, Salomaa V, Karhapää P, Tuomilehto J, Gröhangen-Riska C, Jousilahti P, Finne P. Risk factors for end-stage renal disease in a community-based population: 26-year follow-up of 25,821 men and women in Eastern Finland. J Intern Med. 2009;267:612–20.
17. Reynolds K, Gu D, Muntner P, Kusek JW, Chen J, Wu X, Duan X, Chen CS, Klag MJ, Whelton PK, He J. A population-based prospective study of blood pressure and risk for end-stage renal disease in China. J Am Soc Nephrol. 2007;18:1928–35.
18. Munkhaugen J, Lydersen S, Wilderoe TE, Hallan S. Prehypertension, obesity and risk of kidney disease: 20-year follow-up of the HUNT 1 study in Norway. Am J Kidney Dis. 2009;54:638–46.
19. Appel LJ, Brands MW, Daniels SR, Karanja N, Elmer PJ, Sacks FM. Dietary approaches to prevent and treat hypertension: a scientific statement from the American Heart Association. Hypertension. 2006;47:296–308.
20. Appel LJ, Giles TD, Black HR, Izzo Jr JL, Materson BJ, Oparil S, Weber MA. ASH position paper: dietary approaches to lower blood pressure. J Am Soc Hypertens. 2010;4:79–89.
21. Brook RD, Appel LJ, Rubenfire M, Ogedegbe G, Bisognano JD, Elliott WJ, Fuchs FD, Hughes JW, Lackland DT, Staffileno BA, Townsend RR, Rajagopalan S. Beyond medications and diet: alternative approaches to lowering blood pressure: a scientific statement from the American Heart Association. Hypertension. 2013;61:1360–83.
22. Hu G, Barengo NC, Tuomilehto J, Lakka TA, Nissinen A, Jousilahti P. Relationship of physical activity and body mass index to the risk of hypertension: a prospective study in Finland. Hypertension. 2004;43:25–30.
23. Tuomilehto J, Lindström J, Eriksson JG, Valle TT, Hämäläinen H, Ilanne-Parikka P, Keinänen-Klukaanniemi S, Laakso M, Louheranta A, Rastas M, Salminen V, Uusitupa M, for the Finnish Diabetes Prevention Study Group. Prevention of type 2 diabetes mellitus by changes in lifestyle modification among subjects with impaired glucose tolerance. N Engl J Med. 2001;344:1343–50.
24. Elliott WJ, Meyer PM. Incident diabetes in clinical trials of antihypertensive drugs: a network meta-analysis. Lancet. 2007;369:201–7. Erratum in Lancet. 2007;369(9572):1518.
25. Elliott WJ, Meyer PM, Basu S. Incident diabetes with antihypertensive drugs: updated network and Bayesian meta-analyses of clinical trial data. J Clin Hypertens (Greenwich). 2011;13 Suppl 1:A82.
26. Staessen JA, Richart T, Wang Z, Thijs L. Implications of recently published trials of blood pressure-lowering drugs in hypertensive or high-risk patients. Hypertension. 2010;55:819–31.

27. Eberly LE, Cohen JD, Prineas R, Yang L. Impact of incident diabetes and incident nonfatal cardiovascular disease on 18-year mortality: the multiple risk factor intervention trial experience. Diabetes Care. 2003;26:848–54.
28. Qiao Q, Jousilahti P, Eriksson J, Tuomilehto J. Predictive properties of impaired glucose tolerance for cardiovascular risk are not explained by the development of overt diabetes during follow-up. Diabetes Care. 2003;26:2910–4.
29. Barzilay JI, Davis BR, Cutler JA, Pressel SL, Whelton PK, Basile J, Margolis KL, Ong St, Sadler LS, Summerson J, for the ALLHAT Collaborative Research Group. Fasting glucose levels and incident diabetes mellitus in older nondiabetic adults randomized to receive 3 different classes of antihypertensive treatment: a report from the Antihypertensive and Lipid-Lowering Treatment to Prevent Heart Attack Trial (ALLHAT). Arch Intern Med. 2006;166:2191–201.
30. Kostis JB, Wilson AC, Freudenberger RS, Cosgrove NM, Pressel SL, Davis BR. Long-term effect of diuretic-based therapy on fatal outcomes in subjects with isolated systolic hypertension with and without diabetes. Am J Cardiol. 2005;95:29–35.
31. Verdecchia P, Reboldi G, Angeli F, Borgioni C, Gattobigio R, Filippucci L, Norgiolini S, Bracco C, Porcellati C. Adverse prognostic significance of new diabetes in treated hypertensive subjects. Hypertension. 2004;43:963–9.
32. Almgren T, Wilhelmsen L, Samuelsson O, Himmelmann A, Rosengren A, Andersson OK. Diabetes in treated hypertension is common and carries a high cardiovascular risk: results from a 28-year follow-up. J Hypertens. 2007;25:1311–7.
33. Fox CS, Sullivan L, D'Agostino RB, Sr, Wilson PW, for the Framingham Heart Study. The significant effect of diabetes duration on coronary heart disease mortality: the Framingham Heart Study. Diabetes Care. 2004;27:704–8.
34. Aksnes TA, Kjeldsen SE, Rostrup M, Omvik P, Hua TA, Julius S. Impact of new-onset diabetes mellitus on cardiac outcomes in the Valsartan Antihypertensive Long-term Use Evaluation (VALUE) trial population. Hypertension. 2007;50:467–73.
35. Cushman WC, Evans GW, Byington RP, Goff Jr JC, Grim Jr RH, Cutler JA, Simons Morton DG, Basile JN, Corson MA, Probstfield JL, Katz L, Peterson KA, Friedewald WA, Buse JB, Bigger JT, Gerstein HC, Ismail-Bigi F, on behalf of The Action to Control Cardiovascular Risk in Diabetes (ACCORD) Study Group. Effects of intensive blood-pressure control in type 2 diabetes mellitus. N Engl J Med. 2010;362:1575–85.
36. Lindholm L, Ibsen H, Dahlöf B, Devereux RB, Beevers G, de Faire U, Fyhrquist F, Julius S, Kjeldsen SE, Kristiansson K, Lederballe-Pedersen O, Nieminen MS, Omvik P, Oparil S, Wedel H, Aurup P, Edelman J, Snapinn S, et al., for the LIFE Study Group. Cardiovascular morbidity and mortality in patients with diabetes in the Losartan Intervention For Endpoint reduction in hypertension study (LIFE): a randomised trial against atenolol. Lancet. 2002;359:1004–10.
37. Carlberg B, Samuelsson O, Lindholm LH. Atenolol in hypertension: is it a wise choice? Lancet. 2004;364:1684–9.
38. Sever PS, Poulter NR. Blood pressure reduction is not the only determinant of outcome. Circulation. 2006;113:2754–63.
39. Elliott WJ, Jonsson C, Black HR. It is not beyond the blood pressure; it is the blood pressure. Circulation. 2006;113:2763–74.
40. Mancia G, Laurent S, Agabiti-Rosei E, Ambrosioni E, Burner M, Caulfield MJ, Cifkova R, Clément D, Coca A, Dominiczak A, Erdine S, Fagard R, Farsang C, Grassi G, Haller H, Heagerty A, Kjeldsen SE, Kiowski W, Mallion JM, Manolis A, Narkiewicz K, Nilsson P, Olsen MH, Rahn KH, Redon J, Rodicio J, Ruilope L, Schmieder RE, Strujker-Boudier HA, van Zwieten PA, Viigimaa M, Zanchetti A. Reappraisal of European guidelines on hypertension management: a European Society of Hypertension Task Force document. J Hypertens. 2009;27:2121–58.
41. Lewis EJ, Hunsicker LG, Clarke WR, Berl T, Pohl MA, Lewis JB, Ritz E, Atkins RC, Rohde R, Raz I; Collaborative Study Group. Renoprotective effect of the angiotensin-receptor antagonist irbesartan in patients with nephropathy due to type 2 diabetes. N Engl J Med. 2001;345:851–60.
42. Brenner BM, Cooper ME, de Zeeuw D, Keane WF, Mitch WE, Parving HH, Rumuzzi G, Snapinn SM, Zhange G, Shahinfar S. Effects of losartan on renal and cardiovascular outcomes in patients with Type 2 diabetes and nephropathy. Reduction of Endpoints in Non-Insulin Dependent Diabetes Mellitus with the Angiotensin II Antagonist Losartan (RENAAL) Study Group. N Engl J Med. 2001;345:861–9.
43. Boersma C, Atthobari J, Gansevoort RT, de Jong-Van den Berg LT, de Jong PE, de Zeeuw D, Annemans LJ, Postma MJ. Pharmacoeconomics of angiotensin II antagonists in type 2 diabetic patients with nephropathy: implications for decision making. Pharmacoeconomics. 2006;24:523–35.
44. Parving H-H, Lehnert H, Brochner-Mortensen J, Gomis R, Andersen S, Arner P; The Irbesartan in Patients with Type 2 Diabetes and Microalbuminuria Study Group. The effect of irbesartan on the development of diabetic nephropathy in patients with type 2 diabetes. N Engl J Med. 2001;345:870–8.
45. Hirst JA, Taylor KS, Stevens RJ, Blacklock CL, Roberts NW, Pugh CW, Farmer AJ. The impact of renin-angiotensin-aldosterone system inhibitors on type 1 and type 2 diabetic patients with and without early diabetic nephropathy. Kidney Int. 2012;81:674–83.
46. Lurbe E, Redon J, Kesani A, Pascual JM, Tacons J, Alvarez V, Battle D. Increase in nocturnal blood pressure and progression to microalbuminuria in type 1 diabetes. N Engl J Med. 2002; 347:797–805.
47. Haller H, Ito S, Izzo Jr JL, Januszewicz A, Katayama S, Menne J, Mimran A, Rabelinki TJ, Ritz E, Ruilope LM, Rump LC, Viberti G, for the ROADMAP Trial Investigators. Olmesartan for the delay or prevention of microalbuminuria in type 2 diabetes. N Engl J Med. 2011;364;907–17.
48. Stevens PE, Levin A, for the Kidney Disease: Improving Global Outcomes Chronic Kidney Disease Guideline Development Work Group Members. Evaluation and management of chronic kidney disease: synopsis of the kidney disease: improving global outcomes 2012 clinical practice guideline. Ann Intern Med. 2013;158: 825–30.
49. Lewis EJ, Hunsicker LG, Bain RP, Rohde RD; The Captopril Collaborative Study Group. The effect of angiotensin-converting-enzyme inhibition on diabetic nephropathy. N Engl J Med. 1993;329:1456–62.
50. Barnett AH, Bain SC, Bouter P, Karlberg B, Madsbad S, Jervell J, Mustonen J, for the Diabetics Exposed to Telmisartan and Enalapril Study Group. Angiotensin-receptor blockade versus converting-enzyme inhibition in type 2 diabetes and nephropathy. N Engl J Med. 2004;351:1952–61.
51. Jafar TH, Stark PC, Schmid CH, Landa M, Maschio G, de Jong PE, de Zeeuw D, Shahinfar S, Toto R, Levey AS. Progression of chronic kidney disease: the role of blood pressure control, proteinuria, and angiotensin-converting enzyme inhibition: a patient-level meta-analysis. Ann Intern Med. 2003;139:244–52.
52. Effects of ramipril on cardiovascular and microvascular outcomes in people with diabetes mellitus: The HOPE study and MICRO-HOPE substudy. Heart Outcomes Prevention Evaluation (HOPE) Study Investigators. Lancet. 2000;355:253–9.
53. Whelton PK, Barzilay J, Cushman WC, Davis BR, Iliamathi E, Kostis JB, Leenen FH, Louis GT, Margolis KL, Mathis DE, Moloo J, Nwachuku C, Panebianco D, Parish DC, Parish DC, Pressel S, Simmons DL, Thadani U, for the ALLHAT Collaborative Research Group. Clinical outcomes in antihypertensive treatment of type 2 diabetes, impaired fasting glucose concentration, and normoglycemia: Antihypertensive and Lipid-Lowering Treatment to Prevent Heart Attack Trial (ALLHAT). Arch Intern Med. 2005;165: 1401–9.

54. Mogensen CE, Neldam S, Tikkanen I, Oren S, Viskoper R, Watts RW, Cooper ME. Randomised controlled trial of dual blockade of renin-angiotensin system in patients with hypertension, microalbuminuria, and non-insulin dependent diabetes: the Candesartan and Lisinopril Microalbuminuria (CALM) study. BMJ. 2000;321:1440–4.
55. McMurray JJV, Östergren J, Swedberg K, Granger CG, Held P, Michelson EL, Olofsson B, Yusuf S, Pfeffer MA; CHARM Investigators and Committees. Effects of candesartan in patients with chronic heart failure and reduced left-ventricular systolic function taking angiotensin-converting-enzyme inhibitors: the CHARM-Added trial. Lancet. 2003;362:767–71.
56. ONTARGET Investigators. Telmisartan, ramipril or both in patients at high risk for vascular events. N Engl J Med. 2008;358:1547–59.
57. Mann JFE, Schmieder RE, McQueen M, on behalf of the ONTARGET Investigators. Renal outcomes with telmisartan, ramipril, or both, in people at high vascular risk (the ONTARGET study): A multicentre, randomised, double-blind, controlled trial. Lancet. 2008;372:547–53.
58. Fried LF, Emanuele N, Zhang JH, Brophy M, Conner TA, Duckworth W, Leehey DJ, McCullough PA, O'Connor T, Palevsky PM, Reilly RF, Seliger SL, Warren SR, Watnick S, Peduzzi P, Guarino P, for the VA NEPHRON-D Investigators. Combined angiotensin inhibition for the treatment of diabetic nephropathy. N Engl J Med. 2013;369:1892–903.
59. Parving H-H, Persson F, Lewis JB, Lewis EJ, Hollenberg NK, for the AVOID Study Investigators. Aliskiren combined with losartan in type 2 diabetes and nephropathy. N Engl J Med. 2008;358:2433–46.
60. Parving H-H, Brenner BM, McMurray JJV, de Zeeuw D, Haffner SM, Solomon SD, Chaturvedi N, Persson F, Desai AS, Nicolaides M, Richard A, Xiang Z, Brunel P, Pfeffer MA, for the ALTITUDE Investigators. Cardiorenal end points in a trial of aliskiren for type 2 diabetes. N Engl J Med. 2012;367:2204–13.
61. Mann JFE, Anderson C, Gao P, Gerstein HC, Boehm M, Rydén L, Sleight P, Teo KK, Yusuf S, on behalf of the ONTARGET Investigators. Dual inhibition of the renin-angiotensin system in high-risk diabetes and risk for stroke and other outcomes: results of the ONTARGET trial. J Hypertens. 2013;31:414–21.
62. Östergren J, Poulter NR, Sever PS, Dahlöf B, Wedel H, Beevers G, Caulfield M, Collins R, Kjeldsen SE, Kristinsson A, McInnes GT, Mehlsen J, Nieminen M, O'Brien E, for the ASCOT Investigators. The Anglo-Scandinavian Cardiac Outcomes Trial: Blood pressure-lowering limb: Effects in patients with type 2 diabetes. J Hypertens. 2008;26:2103–11.
63. Weber MA, Bakris GL, Jamerson K, Weir M, Kjeldsen SE, Devereux RB, Velazquez EJ, Dahlöf B, Kelly RY, Hua TA, Hester A, Pitt B, for the ACCOMPLISH Investigators. Cardiovascular events during differing hypertension therapies in patients with diabetes. J Am Coll Cardiol. 2010;56:77–85.
64. Efficacy of atenolol and captopril in reducing the risk of macrovascular and microvascular complications in type 2 diabetes: UKPDS 39. UK Prospective Diabetes Study Group. BMJ. 1998;317:713-720.
65. Curb JD, Pressel SL, Cutler JA, Savage PJ, Applegate WB, Black H, Camel G, Davis BR, Frost PH, Gonzalez N, Guthrie G, Oberman A, Ruttan GH, Stamler J, for the Systolic Hypertension in the Elderly Program Cooperative Research Group. Effect of diuretic-based antihypertensive treatment on cardiovascular disease risk in older diabetic patients with isolated systolic hypertension. JAMA. 1996;276;1886–92.
66. Lièvre M, Gueyffier F, Ekbom T, Fagard R, Cutler J, Schron E, Marre M, Boissel JP. Efficacy of diuretics and beta-blockers in diabetic hypertensive patients. Results from a meta-analysis. The INDANA Steering Committee. Diabetes Care. 2000;23 Suppl 2:B65–71.
67. Roush GC, Holford TR, Guddati AK. Chlorthalidone compared with hydrochlorothiazide in reducing cardiovascular events: systematic review and network meta-analysis. Hypertension. 2012;59:1110–7.
68. Psaty BM, Lumley T, Furberg CD. Meta-analysis of health outcomes of chlorthalidone-based vs nonchlorthalidone-based low dose diuretic therapies [research letter]. JAMA. 2004;292:43–4.
69. Elliott WJ, Childers WK, Meyer PM, Basu S. Outcomes with different diuretics in clinical trials in hypertension: Results of network and Bayesian meta-analyses [abstract]. J Clin Hypertens (Greenwich). 2012;14 Suppl 1:A58–9.
70. Elliott WJ, Basu S, Meyer PM. Network meta-analysis of heart failure prevention by antihypertensive drugs [letter]. Arch Intern Med. 2011;171:472–3.
71. Barzilay JL, Davis BR, Bettencourt J, Margolis KL, Goff Jr DC, Black H, Habib G, Ellsworth A, Force RW, Wiegmann T, Ciocon JO, Basile JN, for the ALLHAT Collaborative Research Group. Cardiovascular outcomes using doxazosin vs. chlorthalidone for the treatment of hypertension in older adults with and without glucose disorders: a report from the ALLHAT Study. J Clin Hypertens (Greenwich). 2004;6:116–25.
72. Tight blood pressure control and risk of macrovascular and microvascular complications in type 2 diabetes: UKPDS 38: UK Prospective Diabetes Study Group. BMJ. 1998;317:703–13.
73. Raikou M, Gray A, Briggs A, Stevens R, Cull C, McGuire A, Feen P, Stratton I, Holman R, Turner R. Cost-effectiveness analysis of improved blood pressure control in hypertensive patients with type 2 diabetes: UKPDS 40. UK Prospective Diabetes Study Group. BMJ. 1998;317:720–6.
74. Elliott WJ, Weir DR, Black HR. Cost-effectiveness of lowering treatment goal of JNC VI for diabetic hypertensives. Arch Intern Med. 2000;160:1277–83.
75. Hansson L, Zanchetti A, Carruthers SG, Dahlöf B, Elmfeldt D, Julius S, Ménard J, Rahn KH, Wedel H, Westerling S. Effects of intensive blood pressure lowering and low-dose aspirin in patients with hypertension: Principal results of the Hypertension Optimal Treatment (HOT) randomised trial: The HOT Study Group. Lancet. 1998;351:1755–62.
76. Gaede P, Vedel P, Larsen N, Jensen GVH, Parving HH, Pedersen O. Multifactorial intervention and cardiovascular disease in patients with type 2 diabetes. N Engl J Med. 2003;348:383–93.
77. Gaede P, Lund-Andersen H, Parving HH, Pedersen O. Effect of a multifactorial intervention on mortality in type 2 diabetes. N Engl J Med. 2008;358:580–91.

Cardiovascular Disease in Diabetic Nephropathy

11

L. Lee Hamm, Tina K. Thethi, and Kathleen S. Hering-Smith

Diabetes and chronic kidney disease (CKD) lead to excess cardiovascular disease. Together these two entities have even more cardiovascular risk leading to excess morbidity and mortality. In fact, adverse cardiovascular outcomes are significantly more likely than end stage renal disease (ESRD) in patients with diabetic nephropathy. These diseases (diabetes, CKD, and cardiovascular diseases) are growing major public health problems as illustrated by the prevalence and costs illustrated in Fig. 11.1. This chapter will review selected aspects of cardiovascular disease in patients with diabetic nephropathy. Because there is abundant literature in these areas, references are only selective and representative.

Cardiovascular Disease in Diabetes

Diabetes is well known to cause excess cardiovascular disease in general [1]. This has been most examined in terms of the incidence of coronary heart disease leading to myocardial infarction. In fact, diabetes has been considered a coronary heart disease equivalent by the National Cholesterol Education Program [2, 3]. This consideration as a coronary heart disease equivalent is derived from the fact that patients with type 2 diabetes are at the same risk for a myocardial infarction as those that have had a previous myocardial infarction. Many studies have examined this relationship and various aspects. Both the Framingham Heart Study and the Multiple Risk Factor Intervention Trial (MRFIT) suggested that the risk for cardiovascular disease is twofold or threefold higher in men and women respectively even after adjusting for age and the presence of other risk factors such as hypertension, smoking, hyperlipidemia, and left ventricular hypertrophy [4, 5]. This risk is probably higher in those with type 1 diabetes, but the prevalence of type 2 diabetes is much higher and therefore the greatest public health impact is with type 2 diabetes.

Glucose intolerance even in the absence of overt diabetes is also associated with excess cardiovascular risk, for example [6]. In addition to the risk directly from diabetes and impaired glucose tolerance, patients with diabetes also have a greater incidence of other cardiovascular risk factors such as hypertension, obesity, hyperlipidemia, and elevated fibrinogen. The combination of obesity, hypertension, diabetes, and hyperlipidemia has been labeled the metabolic syndrome, and also referred to as syndrome X [7]. Obesity-related inflammation may be one of the mechanistic links in these relationships [8]. Microalbuminuria, which occurs early in diabetic nephropathy, is associated with increased cardiovascular disease in both diabetic and non-diabetic patients. This has been demonstrated in numerous studies, including the HOPE (Heart Outcomes Prevention Evaluation) trial [9]. The risk increases progressively with increasing levels of microalbuminuria. This was also seen in the United Kingdom Prospective Diabetes Studies (UKPDS) [10]. Several studies have suggested that microalbuminuria and reduced glomerular filtration rate (GFR) are independent risk factors for cardiovascular disease and diabetics [11].

Traditional cardiovascular risk factors do not fully explain the cardiovascular risks associated with diabetes and obesity. A variety of mechanisms in addition to the effects of hypertension and altered lipid metabolism may contribute to the cardiovascular disease risk in diabetes. These potential mechanisms include endothelial dysfunction, inflammation, platelet activation, and other coagulation abnormalities.

From a clinical standpoint, these considerations have led to the general approach that patients with diabetes have to be considered to have a very high likelihood of having heart

L.L. Hamm, M.D. (✉)
Dean's Office, Tulane Medical School, New Orleans, LA, USA
e-mail: lhamm@tulane.edu

T.K. Thethi, M.D., M.P.H.
Section of Endocrinology, Department of Medicine, Tulane University Health Sciences Center, New Orleans, LA, USA

Southeast Louisiana Veterans Health Care, New Orleans, LA, USA

K.S. Hering-Smith, M.S., Ph.D.
Section of Nephrology and Hypertension, Department of Medicine, Tulane University Health Sciences Center, New Orleans, LA, USA

E.V. Lerma and V. Batuman (eds.), *Diabetes and Kidney Disease*,
DOI 10.1007/978-1-4939-0793-9_11, © Springer Science+Business Media New York 2014

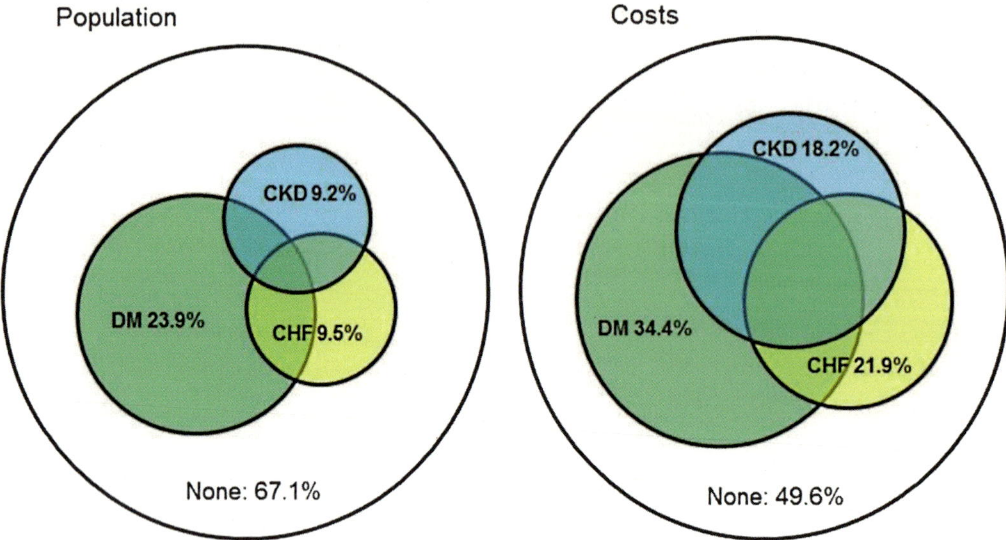

Fig. 11.1 Point prevalence distribution and annual costs of Medicare (fee-for-service) patients, age 65 and older, with diagnosed diabetes, CHF, and CKD, 2011. Adapted from the 2013 USRDS report, [39]. Populations were estimated from a 5 % Medicare sample using a point prevalent model. Population was further restricted to patients aged 65 and older, without ESRD. Diabetes, CHF, and CKD determined from claims data; costs were for calendar year 2011

disease and treated aggressively. In addition, there is recognition that diabetic patients often have less symptoms with coronary events than patients without diabetes, in large part secondary to autonomic denervation of the heart.

Cardiovascular Disease in Chronic Kidney Disease

CKD is also independently associated with increased cardiovascular disease. This can again be illustrated by USRDS (United States Renal Data System) data, Fig. 11.2. Numerous studies over the last decade have documented that cardiovascular disease incidence and mortality are increased in association with both decreased GFR and separately with increased urinary albumin, e.g., [12, 13]. This holds true both for patients without diabetes and have with diabetes. The increased cardiovascular disease have been well known in dialysis patients for decades but the data for CKD only began accumulating some 10–12 years ago. This increased cardiovascular disease has been noted for both coronary artery disease and overall cardiovascular mortality [12]. The increased mortality appears to begin as GFR decreases below 60 mL/min/1.73 m^2 [12, 14]. In fact, mortality, mostly cardiovascular mortality, is a "competing risk" to ESRD for patients with CKD—many patients with CKD including those with diabetes die without reaching ESRD [15, 16]; this is particularly true in older individuals. Most of the patients with CKD have several other cardiovascular risk factors and so analysis has to accurately account for the other risk factors. And these other risk factors such as hypertension, metabolic syndrome, diabetes, dyslipidemia, etc. correlate with the severity of the kidney disease. In addition, a variety of non-traditional risk factors are prevalent in both CKD and CV diseases; such factors include mediators or markers of inflammation, oxidative stress, endothelial dysfunction, coagulation, defects microalbuminuria, etc.

Patients with kidney disease also have worse prognosis after many cardiovascular events such as myocardial infarction and percutaneous coronary procedures [13, 17]. The reasons for these worse outcomes are likely multiple including other comorbid conditions. Unfortunately, there are also data that demonstrate that patients with kidney disease are less likely to be treated aggressively preventively prior to cardiovascular events. Part of this under-treatment may be that patients with kidney disease have been excluded from many clinical trials, and also some therapeutic nihilism (perceptions that treatments would be ineffective in these complicated patients) may exist.

Despite these clear associations between CKD and cardiovascular disease, incorporation of kidney disease into the risk assessment of patients for cardiovascular disease has not occurred at many levels. CKD definitions and measurements or estimations of GFR differ between studies. Therefore the full acceptance of CKD as a risk factor for cardiovascular disease has remained somewhat limited without incorporation into most general models of risk prediction such as the Framingham score.

Another factor which complicates incorporation of renal function into risk assessment is that measurement of renal function is complicated. Currently renal function is best assessed by estimating equations of GFR. The most common

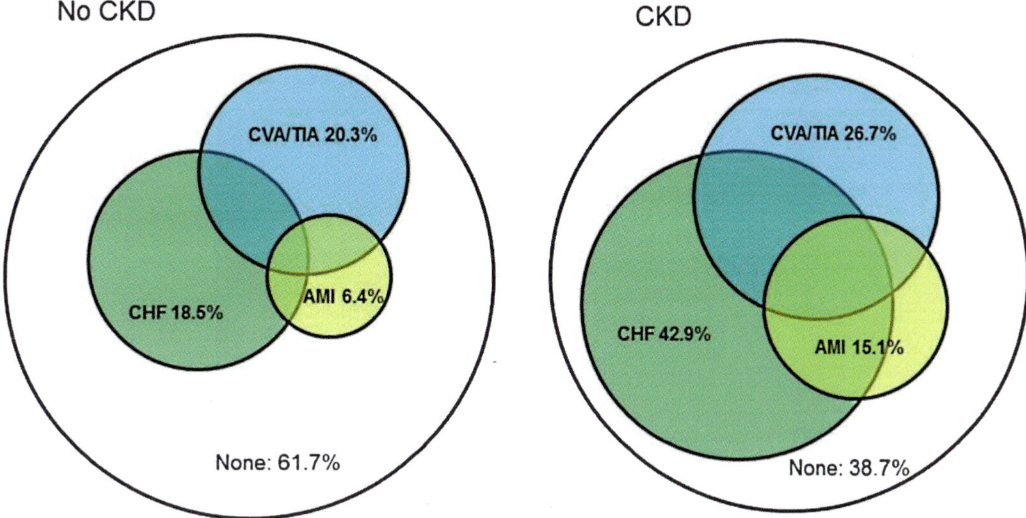

Fig. 11.2 Cardiovascular disease in patients with or without CKD. Point prevalence Medicare enrollees with CVD, age 66 and older, with fee-for-service coverage for the entire calendar year of 2011. Adapted from the 2013 USRDS report, [39]

equation used is the MDRD (Modification of Diet in Renal Disease) equation which uses a function of the inverse of serum creatinine, age, sex, and ethnicity to estimate GFR; unfortunately this equation has a variety of limitations including inaccuracies particularly in the high range of GFR. The Chronic Kidney Disease Epidemiology collaboration (CKD-EPI) equation is a more recently developed estimating equation again based on creatinine but with some more precision [18]. Recently, several studies have demonstrated that cystatin C may be a better marker of decreased GFR (or at least the CV risk associated with CKD) than other methods of estimation of GFR, e.g., [19, 20]. In other studies, formula or predictive models incorporating cystatin C with other parameters achieve the best estimation of subsequent events (such as ESRD or mortality) associated with CKD [21].

Cardiovascular Disease in Diabetic Nephropathy

The preceding discussion indicated that both diabetes and CKD are associated with increased cardiovascular morbidity and mortality. Together diabetes and CKD, specifically in most cases from diabetic nephropathy, lead to substantially increased morbidity and mortality from cardiovascular disease. Some 40 % of diabetic patients (known and those undiagnosed) in the United States have CKD [22]. And CKD essentially doubles the risk of cardiovascular disease events and death in patients with type 2 diabetes [23]. This additive or even multiplier effect is illustrated in Fig. 11.3. In fact some recent data suggest that much of the increased cardiovascular risk with diabetes is accounted for by the patients that have CKD [24–26]. These data suggest that this holds for both type 1 and type 2 diabetes. In other words, diabetes per se in the absence of kidney disease is not associated with nearly the increased cardiovascular risk as that associated with the combination of diabetes and CKD. Several studies have indicated that decreased GFR and increased urinary albumin are independent risk factors [11, 12, 24, 27, 28]. There also is a detrimental compound effect such that the presence of both decreased GFR and increased urinary albumin has more than an additive effect to increase cardiovascular risk [24].

The mechanisms by which kidney disease increases cardiovascular disease clearly include such associated risk factors as hypertension, insulin resistance, endothelial dysfunction, oxidative stress, and inflammation. But there are likely other aspects that relate specifically to renal dysfunction. One candidate for such a renal specific effect to increase cardiovascular disease is FGF-23 which has clearly been shown to be associated with excess cardiovascular disease in both patients with CKD and ESRD [29–31]. And FGF-23 is one of the earliest abnormalities in the hormonal disorders associated with mineral metabolism arrangements in early CKD [29]. FGF-23 is associated particularly with congestive heart failure but is also associated with increased atherosclerosis [29]. FGF-23 may directly lead to cardiac abnormalities [32]. Additionally, in patients with diabetes with CKD, compared to those without diabetes in CKD, the abnormalities in FGF 23 are more severe [33]. There may also be other factors as well that lead to increased cardiovascular disease in patients with CKD and end-stage renal disease, but these have not yet been clearly identified in both experimental models and humans.

The preventive treatment of the cardiovascular risks in patients with diabetic nephropathy include control of blood

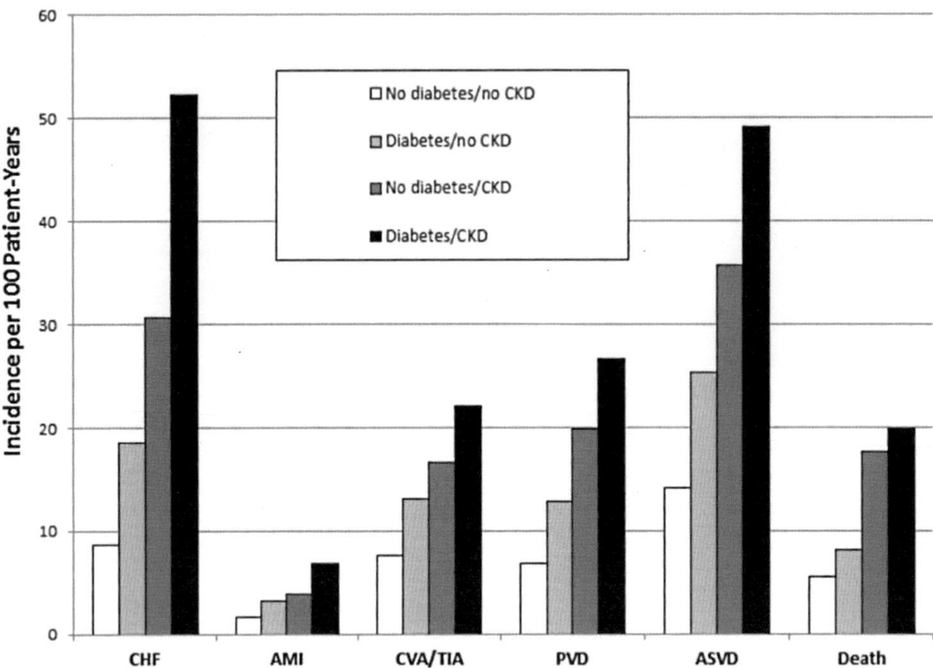

Fig. 11.3 Relative rates of atherosclerotic vascular disease, congestive heart failure, renal replacement therapy, and death compared in a 5 % sample of the United States Medicare population in 1998 and 1999 (n = 1,091,201). Derived from data in Foley RN, et al. J Am Soc Nephrol. 2005;16:489–495 [23]. *CHF* congestive heart failure, *AMI* acute myocardial infarction, *VA/TIA* cerebrovascular accident/transient ischemic attack, *PVD* peripheral vascular disease, *ASVD* atherosclerotic vascular disease. ASVD defined as the first occurrence of AMI, CVD/TIA, or PVD

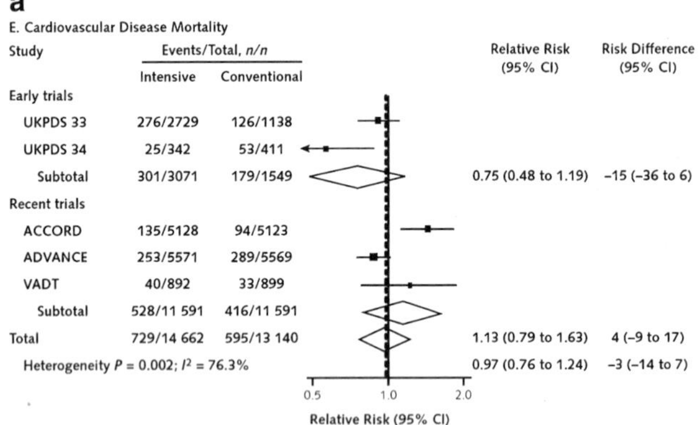

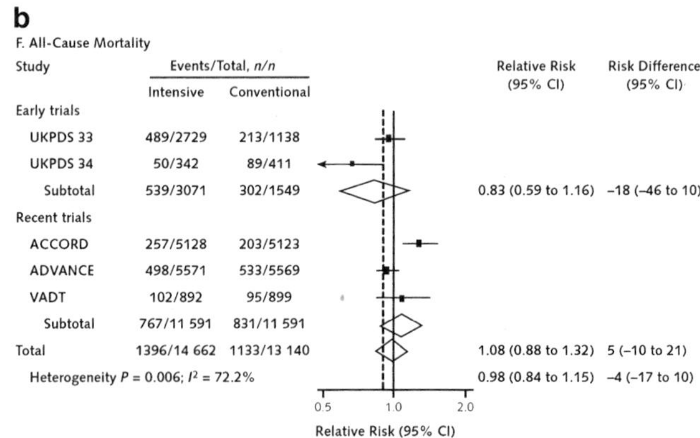

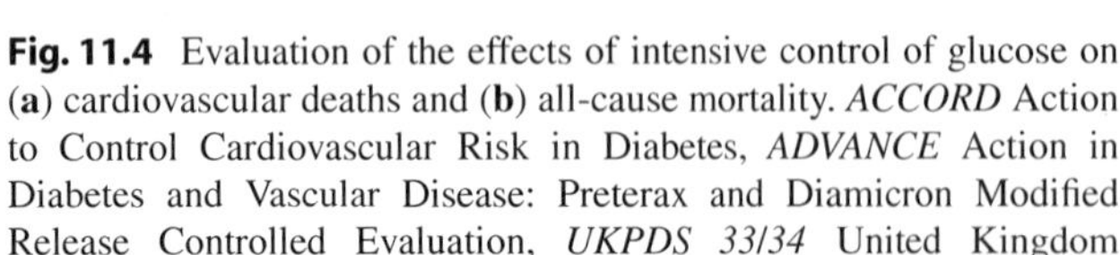

Fig. 11.4 Evaluation of the effects of intensive control of glucose on (**a**) cardiovascular deaths and (**b**) all-cause mortality. *ACCORD* Action to Control Cardiovascular Risk in Diabetes, *ADVANCE* Action in Diabetes and Vascular Disease: Preterax and Diamicron Modified Release Controlled Evaluation, *UKPDS 33/34* United Kingdom Prospective Diabetes Study, *VADT* Veterans Affairs Diabetes Trial. From Kelly TN, Bazzano LA, Fonseca VA, Thethi TK, Reynolds K, He J. Systematic review: glucose control and cardiovascular disease in type 2 diabetes. Ann Intern Med 2009; 151(6):394–403. Reprinted with permission from The American College of Physicians

glucose, treatment of dyslipidemia, smoking cessation, antiplatelet therapy, and control of blood pressure using inhibition of the renin-angiotensin system. Aldosterone antagonists may also have a role but have not been as well studied. The benefits of statins in CKD have not been as clear cut as in patients without CKD, and the role if any in most ESRD patients is limited [34]. Some therapies (glucose and blood pressure control) have clearly been shown to slow the progression of the microvascular complications of diabetes (e.g., retinal disease, neuropathy) and the progression of the kidney disease. However, recent trials of intensive glucose control have failed to demonstrate prevention of macrovascular complications of diabetes. For instance, analyses of multiple studies of intensive lowering of glucose in type 2 diabetes failed to demonstrate a benefit on all-cause mortality or cardiovascular mortality [35, 36], Fig. 11.4; some benefits in some specific cardiovascular outcomes were found to be counterbalanced by increased risk of severe hypoglycemia. In fact, some agents are possibly associated with worse cardiovascular outcomes (e.g., sulfonylureas, rosiglitazone, insulin). But some trials have found benefit, such as with metformin in the UKPDS study [37]. Recently in the Look AHEAD study, weight loss and increased exercise did not improve the rate of cardiovascular events [38]. Undoubtedly, some, and perhaps most, of the lack of benefit derives from interventions being started long after disease processes began. Fortunately, there are many on-going large, well-powered trials that may yield additional insight into newer therapeutic modalities to control glucose and alter cardiovascular outcomes.

In sum, cardiovascular disease is a frequent cause of morbidity and mortality in patients with diabetic nephropathy. Understanding the intertwined mechanisms and optimal therapies are still under intense investigation particularly considering the significant health consequences and the large population health implications.

References

1. Seshasai SR, Kaptoge S, Thompson A, Di AE, Gao P, Sarwar N, et al. Diabetes mellitus, fasting glucose, and risk of cause-specific death. N Engl J Med. 2011;364(9):829–41.
2. Third Report of the National Cholesterol Education Program (NCEP) Expert Panel on Detection, Evaluation, and Treatment of High Blood Cholesterol in Adults (Adult Treatment Panel III) final report. Circulation 2002;106(25):3143–421.
3. De BG, Ambrosioni E, Borch-Johnsen K, Brotons C, Cifkova R, Dallongeville J, et al. European guidelines on cardiovascular disease and prevention in clinical practice. Atherosclerosis. 2003; 171(1):145–55.
4. Kannel WB, McGee DL. Diabetes and cardiovascular risk factors: the Framingham study. Circulation. 1979;59(1):8–13.
5. Stamler J, Vaccaro O, Neaton JD, Wentworth D. Diabetes, other risk factors, and 12-yr cardiovascular mortality for men screened in the Multiple Risk Factor Intervention Trial. Diabetes Care. 1993; 16(2):434–44.
6. Coutinho M, Gerstein HC, Wang Y, Yusuf S. The relationship between glucose and incident cardiovascular events. A metaregression analysis of published data from 20 studies of 95,783 individuals followed for 12.4 years. Diabetes Care. 1999;22(2):233–40.
7. Laguardia HA, Hamm LL, Chen J. The metabolic syndrome and risk of chronic kidney disease: pathophysiology and intervention strategies. J Nutr Metab. 2012;2012:652608. doi:10.1155/2012/652608. Epub@2012 Feb 22.:652608.
8. DeBoer MD. Obesity, systemic inflammation, and increased risk for cardiovascular disease and diabetes among adolescents: a need for screening tools to target interventions. Nutrition. 2013;29(2):379–86.
9. Gerstein HC, Mann JF, Yi Q, Zinman B, Dinneen SF, Hoogwerf B, et al. Albuminuria and risk of cardiovascular events, death, and heart failure in diabetic and nondiabetic individuals. JAMA. 2001; 286(4):421–6.
10. Adler AI, Stevens RJ, Manley SE, Bilous RW, Cull CA, Holman RR. Development and progression of nephropathy in type 2 diabetes: the United Kingdom Prospective Diabetes Study (UKPDS 64). Kidney Int. 2003;63(1):225–32.
11. Ninomiya T, Perkovic V, de Galan BE, Zoungas S, Pillai A, Jardine M, et al. Albuminuria and kidney function independently predict cardiovascular and renal outcomes in diabetes. J Am Soc Nephrol. 2009;20(8):1813–21.
12. Matsushita K, van der Velde M, Astor BC, Woodward M, Levey AS, de Jong PE, et al. Association of estimated glomerular filtration rate and albuminuria with all-cause and cardiovascular mortality in general population cohorts: a collaborative meta-analysis. Lancet. 2010;375(9731):2073–81.
13. Sarnak MJ, Levey AS, Schoolwerth AC, Coresh J, Culleton B, Hamm LL, et al. Kidney disease as a risk factor for development of cardiovascular disease: a statement from the American Heart Association Councils on Kidney in Cardiovascular Disease, High Blood Pressure Research, Clinical Cardiology, and Epidemiology and Prevention. Circulation. 2003;108(17):2154–69.
14. Go AS, Chertow GM, Fan D, McCulloch CE, Hsu CY. Chronic kidney disease and the risks of death, cardiovascular events, and hospitalization. N Engl J Med. 2004;351(13):1296–305.
15. Keith DS, Nichols GA, Gullion CM, Brown JB, Smith DH. Longitudinal follow-up and outcomes among a population with chronic kidney disease in a large managed care organization. Arch Intern Med. 2004;164(6):659–63.
16. Patel UD, Young EW, Ojo AO, Hayward RA. CKD progression and mortality among older patients with diabetes. Am J Kidney Dis. 2005;46(3):406–14.
17. Reinecke H, Trey T, Matzkies F, Fobker M, Breithardt G, Schaefer RM. Grade of chronic renal failure, and acute and long-term outcome after percutaneous coronary interventions. Kidney Int. 2003;63(2):696–701.
18. Levey AS, Coresh J. Chronic kidney disease. Lancet. 2012; 379(9811):165–80.
19. Shlipak MG, Sarnak MJ, Katz R, Fried LF, Seliger SL, Newman AB, et al. Cystatin C and the risk of death and cardiovascular events among elderly persons. N Engl J Med. 2005;352(20):2049–60.
20. Astor BC, Shafi T, Hoogeveen RC, Matsushita K, Ballantyne CM, Inker LA, et al. Novel markers of kidney function as predictors of ESRD, cardiovascular disease, and mortality in the general population. Am J Kidney Dis. 2012;59(5):653–62.
21. Shlipak MG, Matsushita K, Arnlov J, Inker LA, Katz R, Polkinghorne KR, et al. Cystatin C versus creatinine in determining risk based on kidney function. N Engl J Med. 2013;369(10):932–43.
22. Plantinga LC, Crews DC, Coresh J, Miller III ER, Saran R, Yee J, et al. Prevalence of chronic kidney disease in US adults with undiagnosed diabetes or prediabetes. Clin J Am Soc Nephrol. 2010;5(4):673–82.
23. Foley RN, Murray AM, Li S, Herzog CA, McBean AM, Eggers PW, et al. Chronic kidney disease and the risk for cardiovascular disease, renal replacement, and death in the United States Medicare population, 1998 to 1999. J Am Soc Nephrol. 2005;16(2):489–95.
24. Afkarian M, Sachs MC, Kestenbaum B, Hirsch IB, Tuttle KR, Himmelfarb J, et al. Kidney disease and increased mortality risk in type 2 diabetes. J Am Soc Nephrol. 2013;24(2):302–8.
25. Groop PH, Thomas MC, Moran JL, Waden J, Thorn LM, Makinen VP, et al. The presence and severity of chronic kidney disease predicts all-cause mortality in type 1 diabetes. Diabetes. 2009;58(7): 1651–8.
26. Orchard TJ, Secrest AM, Miller RG, Costacou T. In the absence of renal disease, 20 year mortality risk in type 1 diabetes is comparable to that of the general population: a report from the Pittsburgh Epidemiology of Diabetes Complications Study. Diabetologia. 2010;53(11):2312–9.
27. Hemmelgarn BR, Manns BJ, Lloyd A, James MT, Klarenbach S, Quinn RR, et al. Relation between kidney function, proteinuria, and adverse outcomes. JAMA. 2010;303(5):423–9.
28. van der Velde M, Matsushita K, Coresh J, Astor BC, Woodward M, Levey A, et al. Lower estimated glomerular filtration rate and higher albuminuria are associated with all-cause and cardiovascular

mortality. A collaborative meta-analysis of high-risk population cohorts. Kidney Int. 2011;79(12):1341–52.

29. Scialla JJ, Xie H, Rahman M, Anderson AH, Isakova T, Ojo A, et al. Fibroblast growth factor-23 and cardiovascular events in CKD. J Am Soc Nephrol. 2014;25(2):349–60.
30. Isakova T, Xie H, Yang W, Xie D, Anderson AH, Scialla J, et al. Fibroblast growth factor 23 and risks of mortality and end-stage renal disease in patients with chronic kidney disease. JAMA. 2011;305(23):2432–9.
31. Gutierrez OM, Mannstadt M, Isakova T, Rauh-Hain JA, Tamez H, Shah A, et al. Fibroblast growth factor 23 and mortality among patients undergoing hemodialysis. N Engl J Med. 2008;359(6):584–92.
32. Faul C, Amaral AP, Oskouei B, Hu MC, Sloan A, Isakova T, et al. FGF23 induces left ventricular hypertrophy. J Clin Invest. 2011;121(11):4393–408.
33. Wahl P, Xie H, Scialla J, Anderson CA, Bellovich K, Brecklin C, et al. Earlier onset and greater severity of disordered mineral metabolism in diabetic patients with chronic kidney disease. Diabetes Care. 2012;35(5):994–1001.
34. Slinin Y, Ishani A, Rector T, Fitzgerald P, MacDonald R, Tacklind J, et al. Management of hyperglycemia, dyslipidemia, and albuminuria in patients with diabetes and CKD: a systematic review for a KDOQI clinical practice guideline. Am J Kidney Dis. 2012;60(5):747–69.
35. Boussageon R, Bejan-Angoulvant T, Saadatian-Elahi M, Lafont S, Bergeonneau C, Kassai B, et al. Effect of intensive glucose lowering treatment on all cause mortality, cardiovascular death, and microvascular events in type 2 diabetes: meta-analysis of randomised controlled trials. BMJ. 2011;343:d4169. doi:10.1136/bmj.d4169.:d4169.
36. Kelly TN, Bazzano LA, Fonseca VA, Thethi TK, Reynolds K, He J. Systematic review: glucose control and cardiovascular disease in type 2 diabetes. Ann Intern Med. 2009;151(6):394–403.
37. Holman RR, Paul SK, Bethel MA, Matthews DR, Neil HA. 10-year follow-up of intensive glucose control in type 2 diabetes. N Engl J Med. 2008;359(15):1577–89.
38. Wing RR, Bolin P, Brancati FL, Bray GA, Clark JM, Coday M, et al. Cardiovascular effects of intensive lifestyle intervention in type 2 diabetes. N Engl J Med. 2013;369(2):145–54.
39. Collins AJ, Foley RN, Herzog C, Chavers B, Gilbertson D, Herzog C, et al. US renal data system 2012 annual data report. Am J Kidney Dis. 2013;61(1 Suppl 1):A7, e1-A7, 476.

Dyslipidemia in Diabetes Mellitus and Chronic Kidney Disease

12

Armand Krikorian and Joumana T. Chaiban

Introduction

Patients with chronic kidney disease (CKD) and Diabetes Mellitus (DM) are at particularly high risk for developing Cardiovascular (CV) events. CKD is common among adults in the United States. It is estimated that more than 10 % of people aged 20 years or older in the United States have CKD (http://www.cdc.gov/diabetes/pubs/factsheets/kidney.htm). Premature death both from cardiovascular disease (CVD) and all causes is higher in adults with CKD compared to those without. Individuals with CKD are 16–40 times more likely to die than reach End Stage Renal Disease (ESRD) (CDC, www.cdc.gov). On the other hand, more than 35 % of people aged 20 years or older with diabetes have CKD. DM is the leading cause of kidney failure and ESRD (www.cdc.gov) [1]. It is associated with high risks of cardiovascular morbidity and mortality that are greatly increased in the presence of CKD [2] and leads to a substantial personal and economic cost [United States Renal Data System 2012 Annual Data Report (ADR) Atlas 2012, available from www.usrds.org, accessed August 7, 2013]. An aging population with increasing prevalence of diabetes [3] and an alarming rise in the incidence of CKD in the USA [4] will increase even further the burden of diabetic renal disease.

High LDL, low HDL, and hypertriglyceridemia are all known risk factors for coronary artery disease (CAD). In the general population, there is a continuous strong positive correlation between the plasma levels of LDL and the risk of CAD and coronary mortality [5]. This chapter aims to define the pathophysiology of dyslipidemia in patients with DM and CKD and explore its impact on CV mortality. Guidelines for evaluation and assessment as well as therapeutic modalities will be outlined.

A. Krikorian, M.D., F.A.C.E. (✉)
Internal Medicine, Endocrinology and Metabolism, Advocate Christ Medical Center, 4440 West 95th Street, Oak Lawn, IL 60453, USA
e-mail: Armand.Krikorian@advocatehealth.com

J.T. Chaiban, M.D.
Internal Medicine, Endocrinology and Metabolic Diseases, Saint Vincent Charity Medical Center, Cleveland, OH, USA

Case Western Reserve University, Cleveland, OH, USA
e-mail: joumanachaiban@yahoo.com

Pathophysiology

The spectrum of lipid abnormalities in patients with CKD appears to be related to the degree of renal dysfunction as well as the degree of proteinuria (Table 12.1) [6]. In patients with coexisting diabetes, a large body of evidence suggests a central role for lipids contributing to CVD, a pattern termed diabetic dyslipidemia. In addition, there is a proinflammatory milieu at the level of the vascular endothelium due to the accumulation of advanced glycation end products that stimulates accelerated atherosclerosis. Considerable work has demonstrated that the diabetic lipid profile possesses an intrinsic atherogenicity that is not present in those without diabetes [7].

Hypertriglyceridemia is common to both patients with type 2 DM and those with proteinuric dyslipidemia. In type 2 DM, it is mainly due to increased availability of circulating glucose and FFAs (free fatty acids) as well as decreased lipolysis of VLDL. In CKD, the mechanism of hypertriglyceridemia appears to be multifactorial and affected by the presence or absence of proteinuria. LPL (Lipoprotein lipase) activity is significantly reduced, partially due to the presence of circulating inhibitors [8]. ApoC-III, an inhibitor of LPL in humans [9], has increased levels in patients with CKD due to decreased degradation [10]. Recent evidence also points to the down-regulation of glycosylphosphatidylinositol-anchored high density lipoprotein-binding protein-1 (GPIHBP1) molecules, responsible of anchoring LPL to the endothelium and chylomicrons [11]. Two studies have suggested that elevated parathyroid hormone level contributes to elevated triglycerides (TG) in CKD [12, 13], an effect that seems to be found also in patients with primary hyperparathyroidism [14].

E.V. Lerma and V. Batuman (eds.), *Diabetes and Kidney Disease*,
DOI 10.1007/978-1-4939-0793-9_12, © Springer Science+Business Media New York 2014

Table 12.1 Lipid abnormalities in patients with CKD with and without proteinuria

	CKD stage 1–2		CKD stage 3		CKD stage 4–5	
	Without proteinuria	With proteinuria	Without proteinuria	With proteinuria	Without proteinuria	With proteinuria
Total cholesterol	Normal	Increased	Normal	Increased	Normal	Increased
LDL	Nl or reduced	Increased	Nl or reduced	Increased	Nl or reduced	Increased
HDL	Nl to low	Nl to low	Low	Nl to low	Low	low
TGs	Nl to increased	Increased	Increased	Increased	Increased	Increased

Table 12.2 Dyslipidemia in patients with DM and/or CKD versus the general population

	Dyslipidemia without DM or CKD	Diabetic dyslipidemia	Dyslipidemia in CKD	Dyslipidemia in CKD and DM
Total cholesterol	Normal or increased	Normal or increased	Normal or decreased	Increased
LDL-C	Increased	Increased	Normal	Increased
HDL-C	Decreased	Decreased	Decreased	Decreased
Triglycerides	Normal	Increased	Increased	Increased

HDL levels appear to be uniformly decreased in patients with CKD as compared to controls. Serum apoA-1 and A-2, two of the main lipoprotein component particles of HDL, are reduced in diabetic patients with CKD [15]. Serum levels of LCAT (lecithin cholesterol acyltransferase), the enzyme responsible for the maturation of HDL via the disposal of oxidized fatty acids, are also decreased [6]. More recent evidence points to an impairment in the functionality of available HDL in patients with ESRD [16].

LDL-cholesterol is reported to remain normal through the different stages of CKD [17, 18]. Nevertheless, the composition of LDL is markedly altered, with a predominance of small dense LDL [19, 20], suggesting a more relevant role for the measurement of small LDL instead of regular LDL for CVD assessment. The conversion of IDL to LDL is also impaired due to the reduced activity of hepatic lipase in CKD [21]. Several studies point to the increased prevalence of elevated Lp(a) levels in patients with CKD [22, 23].

The presence of nephrotic syndrome markedly alters the lipid profile of individuals with CKD. In addition, diabetic patients with proteinuria exhibit higher rates of dyslipidemia than those without proteinuria [24]. In a study of patients with nephrotic syndrome without complicating DM, Joven et al. confirmed the presence of increased VLDL and LDL as well as normal levels of HDL [25]. They also demonstrated elevated levels of apo CIII, further suggesting the inhibition of LPL as a factor for decreased catabolism of VLDL and elevated TG levels. In a more recent study on rats with the nephrotic syndrome, the increased synthesis of fatty acids was found to be of hepatic origin, with up-regulation of fatty acid synthase and acyl-CoA carboxylase [26].

In ESRD, the resultant decrease in proteinuria may contribute to the return to the typical profile of dyslipidemia of CKD. In these patients, several additional factors seem to contribute to dyslipidemia. HDL particles are dysfunctional in both their capacity to act as reverse cholesterol transporters and their anti-inflammatory properties [16]. Pre-beta-HDL, an inhibitor of serum LPL that is not cleared in uremic patients, also contributes to hypertriglyceridemia [8].

Patients undergoing peritoneal dialysis (PD) have several lipid abnormalities different from those on hemodialysis (HD). The glucose found in high concentration in PD fluids acts as a substrate for further cholesterol synthesis [27]. Continuous protein clearance in PD patients, as compared to HD-dependent patients, contributes to a lipid profile similar to those with the nephrotic syndrome [28].

The presence of insulin resistance (IR), whether intrinsic to CKD or secondary to Type 2 DM, further exacerbates lipid abnormalities. IR has been described in patients with non-DM induced CKD [29] and is thought to be secondary to post-receptor defects [30]. An additional contribution from secondary hyperparathyroidism to the etiology of IR in CKD may also be possible [31]. The effect of IR on lipid metabolism is obviously more pronounced in patients with Type 2 DM, with resulting high TGs, low HDL, increased small dense LDL and apo-B, as well as slightly increased LDL (Table 12.2) [32].

While most studies focus on CKD in patients with Type 2 diabetes, an analysis of the lipid profile of the CCT/EDIC cohort of patients with Type 1 diabetes demonstrated a specific profile of CKD that is characterized by high TG levels, predominantly in the VLDL subclasses [2].

Dyslipidemia, CKD, DM, and Cardiovascular Risk

The Third Report of the Expert Panel on Detection, Evaluation and Treatment of High Blood Cholesterol in Adults (Adult Treatment Panel III, or ATP III) from the National Cholesterol Education Program (NCEP) considers DM as a CAD equivalent [33]. Death from CVD is two to three times more common in diabetic patients than in the non-diabetic population [34]. DM has been defined as a CAD risk equivalent because the likelihood of future events may approach that of people without diabetes who have already had a myocardial infarction [33]. An almost similar risk appears to be induced by the presence of CKD [35]. Although the Framingham Study [36] did not show an association between baseline renal function and incident CVD events and the results of the First National Health and Nutrition Evaluation Survey [37] did not support moderate renal insufficiency as an independent risk factor for CVD, there is a large body of evidence suggesting the opposite, namely that CKD (defined as serum creatinine greater than 1.5 mg/dL [133 μmol/L] and a glomerular filtration rate (GFR) less than 60 mL/min per 1.73 m^2) constitutes a risk factor for CVD. Numerous observational studies have shown that both a reduced GFR and proteinuria are independently associated with an increased risk of cardiovascular events in community-based populations [38–42]. Rashidi et al. showed that the 9-year rates of cardiovascular death among 1,899 individuals were 15.7 %, 15.8 %, and 13 % respectively in those with history of myocardial infarction but no diabetes or CKD, history of diabetes but no myocardial infarction or CKD, history of CKD but no myocardial infarction or diabetes [43]. A serum creatinine level greater than 133 μmol/L (1.5 mg/dL) was associated with a 70 % increase in risk of all-cause mortality in participants followed up for 5 years in the Cardiovascular Health Study [44]. In the TNT (Treating to New Targets) Study, 17.4 % of patients with Type 2 DM and CKD experienced a major CV event versus 13.4 % of patients with type 2 DM with normal eGFR [45]. This, in addition to several other studies [38, 46] has led the National Kidney Foundation and the American College of Cardiology (ACC)/American Heart Association (AHA) to recommend that CKD be also considered as a CAD risk equivalent [47, 48].

When DM is complicated by CKD the cardiovascular risk increases dramatically. An increase in this risk is noted already in the early stages of microalbuminuria [40]. People with diabetes and microalbuminuria have twice the CVD risk of those with normoalbuminuria, and as albuminuria progresses and GFR deteriorates, CVD risk increases progressively [2]. Death from CVD in patients with CKD is substantially more frequent than progression to ESRD [38, 49, 50]. Chang et al. showed a multiplicatively synergistic effect of diabetes and ESRD for CV-related risks, especially for acute myocardial infarction and stroke, of which the adjusted hazard ratios (aHRs) [95 % confidence intervals] were 5.24 [4.83–5.68] and 2.43 [2.32–2.55], respectively in comparison with people without diabetes or ESRD [51]. New-onset diabetes after ESRD had similar effects with aHRs of 4.12 [3.49–4.87] and 1.75 [1.57–1.95], respectively [51]. Moreover, dyslipidemia in patients with both DM and CKD may also increase albuminuria and accelerate progression of diabetic kidney disease [2].

Statin therapy is widely used because it has been proved to reduce the incidence of CV events and mortality in diverse patient populations at increased risk [52–54]. Data regarding the treatment of dyslipidemia and use of statins in patients with CKD and DM relies mainly on post hoc and subgroup analysis of large statin trials conducted in the general population.

The Kidney Disease Outcomes Quality Initiative (KDOQI) Clinical Practice Guidelines for treating patients with renal disease and dyslipidemia were introduced by the National Kidney Foundation in an effort to guide management of dyslipidemia in people with kidney disease. The recent updated KDIGO (Kidney Disease Improving Global Outcomes) guidelines emphasized that adverse events related to appropriate statin regimens do not occur in higher frequency in patients with CKD. Yet, it is not uncommon that the medical community, while acknowledging that these patients are at very high risk for macrovascular complications, is reluctant to treat these patients for concerns of medication side effects and efficacy.

Several studies have shown a beneficial effect of statins on kidney function. CARDS (Collaborative Atorvastatin Diabetes Study) showed a modest positive effect of atorvastatin therapy on eGFR [55]. In the HPS (Heart Protection Study), GFR decreased less in patients with T2DM on simvastatin therapy during a mean 4.8 years of follow-up compared to those not taking statins [56]. In the GREACE (Greek Atorvastatin and Coronary Heart Disease Evaluation) trial, atorvastatin treatment was associated with an improvement in creatinine clearance [57]. In a combined analysis across the WOSCOPS (West of Scotland Coronary Prevention Study), CARE (Cholesterol and Recurrent Events), and LIPID (Long-term Intervention with Pravastatin in Ischemic Disease) trials, pravastatin was associated with a significant small net benefit in eGFR [58]. In the TNT (Treating to New Targets) Study, there was consistently greater improvement in eGFR on 80 mg versus 10 mg of atorvastatin in diabetic participants as well as all participants [45, 59, 60]. A subsequent cohort analysis from the large Veterans Integrated Service Network database (VISN 16) showed that statin therapy resulted in 13 % decrease in the odds of developing kidney dysfunction during 3 years of follow up [61]. Such an effect was not reproduced by others. In the ALLHAT (Antihypertensive and Lipid Lowering Therapy to Prevent Heart Attack Trial), there was no effect of pravastatin, on eGFR [62]. In a meta-analysis by Strippoli et al. [63], no significant effect of statin therapy on creatinine clearance was demonstrated. These conflicting results may have been due to the different use of antihypertensive agents, mainly angiotensin- converting enzyme inhibitors, in these clinical trials. This has led the KDOQI work group to conclude that it is uncertain whether treatment with statins does slow the progression of diabetic kidney disease [2].

The literature on the beneficial effect of statins and their cardiovascular protection in the general population is extensive. However, as mentioned earlier, data on their beneficial effect in patients with diabetes and CKD still relies on subgroup analysis of the large clinical trials. In CARDS, there was an impressive decrease in cardiovascular deaths in people with Type 2 DM on atorvastatin in the absence of markedly decreased kidney function [55]. The CARDS investigators found that patients with an eGFR of 30–60 mL/min/1.73 m^2 (i.e., stage 3 CKD) experienced the same substantial decreases in CVD end points with atorvastatin therapy as seen in the trial overall. Treatment of 26 such patients during 4 years would prevent 1 first major CVD event, and 38 events would be avoided for every 1,000 patients treated for 4 years [55]. Other studies also support the efficacy of statin therapy for preventing CVD in the presence of impairment of kidney function, including the Pravastatin Pooling Project (PPP) [64], the TNT Study [45] and the 4S (Scandinavian Simvastatin Survival Study) [65]. In patients with CKD, treatment with high dose atorvastatin (80 mg) resulted in significant reductions in the risk of cardiovascular event, cerebrovascular event, and congestive heart failure with hospitalization compared to lower dose atorvastatin (10 mg) [45]. Patients in the HPS with diabetes and CVD received the greatest benefit from statin therapy. Data from the HPS and the Pravastatin Pooling study [56, 64] showed that among diabetic patients without occlusive arterial disease, 5 years of treatment would be expected to prevent about 45 people per 1,000 from having at least one major vascular event (and, among these 45 people, to prevent about 70 first or subsequent events during this treatment period) [56]. The authors suggested statin therapy to be considered routinely for all diabetic patients at sufficiently high risk of major vascular events, irrespective of their initial cholesterol concentrations [56]. In that study, the incidence of the primary outcome was lowest in individuals with neither CKD nor diabetes (15.2 %), intermediate in individuals with either only CKD (18.6 %) or diabetes (21.3 %), and highest in individuals with both (27.0 %) [64]. Pravastatin reduced the relative likelihood of the primary outcome to a similar extent in subgroups defined by the presence or absence of CKD and diabetes. It was associated with a significant reduction in the relative risk of the primary outcome by 25 % in patients with CKD and concomitant diabetes and by 24 % in individuals with neither characteristic. However, the absolute reduction in the risk of the primary outcome as a result of pravastatin use was highest in patients with both CKD and diabetes (6.4 %) and lowest in individuals with neither (3.5 %) [64].

Initial results of cardiovascular outcome trials in patients with advanced or end-stage kidney disease raised safety concerns related to potential toxic effects of high-dose statins in patients with reduced renal clearance and may have limited the use of statins in the CKD population [60]. However, most studies so far support the concept that the incidence of non-cardiovascular deaths, rhabdomyolysis, and abnormal liver function test results are not increased with statins and that statins, at reduced doses, are generally safe in patients with renal disease [2, 66]. The KDOQI clinical practice guidelines for diabetes and CKD advises that people with DM and CKD (other than stage 5) should receive LDL-C lowering therapy and recommends against routine liver function tests or muscle enzymes *for patients with type 2 diabetes who are taking statins, except in specific circumstances* [2]. The more recent update to the guidelines by KDIGO reaffirms that routine monitoring with liver function tests or CPK in asymptomatic patients is not backed by evidence from clinical trials [66].

After the publication of the KDOQI guidelines, Slinin et al., in 2012, published a systematic review of clinical trials providing evidence for the management of hyperglycemia, dyslipidemia, and albuminuria in individuals with diabetes [67]. They identified 11 studies ($n=7,539$) that assessed lipid management in patients with DM and kidney disease. They concluded that: (1) overall statins did not reduce all-cause mortality or stroke compared to placebo in adults with both diabetes and CKD and they found insufficient evidence to judge the efficacy of statins for other clinical cardiovascular and kidney outcomes (2) high-dose statin therapy did not decrease all-cause mortality, stroke, or the risk of major cardiovascular events compared to lower dose statin therapy in participants with diabetes and CKD (3) in patients with diabetes and albuminuria, fenofibrate increased regression of microalbuminuria to normoalbuminuria compared to placebo (4) none of the trials reported adverse events or withdrawals for the subgroup of participants with CKD and diabetes. However, they again noted that patients with kidney disease and diabetes constituted subgroup or post hoc analyses in most of these studies.

Patients undergoing maintenance hemodialysis (HD) constitute a separate category and have a greatly increased risk of premature CVD and myocardial infarction. Based on data from US Renal Data System Coordinating Center Case-Mix Adequacy Study, the prevalence of clinical CAD in HD patients is 40 % and CVD mortality is 10–30 times higher than in the general population [68]. The pattern of death from CVD in such patients differs from that in the general population. Multiple factors get into play including sudden cardiac death (from electrolyte abnormalities and arrhythmias) [69] as well as heart failure and cardiomyopathy from volume overload [70–72]. The average annual incidence of myocardial infarction or death from CAD in patients receiving HD and who have type 2 DM is 8.2 % according to the 4D trial [73]. In dialysis patients, observational studies, such as the US Renal Data System Dialysis Morbidity and

Mortality Wave 2 study [74] and the Dialysis Outcomes and Practice Patterns Study (DOPPS I) [75], showed that statin use was associated with a reduction in mortality. These results were not confirmed by large randomized, controlled statin trials in hemodialysis patients. The 4D study [73] is the only randomized controlled trial that included solely patients with T2DM and ESRD on HD and compared atorvastatin 20 mg to placebo. It showed that atorvastatin was associated with a non-significant decrease in the primary end point of major CVD in type 2 DM on HD [73]. Furthermore, no increase in the rate of serious adverse events was found, but investigators noted a significant increase in fatal stroke. It was the first large scale cardiovascular outcome trial that did not show overall benefit from administration of a potent dose of a statin and did not confirm the generally accepted assumption that for every 30-mg/dL change in LDL-C level, the RR of CAD is changed in proportion by about 30 % [2]. This study has led the KDOQI to label the evidence that "Atorvastatin treatment in patients with type 2 diabetes on maintenance hemodialysis treatment does not improve cardiovascular outcomes" as "Strong." Two other randomized controlled trials studied patients on HD, both with and without diabetes: AURORA [76] and SHARP [77]. In Aurora (A Study to Evaluate the Use of Rosuvastatin in Subjects on Regular Hemodialysis: An Assessment of Survival and Cardiovascular Events) [76], investigators studied the effect of rosuvastatin 10 mg versus placebo and included only patients on HD, 731 of which had Type 2 DM. Similarly to 4D, they reported no effect of rosuvastatin on a composite cardiovascular and cerebrovascular endpoint for the overall trial population [78]. The SHARP study (Study of Heart and Renal Protection) evaluated the combination of Simvastatin 20 mg and ezetimibe 10 mg versus placebo and included 9,270 patients with CKD, 3,023 of them on HD and 2,094 with Type 2 DM. It is the largest randomized clinical study of cholesterol lowering agents in patients with CKD and its results were published after the publication of the KDOQI guidelines. It showed that, in patients with both CKD and Type 2 DM, LDL cholesterol lowering (achieved difference of 32 mg/dL) reduced by 22 % a composite outcome of major atherosclerotic events (defined as nonfatal MI, any cardiac death, non-hemorrhagic stroke, or arterial revascularization excluding dialysis access), in patients with or without ESRD. The lack of therapeutic effect likely emphasizes the fact that the benefit of statins is limited when their use is postponed until patients have already reached ESRD. This body of evidence led the KDIGO group to reaffirm that while statin therapy with or without ezetimibe may be continued in ESRD patients on hemodialysis, their continued use will depend on periodic risk/benefit assessment [66].

In order to maximize benefit, statin therapy should be initiated early in the course of the kidney disease and diabetes [55]. Because concomitant CKD and diabetes occur in nearly 40 % of incident dialysis patients in the United States [56, 64], prescription of statins at earlier stages of renal impairment might reduce the burden of CVD among people with ESRD [56].

The use of omega-3 fatty acids in patients on chronic hemodialysis is currently not supported. The OPACH study (Omega-3 Fatty Acids as Secondary Prevention Against Cardiovascular Events in Patients Who Undergo Chronic Hemodialysis) was a randomized, double-blind, placebo controlled trial in 206 chronic HD patients who received either 1.7 g/day of omega-3 fatty acids or placebo [79]. Although no significant reduction was seen in the combined primary end point of cardiovascular events or death, there was a 70 % (95 % CI 0.10–0.92; $p=0.036$) relative risk reduction in the risk of myocardial infarction, with no difference in the incidence of adverse events.

Recipients of kidney transplants constitute a separate category of patients that also need special consideration. Many transplant recipients have either pre-existing CVD or multiple CV risk factors at the time of transplantation. Additional risk factors (including diabetes, hypertension, and hyperlipidemia) may develop, or be aggravated by immunosuppressive therapy following transplantation [80]. Many of the commonly used statin drugs share the metabolism by the microsomal enzyme system CyP 3A4, resulting in greatly increased statin levels and higher potential for adverse effects. Fluvastatin does not share this interaction [81] permitting its safe use in transplant recipients (Table 12.3). In the ALERT study, investigators conducted a large interventional trial in renal transplant patients studying the effect of Fluvastatin on cardiac death or definite nonfatal myocardial infarction [82]. Out of 2,012 total patients, the ALERT study included 396 (18.8 %) with diabetes and showed that renal transplant patients benefit from Fluvastatin therapy with a reduction in cardiac death and nonfatal myocardial infarction. The authors estimated that it would be necessary to treat 31 renal transplant patients for 5 years to prevent a cardiac death or nonfatal myocardial infarction [82].

Trials assessing fibrate therapy in CKD are not as common as ones with statins. In the FIELD study, Davis et al. demonstrated that fenofibrate reduces the progression of albuminuria and the decline of GFR in type 2 DM, despite a small initial rise in plasma creatinine [83]. Another large, double-blind randomized placebo controlled clinical trial, the Action to Control Cardiovascular Risk in Diabetes (ACCORD), also showed an early, sustained rise in serum creatinine with fenofibrate in patients with type 2 diabetes [84]. In both trials, fenofibrate remained safe and well tolerated, but with a small increase in rates of pancreatitis and pulmonary embolism in FIELD [84, 85]. The benefits of fenofibrate may not be solely lipid-mediated but also reflect antioxidant and anti-inflammatory effects [86]. Indeed, triacylglycerols have been linked to nephropathy through mesangial cell uptake of VLDL,

Table 12.3 Safety of statins and fibrates in patients with CKD

Medication	CYP 450 metabolism	Gemfibrozil[a] interaction	Fenofibrate[a] interaction	Dose adjustment		
				GFR 60–90 mL/min	GFR 15–59 mL/min	GFR <15 mL/min
Rosuvastatin	No	Yes	No	No	5–10 mg	5–10 mg
Atorvastatin	Yes	Yes	No	No	No	No
Simvastatin	Yes	Yes	No	No	No	5 mg
Lovastatin	Yes	Yes	Not available	No	Decrease by 50 %	Decrease by 50 %
Pravastatin	No	Yes	No	No	No	No
Fluvastatin	No	No	No	No	Not defined	Not defined
Gemfibrozil	Yes	NA	NA	No	No	No
Fenofibrate	No	NA	NA	Decrease by 50 %	Decrease by 75 %	Avoid

Modified from Harper CR, Jacobson TA. Managing dyslipidemia in chronic kidney disease. J. Am. Coll. Cardiol. [Internet]. 2008 Jun 24 [cited 2013 Oct 25];51(25):2375–84. Available from: http://www.ncbi.nlm.nih.gov/pubmed/18565393

[a]Fibrates may cause a moderate reversible increase in serum creatinine. Gemfibrozil is less likely to cause this increase but is more likely to cause rhabdomyolysis when combined with a statin (Harper et al)

inducing foam cell formation [87] and through VLDL induction of plasminogen activating inhibitor-1 (PAI-1) with up-regulated coagulation and intra-renal microthrombi [88]. HDL does not greatly alter PAI-1 release [89] but has been shown in humans to be renoprotective [90], perhaps through suppression of inflammatory cell adhesion molecules, anti-oxidant effects, and reverse cholesterol transport [91]. Peroxisome-proliferator-alpha receptor agonists such as fenofibrate have positive effects on both HDL and TG and may exert some of their benefits through many of these mechanisms [83, 86].

Evaluation and Assessment

In people with diabetes and CKD, a complete lipid profile (total cholesterol, HDL-C, and triglycerides) should be measured and LDL-C calculated from these values as recommended by the KDOQI 2007 and the ATP III Guidelines [2, 33]. The recent statement by the KDIGO Work Group also recommend an initial assessment of LDL levels but are against the routine measurement of follow-up LDL-levels, since LDL levels tend to be lower in patients with CKD and less significantly correlated with CVD risk [66]. Dyslipidemia associated with diabetes and CKD may occur without an elevated LDL-C level due to increased lipoprotein remnants, hence measuring Non-HDL-C (total cholesterol – HDL-C) is clinically important.

Patients with Type 2 DM or insulin resistance are considered to have predominantly small LDL [92]. A consensus statement endorsed by the American Diabetes Association and the American College of Cardiology advocates for measuring atherogenic particle concentration either as apolipoprotein B (apoB) or LDL particle concentration in subjects at high risk for cardiometabolic disorders for assessing CVD risk and guiding therapy, in conjunction with using LDL and non-HDL cholesterol and suggests the following targets for those at highest risk: LDL cholesterol <70 mg/dL, non-HDL cholesterol <100 mg/dL, apoB <80 mg/dL [93]. A variety of lipoprotein assays are available to subfractionate lipoprotein particles according to size, density, or charge and have been proposed for improving assessment of risk of CVD and for guiding lipid-lowering therapies especially in individuals with low or normal LDL cholesterol [92]. They can detect atherogenic lipoprotein particle concentrations (e.g., apoB or LDL particle concentration) and small dense LDL particles, which are believed to be more atherogenic than larger LDL particles. However, the lack of standardization and the absence of a "gold standard" technique have slowed the adoption of these assays and their utilization. They are currently mostly used in specialized lipid clinics or research studies [92]. Based on current guidelines, LDL-C and non HDL-C remain the primary targets in reducing lipid-based risk in patients with diabetes [33].

Management

Most clinicians consider the decrease in cardiovascular risk as the ultimate goal of lipid lowering therapy. Clinical trials in the general population have shown that LDL-cholesterol lowering in moderate to high-risk patients leads to a reduction in cardiovascular event and is one of the major modifiable risk factors for CVD [94]. Based upon data from the Framingham Heart Study, the risk for myocardial infarction is also estimated to increase by about 25 % for every 5 mg/dL (0.13 mmol/L) decrease in HDL level below median values for men (45 mg/dL) and women (55 mg/dL) and a high HDL (>60 mg/dL or 1.6 mmol/L) is considered to be cardioprotective [95]. The cardiovascular risk of low HDL is more exaggerated in patients with diabetes [96]. Hypertriglyceridemia itself is also associated with an increased risk for CVD [97]. The new ACC/AHA guidelines for the treatment of dyslipidemia highlight the importance of risk factors and suggest a shift from target LDL and non-HDL-cholesterol levels to the

Table 12.4 Target lipid levels in patients with DM and CKD*

		LDL goal	TG goal	Non HDL goal
General population	0–1 risk factors	<160 mg/dL	<150 mg/dL	<190 mg/dL
	2+ risk factors	<130 mg/dL		<160 mg/dL
	CAD or CAD equivalent (10 year risk >20 %)	<100 mg/dL		<130 mg/dL
Diabetes		<100 mg/dL in patients without overt CVD <70 mg/dL in patients with overt CVD	If ≥500 mg/dL start therapeutic lifestyle changes and Fibrates or Niacin	<130 mg/dL
Diabetes and CKD stage 1–4		<100 mg/dL <70 mg/dL (optional)	If ≥500 mg/dL start therapeutic lifestyle changes and Fibrates if needed (use with caution)	<130 mg/dL
Diabetes on maintenance hemodialysis		<100 mg/dL	If ≥500 mg/dL start therapeutic lifestyle changes and fibrates if needed	<130 mg/dL

*Recent ACC/AHA and KDIGO recommendations do not advocate the use of targets of therapy but rather a 'fire and forget' approach

intensity of statin therapy, with higher intensity targeting patients at high risk of CVD [98]. The KDIGO Clinical Practice Guidelines also recommend against the use of LDL-cholesterol levels as a target of therapy in patients with CKD [66]. The intensification of treatment in patients with CKD does raise the risk of statin-related side effects with higher doses and clinicians need to proceed with caution [66]. Since both CKD and DM are considered risk factors for CVD, high-intensity treatment appears justified in patients with both disease entities. While the KDIGO recommendations did advocate for the use of statins in patients with CKD younger than 50 years of age with coexisting diabetes mellitus [66], more research is needed to establish optimal target LDL cholesterol levels, if any, and the effect of lipid lowering therapy in this population. Suggestions from the available evidence regarding therapeutic targets for patients with both CKD and Type 2 DM are summarized in Table 12.4. Treatment with a statin should not be initiated in patients with type 2 diabetes on maintenance HD who do not have a specific cardiovascular indication for treatment [2].

As in the general population, statins are beneficial in patients with CKD [68]. Assessing drug interactions (with macrolide antibiotics, azole antifungal agents, dihydropyridine calcium channel blockers, and cyclosporine A) is important for safety. Acute and chronic liver disease should be excluded before initiation of a statin, but it is not necessary to obtain routine liver enzymes to screen for hepatotoxicity thereafter. Different statins and other anti-hyperlipidemic medications are available on the market and their safe dosage varies for patients with CKD (Table 12.3). The US FDA warned against using high dose Simvastatin (80 mg) due to the risk of myopathy and serious drug interaction (US Food and drug Administration website. http://www.fda.gov/drugs/drugsafety/ucm256581.htm). Other than improving lipid profile, it is important to remember that statins may have additional pleiotropic effects, including improved endothelial function and plaque stabilization [4].

Treating elevated TG becomes a primary goal only in the small number of patients with very-high TG (>500 mg/dL or 5.65 mmol/L) since severe hypertriglyceridemia can be associated with acute pancreatitis [99]. Hypertriglyceridemia is usually treated first with weight reduction, diet, and exercise. Guidelines recommend low-fat diet, medium-chain TG and fish oils for treatment of hypertriglyceridemia [100]. Pharmacotherapy with fibrates and nicotinic acid is added only when the response to lifestyle interventions is not adequate [100]. Secondary causes of hypertriglyceridemia, such as poorly controlled diabetes, excessive alcohol consumption, hypothyroidism, liver disease, nephritic syndrome, immunosuppressive agents (corticosteroids, cyclosporine, and sirolimus), anabolic steroids and other medications (13-*cis*-retinoic acid, anticonvulsants, highly active retroviral therapy, diuretics, beta blockers and oral contraceptives) should be sought. Fibrates should be used cautiously in patients with CKD and they may cause a reversible increase in serum creatinine [68]. The dose of fibrates should be reduced in patients with stage 2–4 CKD, and most should be avoided in stage 5 CKD patients treated with dialysis (Table 12.3). Although gemfibrozil is the NKF fibrate of choice, fenofibrate is the preferred option when combining with a statin [68]. Nevertheless, the risk of side effects from the combination of statins and fibrates has led the KDIGO Work Group to recommend avoiding their combination in patients with CKD [66].

Bile acid sequestrants or ezetimibe (cholesterol absorption inhibitor) could be added to statin therapy if needed. Ezetimibe has fewer gastrointestinal adverse effects than bile acid sequestrants and is safe and well tolerated in moderate to severe CKD without dosing modification for reduced GFR [68]. Its use in monotherapy is not recommended but in combination therapy, it may lead to a lower dose of statin, and hence potentially less side effects from statin use [66]. The bile acid sequestrants, including colesevelam, cholestyramine, and sevelamer which works like a bile acid sequestrant, are generally safe to use in CKD due to their lack of systemic absorption; however, they can increase TG and are hence contraindicated in patients with marked elevated TG [68]. Nicotinic acid can also be used, but the data is limited on the efficacy and safety of nicotinic acid in CKD [68].

Special Considerations

Kidney Transplant Recipients

These patients are especially vulnerable to myopathies because they may be receiving other medications that increase statins toxicity (e.g., Cyclosporine A, Tacrolimus, macrolide antibiotics, azole antifungal agents, fibrates, amiodarone, nefazodone, dihydropyridine calcium blockers). Statin dose should be reduced by 50 % in patients treated with cyclosporine, and additional agents that may increase statin blood levels should be avoided if possible. Much of the high prevalence of dyslipidemias in kidney transplantation recipients is caused by the use of corticosteroids, cyclosporine A, and sirolimus [17].

Angiotensin System Inhibitors and Dyslipidemia

Hypercholesterolemia stimulates the expression of several components of the renin angiotensin system in tissues with pivotal roles in the development of atherosclerosis. It can stimulate circulating angiotensin II as well as angiotensin 2 Type 1 receptor expression [101]. Early studies supported an ability of LDL cholesterol to increase angiotensin 2 Type 1 receptor gene expression in vascular smooth muscle cells [102]. Oxidized LDL can also increase its expression in human coronary artery endothelial cells [103]. These effects may contribute to the beneficial action of 3-hydroxy-3-methylglutaryl-CoA reductase inhibition on atherosclerotic burden. Conversely, the Losartan Intervention for Endpoint reduction in hypertension (LIFE) trial showed that the use of an angiotensin receptor blocker was associated with a reduction in total cholesterol and non-HDL levels. Another angiotensin receptor blocker, Irbesartan, was also found to significantly reduce TG levels and increase HDL levels with the effects being much more pronounced in patients with the metabolic syndrome [104].

Oral Hypoglycemic Agents and Lipids

Improving glycemic control in patients with Type 2 DM generally leads to a reduction in plasma TG levels. Some studies have also demonstrated beneficial effect of certain oral hypoglycemic agents on the lipid profile. A metaanalysis by Monami et al. [105] concluded that DPP-4 (dipeptidyl peptidase 4) inhibitors, sulfonylureas and pioglitazone were all associated with a significant reduction in total cholesterol and that acarbose, pioglitazone as well as DPP-4 inhibitors were associated with a significant reduction in TG. HDL levels were increased by acarbose and pioglitazone and decreased by sulfonylureas [105]. Metformin, which is known to improve insulin resistance, has been shown to decrease cholesterol and TG levels while increasing HDL [106]. It is also thought to prevent plaque progression through a mechanism mediated by AMP-kinase activation which leads to inhibition of HMG CoA reductase activity [107].

Conclusion

The co-management of two complicated diseases, diabetes, and renal insufficiency, is a challenge faced by clinicians tasked with delivering comprehensive evidence-based therapy on a daily basis. Dyslipidemia in individuals with diabetes and CKD is one of the facets of disease management where attention to details, and application of guidelines helps prevent gaps in the delivery of care and improve outcomes.

References

1. Collins AJ, Foley RN, Herzog C, Chavers B, Gilbertson D, Ishani A, et al. US renal data system 2010 annual data report. Am J Kidney Dis. 2011;57(1 Suppl 1):A8, e1–526. http://www.ncbi.nlm.nih.gov/pubmed/21184928. Accessed 31 Oct 2013
2. KDOQI. KDOQI clinical practice guidelines and clinical practice recommendations for diabetes and chronic kidney disease. Am J Kidney Dis. 2007;49(2 Suppl 2):S12–154. http://www.ncbi.nlm.nih.gov/pubmed/17276798. Accessed 12 Oct 2013.
3. Cooper ME, Jandeleit-Dahm K, Thomas MC. Targets to retard the progression of diabetic nephropathy. Kidney Int. 2005;68(4):1439–45. http://www.ncbi.nlm.nih.gov/pubmed/16164619. Accessed 12 Oct 2013.
4. Olyaei A, Steffl JL, Maclaughlan J, Trabolsi M, Quadri SP, Abbasi I, et al. HMG-CoA Reductase Inhibitors in Chronic Kidney Disease. Am J Cardiovasc Drugs. 2013;13(6):385–98. http://www.ncbi.nlm.nih.gov/pubmed/23975627. Accessed 31 Oct 2013.
5. Lewington S, Whitlock G, Clarke R, Sherliker P, Emberson J, Halsey J, et al. Blood cholesterol and vascular mortality by age, sex, and blood pressure: a meta-analysis of individual data from 61 prospective studies with 55,000 vascular deaths. Lancet. 2007;370(9602):1829–39. http://www.ncbi.nlm.nih.gov/pubmed/18061058. Accessed 26 Nov 2013.
6. Vaziri ND, Norris K. Lipid disorders and their relevance to outcomes in chronic kidney disease. Blood Purif. 2011;31(1–3):189–96. http://www.ncbi.nlm.nih.gov/pubmed/21228589. Accessed 23 Jul 2013.
7. Moin DS, Rohatgi A. Clinical applications of advanced lipoprotein testing in diabetes mellitus. Clin Lipidol. 2011;6(4):371–87.
8. Cheung AK, Parker CJ, Ren K, Iverius PH. Increased lipase inhibition in uremia: identification of pre-beta-HDL as a major inhibitor in normal and uremic plasma. Kidney Int. 1996;49(5):1360–71. http://www.ncbi.nlm.nih.gov/pubmed/8731101. Accessed 12 Oct 2013.

9. Ginsberg HN, Le NA, Goldberg IJ, Gibson JC, Rubinstein A, Wang-Iverson P, et al. Apolipoprotein B metabolism in subjects with deficiency of apolipoproteins CIII and AI. Evidence that apolipoprotein CIII inhibits catabolism of triglyceride-rich lipoproteins by lipoprotein lipase in vivo. J Clin Invest. 1986;78(5):1287–95. http://www.pubmedcentral.nih.gov/articlerender.fcgi?artid=423815&tool=pmcentrez&rendertype=abstract. Accessed 16 Nov 2013.
10. Ooi EMM, Chan DT, Watts GF, Chan DC, Ng TWK, Dogra GK, et al. Plasma apolipoprotein C-III metabolism in patients with chronic kidney disease. J Lipid Res. 2011;52(4):794–800. http://www.pubmedcentral.nih.gov/articlerender.fcgi?artid=3284168&tool=pmcentrez&rendertype=abstract. Accessed 16 Nov 2013.
11. Vaziri ND, Yuan J, Ni Z, Nicholas SB, Norris KC. Lipoprotein lipase deficiency in chronic kidney disease is accompanied by down-regulation of endothelial GPIHBP1 expression. Clin Exp Nephrol. 2012;16(2):238–43. http://www.pubmedcentral.nih.gov/articlerender.fcgi?artid=3417131&tool=pmcentrez&rendertype=abstract. Accessed 12 Oct 2013.
12. Akmal M, Kasim SE, Soliman AR, Massry SG. Excess parathyroid hormone adversely affects lipid metabolism in chronic renal failure. Kidney Int. 1990;37(3):854–8. http://www.ncbi.nlm.nih.gov/pubmed/2313975. Accessed 16 Nov 2013.
13. Vaziri ND, Wang XQ, Liang K. Secondary hyperparathyroidism downregulates lipoprotein lipase expression in chronic renal failure. Am J Physiol. 1997;273(6 Pt 2):F925–30. http://www.ncbi.nlm.nih.gov/pubmed/9435681. Accessed 16 Nov 2013.
14. Hagström E, Lundgren E, Rastad J, Hellman P. Metabolic abnormalities in patients with normocalcemic hyperparathyroidism detected at a population-based screening. Eur J Endocrinol. 2006;155(1):33–9. http://www.ncbi.nlm.nih.gov/pubmed/16793947. Accessed 16 Nov 2013.
15. Attman PO, Knight-Gibson C, Tavella M, Samuelsson O, Alaupovic P. The compositional abnormalities of lipoproteins in diabetic renal failure. Nephrol Dial Transplant. 1998;13(11):2833–41. http://www.ncbi.nlm.nih.gov/pubmed/9829487. Accessed 1 Nov 2013.
16. Yamamoto S, Yancey PG, Ikizler TA, Jerome WG, Kaseda R, Cox B, et al. Dysfunctional high-density lipoprotein in patients on chronic hemodialysis. J Am Coll Cardiol. 2012;60(23):2372–9. http://www.ncbi.nlm.nih.gov/pubmed/23141484. Accessed 12 Oct 2013.
17. Farbakhsh K, Kasiske BL. Dyslipidemias in patients who have chronic kidney disease. Med Clin North Am. 2005;89:689–99.
18. Tsimihodimos V, Dounousi E, Siamopoulos KC. Dyslipidemia in chronic kidney disease: an approach to pathogenesis and treatment. Am J Nephrol. 2008;28(6):958–73. http://www.ncbi.nlm.nih.gov/pubmed/18612199. Accessed 16 Nov 2013.
19. Rajman I, Harper L, McPake D, Kendall MJ, Wheeler DC. Low-density lipoprotein subfraction profiles in chronic renal failure. Nephrol Dial Transplant. 1998;13(9):2281–7. http://www.ncbi.nlm.nih.gov/pubmed/9761510. Accessed 16 Nov 2013.
20. Chu M, Wang AYM, Chan IHS, Chui SH, Lam CWK. Serum small-dense LDL abnormalities in chronic renal disease patients. Br J Biomed Sci. 2012;69(3):99–102. http://www.ncbi.nlm.nih.gov/pubmed/23057155. Accessed 16 Nov 2013.
21. Klin M, Smogorzewski M, Ni Z, Zhang G, Massry SG. Abnormalities in hepatic lipase in chronic renal failure: role of excess parathyroid hormone. J Clin Invest. 1996;97(10):2167–73. http://www.pubmedcentral.nih.gov/articlerender.fcgi?artid=507295&tool=pmcentrez&rendertype=abstract. Accessed 1 Nov 2013.
22. Bairaktari E, Elisaf M, Tsolas O, Siamopoulos KC. Serum Lp(a) levels in patients with moderate renal failure. Nephron 1998;79(3):367–8. http://www.ncbi.nlm.nih.gov/pubmed/9678450. Accessed 1 Nov 2013.
23. Haffner SM, Gruber KK, Aldrete G, Morales PA, Stern MP, Tuttle KR. Increased lipoprotein(a) concentrations in chronic renal failure. J Am Soc Nephrol. 1992;3(5):1156–62. http://www.ncbi.nlm.nih.gov/pubmed/1482754. Accessed 1 Nov 2013.
24. Mattock M, Cronin N, Cavallo-Perin P, Idzior-Walus B, Penno G, Bandinelli S, et al. Plasma lipids and urinary albumin excretion rate in type 1 diabetes mellitus: The EURODIAB IDDM Complications Study. Diabet Med. 2001;18:59–67. http://discovery.ucl.ac.uk/26964/
25. Joven J, Villabona C, Vilella E, Masana L, Albertí R, Vallés M. Abnormalities of lipoprotein metabolism in patients with the nephrotic syndrome. N Engl J Med. 1990;323(9):579–84. http://www.ncbi.nlm.nih.gov/pubmed/2381443. Accessed 12 Oct 2013.
26. Han S, Vaziri ND, Gollapudi P, Kwok V, Moradi H. Hepatic fatty acid and cholesterol metabolism in nephrotic syndrome. Am J Transl Res. 2013;5:246–53. http://www.ncbi.nlm.nih.gov/pubmed/23573368
27. Johansson AC, Samuelsson O, Attman PO, Haraldsson B, Moberly J, Knight-Gibson C, et al. Dyslipidemia in peritoneal dialysis—relation to dialytic variables. Perit Dial Int. 2000;20(3):306–14. http://www.ncbi.nlm.nih.gov/pubmed/10898048. Accessed 12 Oct 2013.
28. Kagan A, Bar-Khayim Y, Schafer Z, Fainaru M. Kinetics of peritoneal protein loss during CAPD: II. Lipoprotein leakage and its impact on plasma lipid levels. Kidney Int. 1990;37(3):980–90. http://www.ncbi.nlm.nih.gov/pubmed/2313985. Accessed 12 Oct 2013.
29. Alvestrand A. Carbohydrate and insulin metabolism in renal failure. Kidney Int Suppl. 1997;62:S48–52. http://www.ncbi.nlm.nih.gov/pubmed/9350680. Accessed 12 Oct 2013.
30. Mak RH, DeFronzo RA. Glucose and insulin metabolism in uremia. Nephron 1992;61(4):377–82. http://www.ncbi.nlm.nih.gov/pubmed/1501732. Accessed 12 Oct 2013.
31. Mak RH. Insulin secretion in uremia: effect of parathyroid hormone and vitamin D metabolites. Kidney Int Suppl. 1989;27:S227–30. http://www.ncbi.nlm.nih.gov/pubmed/2699996. Accessed 12 Oct 2013.
32. Ginsberg HN, Zhang Y-L, Hernandez-Ono A. Metabolic syndrome: focus on dyslipidemia. Obesity (Silver Spring). 2006;14 Suppl 1:41S–49S. http://www.ncbi.nlm.nih.gov/pubmed/16642962. Accessed 12 Oct 2013.
33. Third Report of the National Cholesterol Education Program (NCEP) Expert Panel on Detection, Evaluation, and Treatment of High Blood Cholesterol in Adults (Adult Treatment Panel III) final report. Circulation 2002;106(25):3143–421. http://www.ncbi.nlm.nih.gov/pubmed/12485966. Accessed 19 Sep 2013.
34. Panzram G. Mortality and survival in type 2 (non-insulin-dependent) diabetes mellitus. Diabetologia 1987;30(3):123–31. http://www.ncbi.nlm.nih.gov/pubmed/3556287. Accessed 16 Sep 2013.
35. Tonelli M, Muntner P, Lloyd A, Manns BJ, Klarenbach S, Pannu N, et al. Risk of coronary events in people with chronic kidney disease compared with those with diabetes: a population-level cohort study. Lancet 2012;380(9844):807–14. http://www.ncbi.nlm.nih.gov/pubmed/22717317. Accessed 10 Oct 2013.
36. Culleton BF, Larson MG, Wilson PW, Evans JC, Parfrey PS, Levy D. Cardiovascular disease and mortality in a community-based cohort with mild renal insufficiency. Kidney Int. 1999;56(6):2214–9. http://www.ncbi.nlm.nih.gov/pubmed/10594797. Accessed 13 Oct 2013.
37. Garg AX, Clark WF, Haynes RB, House AA. Moderate renal insufficiency and the risk of cardiovascular mortality: results from the NHANES I. Kidney Int. 2002;61(4):1486–94. http://www.ncbi.nlm.nih.gov/pubmed/11918756. Accessed 13 Oct 2013.
38. Sarnak MJ, Levey AS, Schoolwerth AC, Coresh J, Culleton B, Hamm LL, et al. Kidney disease as a risk factor for development

of cardiovascular disease: a statement from the American Heart Association Councils on Kidney in Cardiovascular Disease, High Blood Pressure Research, Clinical Cardiology, and Epidemiology and Prevention. Circulation. 2003;108(17):2154–69. http://www.ncbi.nlm.nih.gov/pubmed/14581387. Accessed 25 Sep 2013.

39. Muntner P, He J, Hamm L, Loria C, Whelton PK. Renal insufficiency and subsequent death resulting from cardiovascular disease in the United States. J Am Soc Nephrol. 2002;13(3):745–53. http://www.ncbi.nlm.nih.gov/pubmed/11856780. Accessed 13 Oct 2013.
40. Hallan S, Astor B, Romundstad S, Aasarød K, Kvenild K, Coresh J. Association of kidney function and albuminuria with cardiovascular mortality in older vs younger individuals: The HUNT II Study. Arch Intern Med. 2007;167(22):2490–6. http://www.ncbi.nlm.nih.gov/pubmed/18071172. Accessed 13 Oct 2013.
41. Matsushita K, van der Velde M, Astor BC, Woodward M, Levey AS, de Jong PE, et al. Association of estimated glomerular filtration rate and albuminuria with all-cause and cardiovascular mortality in general population cohorts: a collaborative meta-analysis. Lancet 2010;375(9731):2073–81. http://www.ncbi.nlm.nih.gov/pubmed/20483451. Accessed 1 Oct 2013.
42. Mann JFE, Gerstein HC, Dulau-Florea I, Lonn E. Cardiovascular risk in patients with mild renal insufficiency. Kidney Int Suppl. 2003;(84):S192–6. http://www.ncbi.nlm.nih.gov/pubmed/12694342. Accessed 13 Oct 2013.
43. Rashidi A, Sehgal AR, Rahman M, O'Connor AS. The case for chronic kidney disease, diabetes mellitus, and myocardial infarction being equivalent risk factors for cardiovascular mortality in patients older than 65 years. Am J Cardiol. 2008;102(12):1668–73. http://www.ncbi.nlm.nih.gov/pubmed/19064021. Accessed 13 Oct 2013.
44. Fried LP, Kronmal RA, Newman AB, Bild DE, Mittelmark MB, Polak JF, et al. Risk factors for 5-year mortality in older adults: the Cardiovascular Health Study. JAMA. 1998;279(8):585–92. http://www.ncbi.nlm.nih.gov/pubmed/9486752. Accessed 13 Oct 2013.
45. Shepherd J, Kastelein JJP, Bittner V, Deedwania P, Breazna A, Dobson S, et al. Intensive lipid lowering with atorvastatin in patients with coronary heart disease and chronic kidney disease: the TNT (Treating to New Targets) study. J Am Coll Cardiol. 2008;51:1448–54. http://www.ncbi.nlm.nih.gov/pubmed/18402899
46. Clase CM, Gao P, Tobe SW, McQueen MJ, Grosshennig A, Teo KK, et al. Estimated glomerular filtration rate and albuminuria as predictors of outcomes in patients with high cardiovascular risk: a cohort study. Ann Intern Med. 2011;154(5):310–8. http://www.ncbi.nlm.nih.gov/pubmed/21357908. Accessed 13 Oct 2013.
47. National Kidney Foundation. K/DOQI clinical practice guidelines for chronic kidney disease: evaluation, classification, and stratification. Am J Kidney Dis. 2002;39(2 Suppl 1):S1–266. http://www.ncbi.nlm.nih.gov/pubmed/11904577. Accessed 21 Sep 2013.
48. Antman EM, Anbe DT, Armstrong PW, Bates ER, Green LA, Hand M, et al. ACC/AHA guidelines for the management of patients with ST-elevation myocardial infarction—executive summary: a report of the American College of Cardiology/American Heart Association Task Force on Practice Guidelines (Writing Committee to Revise the 1999 Guidelines for the Management of Patients With Acute Myocardial Infarction). Circulation. 2004;110(5):588–636. http://www.ncbi.nlm.nih.gov/pubmed/15289388. Accessed 20 Sep 2013.
49. Mann JF, Gerstein HC, Pogue J, Bosch J, Yusuf S. Renal insufficiency as a predictor of cardiovascular outcomes and the impact of ramipril: the HOPE randomized trial. Ann Intern Med. 2001;134(8):629–36. http://www.ncbi.nlm.nih.gov/pubmed/11304102. Accessed 16 Oct 2013.
50. Anavekar NS, McMurray JJ, Velazquez EJ, Solomon SD, Kober L, Rouleau J-L, et al. Relation between renal dysfunction and cardiovascular outcomes after myocardial infarction. N Engl J Med. 2004;351(13):1285–95. http://www.ncbi.nlm.nih.gov/pubmed/15385655. Accessed 16 Oct 2013.
51. Chang Y-T, Wu J-L, Hsu C-C, Wang J-D, Sung J-M. Diabetes and end-stage renal disease synergistically contribute to increased incidence of cardiovascular events: a nation-wide follow-up study during 1998-2009. Diabetes Care 2014;37(1):277–85. http://www.ncbi.nlm.nih.gov/pubmed/23920086. Accessed 22 Oct 2013.
52. Baigent C, Keech A, Kearney PM, Blackwell L, Buck G, Pollicino C, et al. Efficacy and safety of cholesterol-lowering treatment: prospective meta-analysis of data from 90,056 participants in 14 randomised trials of statins. Lancet 2005;366(9493):1267–78. http://www.ncbi.nlm.nih.gov/pubmed/16214597. Accessed 27 Sep 2013.
53. Thavendiranathan P, Bagai A, Brookhart MA, Choudhry NK. Primary prevention of cardiovascular diseases with statin therapy: a meta-analysis of randomized controlled trials. Arch Intern Med. 2006;166(21):2307–13. http://www.ncbi.nlm.nih.gov/pubmed/17130382. Accessed 2 Oct 2013.
54. Sever PS, Dahlöf B, Poulter NR, Wedel H, Beevers G, Caulfield M, et al. Prevention of coronary and stroke events with atorvastatin in hypertensive patients who have average or lower-than-average cholesterol concentrations, in the Anglo-Scandinavian Cardiac Outcomes Trial—Lipid Lowering Arm (ASCOT-LLA): a multicentre randomised controlled trial. Lancet. 2003;361(9364):1149–58. http://www.ncbi.nlm.nih.gov/pubmed/12686036. Accessed 2 Oct 2013.
55. Colhoun HM, Betteridge DJ, Durrington PN, Hitman GA, Neil HAW, Livingstone SJ, et al. Effects of atorvastatin on kidney outcomes and cardiovascular disease in patients with diabetes: an analysis from the Collaborative Atorvastatin Diabetes Study (CARDS). Am J Kidney Dis. 2009;54(5):810–9. http://www.ncbi.nlm.nih.gov/pubmed/19540640. Accessed 19 Oct 2013.
56. Collins R, Armitage J, Parish S, Sleigh P, Peto R. MRC/BHF Heart Protection Study of cholesterol-lowering with simvastatin in 5963 people with diabetes: a randomised placebo-controlled trial. Lancet 2003;361(9374):2005–16. http://www.ncbi.nlm.nih.gov/pubmed/12814710. Accessed 19 Oct 2013.
57. Athyros VG, Mikhailidis DP, Papageorgiou AA, Symeonidis AN, Pehlivanidis AN, Bouloukos VI, et al. The effect of statins versus untreated dyslipidaemia on renal function in patients with coronary heart disease. A subgroup analysis of the Greek atorvastatin and coronary heart disease evaluation (GREACE) study. J Clin Pathol. 2004;57(7):728–34. http://www.pubmedcentral.nih.gov/articlerender.fcgi?artid=1770346&tool=pmcentrez&rendertype=abstract. Accessed 19 Oct 2013.
58. Tonelli M, Isles C, Craven T, Tonkin A, Pfeffer MA, Shepherd J, et al. Effect of pravastatin on rate of kidney function loss in people with or at risk for coronary disease. Circulation 2005;112(2):171–8. http://www.ncbi.nlm.nih.gov/pubmed/15998677. Accessed 19 Oct 2013.
59. Shepherd J, Kastelein JP, Bittner VA, Carmena R, Deedwania PC, Breazna A, et al. Intensive lipid lowering with atorvastatin in patients with coronary artery disease, diabetes, and chronic kidney disease. Mayo Clin Proc. 2008;83(8):870–9. http://www.ncbi.nlm.nih.gov/pubmed/18674471. Accessed 19 Oct 2013.
60. Shepherd J, Kastelein JJP, Bittner V, Deedwania P, Breazna A, Dobson S, et al. Effect of intensive lipid lowering with atorvastatin on renal function in patients with coronary heart disease: the Treating to New Targets (TNT) study. Clin J Am Soc Nephrol. 2007;2(6):1131–9. http://www.ncbi.nlm.nih.gov/pubmed/17942759. Accessed 19 Oct 2013.
61. Sukhija R, Bursac Z, Kakar P, Fink L, Fort C, Satwani S, et al. Effect of statins on the development of renal dysfunction. Am J Cardiol. 2008;101(7):975–9. http://www.ncbi.nlm.nih.gov/pubmed/18359317. Accessed 19 Oct 2013.

62. Rahman M, Baimbridge C, Davis BR, Barzilay J, Basile JN, Henriquez MA, et al. Progression of kidney disease in moderately hypercholesterolemic, hypertensive patients randomized to pravastatin versus usual care: a report from the Antihypertensive and Lipid-Lowering Treatment to Prevent Heart Attack Trial (ALLHAT). Am J Kidney Dis. 2008;52(3):412–24. http://www.pubmedcentral.nih.gov/articlerender.fcgi?artid=2897819&tool=pmcentrez&rendertype=abstract. Accessed 19 Oct 2013.
63. Strippoli GFM, Navaneethan SD, Johnson DW, Perkovic V, Pellegrini F, Nicolucci A, et al. Effects of statins in patients with chronic kidney disease: meta-analysis and meta-regression of randomised controlled trials. BMJ. 2008;336(7645):645–51. http://www.pubmedcentral.nih.gov/articlerender.fcgi?artid=2270960&tool=pmcentrez&rendertype=abstract. Accessed 19 Oct 2013.
64. Tonelli M, Keech A, Shepherd J, Sacks F, Tonkin A, Packard C, et al. Effect of pravastatin in people with diabetes and chronic kidney disease. J Am Soc Nephrol. 2005;16(12):3748–54. http://www.ncbi.nlm.nih.gov/pubmed/16251235. Accessed 19 Oct 2013.
65. Chonchol M, Cook T, Kjekshus J, Pedersen TR, Lindenfeld J. Simvastatin for secondary prevention of all-cause mortality and major coronary events in patients with mild chronic renal insufficiency. Am J Kidney Dis. 2007;49(3):373–82. http://www.ncbi.nlm.nih.gov/pubmed/17336698. Accessed 19 Oct 2013.
66. KDIGO clinical practice guideline for lipid management in chronic kidney disease. Kidney Int Suppl. 2013;3(3):271–9. http://dx.doi.org/10.1038/kisup.2013.34. Accessed 1 Dec 2013.
67. Slinin Y, Ishani A, Rector T, Fitzgerald P, MacDonald R, Tacklind J, et al. Management of hyperglycemia, dyslipidemia, and albuminuria in patients with diabetes and CKD: a systematic review for a KDOQI clinical practice guideline. Am J Kidney Dis. 2012;60(5):747–69. http://www.ncbi.nlm.nih.gov/pubmed/22999165. Accessed 28 May 2013.
68. Harper CR, Jacobson TA. Managing dyslipidemia in chronic kidney disease. J Am Coll Cardiol. 2008;51(25):2375–84. http://www.ncbi.nlm.nih.gov/pubmed/18565393. Accessed 25 Oct 2013.
69. Karnik JA, Young BS, Lew NL, Herget M, Dubinsky C, Lazarus JM, et al. Cardiac arrest and sudden death in dialysis units. Kidney Int. 2001;60(1):350–7. http://www.ncbi.nlm.nih.gov/pubmed/11422771. Accessed 25 Oct 2013.
70. Herzog CA. How to manage the renal patient with coronary heart disease: the agony and the ecstasy of opinion-based medicine. J Am Soc Nephrol. 2003;14(10):2556–72. http://www.ncbi.nlm.nih.gov/pubmed/14514733. Accessed 25 Oct 2013.
71. Sarnak MJ. Cardiovascular complications in chronic kidney disease. Am J Kidney Dis. 2003;41(5 Suppl):11–7. http://www.ncbi.nlm.nih.gov/pubmed/12776309. Accessed 26 Oct 2013.
72. Baigent C, Burbury K, Wheeler D. Premature cardiovascular disease in chronic renal failure. Lancet 2000;356(9224):147–52. http://www.ncbi.nlm.nih.gov/pubmed/10963260. Accessed 26 Oct 2013.
73. Wanner C, Krane V, März W, Olschewski M, Mann JFE, Ruf G, et al. Atorvastatin in patients with type 2 diabetes mellitus undergoing hemodialysis. N Engl J Med. 2005;353(3):238–48. http://www.ncbi.nlm.nih.gov/pubmed/16034009
74. Seliger SL, Weiss NS, Gillen DL, Kestenbaum B, Ball A, Sherrard DJ, et al. HMG-CoA reductase inhibitors are associated with reduced mortality in ESRD patients. Kidney Int. 2002;61(1):297–304. http://www.ncbi.nlm.nih.gov/pubmed/11786112. Accessed 26 Oct 2013.
75. Mason NA, Bailie GR, Satayathum S, Bragg-Gresham JL, Akiba T, Akizawa T, et al. HMG-coenzyme a reductase inhibitor use is associated with mortality reduction in hemodialysis patients. Am J Kidney Dis. 2005;45(1):119–26. http://www.ncbi.nlm.nih.gov/pubmed/15696451. Accessed 26 Oct 2013.
76. Fellström B, Holdaas H, Jardine AG, Rose H, Schmieder R, Wilpshaar W, et al. Effect of rosuvastatin on outcomes in chronic haemodialysis patients: baseline data from the AURORA study. Kidney Blood Press Res. 2007;30(5):314–22. http://www.pubmedcentral.nih.gov/articlerender.fcgi?artid=2790755&tool=pmcentrez&rendertype=abstract. Accessed 26 Oct 2013.
77. Baigent C, Landray MJ, Reith C, Emberson J, Wheeler DC, Tomson C, et al. The effects of lowering LDL cholesterol with simvastatin plus ezetimibe in patients with chronic kidney disease (Study of Heart and Renal Protection): a randomised placebo-controlled trial. Lancet 2011;377(9784):2181–92. http://www.pubmedcentral.nih.gov/articlerender.fcgi?artid=3145073&tool=pmcentrez&rendertype=abstract. Accessed 26 Oct 2013.
78. Holdaas H, Holme I, Schmieder RE, Jardine AG, Zannad F, Norby GE, et al. Rosuvastatin in diabetic hemodialysis patients. J Am Soc Nephrol. 2011;22(7):1335–41. http://www.pubmedcentral.nih.gov/articlerender.fcgi?artid=3137581&tool=pmcentrez&rendertype=abstract. Accessed 26 Oct 2013.
79. Svensson M, Schmidt EB, Jørgensen KA, Christensen JH. N-3 fatty acids as secondary prevention against cardiovascular events in patients who undergo chronic hemodialysis: a randomized, placebo-controlled intervention trial. Clin J Am Soc Nephrol. 2006;1(4):780–6. http://www.ncbi.nlm.nih.gov/pubmed/17699287. Accessed 26 Oct 2013.
80. Jardine A. Assessing cardiovascular risk profile of immunosuppressive agents. Transplantation 2001;72(12 Suppl):S81–8. http://www.ncbi.nlm.nih.gov/pubmed/11833146. Accessed 29 Oct 2013.
81. Jardine A, Holdaas H. Fluvastatin in combination with cyclosporin in renal transplant recipients: a review of clinical and safety experience. J Clin Pharm Ther. 1999;24(6):397–408. http://www.ncbi.nlm.nih.gov/pubmed/10651972. Accessed 29 Oct 2013.
82. Jardine AG, Holdaas H, Fellström B, Cole E, Nyberg G, Grönhagen-Riska C, et al. Fluvastatin prevents cardiac death and myocardial infarction in renal transplant recipients: post-hoc subgroup analyses of the ALERT Study. Am J Transplant. 2004;4(6):988–95. http://www.ncbi.nlm.nih.gov/pubmed/15147434. Accessed 29 Oct 2013.
83. Davis TME, Ting R, Best JD, Donoghoe MW, Drury PL, Sullivan DR, et al. Effects of fenofibrate on renal function in patients with type 2 diabetes mellitus: the Fenofibrate Intervention and Event Lowering in Diabetes (FIELD) Study. Diabetologia 2011;54(2):280–90. http://www.ncbi.nlm.nih.gov/pubmed/21052978. Accessed 29 Oct 2013.
84. Ginsberg HN, Elam MB, Lovato LC, Crouse JR, Leiter LA, Linz P, et al. Effects of combination lipid therapy in type 2 diabetes mellitus. N Engl J Med. 2010;362(17):1563–74. http://www.pubmedcentral.nih.gov/articlerender.fcgi?artid=2879499&tool=pmcentrez&rendertype=abstract. Accessed 17 Oct 2013.
85. Keech A, Simes RJ, Barter P, Best J, Scott R, Taskinen MR, et al. Effects of long-term fenofibrate therapy on cardiovascular events in 9795 people with type 2 diabetes mellitus (the FIELD study): randomised controlled trial. Lancet 2005;366(9500):1849–61. http://www.ncbi.nlm.nih.gov/pubmed/16310551. Accessed 24 Oct 2013.
86. Han SH, Quon MJ, Koh KK. Beneficial vascular and metabolic effects of peroxisome proliferator-activated receptor-alpha activators. Hypertension 2005;46(5):1086–92. http://www.ncbi.nlm.nih.gov/pubmed/16230515. Accessed 29 Oct 2013.
87. Anami Y, Kobori S, Sakai M, Kasho M, Nishikawa T, Yano T, et al. Human beta-migrating very low density lipoprotein induces foam cell formation in human mesangial cells. Atherosclerosis. 1997;135(2):225–34. http://www.ncbi.nlm.nih.gov/pubmed/9430372. Accessed 29 Oct 2013.
88. Olufadi R, Byrne CD. Effects of VLDL and remnant particles on platelets. Pathophysiol Haemost Thromb. 2006;35(3-4):281–91. http://www.ncbi.nlm.nih.gov/pubmed/16877877. Accessed 29 Oct 2013.

89. Shen GX. Impact and mechanism for oxidized and glycated lipoproteins on generation of fibrinolytic regulators from vascular endothelial cells. Mol Cell Biochem. 2003;246(1–2):69–74. http://www.ncbi.nlm.nih.gov/pubmed/12841345. Accessed 29 Oct 2013.
90. Muntner P, Coresh J, Smith JC, Eckfeldt J, Klag MJ. Plasma lipids and risk of developing renal dysfunction: the atherosclerosis risk in communities study. Kidney Int. 2000;58(1):293–301. http://www.ncbi.nlm.nih.gov/pubmed/10886574. Accessed 29 Oct 2013.
91. Lopes-Virella MF, Carter RE, Gilbert GE, Klein RL, Jaffa M, Jenkins AJ, et al. Risk factors related to inflammation and endothelial dysfunction in the DCCT/EDIC cohort and their relationship with nephropathy and macrovascular complications. Diabetes Care 2008;31(10):2006–12. http://www.pubmedcentral.nih.gov/articlerender.fcgi?artid=2551645&tool=pmcentrez&rendertype=abstract. Accessed 18 Oct 2013.
92. Mora S. Advanced lipoprotein testing and subfractionation are not (yet) ready for routine clinical use. Circulation 2009;119(17):2396–404. http://www.pubmedcentral.nih.gov/articlerender.fcgi?artid=2735461&tool=pmcentrez&rendertype=abstract. Accessed 29 Oct 2013.
93. Brunzell JD, Davidson M, Furberg CD, Goldberg RB, Howard B V, Stein JH, et al. Lipoprotein management in patients with cardiometabolic risk: consensus conference report from the American Diabetes Association and the American College of Cardiology Foundation. J Am Coll Cardiol. 2008;51(15):1512–24. http://www.ncbi.nlm.nih.gov/pubmed/18402913. Accessed 27 May 2013.
94. Stamler J, Wentworth D, Neaton JD. Is relationship between serum cholesterol and risk of premature death from coronary heart disease continuous and graded? Findings in 356,222 primary screenees of the Multiple Risk Factor Intervention Trial (MRFIT). JAMA. 1986;256(20):2823–8. http://www.ncbi.nlm.nih.gov/pubmed/3773199. Accessed 29 Oct 2013.
95. Castelli WP. Cardiovascular disease and multifactorial risk: challenge of the 1980s. Am Heart J. 1983;106(5 Pt 2):1191–200. http://www.ncbi.nlm.nih.gov/pubmed/6637784. Accessed 29 Oct 2013.
96. Laakso M, Lehto S, Penttilä I, Pyörälä K. Lipids and lipoproteins predicting coronary heart disease mortality and morbidity in patients with non-insulin-dependent diabetes. Circulation 1993;88(4 Pt 1):1421–30. http://www.ncbi.nlm.nih.gov/pubmed/8403288. Accessed 29 Oct 2013.
97. Manninen V, Tenkanen L, Koskinen P, Huttunen JK, Mänttäri M, Heinonen OP, et al. Joint effects of serum triglyceride and LDL cholesterol and HDL cholesterol concentrations on coronary heart disease risk in the Helsinki Heart Study. Implications for treatment. Circulation 1992;85(1):37–45. http://www.ncbi.nlm.nih.gov/pubmed/1728471. Accessed 29 Oct 2013.
98. Stone NJ, Robinson J, Lichtenstein AH, Merz CNB, Blum CB, Eckel RH, et al. 2013 ACC/AHA guideline on the treatment of blood cholesterol to reduce atherosclerotic cardiovascular risk in adults: a report of the American College of Cardiology/American Heart Association Task Force on Practice Guidelines. Circulation 2013. http://www.ncbi.nlm.nih.gov/pubmed/24222016. Accessed 13 Nov 2013.
99. Farbakhsh K, Kasiske BL. Dyslipidemias in patients who have chronic kidney disease. Med Clin North Am. 2005;89(3):689–99. http://www.ncbi.nlm.nih.gov/pubmed/15755473. Accessed 29 Oct 2013.
100. National Kidney Foundation. K/DOQI clinical practice guidelines for managing dyslipidemias in chronic kidney disease. Am J Kidney Dis. 2003;41(4):S1–77.
101. Putnam K, Shoemaker R, Yiannikouris F, Cassis LA. The renin-angiotensin system: a target of and contributor to dyslipidemias, altered glucose homeostasis, and hypertension of the metabolic syndrome. Am J Physiol Heart Circ Physiol. 2012;302(6):H1219–30. http://www.pubmedcentral.nih.gov/articlerender.fcgi?artid=3311482&tool=pmcentrez&rendertype=abstract. Accessed 31 Oct 2013.
102. Nickenig G, Sachinidis A, Michaelsen F, Böhm M, Seewald S, Vetter H. Upregulation of vascular angiotensin II receptor gene expression by low-density lipoprotein in vascular smooth muscle cells. Circulation 1997;95(2):473–8. http://www.ncbi.nlm.nih.gov/pubmed/9008466. Accessed 31 Oct 2013.
103. Li D, Saldeen T, Romeo F, Mehta JL. Oxidized LDL upregulates angiotensin II type 1 receptor expression in cultured human coronary artery endothelial cells: the potential role of transcription factor NF-kappaB. Circulation 2000;102(16):1970–6. http://www.ncbi.nlm.nih.gov/pubmed/11034947. Accessed 31 Oct 2013.
104. Kintscher U, Bramlage P, Paar WD, Thoenes M, Unger T. Irbesartan for the treatment of hypertension in patients with the metabolic syndrome: a sub analysis of the Treat to Target post authorization survey. Prospective observational, two armed study in 14,200 patients. Cardiovasc Diabetol. 2007;6:12. http://www.pubmedcentral.nih.gov/articlerender.fcgi?artid=1853076&tool=pmcentrez&rendertype=abstract. Accessed 31 Oct 2013.
105. Monami M, Vitale V, Ambrosio ML, Bartoli N, Toffanello G, Ragghianti B, et al. Effects on lipid profile of dipeptidyl peptidase 4 inhibitors, pioglitazone, acarbose, and sulfonylureas: meta-analysis of placebo-controlled trials. Adv Ther. 2012;29(9):736–46. http://www.ncbi.nlm.nih.gov/pubmed/22923161. Accessed 31 Oct 2013.
106. Giugliano D, De Rosa N, Di Maro G, Marfella R, Acampora R, Buoninconti R, et al. Metformin improves glucose, lipid metabolism, and reduces blood pressure in hypertensive, obese women. Diabetes Care 1993;16(10):1387–90. http://www.ncbi.nlm.nih.gov/pubmed/8269798. Accessed 31 Oct 2013.
107. Fitch K, Abbara S, Lee H, Stavrou E, Sacks R, Michel T, et al. Effects of lifestyle modification and metformin on atherosclerotic indices among HIV-infected patients with the metabolic syndrome. AIDS. 2012;26(5):587–97. http://www.pubmedcentral.nih.gov/articlerender.fcgi?artid=3675446&tool=pmcentrez&rendertype=abstract. Accessed 12 Oct 2013.

Diabetic Eye Disease

13

Azin Abazari, Nicola G. Ghazi, and Zeynel A. Karcioglu

Diabetes mellitus is a pandemic that has been associated with a significant increase in incidence among all ages, genders, ethnic groups, and regions over the last decade. It is estimated that 366 million will have diabetes worldwide in 2030 [1]. Over 30 % of diabetics have some form of diabetic retinopathy (DR).

Diabetic retinopathy (DR) is the leading cause of preventable blindness among individuals of working age (20–65 years), and a major cause of vision loss in the elderly population. Visual loss occurs secondary to complications of DR such as vitreous hemorrhage, retinal detachment, diabetic macular edema (DME), or macular ischemia.

In 2010, 285 million people had diabetes worldwide. Over one-third of diabetics had signs of DR, and a third of them had vision threatening retinopathy, defined as severe non-proliferative DR (NPDR), proliferative diabetic retinopathy (PDR), or DME [2]. The likelihood of developing retinopathy is strongly related to the duration of diabetes in patients with both type 1 and type 2 diabetes. In the Wisconsin Epidemiologic Study of Diabetic Retinopathy (WESDR), the overall 10-year incidence of retinopathy was 74 %, and among those with retinopathy at baseline, 64 % developed more severe retinopathy and 17 % progressed to develop PDR. After 25 years, the incidence of retinopathy in patients with type 1 diabetes was 97 %. Among those with retinopathy at baseline, 42 % progressed to develop PDR [3], and 17 % developed clinically significant macular edema (CSME) [4]. Although the main purpose of this chapter is to summarize the clinical state of the art in diabetic eye disease, a brief discussion on the relationship of diabetic retinopathy to diabetic nephropathy as well as the pathogenesis of diabetic retinopathy is in order.

Epidemiological evidence exists regarding the correlation of morphologic parameters of diabetic retinopathy and nephropathy, especially early in the disease. The severity of diabetic retinopathy has been proven to correlate with morphologic measures of kidney biopsies, such as glomerular mesangial fractional volume and glomerular basement membrane width in patients with type 1 diabetes [5, 6]. Glomerular and retinal pathology also correlates with the clinical features of patients with type 2 diabetes mellitus and hypertension [7].

The exact mechanism of vascular "degeneration" in the diabetic retina is not known, but the following are blamed for the process: (1) self-destructive biochemical abnormalities within the endothelial cells and pericytes secondarily leading to basement membrane abnormalities, (2) occlusion of the vascular lumen by these dead cells and leukocytes and/or platelets, and (3) additional capillary endothelial cell apoptosis secondary to products generated by other neuroretinal cells (such as ganglion cells or glia) [8].

In addition to the vasculopathy or, according to some, as a result of it, certain inflammatory changes take place in the neuroretina of diabetic animals and patients, and also in cultured retinal cells exposed to elevated concentrations of glucose [9]. The concept that localized neuroretinal inflammatory processes play a role in the development of diabetic retinopathy is relatively new, but the evidence that supports this hypothesis is accumulating rapidly. Research in this field may offer novel targets to inhibit the ocular disease using selective pharmacologic inflammation mediator inhibitors in the early stages of diabetic retinopathy, before it advances to the occlusion of retinal capillaries [10, 11].

Multiple epidemiologic studies have shown that hyperglycemia, hypertension, dyslipidemia, and obesity are risk factors for development and progression of diabetic retinopathy and CSME. The following sections discuss these risk factors in more detail.

A. Abazari, M.D. (✉)
Department of Ophthalmology, Stony Brook University, Stony Brook, NY, USA
e-mail: azin.abazari@stonybrookmedicine.edu

N.G. Ghazi, M.D. (✉)
King Khaled Eye Specialist Hospital, PO Box 7191, Riyadh 11462, Saudi Arabia

University of Virginia, Charlottesville, VA, USA
e-mail: nghazi@kkesh.med.sa

Z.A. Karcioglu, M.D. (✉)
Department of Ophthalmology, University of Virginia, 300 Jefferson Park Avenue, OMS 2783, Charlottesville, VA 22908, USA
e-mail: zak8g@virginia.edu

E.V. Lerma and V. Batuman (eds.), *Diabetes and Kidney Disease*,
DOI 10.1007/978-1-4939-0793-9_13, © Springer Science+Business Media New York 2014

Hyperglycemia

One of the most important risk factors for DR and DME is poor glycemic control. Two large randomized clinical trials, the Diabetes Control and Complications Trial (DCCT) and the United Kingdom Prospective Diabetes Study (UKPDS), provided strong evidence that tighter glycemic control reduces the risk of development and progression of DR in both type 1 and 2 diabetes.

In the DCCT, 1,441 patients with type 1 diabetes were randomly assigned to either conventional or intensive insulin treatment and followed for a period of 4–9 years. In this study, the 3-year risk of development and progression of retinopathy was reduced by 75 and 54 % in the intensive insulin treatment group compared with the standard treatment group. Analysis of data from DCCT demonstrated that the risk of progression of retinopathy reduced by 35–40 % for every 10 % decrease in HbA_1C [12–16]. Later, patients from DCCT were enrolled in the observational 7-year follow-up phase of the study, which demonstrated that the risk reduction of retinopathy progression was maintained in those patients initially randomized for intensive therapy even after cessation of intensive HbA_1C control [17].

The UKPDS and Action to Control Cardiovascular Risk in Diabetes (ACCORD) study confirmed the significant benefit of glycemic control on the development and progression of retinopathy in type 2 diabetics [18–20].

Hypertension

Hypertension is an important risk factor for DR. In the UKPDS, tight blood pressure control (systolic blood pressure <150 mmHg) in patients with type 2 diabetes reduced the risk of progression of retinopathy by 34 %. The UKPDS showed that benefits from tight blood pressure control were present in patients on both beta-blockers and angiotensin converting enzyme (ACE) inhibitors, with no statistically significant difference between the two [21]. However, some clinical trials suggest that ACE inhibitors may have additional beneficial effects on diabetic retinopathy, independent of their blood pressure lowering effect [22–24]. The ACCORD study did not demonstrate a significant advantage of intensive blood pressure control (systolic pressure <120) over standard blood pressure control (systolic pressure <140) in controlling the progression of diabetic retinopathy [20].

Hyperlipidemia

The role of elevated cholesterol and triglyceride in development and progression of DR has been confirmed in several studies. The DCCT showed that severity of retinopathy was associated with elevated triglycerides and inversely related to the level of HDL cholesterol in type 1 diabetes [25]. ACCORD demonstrated that intensive treatment of dyslipidemia with fenofibrate and simvastatin reduced the rate of progression of diabetic retinopathy in type 2 diabetics [20]. Other studies reported that an elevated serum lipid level was independently associated with development of DME [26, 27].

Pregnancy

Diabetic retinopathy may be accelerated during pregnancy because of hormonal or glycemic control changes. In DCCT's ancillary study, some patients had transient worsening of retinopathy during pregnancy, even to the proliferative level. However, at the end of the study, mean levels of retinopathy in subjects who had become pregnant were similar to those patients who had not become pregnant [28]. It is known that pregnancy induces a transient increase in the risk of retinopathy [28–30]; therefore, ophthalmic examination should be performed more frequently during pregnancy and the first year postpartum.

Nephropathy

Multiple studies have demonstrated that proteinuria is associated with increased risk of sight threatening or PDR in type 1 diabetics [3, 31]. Proliferative retinopathy has also been shown to be an independent marker of long-term nephropathy in type 1 diabetes [32].

Other Risk Factors

Several studies suggest a role for other factors, including anemia [33–35], sleep apnea [36], inflammatory markers, homocysteine [37], as well as genetic predisposition [38–41], in development and progression of diabetic retinopathy. In addition, the association between microalbuminuria and the presence/severity of diabetic retinopathy has been reported in several studies [42, 43].

Classification of Diabetic Retinopathy

Diabetic retinopathy is classified into an early stage, NPDR and a more advanced stage, PDR.

Non-proliferative Diabetic Retinopathy

Characteristic retinal findings in NPDR include microaneurysms (Fig. 13.1a), cotton wool spots which represent nerve

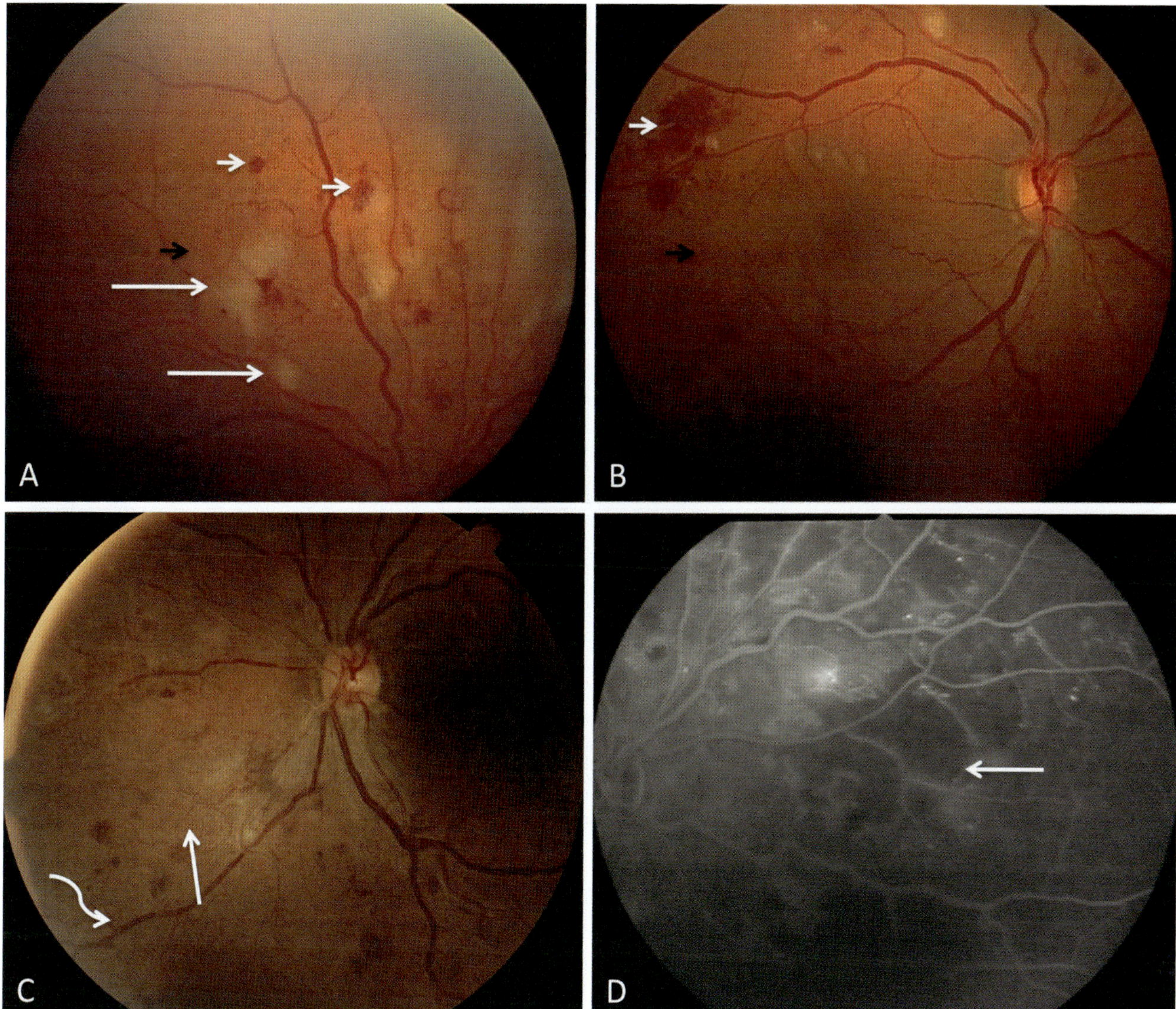

Fig. 13.1 Retinal changes seen in non-proliferative diabetic retinopathy. (**a**, **b**) Fundus photographs illustrating retinal "dot and blot" hemorrhages (*small white arrows*), retinal "cotton wool" spots (*large white arrows*), and clusters of microaneurysms (*small black arrows*). (**c**) Fundus photograph depicting intraretinal microangiopathy (*straight arrow*) and venous beading (*curved arrow*). (**d**) Intravenous fluorescein angiogram (IVFA) disclosing areas of peripheral retinal capillary non-perfusion (*straight arrow*). The scattered white spots are microaneurysms filled with the fluorescein dye; the microaneurysms are usually better seen on IVFA than on fundus examination or photography

fiber layer infarcts (Fig. 13.1a), hard exudates, intraretinal hemorrhages (Fig. 13.1a, b, d), dilation and beading of retinal veins (Fig. 13.1c), intraretinal microvascular abnormalities (IRMA) (Fig. 13.1c), and areas of capillary non-perfusion (Fig. 13.1d).

Non-proliferative retinopathy is further categorized into four levels of severity based on the presence and extent of retinal findings: mild, moderate, severe, and very severe. In the mild-to-moderate non-proliferative categories, there are relatively few intraretinal hemorrhages and microaneurysms. Hard exudates and cotton wool spots can also be seen. The severe non-proliferative retinopathy is clinically detected by evaluating the retina in the four mid peripheral quadrants. Patients with any one of the following features are considered to have severe NPDR: (1) severe intraretinal hemorrhages and microaneurysms in all four quadrants; (2) venous beading in two or more quadrants; or (3) moderate IRMA in at least one quadrant. If any two of these features are present, the retinopathy level is considered to be very severe non-proliferative.

Diabetic Macular Edema

Excessive vascular permeability and loss of blood–retinal barrier result in the leakage of fluid and plasma constituents into the retinal tissue. This is usually most prominent in the

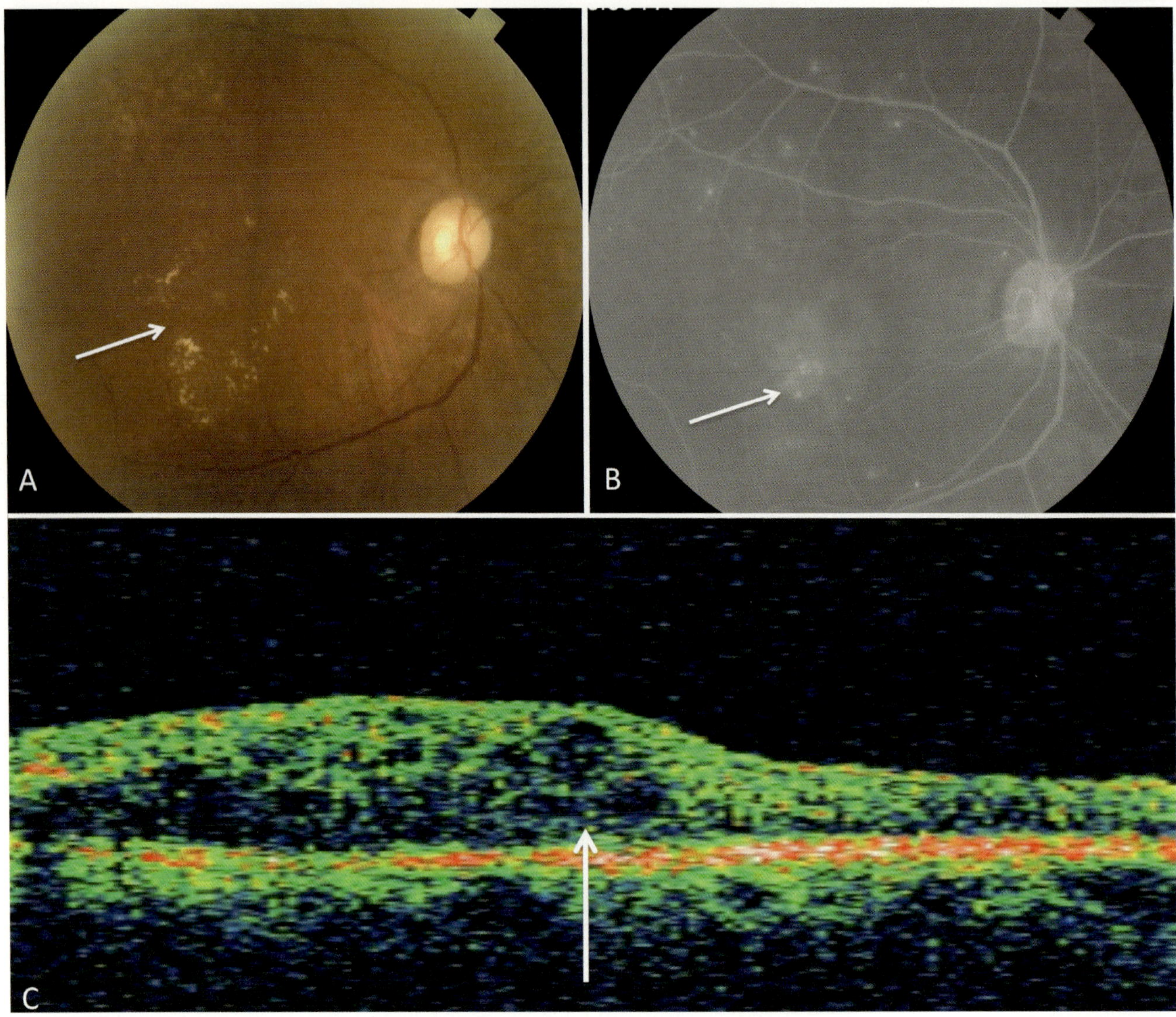

Fig. 13.2 Clinically significant macular edema associated with diabetic retinopathy. (**a**) Fundus photograph illustrating a ring of hard exudates (lipid deposits) that have escaped out of the retinal circulation surrounding an area of retinal swelling (*straight arrow*). Note that the process involves the center of the macula; the corresponding fluorescein angiogram (**b**) discloses a cluster of leaky microaneurysms (*straight arrow*) in the center of the hard exudate ring. (**c**) Optical coherence tomography (OCT) discloses swelling of the involved retina with disruption of the normal foveal contour (*straight arrow*)

macular area of the retina leading to the development of macular edema (Fig. 13.2). DME may be associated with any stage of diabetic retinopathy. It can manifest as focal or diffuse retinal thickening with or without exudates. Macular edema is the most frequent cause of visual impairment in patients with NPDR. In the Early Treatment Diabetic Retinopathy Study (ETDRS), the 3-year risk of moderate visual loss (a doubling of the initial visual angle or loss of 15 letters on a logarithmic visual acuity chart) secondary to macular edema was 32 %. The ETDRS investigators classified macular edema by its severity. It was defined as CSME if any of the following features were present: (1) thickening of the retina at or within 500 μm of the center of the macula; (2) hard exudates at or within 500 μm of the center of the macula, if associated with thickening of the adjacent retina; or (3) a zone of retinal thickening of 1 disc diameter (DD) or larger, any part of which is within one disc diameter of the center of the macula [44]. In addition to optimizing diabetic control, patients with CSME benefit from ocular-specific treatments such as laser photocoagulation or intravitreal injection of pharmacologic agents. This is discussed further in the treatment section. Ancillary tests such as fluorescein angiography (FA) (Figs. 13.1d and 13.2b) and optical coherence tomography (OCT) (Fig. 13.2c) complement the clinical exam and are helpful for detection of DME, guidance of treatment, and monitoring treatment response.

Proliferative Diabetic Retinopathy

Proliferative retinopathy is characterized by formation of new blood vessels and/or fibrous tissue induced by retinal ischemia. Patients can present with neovascularization on the optic disc (Fig. 13.3a), other parts of the retina (Fig. 13.3b), iris (Fig. 13.3c), and/or anterior chamber angle (Fig. 13.3d); pre-retinal and/or vitreous hemorrhages (Fig. 13.4a, b); vitreoretinal traction bands (Fig. 13.4c, d); or tractional retinal detachment (Fig. 13.4c, d). PDR is considered high risk if neovascularization is accompanied by vitreous/pre-retinal hemorrhage or if it is located on the optic disc and occupies at least 1/3 the disc area even in the absence of vitreous hemorrhage. Neovascular glaucoma, a potentially irreversible and blinding complication, can result from new vessel

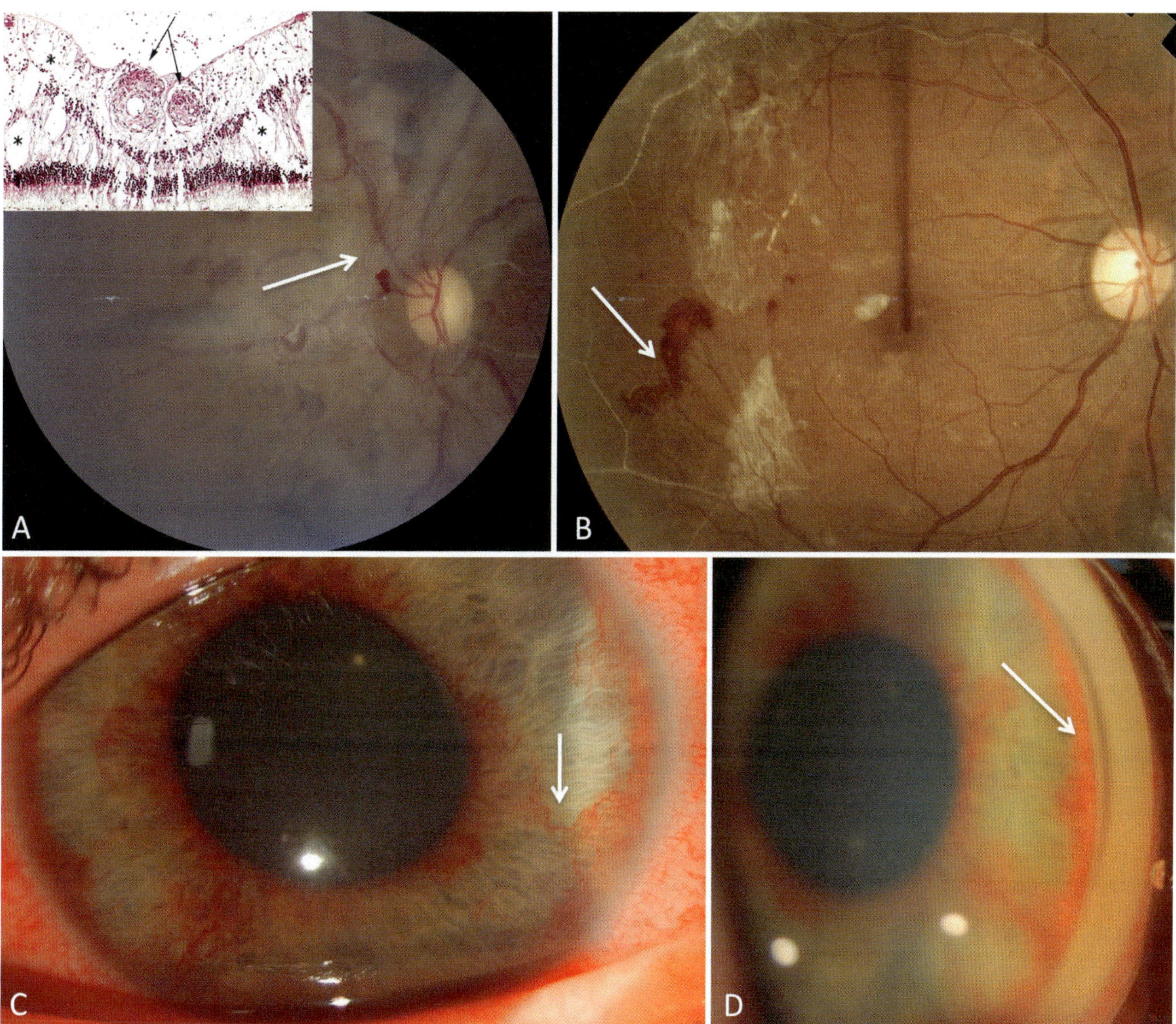

Fig. 13.3 Types of neovascularization seen in proliferative diabetic retinopathy. (**a**) Fundus photograph illustrating neovascularization at the disc (NVD) (*white arrow*). Scattered hemorrhages and laser scars (*black spots*) are also seen. *Inset*: Histopathologic appearance of retinal neovascularization, forming vascular tufts (*black arrows*) in neuroretina. Note the substantial loss of retinal structural integrity secondary to fluid (*asterisk*) leaking from newly formed abnormal vascular structures. Edema (*asterisk*) is seen in all layers of retina including the perivascular space surrounding the vascular tufts. The internal limiting membrane (ILM) is thickened, pushed inward, and is barely intact over the larger tuft. (**b**) Fundus photograph illustrating neovascularization affecting other parts of the retina (neovascularization elsewhere (NVE), *white arrow*). The scattered whitish tissue also represents NVEs that are primarily composed of fibrous rather than vascular tissue. (**c**) Slit-lamp photograph showing neovascularization of the iris (*white arrow*). (**d**) Photograph of the anterior chamber angle, depicting neovascularization (*white arrow*). The patient developed neovascular glaucoma, a serious complication of proliferative diabetic retinopathy that may lead to irreversible loss of vision in the involved eye

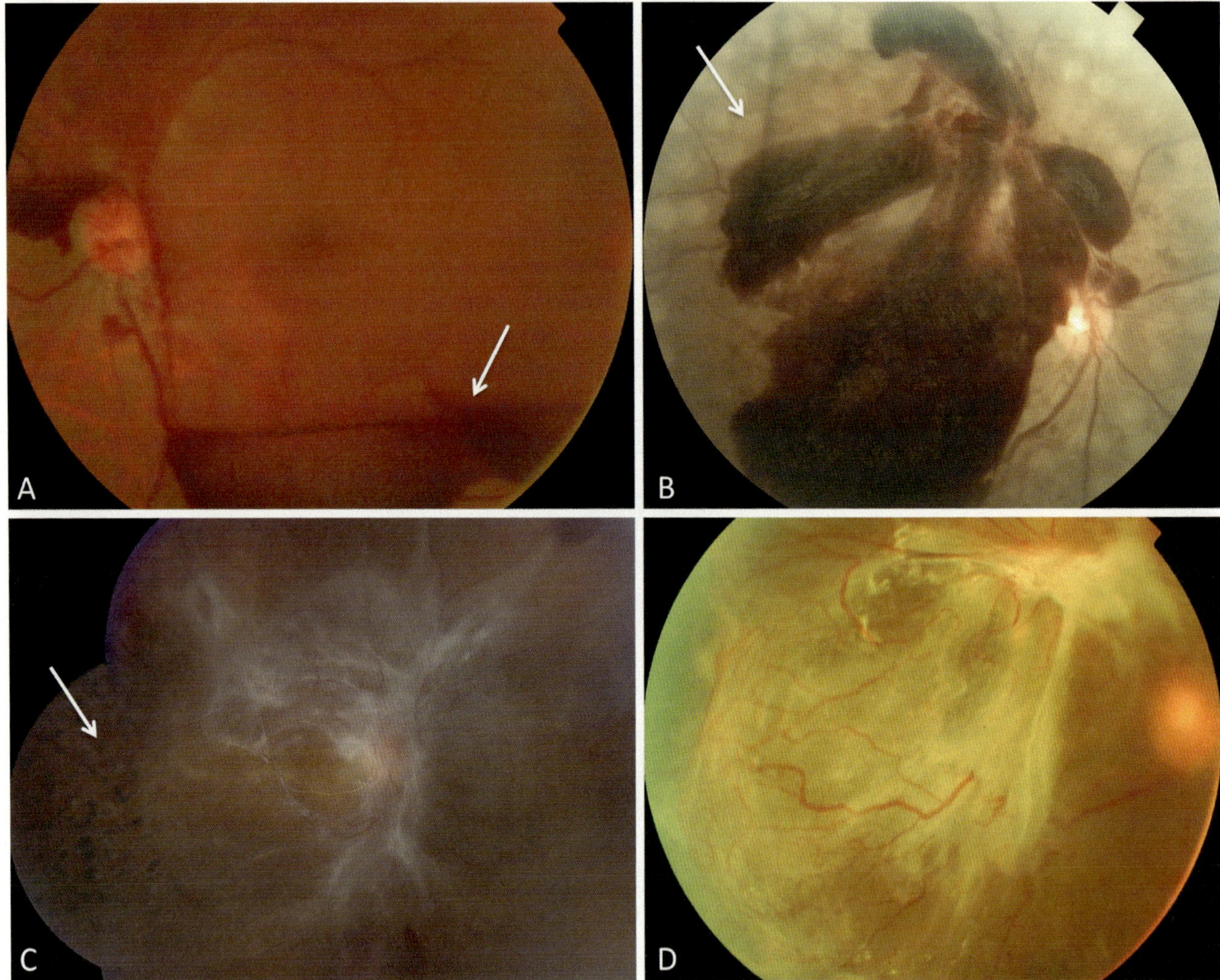

Fig. 13.4 Fundus photographs illustrating sight threatening complications of proliferative diabetic retinopathy. (**a**) Vitreous and pre-retinal or subhyaloid (*white arrow*) hemorrhages. The hemorrhage may sometimes be very dense, obscuring visualization of the underlying retina. (**b**) Large subhyaloid hemorrhage covering the entire posterior pole and macula. Note also the scars of previous panretinal laser photocoagulation (PRP, *white arrow*). (**c**, **d**) Massive proliferation of fibrous bands and fibrovascular tissue leading to traction and retinal detachment of the macula. Note also the scars of previous panretinal laser photocoagulation (PRP, *white arrow* in (**c**))

formation on the iris and anterior chamber angle structure (Fig. 13.3c, d). Patients with high-risk PDR or neovascularization of iris/angle require prompt panretinal laser photocoagulation (PRP) to reduce the chance of severe visual loss.

Screening for Diabetic Retinopathy

As diabetic retinopathy can progress with relatively few visual symptoms, the importance of regular eye screening and subsequent early intervention is essential for all diabetic patients. In patients with type 1 diabetes screening eye examination can be delayed until 3–5 years after diagnosis of diabetes as prevalence of retinopathy during first 4 years after diagnosis is reported to be 1 % [45, 46]. On the other hand, the time of onset of type 2 diabetes is often difficult to determine and may precede the diagnosis by number of years. Therefore, type 2 diabetics should be referred for eye exam at the time of diagnosis. Table 13.1 summarizes the recommended frequency of eye exam by the American Academy of Ophthalmology [47].

Table 13.1 The American Academy of Ophthalmology recommendations on the frequency of eye examinations for different stages of diabetic retinopathy

Status of retinopathy	Frequency of follow-up (months)
No retinopathy	12
Mild-to-moderate NPDR without macular edema	6–12
Mild/moderate NPDR with CSME	2–4
Severe/very severe NPDR	2–4
PDR	2–4
Inactive/involuted PDR without macular edema	6–12

Treatment of Diabetic Retinopathy

Large, randomized trials have shown the benefits of systemic therapies for the prevention and treatment of diabetic retinopathy. The DCCT showed that intensive metabolic control in type 1 diabetics reduced the risk of developing retinopathy by 76 %, and slowed progression of retinopathy by 54 %. Furthermore, intensive glycemic control was associated with reduction in the incidence of macular edema, and the need for panretinal and focal laser photocoagulation [16]. UKPDS showed that intensive blood glucose and blood pressure control slowed progression of retinopathy in type 2 diabetics [18].

Multiple studies have demonstrated that ACE inhibitors reduce the incidence and risk of progression of diabetic retinopathy in patients with type 1 diabetes [22–24, 48].

As mentioned before, two large clinical trials, the Fenofibrate Intervention and Event Lowering in Diabetes (FIELD) [49] and ACCORD [20] trials, demonstrated that hyperlipidemia control with fenofibrate reduces the risk of progression of retinopathy by up to 40 %.

In addition to optimizing metabolic status, and blood pressure control, eye-specific treatments are needed in patients with vision threatening complications of diabetes (PDR and macular edema). The Diabetic Retinopathy Study (DRS) was a prospective, randomized clinical trial evaluating laser panretinal photocoagulation (PRP) treatment (Fig. 13.4b, c) to one eye of patients with advanced NPDR or PDR in both eyes. The primary outcome measurement was severe visual loss, defined as visual acuity of less than 5/200 on two consecutive follow-up examinations 4 months apart. The DRS demonstrated a 50 % or greater reduction in the rate of severe visual loss in eyes treated with PRP compared to untreated control eyes during a follow-up of over 5 years [50]. In this study, treated eyes with high-risk PDR achieved the greatest benefit.

The ETDRS showed that focal/grid laser photocoagulation for clinically significant diabetic macular edema (CSME) substantially reduced the risk of moderate visual loss. In addition, it increased the chance of visual improvement, decreased the frequency of persistent macular edema, and caused only minor visual field loss [44].

A large body of scientific evidence has implicated vascular endothelial growth factor (VEGF) in the pathophysiology of DME. Multiple studies have shown that intravitreal injection of the anti-VEGF antibodies, bevacizumab and ranibizumab, alone or in combination with other treatments, improves visual acuity by an average of one to two lines on a Snellen chart, with an improvement of three or more lines in 25–45 % of patients over a period of 2 years. These results are significantly better than the outcome of laser treatment alone [51–55].

Glucocorticoids are known to reduce retinal inflammation and may have a role in restoring the integrity of the blood–retina barrier. Therefore, intravitreal injection of steroids has been tried for treatment of DME in multiple studies. Intravitreal injection of triamcinolone has been associated with equivocal results in treatment of DME [56–58]. Fluocinolone acetonide intravitreal implant has been shown to be effective in improving vision and resolution of macular retinal thickening in patients with refractory DME [59–61]. However, during a 4-year follow-up, more than 60 % of implanted eyes developed glaucoma of whom half required glaucoma surgery. In addition, more than 90 % of patients developed visually significant cataract that required cataract extraction [59]. A dexamethasone intravitreous drug delivery system has also been shown to be effective in improvement of vision, and reduction of central retinal thickness in eyes with persistent DME with a lower side effect profile [62].

In addition to laser and pharmacotherapy, a group of patients with diabetic retinopathy will require surgical management to restore vision or prevent further visual loss. Pars plana vitrectomy, which involves surgical removal of vitreous opacities and proliferative retinal tractional membranes, is indicated in patients with dense, non-clearing vitreous hemorrhage, tractional retinal detachment involving the macula, diffuse DME associated with vitreomacular traction, or combined tractional and rhegmatogenous (derived from the Greek *rhegma*, which means a rupture or break) retinal detachment (RRD). RRD is the most common type of RD that arises when a tear in the retina occurs and leads to fluid accumulation between the neurosensory retina and the underlying retinal pigment epithelium.

Other Ocular Manifestations

In addition to the retina, diabetes can affect other parts of the eye, including the conjunctiva, tear film, cornea, and iris. Patients can present with conjunctival microaneurysms, dry eye, decreased corneal sensation, poor corneal wound healing, as well as neovascularization of iris/anterior chamber angle.

Dry eye syndrome is more common in diabetics secondary to decreased tear film, abnormal tear lipid layer, higher tear osmolarity, and glucose level [63, 64]. Worsening of dry eye symptoms may correlate with the severity of diabetic retinopathy [65].

Diabetics have reduced corneal sensation as part of diabetic polyneuropathy. As corneal innervation provides protective and trophic functions, diabetics can develop neurotrophic keratopathy. Confocal biomicroscopy studies in vivo have confirmed the reduction in the number and branching of corneal nerves as well as increase in the tortuosity of subbasal corneal nerve plexus [66, 67]. Changes in subbasal nerve plexus of diabetic corneas appear to be related to progression of diabetic retinopathy and peripheral neuropathy. Therefore, corneal confocal microscopy can be used as an adjuvant technique for the early diagnosis and assessment of diabetic neuropathy [68].

Last but not least, the diabetic papillopathy, a relatively rare and benign ocular complication of diabetes mellitus, is worth mentioning here [69, 70]. Ischemia of the optic nerve is considered to be a likely mechanism for this pathology; however, this process is independent of the ischemia of DR [70]. Optic disc edema may vary from minimal to extensive with hemorrhages and exudates even to the degree of forming a "macular star." Papillopathy of diabetes may be a bothersome entity to detect because it mimics both papilledema due to raised intracranial pressure and anterior ischemic optic neuropathy (AION). The setting and absence of systemic findings associated with increased intracranial pressure such as headache and rushing noise help differentiate the papilledema from diabetic papillopathy. When diabetic papillopathy is bilateral or detected in a juvenile diabetic patient as conventionally occurs, it is not likely to be mistaken for AION [69]. However, some cases may present unilaterally or asymmetrically in older patients and the differentiation in such cases may be challenging. During the acute phase there may be loss of central vision, enlarged blind spots, or other field defects. However, unlike AION, these usually resolve and the prognosis is good without chronic impairment of vision. The prognosis might be poorer in older patients with type 2 diabetes [71].

References

1. Ho AC, Scott IU, Kim SJ, et al. Anti-vascular endothelial growth factor pharmacotherapy for diabetic macular edema: a report by the American Academy of Ophthalmology. Ophthalmology. 2012;119: 2179–88.
2. Cheung N, Mitchell P, Wong TY. Diabetic retinopathy. Lancet. 2010;376:124–36.
3. Klein R, Knudtson MD, Lee KE, Gangnon R, Klein BE. The Wisconsin Epidemiologic Study of Diabetic Retinopathy: XXII the twenty-five-year progression of retinopathy in persons with type 1 diabetes. Ophthalmology. 2008;115:1859–68.
4. Klein R, Knudtson M, Lee K, Gangnon R, Klein B. The Wisconsin Epidemiologic Study of Diabetic Retinopathy XXIII: the twenty-five-year incidence of macular edema in persons with type 1 diabetes. Ophthalmology. 2009;116:497–503.
5. Klein R, Zinman B, Gardiner R, et al. The relationship of diabetic retinopathy to preclinical diabetic glomerulopathy lesions in type 1 diabetic patients: the Renin-Angiotensin System Study. Diabetes. 2005;54:527–33.
6. Klein R, Knudtson MD, Klein BE, et al. The relationship of retinal vessel diameter to changes in diabetic nephropathy structural variables in patients with type 1 diabetes. Diabetologia. 2010;53:1638–46.
7. Schwartz MM, Lewis EJ, Leonard-Martin T, Lewis JB, Batlle D. Renal pathology patterns in type II diabetes mellitus: relationship with retinopathy. The Collaborative Study Group. Nephrol Dial Transplant. 1998;13:2547–52.
8. Kern TS. Contributions of inflammatory processes to the development of the early stages of diabetic retinopathy. Exp Diabetes Res. 2007;2007:95103.
9. Kern T, Mohr S. Nonproliferative stages of diabetic retinopathy: animal models and pathogenesis. In: Joussen AM, Gardner GM, Kirchhof B, Ryan SJ, editors. Retinal vascular disease. New York: Springer; 2007. p. 303–11.
10. Hammes HP, Federoff HJ, Brownlee M. Nerve growth factor prevents both neuroretinal programmed cell death and capillary pathology in experimental diabetes. Mol Med. 1995;1:527–34.
11. Barber AJ, Lieth E, Khin SA, Antonetti DA, Buchanan AG, Gardner TW. Neural apoptosis in the retina during experimental and human diabetes. Early onset and effect of insulin. J Clin Invest. 1998;102:783–91.
12. Reichard P, Nilsson BY, Rosenqvist U. The effect of long-term intensified insulin treatment on the development of microvascular complications of diabetes mellitus. N Engl J Med. 1993;329:304–9.
13. The absence of a glycemic threshold for the development of long-term complications: the perspective of the Diabetes Control and Complications Trial. Diabetes. 1996;45:1289–98.
14. The relationship of glycemic exposure (HbA1c) to the risk of development and progression of retinopathy in the Diabetes Control and Complications Trial. Diabetes. 1995;44:968–83.
15. The effect of intensive diabetes treatment on the progression of diabetic retinopathy in insulin-dependent diabetes mellitus. The Diabetes Control and Complications Trial. Arch Ophthalmol. 1995;113:36–51.
16. The effect of intensive treatment of diabetes on the development and progression of long-term complications in insulin-dependent diabetes mellitus. The Diabetes Control and Complications Trial Research Group. N Engl J Med. 1993;329:977–86.
17. Writing Team for the Diabetes Control and Complications Trial/Epidemiology of Diabetes Interventions and Complications Research Group. Effect of intensive therapy on the microvascular complications of type 1 diabetes mellitus. JAMA. 2002;287:2563–9.
18. Effect of intensive blood-glucose control with metformin on complications in overweight patients with type 2 diabetes (UKPDS 34). UK Prospective Diabetes Study (UKPDS) Group. Lancet 1998; 352:854–65.
19. Intensive blood-glucose control with sulphonylureas or insulin compared with conventional treatment and risk of complications in patients with type 2 diabetes (UKPDS 33). UK Prospective Diabetes Study (UKPDS) Group. Lancet 1998;352:837–53.
20. Chew EY, Ambrosius WT, Davis MD, et al. Effects of medical therapies on retinopathy progression in type 2 diabetes. N Engl J Med. 2010;363:233–44.
21. Tight blood pressure control and risk of macrovascular and microvascular complications in type 2 diabetes: UKPDS 38. UK Prospective Diabetes Study Group. BMJ. 1998;317:703–13.
22. Mitchell P, Wong TY. DIRECT new treatments for diabetic retinopathy. Lancet. 2008;372:1361–3.
23. Chaturvedi N, Porta M, Klein R, et al. Effect of candesartan on prevention (DIRECT-Prevent 1) and progression (DIRECT-Protect 1) of retinopathy in type 1 diabetes: randomised, placebo-controlled trials. Lancet. 2008;372:1394–402.
24. Mauer M, Zinman B, Gardiner R, et al. Renal and retinal effects of enalapril and losartan in type 1 diabetes. N Engl J Med. 2009;361: 40–51.
25. Lyons TJ, Jenkins AJ, Zheng D, et al. Diabetic retinopathy and serum lipoprotein subclasses in the DCCT/EDIC cohort. Invest Ophthalmol Vis Sci. 2004;45:910–8.
26. Raman R, Rani PK, Kulothungan V, Rachepalle SR, Kumaramanickavel G, Sharma T. Influence of serum lipids on clinically significant versus nonclinically significant macular edema: SN-DREAMS report number 13. Ophthalmology. 2010;117:766–72.
27. Benarous R, Sasongko MB, Qureshi S, et al. Differential association of serum lipids with diabetic retinopathy and diabetic macular edema. Invest Ophthalmol Vis Sci. 2011;52:7464–9.
28. The Diabetes Control and Complications Trial Research Group. Effect of pregnancy on microvascular complications in the Diabetes Control and Complications Trial. Diabetes Care 2000;23:1084–91.
29. Rasmussen KL, Laugesen CS, Ringholm L, Vestgaard M, Damm P, Mathiesen ER. Progression of diabetic retinopathy during pregnancy in women with type 2 diabetes. Diabetologia. 2010;53:1076–83.

30. Vestgaard M, Ringholm L, Laugesen CS, Rasmussen KL, Damm P, Mathiesen ER. Pregnancy-induced sight-threatening diabetic retinopathy in women with Type 1 diabetes. Diabet Med. 2010;27:431–5.
31. Romero-Aroca P, Baget-Bernaldiz M, Reyes-Torres J, et al. Relationship between diabetic retinopathy, microalbuminuria and overt nephropathy, and twenty-year incidence follow-up of a sample of type 1 diabetic patients. J Diabetes Complications. 2012;26:506–12.
32. Karlberg C, Falk C, Green A, Sjolie AK, Grauslund J. Proliferative retinopathy predicts nephropathy: a 25-year follow-up study of type 1 diabetic patients. Acta Diabetol. 2012;49:263–8.
33. Berman DH, Friedman EA. Partial absorption of hard exudates in patients with diabetic end-stage renal disease and severe anemia after treatment with erythropoietin. Retina. 1994;14:1–5.
34. Qiao Q, Keinanen-Kiukaanniemi S, Laara E. The relationship between hemoglobin levels and diabetic retinopathy. J Clin Epidemiol. 1997;50:153–8.
35. Shorb SR. Anemia and diabetic retinopathy. Am J Ophthalmol. 1985;100:434–6.
36. West SD, Groves DC, Lipinski HJ, et al. The prevalence of retinopathy in men with Type 2 diabetes and obstructive sleep apnoea. Diabet Med. 2010;27:423–30.
37. Nguyen TT, Alibrahim E, Islam FM, et al. Inflammatory, hemostatic, and other novel biomarkers for diabetic retinopathy: the multi-ethnic study of atherosclerosis. Diabetes Care. 2009;32:1704–9.
38. Sobrin L, Green T, Sim X, et al. Candidate gene association study for diabetic retinopathy in persons with type 2 diabetes: the Candidate gene Association Resource (CARe). Invest Ophthalmol Vis Sci. 2011;52:7593–602.
39. Abhary S, Hewitt AW, Burdon KP, Craig JE. A systematic meta-analysis of genetic association studies for diabetic retinopathy. Diabetes. 2009;58:2137–47.
40. Arar NH, Freedman BI, Adler SG, et al. Heritability of the severity of diabetic retinopathy: the FIND-Eye study. Invest Ophthalmol Vis Sci. 2008;49:3839–45.
41. Liew G, Klein R, Wong TY. The role of genetics in susceptibility to diabetic retinopathy. Int Ophthalmol Clin. 2009;49:35–52.
42. Cruickshanks KJ, Ritter LL, Klein R, Moss SE. The association of microalbuminuria with diabetic retinopathy. The Wisconsin Epidemiologic Study of Diabetic Retinopathy. Ophthalmology. 1993;100:862–7.
43. Nwanyanwu KH, Talwar N, Gardner TW, Wrobel JS, Herman WH, Stein JD. Predicting development of proliferative diabetic retinopathy. Diabetes Care. 2013;36(6):1562–8.
44. Photocoagulation for diabetic macular edema. Early Treatment Diabetic Retinopathy Study report number 1. Early Treatment Diabetic Retinopathy Study Research Group. Arch Ophthalmol. 1985;103:1796–806.
45. Frank RN, Hoffman WH, Podgor MJ, et al. Retinopathy in juvenile-onset type I diabetes of short duration. Diabetes. 1982;31:874–82.
46. Frank RN, Hoffman WH, Podgor MJ, et al. Retinopathy in juvenile-onset diabetes of short duration. Ophthalmology. 1980;87:1–9.
47. American Academy of Ophthalmology. Preferred practice pattern. Diabetic retinopathy. San Francisco: AAO; 2008.
48. Chaturvedi N, Sjolie AK, Stephenson JM, et al. Effect of lisinopril on progression of retinopathy in normotensive people with type 1 diabetes. The EUCLID Study Group. EURODIAB Controlled Trial of Lisinopril in Insulin-Dependent Diabetes Mellitus. Lancet. 1998;351:28–31.
49. Keech AC, Mitchell P, Summanen PA, et al. Effect of fenofibrate on the need for laser treatment for diabetic retinopathy (FIELD study): a randomised controlled trial. Lancet. 2007;370:1687–97.
50. Photocoagulation treatment of proliferative diabetic retinopathy: the second report of diabetic retinopathy study findings. Ophthalmology 1978;85:82–106.
51. Elman MJ, Aiello LP, Beck RW, et al. Randomized trial evaluating ranibizumab plus prompt or deferred laser or triamcinolone plus prompt laser for diabetic macular edema. Ophthalmology. 2010; 117:1064–77.e35.
52. Googe J, Brucker AJ, Bressler NM, et al. Randomized trial evaluating short-term effects of intravitreal ranibizumab or triamcinolone acetonide on macular edema after focal/grid laser for diabetic macular edema in eyes also receiving panretinal photocoagulation. Retina. 2011;31:1009–27.
53. Michaelides M, Kaines A, Hamilton RD, et al. A prospective randomized trial of intravitreal bevacizumab or laser therapy in the management of diabetic macular edema (BOLT study) 12-month data: report 2. Ophthalmology. 2010;117:1078–86.e2.
54. Mitchell P, Bandello F, Schmidt-Erfurth U, et al. The RESTORE study: ranibizumab monotherapy or combined with laser versus laser monotherapy for diabetic macular edema. Ophthalmology. 2011;118:615–25.
55. Nguyen QD, Brown DM, Marcus DM, et al. Ranibizumab for diabetic macular edema: results from 2 phase III randomized trials: RISE and RIDE. Ophthalmology. 2012;119:789–801.
56. Beck RW, Edwards AR, Aiello LP, et al. Three-year follow-up of a randomized trial comparing focal/grid photocoagulation and intravitreal triamcinolone for diabetic macular edema. Arch Ophthalmol. 2009;127:245–51.
57. Gillies MC, McAllister IL, Zhu M, et al. Pretreatment with intravitreal triamcinolone before laser for diabetic macular edema: 6-month results of a randomized, placebo-controlled trial. Invest Ophthalmol Vis Sci. 2010;51:2322–8.
58. Gillies MC, Sutter FK, Simpson JM, Larsson J, Ali H, Zhu M. Intravitreal triamcinolone for refractory diabetic macular edema: two-year results of a double-masked, placebo-controlled, randomized clinical trial. Ophthalmology. 2006;113:1533–8.
59. Pearson PA, Comstock TL, Ip M, et al. Fluocinolone acetonide intravitreal implant for diabetic macular edema: a 3-year multicenter, randomized, controlled clinical trial. Ophthalmology. 2011;118:1580–7.
60. Campochiaro PA, Brown DM, Pearson A, et al. Sustained delivery fluocinolone acetonide vitreous inserts provide benefit for at least 3 years in patients with diabetic macular edema. Ophthalmology. 2012;119:2125–32.
61. Campochiaro PA, Brown DM, Pearson A, et al. Long-term benefit of sustained-delivery fluocinolone acetonide vitreous inserts for diabetic macular edema. Ophthalmology. 2011;118: 626–35.e2.
62. Haller JA, Kuppermann BD, Blumenkranz MS, et al. Randomized controlled trial of an intravitreous dexamethasone drug delivery system in patients with diabetic macular edema. Arch Ophthalmol. 2010;128:289–96.
63. Inoue K, Kato S, Ohara C, Numaga J, Amano S, Oshika T. Ocular and systemic factors relevant to diabetic keratoepitheliopathy. Cornea. 2001;20:798–801.
64. Dogru M, Katakami C, Inoue M. Tear function and ocular surface changes in noninsulin-dependent diabetes mellitus. Ophthalmology. 2001;108:586–92.
65. Nepp J, Abela C, Polzer I, et al. Is there a correlation between the severity of diabetic retinopathy and keratoconjunctivitis sicca? Cornea. 2000;19:487–91.
66. Kallinikos P, Berhanu M, O'Donnell C, et al. Corneal nerve tortuosity in diabetic patients with neuropathy. Invest Ophthalmol Vis Sci. 2004;45:418–22.
67. Midena E, Brugin E, Ghirlando A, et al. Corneal diabetic neuropathy: a confocal microscopy study. J Refract Surg. 2006;22: S1047–52.
68. Nitoda E, Kallinikos P, Pallikaris A, et al. Correlation of diabetic retinopathy and corneal neuropathy using confocal microscopy. Curr Eye Res. 2012;37:898–906.
69. Vaphiades MS. The disk edema dilemma. Surv Ophthalmol. 2002;47(2):183.
70. Pavan PR, Aiello LM, Wafai MZ, et al. Optic disc edema in juvenile-onset diabetes. Arch Ophthalmol. 1980;98(12):2193–7.
71. Bayraktar Z, Alacali N. Bayraktar: diabetic papillopathy in type II diabetic patients. Retina. 2002;22(6):752.

14 Pregnancy and Diabetic Nephropathy

N. Kevin Krane, Radha Pasala, and Adrian Baudy IV

Introduction

Women who become pregnant with chronic kidney disease (CKD) may have increased maternal and fetal morbidity and mortality, including the risk of increasing the progression of the underlying renal disease. Pregnancy in women with diabetes mellitus can therefore be of significant concern, especially because diabetes mellitus (DM) is the most common cause of CKD leading to end-stage renal failure and the prevalence of DM continues to increase [1, 2]. While most of these patients are older and have type 2 DM and multiple comorbidities, many women of child-bearing age are affected by this disease. It has been estimated that 13 % of the US population aged 20 years or older have a hyperglycemic condition, with Hispanic and African-Americans disproportionately affected. In addition, Jovanovic and Pettitt in 2001 reported that gestational diabetes (GD) affects up to 14 % of all pregnancies, and the prevalence continues to increase [3, 4]. Hyperglycemic disorders of pregnancy are therefore common and bring unique concerns for both maternal and fetal outcomes. Pregnancy in women with established diabetic nephropathy (DN) raises even greater concerns about further increasing maternal and fetal morbidity and mortality, as well as the concern that pregnancy itself may accelerate renal functional deterioration. Since the initial reports from the 1950s of grave consequences of diabetic women who became pregnant, significant progress has been made not only in the diagnosis, management, and treatment of diabetes but also in the management of high-risk pregnant women [5–7]. While all women should receive optimal prenatal care, women with diabetic nephropathy should also receive preconception counseling that may often result in important changes in their care to optimize pregnancy outcomes for both mother and fetus [8]. The goal of this chapter is to provide an understanding of issues associated with pregnancy in diabetic nephropathy so that physicians providing care for these women can do so with a comprehensive understanding of the risks and potential complications to provide evidence-based counseling and care for these women.

Previous studies have shown that hyperglycemia in pregnancy may increase the risk of increased birth weight and increased cord blood serum C-peptide levels [9]. Pregnancy in women with diabetes mellitus increases risks for preeclampsia, preterm delivery, congenital malformations, and both maternal and fetal mortality [10] though these complications may be reduced for women with type 2 diabetes compared to those with type 1 [11]. Pregnancy in women diagnosed with diabetic nephropathy (DN) raises additional concerns. In normal pregnancy, glomerular filtration rises immediately after conception reaching its highest values during the second trimester and returning to about 20 % during the third trimester and returning to normal within 3 months after delivery. These changes are also associated with a significant increase in renal blood flow, increased sodium retention, decreased peripheral vascular resistance, and resistance to the action of angiotensin II [12]. Pregnancy may also be associated with a small increase in protein excretion and even renal glycosuria. Pregnancy in women with underlying CKD is often complicated by increased proteinuria, hypertension, and a reduced glomerular filtration rate, all of which depend more on the severity of the underlying kidney disease rather than the etiology [13, 14]. One of the bigger challenges in the management of these women is differentiating superimposed

N.K. Krane, M.D. (✉)
Department of Medicine, Section of Nephrology and Hypertension, Tulane University School of Medicine, 1430 Tulane Avenue, #8020, New Orleans, LA 70112, USA
e-mail: kkrane@tulane.edu

R. Pasala M.D.
Section of Nephrology and Hypertension, Tulane University School of Medicine, 1430 Tulane Avenue, SL 45, New Orleans, LA 70112, USA
e-mail: rpasala@tulane.edu

A. Baudy IV, M.D.
Section of Nephrology and Hypertension, Tulane Medical Center, 1430 Tulane Avenue, SL 45, New Orleans, LA 70112, USA
e-mail: abaudy@tulane.edu

E.V. Lerma and V. Batuman (eds.), *Diabetes and Kidney Disease*,
DOI 10.1007/978-1-4939-0793-9_14, © Springer Science+Business Media New York 2014

preeclampsia from the changes associated with the underlying disease, though new tests based on recent developments in our understanding of the pathogenesis of preeclampsia hold great promise for advanced diagnostic studies [15, 16]. Fortunately, in women with mild underlying CKD, many of these complications reverse after delivery. Given the challenges of managing women with CKD in pregnancy, those with underlying diabetic nephropathy carry significant concern. A review of the risks and concerns for physicians who provide care to women with diabetic nephropathy so that they can provide appropriate counsel prior to conception and during and after pregnancy is provided.

Overview of Diabetic Nephropathy

The clinical hallmark of diabetic nephropathy is proteinuria. DN has both a subclinical phase that begins with microalbuminuria and a clinical phase in which macroalbuminemia and reduced glomerular filtration rate are present. The initial finding in the subclinical phase is microalbuminuria and all patients with diabetes should be screened for diabetic nephropathy by determining urinary albumin excretion using a spot urine sample and measuring urine protein and creatinine [17]. Microalbuminuria is defined as an elevated urine albumin to creatinine ratio (ACR) of greater than 30 mg/g in two out of three samples without known other CKD. In those diabetic patients who have CKD, the etiology can be attributed to diabetes if there is an ACR greater than 300 mg/g (macroalbuminuria) or ACR 30–300 mg/g (microalbuminuria) in the presence of diabetic retinopathy and type 1 diabetes of at least 10 years' duration [18]. In progressive disease, microalbuminuria increases to levels of macroalbuminuria, and then overt nephrotic syndrome may develop. During this period of time, without treatment, hypertension may develop, and the glomerular filtration rate begins to fall with patients developing end-stage renal disease (ESRD) over several years. The goal of therapy is to either prevent or slow the development and progression of clinical disease. Mainstays of therapy in nonpregnant patients with DN are tight control of blood glucose, angiotensin converting enzyme (ACE) inhibitors or angiotensin receptor blockers (ARBs), and strict control of hypertension. Supportive therapy includes dietary therapy, management of hyperlipidemia, and smoking cessation. The pathogenesis of DN is dependent on glomerular hyperfiltration, hyperglycemia, and advanced glycosylation end-products [19–22]. Other mechanisms that play a role include cytokine activation and impaired renal nephrin expression [23, 24]. This raises concerns unique to DN because normal pregnancy is already associated with hyperfiltration.

There is evidence from the Diabetes Control Complications Trial Research Group and Epidemiology of Diabetes Interventions and Complications that achieving a hemoglobin A1c (HbA1c) level of approximately 7.0 % is able to mitigate some of the renal complication of diabetes [25, 26]. Studies have shown that in both type 1 and type 2 diabetes, improved glycemic control and agents that reduce glomerular capillary pressure by interfering with the actions of angiotensin II are associated with reduced incidence of microalbuminuria and prevent or slow the development of overt diabetic nephropathy [27–31]. Mainstays of management in diabetes to prevent kidney disease are therefore monitoring the glomerular filtration rate, monitoring for the presence of microalbuminuria using ACE inhibitors or ARBs (contraindicated in pregnant women), as well as lipid management and smoking cessation if necessary. The approach to diabetic women who wish to conceive or are pregnant may be different.

Pre-pregnancy Risks and Counseling

All women with diabetes should receive pre-pregnancy counseling [8, 32–34]. Women with diabetes and particularly diabetic nephropathy need to be counseled as to the safety of conceiving and the likelihood of a successful pregnancy if they do. Therefore physicians who care for diabetics who desire families must have a complete understanding of clinical guidelines and the relevant literature to provide the necessary information from which decisions can be made on an individual basis. For many years, women with diabetes were discouraged from becoming pregnant. Despite an increased risk of complications, with improved care and careful monitoring, studies have shown that diabetic women can safely and successfully have children [35, 36].

Counseling prior to conception for diabetics should include a discussion of potential maternal or fetal health risks with an obstetrician and other appropriate physicians before deciding on pregnancy. If they have not received an evaluation for proteinuria and renal function within the past 12 months, it should be performed at the initial visit [8]. The major concerns discussed in this chapter focus on hypertension and diabetic nephropathy, but women with long-standing diabetes may also have other comorbidities that must be considered. In addition, these women, especially those with hypertension and/or microalbuminuria, must have a thorough review of their medications because they may be receiving ACE inhibitors, ARBs, or other drugs that are potentially harmful in pregnancy [37, 38].

Although ACE inhibitors and ARBs are mainstays for the treatment of both type 1 and type 2 diabetic nephropathy, this group of drugs is unfortunately contraindicated in pregnant women [39]. In a recent meta-analysis of 49 randomized controlled trials, ACE inhibitors and ARBs were found to not only prevent progression but also reverse microalbuminuria [31]. However, ACE inhibitors and ARBs are contraindicated in pregnancy because of the risk of fetal malformations; therefore, modification of antihypertensives in patients considering pregnancy is very important [40–42]. Reported fetal effects include severe oligohydramnios, renal failure, arterial hypotension, intrauterine growth retardation (IUGR), respiratory distress syndrome, pulmonary hypoplasia, hypocalvaria, limb defects, persistent patent ductus arteriosus, cerebral complications, and death [40]. Therefore, discontinuing ACE inhibitors or ARBs is an essential part of the preconception evaluation. Similarly, these drugs should be discontinued immediately when pregnancy is confirmed in women receiving either of these agents. When these drugs are discontinued and antihypertensive therapy is required, several agents such as methyldopa or labetalol can be started as they have an excellent safety profile in pregnancy [41]. Women with mild hypertension, particularly in early pregnancy, may require no other therapy because of the physiologic decrease in blood pressure that occurs [42]. Therapy must be individualized but can be guided by consensus statements including those that suggest that certain patients should be started on antihypertensives, particularly those with a systolic pressure of 140 mmHg or a diastolic pressure of 90 mmHg in women with gestational hypertension without proteinuria or preexisting hypertension before 28 weeks' gestation, those with gestational hypertension and proteinuria or symptoms at any time during the pregnancy, those with preexisting hypertension and underlying conditions or target-organ damage, and those with preexisting hypertension and superimposed gestational hypertension [42–44].

Women with diabetic nephropathy are also more likely to have other significant medical problems such as ischemic cardiovascular disease or diabetic gastroparesis [45]. In addition, all women with diabetes are at risk for the development of either gestational hypertension or preeclampsia, though the risk is greater in those with preexisting hypertension and diabetic nephropathy [46].

Counseling women with preexisting diabetic nephropathy needs to be very individualized. Within this population of women, risks and outcomes may differ between those with only microalbuminuria, and those with overt clinical diabetic nephropathy as manifested by proteinuria and/or a decreased glomerular filtration rate. For all these women, understanding not only the maternal and fetal risks but also the risk of accelerating the progression of underlying renal disease is essential. The following discussion focuses on the reported outcomes of pregnancy in women with diabetic nephropathy over the past 30 years.

Gestational Diabetes Mellitus

Gestational diabetes mellitus (GDM) is another problem associated with impaired glucose tolerance that may occur during pregnancy. The International Association of Diabetes and Pregnancy Study Group (IADPSG) defines GDM as a fasting plasma glucose ≥92 mg/dL but <126 mg/dL or at least one abnormal result with the 75 g oral glucose tolerance test (GTT) at 24- to 28-week gestation, fasting glucose ≥92 but <126 mg/dL or 1 h glucose ≥180 mg/dL or 2 h glucose is > 153 mg/dl. If the fasting plasma glucose is ≥126 md/dL or random glucose ≥200 mg/dL or the HbA1c≥6.5 then overt diabetes can be diagnosed [47].

According to National Diabetes Statistics in 2011, GDM is seen in about 2–10 % of pregnant women [48]. Increasing maternal age, lower socioeconomic status, African-Americans or Hispanics ethnicity, obesity, and family history of diabetes are associated with an increased risk of developing GDM, with a higher prevalence in the United States [49].

Identifying women with gestational diabetes is important because the Hyperglycemia and Adverse Pregnancy Outcome (HAPO) study showed a direct association between increasing levels of fasting, 1-h, and 2-h plasma glucose post a 75 g oral GTT and adverse maternal and fetal outcomes including preeclampsia, abnormal birth weight, cord blood serum C-peptide level, primary cesarean delivery, clinical neonatal hypoglycemia, premature delivery, and shoulder dystocia. There is an increased risk of developing overt diabetes in women with GDM and a concern for impaired glucose tolerance and development of obesity and diabetes in the babies born to women with GDM [50].

GDM can have significant adverse affects on the fetus. Elevated glucose levels can stimulate insulin release by the fetus and may also lead to respiratory distress in the infant after delivery due to the inhibition of fetal lung maturation. Women with GDM commonly have large for gestational age babies as the fetus is exposed to the excess glucose. This results in conversion of the glucose to fat and deposition of adipose tissue. Delivery may then be complicated by increased rates of cesarean sections, and birth injuries including shoulder dystocia, and nerve palsies. Hypoglycemia is another significant complication that can occur in the newborn baby [51].

The management and treatment of gestational diabetes include dietary modification, exercise, self-monitoring of blood glucose, and if necessary, hypoglycemic therapy. In a large randomized control trial of 958 women, treatment of mild GDM decreased the risk of perinatal problems like preeclampsia, gestational hypertension, macrosomia, and shoulder dystocia compared to the control group though there was no significant decrease in stillbirths or perinatal death [52]. In a randomized clinical trial, Crowther et al. showed there was a significant decrease in the rate of serious perinatal outcomes (i.e., death, shoulder dystocia, bone fracture, and nerve palsy) from 4 to 1 % in women with gestational diabetes who received intervention with dietary advice, blood glucose monitoring, and insulin therapy compared to those who received routine care. The women in the intervention group also reported better quality of life and general health status postpartum [53].

Exercise along with diet was found to lower the glucose concentration and HbA1c levels more in women with GDM when compared to diet alone and can help avoid the need for insulin treatment [54]. The American Diabetes Association (ADA) recommends that nutrition therapy for women with GDM should aim at achieving normal blood glucose levels and also provide adequate energy levels to promote both maternal and fetal well-being and allow for appropriate weight gain during pregnancy. Diet should be tailored to meet individual nutrition needs and blood glucose levels and ketosis. They recommended that the required carbohydrates be provided in small-to-moderate-sized meals and snacks throughout the day [55].

In a retrospective cohort study Chen et al. examined the association between gestational weight gain and perinatal outcomes in 31,074 women with GDM. They found that women who had gestational weight gain above the Institute of Medicine (IOM) guidelines had a higher risk of having large for gestational age neonates, preterm delivery, and primary cesarean delivery when compared to women who gained weight within the IOM guidelines. They also reported that women who had gestational weight gain below the IOM guidelines had a higher risk of having small for gestational age neonates and lower odds of having large for gestational age neonates but these women were able to maintain diet-controlled GDM [55]. Others have also reported that excessive weight gain may increase the risk of large for gestational age infants [56–60].

Insulin therapy should be initiated in women with GDM who have uncontrolled glucose levels with diet and exercise. The ADA recommends that insulin should be initiated in women with GDM who fail to achieve fasting blood glucose level less than or equal to 105 mg/dL or the 1 h postprandial glucose level ≤155 mg/dL or the 2 h postprandial glucose level ≤130 mg/dL. Insulin treatment should be administered in divided doses with the risk of perinatal complications being lowest when insulin was administered four times daily compared to twice daily insulin [61]. The use of oral antihyperglycemic agents is not recommended by the ADA and ACOG (The American College of Obstetricians and Gynecologists' Committee on Obstetric Practice) during pregnancy. Metformin carries a Category B warning and glyburide has a Category C warning by the FDA.

Women with GDM have up to a 41 % increased risk of recurrence of GDM during subsequent pregnancies and there is an increased risk of development of subsequent type 2 diabetes and cardiovascular disease [62–64]. Women with GDM also require long-term follow-up. The ACOG recommends that all women with GDM should undergo screening for diabetes at 6–12 weeks postpartum [65].

The goal of treatment in women with GDM is to provide excellent support to assure successful outcomes. The ADA recommends that the nutrition therapy for women with GDM should aim at achieving normal blood glucose levels and also provide adequate energy levels to promote both maternal and fetal well-being and allow for appropriate weight gain during pregnancy. Diet should be tailored to meet individual nutrition needs and blood glucose levels and ketosis. They recommended providing the required carbohydrates in small-to-moderate-sized meals and snacks throughout the day [55]. However, diet alone may not achieve optimal glycemic control. Insulin is the standard against which all therapies are measured; a recent study reviewed eight randomized control trials published since 2009 that compared the use of the oral agents metformin and glyburide with insulin [66]. While these agents are effective, there were some differences between agents in individual studies, but they found few adverse events occurred overall. The authors concluded that larger, prospective studies to fully evaluate the long-term safety of oral hypoglycemic agents are necessary.

The Pregnant Diabetic

Early Diabetic Nephropathy: Microalbuminuria

Pregnancy in women with diabetic nephropathy poses additional theoretical challenges because of the physiologic hyperfiltration though there is little evidence of increased intraglomerular pressure [67, 68]. However proteinuria is of real concern, given that proteinuria increases in pregnancy. An important question is whether or not proteinuria, including microalbuminuria, predicts adverse outcomes in these women? Twenty years ago, Combs et al. looked at the impact of proteinuria on pregnancy in diabetic women. They showed that the risk of preeclampsia was 7 % when early pregnancy proteinuria was less than 190 mg/24 h, increased to 31 % when proteinuria was 190–499 mg/24 h, and was 38 % when proteinuria exceeded 500 mg/24 h [68]. Ten years later, Eckbom et al. also reviewed outcomes in diabetic pregnancies that correlated urinary albumin excretion with outcomes of proteinuria. They showed there were increasing rates of preterm delivery, small for gestational age infants, and preeclampsia depending on whether there was normoalbuminuria, microalbuminuria, or overt nephropathy with proteinuria greater than 300 mg/24 h [70]. Thirty-five percent of women with microalbuminuria prior to pregnancy had preterm delivery due to preeclampsia, which was also associated with a higher HbA1c at 2–6 weeks of gestation. In addition, many of these women also developed nephrotic range proteinuria. These findings are also consistent with those reported by Biesenbach et al. They compared urinary albumin excretion during and after pregnancy in women with type 1 DM; 30 women had normoalbuminuria and 12 women had microalbuminuria prior to conception. In both groups of patients the urinary albumin excretion reached a peak during the third trimester with a greater increase in microalbuminuria in diabetic women with preexisting microalbuminuria (almost sevenfold) compared to those with normoalbuminuria (fourfold) though normalization occurred within 12 weeks after delivery in both patient groups. Renal function remained normal during pregnancy in both of the groups [71].

Using logistic regression analysis, Ekbom et al. reported that the relative risk for preeclampsia in insulin-dependent diabetic women with microalbuminuria was 16. Six of ten women with microalbuminuria compared to 2 of 54 normoalbuminuric diabetic women developed preeclampsia [72]. Similarly, in a prospective study of 846 diabetic women, Jensen et al. also reported a significantly higher incidence of preeclampsia (odds ratio 4.0) in diabetic women with microalbuminuria compared to those with normoalbuminuria [73]. Nielsen et al. however reported no cases of preeclampsia in five of ten women with microalbuminuria who received intensive blood pressure and glycemic control [74].

Women with early diabetic nephropathy, manifested as "only" microalbuminuria, are at increased risk for the development of preeclampsia, preterm delivery, and significant increases in urinary albumin excretion during pregnancy. Pregnancy, however, has not been found to be a risk factor for the development of microalbuminuria or long-term progression of nephropathy in women with no nephropathy or only microalbuminuria at baseline [74, 75]. Intensive therapy may reduce these complications.

Clinical Diabetic Nephropathy: Proteinuria

When pregnancy occurs in women with clinical diabetic nephropathy, either proteinuria >300 mg/24 h or reduced glomerular filtration rate, there is increased concern regarding maternal morbidity and mortality and fetal outcomes, and the affect of the pregnancy on the progression of the underlying kidney disease. Early reports from the 1950s of pregnant diabetic women with kidney disease describe difficult pregnancies with significant maternal morbidity and fetal mortality [5–7] and therefore pregnancy was strongly discouraged. By the time Hare and White reviewed a series of patients in 1977, the fetal survival rate had improved to 72 % in diabetic nephropathy, but it was still lower than the survival rate for diabetics without kidney disease [76]. In 1986, Grenfell et al. reported the outcomes of 22 pregnancies in 20 women from 1974 to 1984 with proteinuria during or before pregnancy and compared them to diabetic women without proteinuria. Four women had elevated serum creatinine. The proteinuria diabetic women had a higher rate of preterm delivery and small for gestational age infants but all pregnancies were successful. One patient subsequently died of renal failure and three had further deterioration of renal function. The authors concluded that pregnancy should be discouraged in these patients because of poor long-term maternal outcome [77].

Fortunately, there have been significant improvements in both obstetric and neonatal care since that time, as well as significant advances in the management of diabetes, hypertension, and specifically diabetic nephropathy over this time contributing to the improved outcomes. It is essential however for physicians, both obstetricians and nephrologists, who provide care to women with diabetic nephropathy to know what outcomes are most likely to occur in an individual patient, based on the many reports published in the literature so that they can best counsel and advise diabetic women as to risks to the mother and fetus, as well as the risk of causing irreversible renal damage. Armed with this knowledge, one can provide appropriate expectations and guidelines that can help patients make an informed decision as to the likelihood of safe and successful outcomes, and also increase awareness of potential problems for the patient and the physicians providing care.

In 1981, Kitzmiller et al. described one of the first series on pregnancy in women with diabetic nephropathy in which outcomes were significantly improved. As in many early studies, the abortion rate, both spontaneous and planned, was high (25.7 %). Of the remaining pregnancies, proteinuria increased in most women and both hypertension and reduced renal function were present in the third trimester in approximately 75 % of women. While early delivery (prior to 37 weeks) occurred in 71 %, with low birth weights correlating with maternal blood pressure and proteinuria, fetal survival was 89 %. Proteinuria improved after delivery in 65 % of cases, and hypertension resolved in 43.5 %. They reported that creatinine clearance decreased by a rate of 0.81 mL/min/month in women following delivery, no different than non-pregnant women with diabetic nephropathy [78]. Later, Reece et al. described 31 pregnancies in women with diabetic nephropathy over a nearly 10-year period from the Yale-New Haven Hospital. Initially, 39 % of women had a serum creatinine greater than 1.2 mg/dL, increasing to 45 % of women during pregnancy; there was an increase in heavy proteinuria (>3.0 g/day) from 26 to 71 % and hypertension increased from 26 to 58 %. Following delivery, proteinuria returned nearly to prepartum values with no evidence of adverse affect on underlying renal function with an infant survival rate of 94 %. Of note, the creatinine clearance, measured in the first or second trimester, was below 50 in only four women. They too reported rates of renal functional decline following pregnancy in diabetic nephropathy to be similar to those reported by Kitzmiller, and not different than those patients with nephropathy who did not get pregnant [79]. They concluded that the likelihood of successful outcome in their patients with diabetic nephropathy was comparable to other insulin-dependent diabetics. Two years later, Reece provided follow-up data on 11 women, with mild-to-moderate diabetic nephropathy who did not seem to develop an accelerated rate of decline in renal function. Although all of these patients were hypertensive and had increased proteinuria during pregnancy, the mean serum creatinine just prior to conception (1.3 mg/dL) and the last follow-up value (1.2 mg/dL) were not significantly different. The observed rate of decline in renal function appeared to be consistent with the expected natural course of diabetic nephropathy in the absence of pregnancy [80]. In a subsequent review, Reece reported successful pregnancy outcomes in >95 % of 27 pregnant women with diabetic nephropathy (>300 mg proteinuria/24 h). Care included stringent metabolic control of glucose and management of hypertension. While chronic hypertension and preeclampsia were common maternal complications, there were no fetal deaths [81]. Based on Kitzmiller and Reece's data, it is suggested that while the risk of complications that occur during pregnancy, i.e., preeclampsia, preterm delivery, and small for gestational age baby, may be greater in women with early diabetic nephropathy, the likelihood of a successful pregnancy is very high without increasing the risk of renal functional decline. Although numbers of patients were small, this finding is consistent with a report from Pittsburgh that followed patients over a 2-year period to determine if pregnancy accelerated progression of diabetic complications [82].

However, in diabetic women with more severe disease, outcomes in pregnancy may be significantly more variable. Biesenbach et al. reported more rapid progression of renal failure related to pregnancy in five women, four of whom had significant disease with creatinine clearance less than 80 mL/min, proteinuria greater than 2 g/24 h, and hypertension prior to pregnancy. They attributed the advanced progression of the kidney disease to increased hypertension in the third trimester [83]. In contrast, Mackie et al. reported outcomes in a series of 17 women, six of whom had a mean serum creatinine of 1.8, while the remaining women had proteinuria with preserved renal function. The mean gestational age was 31 weeks in the former group and 36 in the latter with only one neonatal death. They found no long-term effect on maternal renal function and concluded that their favorable outcomes were largely due to improved neonatal care [84].

In a larger series from Germany, Kimmerle et al. described outcomes in 40 pregnancies in 22 women with diabetic nephropathy and compared outcomes to 110 pregnancies in 91 women at their center who were diabetic without nephropathy. Four pregnancies were terminated early because of worsening renal function and severe hypertension. Of the remaining pregnancies, there was no maternal mortality but early delivery occurred in 34 % and one-fourth of newborns had respiratory distress, complications not seen in diabetics with normal kidney function. Proteinuria increased and reached the nephrotic range in 53 % of pregnancies. While pregnancy did not seem to accelerate the progression of kidney disease, those women with more significant proteinuria or kidney dysfunction when they became pregnant appear to be at greater risk for increased morbidity [85]. Gordon et al. followed 46 pregnancies in 45 women at their center in Columbus, Ohio, and while perinatal survival was 100 %, the risk of early delivery was higher in women with initial serum creatinine greater than 1.5 mg/dL, or more than 3 g proteinuria/24 h. More than half their patients developed preeclampsia and in over one-third, the creatinine clearance decreased more than 15 %. In those women in whom follow-up was available for a mean of 2.8 years, renal functional decline was greater for those women with initial creatinine clearance less than 90 mL/min and proteinuria greater than 1 g/day and almost one-fourth of these women continued to have protein excretion greater than 3 g/24 h [86].

In a more recent study of pregnancy in women with diabetic nephropathy, Nielsen and colleagues in Copenhagen followed 117 pregnant women with type 1 diabetes, ten of whom had microalbuminuria and seven had clinical diabetic nephropathy (serum creatinine 0.5–1.1 and urinary albumin excretion rate 450–3,290 mg/24 h). They used an aggressive approach to antihypertensive therapy so that half the patients with microalbuminuria and all patients with diabetic nephropathy received antihypertensive therapy. They reduced the rates of preeclampsia and preterm delivery in women with microalbuminuria resulting in outcomes similar to normoalbuminuric diabetic women. Women with diabetic nephropathy had higher birth weights and later gestational ages, but still delivered early with smaller infants compared to other groups. Three of seven (43 %) women with diabetic nephropathy had preeclampsia, compared to 7 % of the normoalbuminuric patients and none of those with microalbuminuria. The authors concluded that early antihypertensive therapy and strict metabolic control improved pregnancy outcomes [74, 87].

Given these data, one should anticipate that women with diabetic nephropathy are very likely to develop increasing amounts of proteinuria. Diabetics with significant proteinuria may be at increased risk for thrombotic complications and guidelines published by the Royal College of Obstetrics and Gynecology recommend considering the use of thromboprophylaxis for proteinuria >5 g/day [8]. These women are also at risk for the development of preeclampsia. A Cochrane review on the use of antiplatelet agents to prevent preeclampsia concluded that low-dose antiplatelet agents significantly reduced the risk of preeclampsia in high-risk women compared to women at moderate risk [88]. They also concluded that antiplatelet agents, primarily low-dose aspirin, offer moderate benefit. This review however did not focus on diabetic women. Antiplatelet agents were also associated with lower rates of small for gestational age babies, preterm delivery, and fetal or neonatal deaths. Therefore one should strongly consider the use of low-dose aspirin in all women with diabetic nephropathy, particularly those who have reduced glomerular filtration rates and/or proteinuria and are therefore at higher risk for preeclampsia.

The risk of developing worsening renal function however may depend to a great extent on the level of prepartum renal function, with a significant risk of preeclampsia and preterm delivery in all women with clinical diabetic nephropathy. Despite these challenges, the likelihood of a viable neonate is very high. The changes in renal function and worsening proteinuria are consistent with those seen in most pregnant women with other chronic renal diseases, and in most patients, proteinuria improves postpartum, often to baseline levels, as does blood pressure and renal function. The importance of both strict blood pressure and glucose control in achieving successful pregnancies has been emphasized by many investigators [8, 25–29, 81, 86, 87]. Intensive glycemic control however carries the risk of maternal hypoglycemia which can result in impaired glucose counter-regulatory mechanisms. In several studies, an association between maternal hypoglycemia and fetal embryopathy was not established; however, the risk of a teratogenic effect of hypoglycemia in early pregnancy remains unanswered [89]. While counseling individual patients can be challenging, making sure that patients are aware of the potential problems, based on their degree of pre-pregnancy proteinuria and renal function, is essential. It is also important that all physicians involved in the care of women with diabetic nephropathy have the appropriate training and background to provide appropriate supportive and expectant care throughout pregnancy and that they communicate and work effectively as a team to achieve the best outcomes.

Does Pregnancy Accelerate Kidney Disease in Women with Underlying Diabetic Nephropathy?

There has long been concern regarding whether or not pregnancy in diabetic women accelerates diabetic nephropathy and can contribute to earlier development of ESRD. The 11 pregnancies complicated by mild-to-moderate diabetic nephropathy that were described by Reece et al. did not seem to have acceleration of the rate of decline in renal function, despite that fact that all of these patients were hypertensive and had increased proteinuria during pregnancy. Their mean serum creatinine just prior to conception (1.3 ± 0.5 mg/dL) and the last follow-up value (1.2 ± 0.3 mg/dL) were not significantly different. The observed rate of decline in renal function appeared to be consistent with the expected natural course of diabetic nephropathy in the absence of pregnancy [80]. In a series from the University of Cincinnati, Miodovnik et al. reviewed outcomes of 182 pregnant women from their diabetes-in-pregnancy trial, 46 of whom had nephropathy with a minimum of 3-year outcome data. They concluded that while a substantial proportion of these women will eventually develop ESRD, this risk was not attributable to pregnancy and they could not identify significant risk factors for the development of ESRD. As in other studies, women with diabetic nephropathy did however have statistically higher incidences of preterm delivery, hypertension, and preeclampsia than those women without nephropathy [90].

Reece et al., in 1998, reviewed the world literature of pregnancy in women with diabetic nephropathy from 1981 to 1996 and reported the outcomes in 315 patients from this survey [80]. Chronic hypertension was present in 42 % of women, with 60 % becoming hypertensive by the third trimester. Proteinuria and mean arterial pressure significantly increased from the first to the third trimester, and preeclampsia was reported in 41 % of pregnancies. There was an overall perinatal mortality of 5 % with preterm delivery in 22 % and IUGR in 15 %. They noted that both gestational age and birth weight were significantly correlated with first- and third-trimester renal function and third-trimester proteinuria and blood pressure. Though 17 % of the 185 patients available for long-term follow-up (mean 35 months) developed ESRD the authors concluded that pregnancy did not appear to accelerate renal functional deterioration. While many women had transient worsening of renal function, they did note a small, but significant, increase in proteinuria postpartum. They also noted that improved perinatal care contributed to a fetal survival rate of 95 % [81].

Dunne et al. retrospectively reviewed 21 pregnancies in 18 women with diabetic nephropathy, categorized as mild, moderate, or severe based on a serum creatinine of less than 1.1, 1.1–1.7, and greater than 1.7 mg/dL, respectively. The authors did not stratify outcome related to renal function and although there was a 100 % live birth rate, there was a higher rate of neonatal mortality, perinatal mortality, and congenital malformations than a matched population. In addition, there was a significant risk of increased proteinuria and hypertension, though after a 48-month follow-up there was no deterioration of renal function [36]. In 2002, Rossing et al. reported their results from a long-term observational case–control study from Denmark of all diabetics from 1970 to 1989 with at least 10 years of follow-up, and compared the progression of kidney disease in 26 women who became pregnant after the diagnosis of diabetic nephropathy with 67 diabetic women without nephropathy who became pregnant. They compared the slopes of 1/serum creatinine over time between the two groups and found no difference in progression of renal deterioration related to pregnancy. They described a lower rate of functional renal decline, which they attributed to aggressive antihypertensive therapy. Of note, the mean serum creatinine at onset of nephropathy was 0.9 mg/dL with mean proteinuria of 597 mg/24 h and only three women had an elevated serum creatinine at the onset of pregnancy. In women with diabetic nephropathy, proteinuria and hypertension were common and one-third of these women either died or reached ESRD after 10 years. However, the authors concluded that the prognosis for a successful pregnancy was high if renal function was well preserved at the onset of pregnancy [91]. In a recent prospective observational study from Brazil, Young and colleagues followed 43 pregnant women with diabetes, 11 of whom had early diabetic nephropathy. The mean serum creatinine of the women with nephropathy was 0.8 mg/dL with a mean urinary albumin excretion rate of 119 mg/24 h. Though the women with nephropathy had a statistically higher rate of preterm delivery, preeclampsia, and small for gestational age births, the authors concluded that pregnancy was not associated with the development or progression of diabetic nephropathy in women with mild renal dysfunction [92].

While the risks of preeclampsia, preterm delivery, and small for gestational age babies are increased in diabetic women with mild diabetic nephropathy, there does not appear to be an increased risk for accelerating the progression of renal failure when compared to diabetic women with either microalbuminuria or no kidney disease. This does not appear to be true for diabetic women with more significant kidney disease.

Biesenbach et al. described four of five female patients with type 2 diabetes mellitus with preexisting impaired renal function (creatinine clearance less than 80 mL/min), significant proteinuria (greater than 2 g/24 h urine), and hypertension who had a further decline in renal function during pregnancy. The mean decline of the glomerular filtration rate was 1.8 mL/min per month during pregnancy and 1.4 mL/min per month postpartum until the start of dialysis treatment. They suggested that the difference in the progression of diabetic nephropathy during and after pregnancy was due to increased hypertension during pregnancy, particularly in the third trimester, despite an intensified antihypertensive therapy. They concluded that pregnancy in these patients resulted in an earlier requirement for renal replacement therapy than would have been expected without pregnancy [83]. In another series of women with moderate-to-severe diabetic nephropathy, defined as a serum creatinine >1.4 mg/dL, Purdy et al. followed 11 women to determine if pregnancy had an affect on long-term (35–138 months) renal outcome and compared them to pregnancies in diabetic women without nephropathy. Five of these women had permanent deterioration of renal function that was greater than the predicted progression of disease and reached ESRD less than 2 years postpartum. Preeclampsia occurred in three patients. One-fourth of these women had transient reduction in renal function; one-fourth had no change. Consistent with previous reports, preterm delivery and IUGR rates were high in all of the women. The authors concluded there was a greater than 40 % risk of progression of diabetic nephropathy attributable to pregnancy [93]. In a retrospective review of 36 Pakistani women with moderate-to-severe diabetic nephropathy (mean serum creatinine 1.8 mg/dL, all of whom had diabetic retinopathy), Irfan also reported increased progression of kidney disease [94]. Proteinuria increased in 79 %, hypertension worsened in 73 %, and renal function transiently deteriorated in 27 % with 45 % showing a permanent decline. These patients were compared to an equal number of nonpregnant diabetic women with similar renal dysfunction. The authors concluded that in women with diabetic nephropathy, pregnancy was associated with a >40 % risk of increased progression of renal failure.

In summary, women with diabetic nephropathy have a significantly increased risk of preeclampsia and are more likely to experience preterm delivery and IUGR. Increased proteinuria, hypertension, and transient reductions in renal function are common. However, in women with either microalbuminuria or mild renal disease, there does not appear to be an adverse long-term effect on renal function. Pregnancy in women with moderate or more severe diabetic nephropathy is much more likely to accelerate the progression of renal disease. Aggressive treatment of hypertension and hyperglycemia may reduce these risks and are particularly important in the management of pregnancy in women with diabetic nephropathy.

Pregnancy in Diabetic Transplant Patients

Pregnancy in diabetic kidney and kidney–pancreas transplant recipients provides additional challenges in management and care. These women are particularly in need of both preconception counseling and care by those with experience in kidney and kidney–pancreas transplantation. Patients must be counseled regarding not only maternal and fetal risks but also risks related to allograft rejection or failure. Recommendations for pregnancy in renal transplant recipients include excellent and stable graft function, minimal or no proteinuria, well-controlled hypertension on few if any antihypertensives, and discontinuation of both mycophenolate mofetil and rapamycin prior to conception [95]. While outcomes are very good when these guidelines are followed, there is still a higher rate of preterm delivery, low birth weight, and preeclampsia in this population [96–98]. There is a limited but growing body of literature on post-transplant outcomes in diabetic transplant recipients [8, 99, 100]. A 1998 report from the International Pancreas Transplant Registry described outcomes of 19 pregnancies in 17 women. There was the loss of one pancreas transplant due to acute rejection following delivery, and the loss of one kidney transplant 3 months following delivery [99]. While the overall outcomes of pregnancy in women with combined kidney–pancreas transplant are good, a higher incidence of infections and graft loss has been reported [100]. Diabetic transplant recipients who consider pregnancy must therefore be carefully monitored for appropriate immunosuppressive therapy, antihypertensive therapy, and graft function.

Conclusion

How can this reviewed literature be applied to individual diabetic women seeking guidance, ideally, before pregnancy and but also during pregnancy? All pregnant women with diabetic nephropathy have a higher risk of preterm delivery, preeclampsia, and small for gestational age births though this risk may be minimized by excellent glycemic and blood pressure control. Women with preclinical or mild diabetic nephropathy with only microalbuminuria or minimal proteinuria and well-preserved glomerular filtration rate, and normal or only minimally elevated blood pressure may have transient increases in proteinuria and blood pressure. These women do not have significant progression of their renal failure, but in women with moderate diabetic nephropathy and lower creatinine clearances prior to conception renal function may significantly worsen during and after pregnancy without complete recovery [93, 94].

This review provides guidelines for counseling women with diabetes who are considering pregnancy. While all of these women face similar risks and challenges, differences exist between those with microalbuminuria and those with overt proteinuria and/or decreased renal function. Similar risks exist for those women who present already pregnant. Aggressive blood pressure and glycemic control to reduce the risk of preeclampsia and other complications is an essential element in the care of all these women. Aspirin therapy should also be considered in these patients to reduce the risk of preeclampsia. Central to this process is a knowledgeable team of physicians who effectively communicate with each other regarding all aspects of care. Sharing information across disciplines and if necessary, institutions, is particularly important for these patients where input from each team member is necessary to maximize the likelihood of successful fetal and maternal outcomes.

References

1. U.S. Renal Data System, USRDS 2009. Annual data report: atlas of end-stage renal disease in the United States. Bethesda, MD: National Institutes of Health, National Institute of Diabetes and Digestive and Kidney Diseases; 2009.
2. Cowie CC, Rust KF, Byrd-Holt DD, Eberhardt MS, Flegal KM, Engelgau MM, Saydah SH, Williams DE, Geiss LS, Gregg EW. Prevalence of diabetes, impaired fasting glucose, and impaired glucose tolerance in U.S. adults. The Third National Health and Nutrition Examination Survey, 1988–1994. Diabetes Care. 2006;29(6):1263–8.
3. Jovanovic L, Pettitt DJ. Gestational diabetes mellitus. JAMA. 2001;286(20):2516–8.
4. Ferrara A. Increasing prevalence of gestational diabetes mellitus a public health perspective. Diabetes Care. 2007;30:S141–6.
5. White P. In: Joslin EP, Root HF, White P, Marble A, editors. The treatment of diabetes mellitus. 9th ed. London: Kimpton; 1952.
6. Clayton SG. The pregnant diabetic; a report on 200 cases. J Obstet Gynaecol Br Emp. 1956;63(4):532–41.
7. Kelsey HA. Pregnancy associated with diabetic nephropathy. J Obstet Gynaecol Br Emp. 1957;64(5):735–7.
8. National Institute for Health and Clinical Excellence. Diabetes in pregnancy: management of diabetes and its complications from pre-conception to the postnatal period. London: NICE; 2008.
9. Hyperglycemia and Adverse Pregnancy Outcome (HAPO) Study Cooperative Research Group. Hyperglycemia and adverse pregnancy outcomes. N Engl J Med. 2008;358(19):1991–2002.
10. Taylor R, Lee C, Kyne-Grzebalski D, Marshall SM, Davison JM. Clinical outcomes of pregnancy in women with type 1 diabetes. Obstet Gynecol. 2002;99(4):537–41.
11. Murphy HR, Steel SA, Roland JM, Morris D, Ball V, Campbell PJ, Temple RC, East Anglia Study Group for Improving Pregnancy Outcomes in Women with Diabetes (EASIPOD). Obstetric and perinatal outcomes in pregnancies complicated by type 1 and type 2 diabetes: influences of glycaemic control, obesity and social disadvantage. Diabet Med. 2011;28(9):1060–7.
12. Krane NK, Hamrahian M. Pregnancy: kidney diseases and hypertension. Am J Kidney Dis. 2007;49(2):336–45.
13. Imbasciati E, Ponticelli C. Pregnancy and renal disease: predictors for fetal and maternal outcome. Am J Nephrol. 1991;11: 353–62.
14. Imbasciati E, Gregorini G, Cabiddu G, Cammaro L, Ambroso G, Del Giudice A, Ravani P. Pregnancy in CKD stages 3 to 5: fetal and maternal outcomes. Am J Kidney Dis. 2007;49(6):753–62.
15. Sunderji S, Gaziano E, Wothe D, Rogers LC, Sibai B, Karumanchi SA, Hodges-Savola C. Automated assays for sVEGF R1 and PlGF as an aid in the diagnosis of preterm preeclampsia: a prospective clinical study. Am J Obstet Gynecol. 2010;202(1):40.e1–7.
16. Rolfo A, Attini R, Nuzzo AM, Piazzese A, Parisi S, Ferraresi M, Todros T, Piccoli GB. Chronic kidney disease may be differentially diagnosed from preeclampsia by serum biomarkers. Kidney Int. 2013;83(1):177–81.
17. Mogensen CE, Chachati A, Christensen CK, Close CF, Deckert T, Hommel E, Kastrup J, Lefebvre P, Mathiesen ER, Feldt-Rasmussen B, et al. Microalbuminuria: an early marker for renal involvement in diabetes. Uremia Invest. 1985–1986;9(2):85–95.
18. Molitch ME, DeFronzo RA, Franz MJ, Keane WF, Mogensen CE, Parving HH, Steffes MW. American Diabetes Association. Nephropathy in Diabetes. Diabetes Care. 2004;27 (Suppl 1):S79–83.
19. Cherney DZ, Scholey JW, Miller JA. Insights into the regulation of renal hemodynamic function in diabetic mellitus. Curr Diabetes Rev. 2008;4(4):280–90.
20. Anderson S, Vora JP. Current concepts of renal hemodynamics in diabetes. J Diabetes Complications. 1995;9(4):304–7.
21. Mishra R, Emancipator SN, Kern T, Simonson MS. High glucose evokes an intrinsic proapoptotic signaling pathway in mesangial cells. Kidney Int. 2005;67(1):82–93.
22. Bucala R, Vlassara H. Advanced glycosylation endproducts in diabetic renal disease: clinical measurement, pathophysiological significance, and prospects for pharmacological inhibition. Blood Purif. 1995;13(3–4):160–70.
23. Wolf G, Ziyadeh FN. Molecular mechanisms of diabetic renal hypertrophy. Kidney Int. 1999;56(2):393–405.
24. Benigni A, Gagliardini E, Tomasoni S, Abbate M, Ruggenenti P, Kalluri R, Remuzzi G. Selective impairment of gene expression and assembly of nephrin in human diabetic nephropathy. Kidney Int. 2004;65(6):2193–200.
25. The Diabetes Control Complications Trial Research Group. The effect of intensive treatment of diabetes on the development and progression of long-term complications in insulin-dependent diabetes mellitus. N Engl J Med. 1993;329(14):977–86.
26. EDIC Research Group. Retinopathy and nephropathy in patients with type 1 diabetes four years after a trial of intensive therapy. N Engl J Med. 2000;342(6):381–9.
27. The DCCT/EDIC Research Group. Intensive diabetes therapy and glomerular filtration rate in type 1 diabetes. N Engl J Med. 2000;342(6):381–9.

28. Ismail-Beigi F, Craven T, Banerji MA, Basile J, Calles J, Cohen RM, Cuddihy R, Cushman WC, Genuth S, Grimm Jr RH, Hamilton BP, Hoogwerf B, Karl D, Katz L, Krikorian A, O'Connor P, Pop-Busui R, Schubart U, Simmons D, Taylor H, Thomas A, Weiss D, Hramiak I, ACCORD Trial Group. Effect of intensive treatment of hyperglycaemia on microvascular outcomes in type 2 diabetes: an analysis of the ACCORD randomised trial. Lancet. 2010;376(9739):419–30.
29. Duckworth W, Abraira C, Moritz T, Reda D, Emanuele N, Reaven PD, Zieve FJ, Marks J, Davis SN, Hayward R, Warren SR, Goldman S, McCarren M, Vitek ME, Henderson WG, Huang GD, VADT Investigators. Glucose control and vascular complications in veterans with type 2 diabetes. N Engl J Med. 2009;360(2):129–39.
30. Lewis EJ, Hunsicker LG, Bain RP, Rohde RD. The effect of angiotensin-converting-enzyme inhibition on diabetic nephropathy. The Collaborative Study Group. N Engl J Med. 1993;329(20):1456–62.
31. Hirst JA, Taylor KS, Stevens RJ, Blacklock CL, Roberts NW, Pugh CW, Farmer AJ. The impact of renin–angiotensin–aldosterone system inhibitors on type 1 and type 2 diabetic patients with and without early diabetic nephropathy. Kidney Int. 2012;81(7):674–83.
32. Allen VM, Armson BA, Wilson RD, Blight C, Gagnon A, Johnson JA, Langlois S, Summers A, Wyatt P, Farine D, Armson BA, Crane J, Delisle MF, Keenan-Lindsay L, Morin V, Schneider CE, Van Aerde J, Society of Obstetricians and Gynecologists of Canada. Teratogenicity associated with pre-existing and gestational diabetes. J Obstet Gynaecol Can. 2007;29(11):927–44.
33. Kitzmiller JL, Block JM, Brown FM, Catalano PM, Conway DL, Coustan DR, Gunderson EP, Herman WH, Hoffman LD, Inturrisi M, Jovanovic LB, Kjos SI, Knopp RH, Montoro MN, Ogata ES, Paramsothy P, Reader DM, Rosenn BM, Thomas AM, Kirkman MS. Managing preexisting diabetes for pregnancy: summary of evidence and consensus recommendations for care. Diabetes Care. 2008;31(5):1060–79.
34. Metzger SJ. Prepregnancy care: a shared responsibility. Diabetes Care. 2010;33(12):2713–5.
35. Vargas R, Repke JT, Ural SH. Type I diabetes mellitus and pregnancy. Rev Obstet Gynecol. 2010;3(3):92–100.
36. Dunne FP, Chowdhury TP, Hartland A, Smith T, Brydon PA, McConkey C, Nicholson HO. Pregnancy outcome in women with insulin-dependent diabetes mellitus complicated by nephropathy. Q J Med. 1999;92(8):451–4.
37. Quan A. Fetopathy associated with exposure to angiotensin converting enzyme inhibitors and angiotensin receptor antagonists. Early Hum Dev. 2006;82(1):23–8.
38. Godfry LM, Erramouspe J, Cleveland KW. Teratogenic risk of statins in pregnancy. Ann Pharmacother. 2012;46(10):1419–24.
39. Cooper WO, Hernandez-Diaz S, Arbogast PG, Dudley JA, Dyer S, Gideon PS, Hall K, Ray WA. Major congenital malformations after first-trimester exposure to ACE inhibitors. N Engl J Med. 2006;354(23):2443–51.
40. Bullo M, Tschumi S, Bucher BS, Bianchetti MG, Simonetti GD. Pregnancy outcome following exposure to angiotensin-converting enzyme inhibitors or angiotensin receptor antagonists novelty and significance a systematic review. Hypertension. 2012;60(2):444–50.
41. Report of the National High Blood Pressure Education Program Working Group on high blood pressure in pregnancy. Am J Obstet Gynecol. 2000;183(1):S1-22.
42. Abalos E, Duley L, Steyn DW, Henderson-Smart DJ. Antihypertensive drug therapy for mild to moderate hypertension during pregnancy. Cochrane Database Syst Rev. 2007;1:CD002252.
43. Rey E, LeLorier J, Burgess E, Lange IR, Leduc L. Report of the Canadian Hypertension Society Consensus Conference: 3. Pharmacologic treatment of hypertensive disorders in pregnancy. CMAJ. 1997;157(9):1245–54.
44. Brown MA, Hague WM, Higgins J, Lowe S, McCowan L, Oats J, Peek MJ, Rowan JA, Walters BNJ. The detection, investigation and management of hypertension in pregnancy: full consensus statement. Aust N Z J Obstet Gynaecol. 2000;40(2):139–55.
45. Hawthorne G. Maternal complications in diabetic pregnancy. Best Pract Res Clin Obstet Gynaecol. 2011;25(1):77–90.
46. Sullivan SD, Umans JG, Ratner R. Hypertension complicating diabetic pregnancies: pathophysiology, management, and controversies. J Clin Hypertens (Greenwich). 2011;13(4):275–84.
47. International Association of Diabetes and Pregnancy Study Groups Consensus Panel. International association of diabetes and pregnancy study groups recommendations on the diagnosis and classification of hyperglycemia in pregnancy. Diabetes Care. 2010;33(3):676–82.
48. Sacks DA, Hadden DR, Maresh M, Deerochanawong C, Dyer AR, Metzger BE, Lowe LP, Coustan DR, Hod M, Oats JJ, Persson B, Trimble ER, HAPO Study Cooperative Research Group. Frequency of gestational diabetes mellitus at collaborating centers based on IADPSG consensus panel-recommend criteria: the Hyperglycemia and Adverse Pregnancy Outcome (HAPO) Study. Diabetes Care. 2012;35(3):526–8.
49. Anna V, van der Ploeg HP, Cheung NW, Huxley RR, Bauman AE. Sociodemographic correlates of the increasing trend in prevalence of gestational diabetes mellitus in a large population of women between 1995 and 2008. Diabetes Care. 2008;31(12):2288–93.
50. HAPO Study Cooperative Research Group. The Hyperglycemia and Adverse Pregnancy Outcome (HAPO) Study. Int J Gynaecol Obstet. 2002;78(1):69–77.
51. Blank A, Grave GD, Metzger BE. Effects of gestational diabetes on perinatal morbidity reassessed. Report of the international workshop on adverse perinatal outcomes of gestational diabetes mellitus, December 3–4, 1992. Diabetes Care. 1995;18(1):127–9.
52. Landon MB, Spong CY, Thom E, Carpenter MW, Ramin SM, Casey B, Wapner RJ, Varner MW, Rouse DJ, Thorp Jr JM, Sciscione A, Catalano P, Harper M, Saade G, Lain KY, Sorokin Y, Peaceman AM, Tolosa JE, Anderson GB, Eunice Kennedy Shriver National Institute of Child Health and Human Development Maternal-Fetal Medicine Units Network. A multicenter, randomized trial of treatment for mild gestational diabetes. N Engl J Med. 2009;361(14):1339–48.
53. Crowther CA, Hiller JE, Moss JR, McPhee AJ, Jeffries WS, Robinson JS, Australian Carbohydrate Intolerance Study in Pregnant Women (ACHOIS) Trial Group. Effect of treatment of gestational diabetes mellitus on pregnancy outcomes. N Engl J Med. 2005;352(24):2477–86.
54. Jovanovic-Peterson L, Durak EP, Peterson CM. Randomized trial of diet versus diet plus cardiovascular conditioning on glucose levels in gestational diabetes. Am J Obstet Gynecol. 1989;161(2):415–9.
55. Franz MJ, Bantle JP, Beebe CA, Brunzell JD, Chiasson JL, Garg A, Holzmeister LA, Hoogwerf B, Mayer-Davis E, Mooradian AD, Purnell JQ, Wheeler M, American Diabetes Association. Evidence-based nutrition principles and recommendations for the treatment and prevention of diabetes and related complications. Diabetes Care. 2003;26 Suppl 1:S51–61.
56. Cheng YW, Chung JH, Kurbisch-Block I, Inturrisi M, Shafer S, Caughey AB. Gestational weight gain and gestational diabetes mellitus: perinatal outcomes. Obstet Gynecol. 2008;112(5):1015–22.
57. Hedderson MM, Weiss NS, Sacks DA, Pettitt DJ, Selby JV, Quesenberry CP, Ferrara A. Pregnancy weight gain and risk of neonatal complications: macrosomia, hypoglycemia, and hyperbilirubinemia. Obstet Gynecol. 2006;108(5):1153–61.
58. Stotland NE, Hopkins LM, Caughey AB. Gestational weight gain, macrosomia, and risk of cesarean birth in nondiabetic nulliparas. Obstet Gynecol. 2004;104(4):671–7.
59. Rhodes JC, Schoendorf KC, Parker JD. Contribution of excess weight gain during pregnancy and macrosomia to the cesarean delivery rate, 1990–2000. Pediatrics. 2003;111(5 Pt 2):1181–5.
60. Cundy T, Gamble G, Manuel A, Townend K, Roberts A. Determinants of birth-weight in women with established and gestational diabetes. Aust N Z J Obstet Gynaecol. 1993;33(3):249–54.
61. Nachum Z, Ben-Shlomo I, Weiner E, Shalev E. Twice daily versus four times daily insulin dose regimens for diabetes in pregnancy: randomised controlled trial. BMJ. 1999;319(7219):1223–7.

62. Getahun D, Fassett MJ, Jacobsen SJ. Gestational diabetes: risk of recurrence in subsequent pregnancies. Am J Obstet Gynecol. 2010;203(5):467.e1–6.
63. Bellamy L, Casas JP, Hingorani AD, Williams D. Type 2 diabetes mellitus after gestational diabetes: a systematic review and meta-analysis. Lancet. 2009;373(9677):1773–9.
64. Shah BR, Retnakaran R, Booth GL. Increased risk of cardiovascular disease in young women following gestational diabetes mellitus. Diabetes Care. 2008;31(8):1668–9.
65. Committee on Obstetric Practice. ACOG Committee Opinion No. 435: postpartum screening for abnormal glucose tolerance in women who had gestational diabetes mellitus. Obstet Gynecol. 2009;113(6):1419–21.
66. Nicholson W, Baptiste-Roberts K. Oral hypoglycaemic agents during pregnancy: the evidence for effectiveness and safety. Best Pract Res Clin Obstet Gynaecol. 2011;25(1):51–63.
67. Omer S, Shan J, Mulay S, Varma DR, Mulay S. Augmentation of diabetes-associated renal hyperfiltration and nitric oxide production by pregnancy in rats. J Endocrinol. 1999;161(1): 15–23.
68. Sturgiss SN, Dunlop W, Davison JM. Renal haemodynamics and tubular function in human pregnancy. Baillieres Clin Obstet Gynaecol. 1994;8(2):209–34.
69. Combs CA, Rosenn B, Kitzmiller JL, Khoury JC, Wheeler BC, Miodovnik M. Early-pregnancy proteinuria in diabetes related to preeclampsia. Obstet Gynecol. 1993;82(5):802–7.
70. Ekbum P, Damm P, Feldt-Rasmussen B, Feldt-Rasmussen U, Molvig J, Mathiesen ER. Pregnancy outcomes in type I diabetic women with microalbuminuria. Diabetes Care. 2001;24(10):1739–44.
71. Biesenbach G, Zasgornik J, Stoger H, Grafinger P, Hubmann R, Kaiser W, Janko O, Stuby Y. Abnormal increases in urinary albumin excretion during pregnancy in IDDM women with preexisting albuminuria. Diabetologia. 1994;37(9):905–10.
72. Ekbom P, The Copenhagen Pre-eclampsia in Diabetic Pregnancy Study Group. Pre-pregnancy microalbuminuria predicts pre-eclampsia in insulin-dependent diabetes mellitus. Lancet. 1999;353(9150):377.
73. Jensen DM, Damm P, Ovesen P, Mølsted-Pedersen L, Beck-Nielsen H, Westergaard JG, Moeller M, Mathiesen ER. Microalbuminuria, preeclampsia, and preterm delivery in pregnant women with type 1 diabetes: results from a nationwide Danish study. Diabetes Care. 2010;33(1):90–4.
74. Nielsen LR, Damm P, Mathiesen ER. Improved pregnancy outcome in type 1 diabetic women with microalbuminuria or diabetic nephropathy: effect of intensified antihypertensive therapy? Diabetes Care. 2009;32(1):38–44.
75. Chaturvedi N, Stephenson JM, Fuller JH, EURODIAB IDDM Complications Study Group. The relationship between pregnancy and long-term maternal complications in the EURODIAB IDDM complications study. Diabet Med. 1995;12(6):494–9.
76. Hare JW, White P. Pregnancy in diabetes complicated by vascular disease. Diabetes. 1977;26(10):953–5.
77. Grenfell A, Brudenell JM, Doddridge MC, Watkins PJ. Pregnancy in diabetic women who have proteinuria. Q J Med. 1986;59(228): 379–86.
78. Kitzmiller JL, Brown ER, Phillippe M, Stark AR, Acker D, Kaldany A, Singh S, Hare JW. Diabetic nephropathy and perinatal outcome. Am J Obstet Gynecol. 1981;141(7):741–51.
79. Reece EA, Coustan DR, Hayslett JP, Holford T, Coulehan J, O'Connor TZ, Hobbins JC. Diabetic nephropathy: pregnancy performance and fetomaternal outcome. Am J Obstet Gynecol. 1988;159(1):56–66.
80. Reece EA, Winn HN, Hayslett JP, Coulehan J, Wan M, Hobbins JC. Does pregnancy alter the rate of progression of diabetic nephropathy? Am J Perinatol. 1990;7(2):193–7.
81. Reece EA, Leguizamon G, Homko C. Stringent controls in diabetic nephropathy associated with optimization of pregnancy outcomes. J Matern Fetal Med. 1998;7(4):213–6.
82. Hemachandra A, Ellis D, Lloyd CE, Orchard TJ. The influence of pregnancy on IDDM complications. Diabetes Care. 1995;18(7):950–4.
83. Biesenbach G, Stoger H, Zasgornik J. Influence of pregnancy on progression of diabetic nephropathy and subsequent requirement of renal replacement therapy in female type I diabetic patients with impaired renal function. Nephrol Dial Transplant. 1992;7(2):105–9.
84. Mackie AD, Doddridge MC, Gamsu HR, Brudenell JM, Nicolaides KH, Drury PL. Outcome of pregnancy in patients with insulin-dependent diabetes mellitus and nephropathy with moderate renal impairment. Diabet Med. 1996;13(1):90–6.
85. Kimmerle R, Za R-P, Cupisti S, Somville T, Bender R, Pawlowski B, Berger M. Pregnancies in women with diabetic nephropathy: long-term outcome for mother and child. Diabetologia. 1995;38(2):227–35.
86. Gordon M, Landon MB, Samuels P, Hissrich S, Gabbe SG. Perinatal outcome and long-term follow-associated with modern management of diabetic nephropathy. Obstet Gynecol. 1996;87(3):401–9.
87. Nielsen LR, Muller C, Damm P, Mathiesen ER. Reduced prevalence of early preterm delivery in women with type 1 diabetes and microalbuminuria: possible effect of early antihypertensive treatment during pregnancy. Diabet Med. 2006;23(4):426–31.
88. Duley L, Henerson-Smart DJ, Meher S, King JF. Antiplatelet agents for preventing pre-eclampsia and its complications. Cochrane Database Syst Rev. 2007;2:CD004659.
89. ter Braak EWMT, Evers IM, Erkelens DW, Vissar GHA. Maternal hypoglycemia during pregnancy in type 1 diabetes: maternal and fetal consequences. Diabetes Metab Res Rev. 2002;18(2):96–105.
90. Miodovnik M, Rosenn BM, Khoury JC, Grigsby JL, Siddiqi TA. Does pregnancy increase the risk for development and progression of diabetic nephropathy? Am J Obstet Gynecol. 1996;174(4):1180–9; discussion 1189–91.
91. Rossing K, Jacobsen E, Hommel E, Mathiesen A, Svenningsen A, Possing P, Parving H-H. Pregnancy and progression of diabetic nephropathy. Diabetologia. 2002;45(1):36–41.
92. Young EC, Pires MLE, Marques LPJ, de Oliveira JEP, Zajdenerg L. Effects of pregnancy on the onset and progression of diabetic nephropathy and of diabetic nephropathy on pregnancy outcomes. Diabetes Metab Syndr. 2011;5(3):137–42.
93. Purdy LP, Hantsch CE, Molitch ME, Metzger BE, Phelps RL, Dooley SL, Hou S. Effect of pregnancy on renal function in patients with moderate-to-severe diabetic renal insufficiency. Diabetes Care. 1996;19(10):1067–74.
94. Irfan S, Arain TM, Shaukat A, Shahid A. Effect of pregnancy on diabetic nephropathy and retinopathy. J Coll Physicians Surg Pak. 2004;14(2):75–8.
95. Armenti VT, Constantinescu S, Moritz MJ, Davison JM. Pregnancy after transplantation. Transplant Rev (Orlando). 2008;22(4):223–40.
96. Thompson BC, Kingdon EJ, Tuck SM, Fernando ON, Sweny P. Pregnancy in renal transplant recipients: the Royal Free Hospital experience. Q J Med. 2003;96(11):837–44.
97. Coscia LA, Constantinescu S, Moritz MJ, Radomski JS, Gaughan WJ, McGrory CH, Armenti VT, National Transplantation Pregnancy Registry. Report from the National Transplantation Pregnancy Registry (NTPR): outcomes of pregnancy after transplantation. Clin Transpl. 2003;96(11):837–44.
98. Levidiotis V, Chang S, McDonald S. Pregnancy and maternal outcomes among kidney transplant recipients. J Am Soc Nephrol. 2009;20(11):2433–40.
99. Barrou BM, Gruessner AC, Sutherland DE, Gruessner RW. Pregnancy after pancreas transplantation in the cyclosporine era: report from the International Pancreas Transplant Registry. Transplantation. 1998;65(4):524–7.
100. Jain AB, Shapiro R, Scantlebury VP, Potdar S, Jordan ML, Flohr J, Marcos A, Fung JJ. Pregnancy after kidney and kidney-pancreas transplantation under tacrolimus: a single center's experience. Transplantation. 2004;77(6):897–902.

15 Transplantation: Kidney, Kidney–Pancreas Transplant

Rubin Zhang and Anil Paramesh

Transplant Immunology and Immunological Risk Assessment

MHC/HLA Molecules

When a foreign organ is transplanted into a nonidentical individual of the same species, the organ is called allograft. The immune response from recipient to allograft is termed alloimmune response, which is initiated by T-cell recognition of alloantigens (allorecognition) [1–3]. The strongest transplant antigens are coded by the major histocompatibility complex (MHC) genes. In humans, the MHC molecules are called human leukocyte antigens (HLA) and the genetic region is located on the short arm of chromosome 6. Each parent provides a haplotype (a linked set of MHC genes) to each offspring as mendelian codominant inheritance. There are two classes of MHC or HLA molecules. Class I molecules (HLA-A, -B, and -C) are composed of a polymorphic heavy chain (a chain, 44 kDa) and a nonpolymorphic light chain (ß2 microglobulin, 12 kDa). They are expressed on all nucleated cells, and generally present endogenous small antigens (typically 9–11 amino acids), such as viruses and self-protein fragments, in the context of self-MHC to CD8+ T lymphocytes. Class II molecules (HLA-DP, -DQ, and -DR) are composed of polymorphic a chain (35 kDa) and ß chain (31 kDa). They are constitutively expressed only on professional antigen-presenting cells (APC), including dendritic cells, macrophages, and B-cell. But their expression may be upregulated on epithelial and vascular endothelial cells after exposure to pro-inflammatory cytokines. Class II molecules present relatively larger antigens (12–28 amino acids) derived from extracellular proteins to CD4+ T cells [1–4]. The degree of HLA mismatching between donor and recipient plays a role in determining the risk of chronic rejection and graft loss. HLA-A, -B, and -DR (three pairs, six antigens) are traditionally used for typing and matching before kidney and/or pancreas transplant. HLA-Cw, -DP, and -DQ are now increasingly typed and used in many transplant centers. The long-term graft survival is best in HLA-identical living-related kidney transplants. The major impact comes from the match of the DR antigen, and the order of importance for HLA match is DR>B>A [1, 3, 4].

Non-HLA Antigens/Antibodies

Acute and chronic graft rejection can occur in HLA-identical sibling transplants, indicating the presence of immune response to non-HLA antigens. There are several non-HLA antigens and their antibodies derived from either alloimmunity or autoimmunity have been reported [5, 6].

ABO blood group antigens are not only expressed on red blood cells but they are also expressed on vascular endothelial cells and other cells. ABO incompatible organ transplant causes hyperacute rejection due to the presence of the preformed hemagglutinin A and/or B antibody. ABO compatibility between donor and recipient are essential for organ transplant, similar to red blood cell transfusion. Desensitization protocol to remove the preformed hemagglutinin A and/or B from recipient circulation has been used for ABO incompatible kidney transplant [1, 7]. The rhesus (Rh) factor and other red cell antigens are not that relevant to organ transplant as they are not expressed on endothelium.

Minor histocompatibility antigens (*MiHA*) are small endogenous peptides that occupy the antigen-binding site of donor MHC molecules. They are generally recognized by CD8+ cytotoxic T cells in the context of self-MHC, thus

R. Zhang (✉)
Department of Medicine, Tulane University School of Medicine, 1430 Tulane Avenue, SL-45, New Orleans, LA 70112, USA
e-mail: rzhang@tulane.edu

A. Paramesh
Departments of Surgery and Urology, Tulane Abdominal Transplant Institute, Tulane University School of Medicine, New Orleans, LA, USA

E.V. Lerma and V. Batuman (eds.), *Diabetes and Kidney Disease*,
DOI 10.1007/978-1-4939-0793-9_15, © Springer Science+Business Media New York 2014

causing graft rejection. In bone marrow transplant, MiHA play an important role in graft-versus-host (GVH) disease in patients who received HLA-matched cells [8]. H-Y MiHA is encoded by the Y chromosome in males and can induce alloimmune response when a male organ is transplanted into a female recipient [9]. MICA and MICB (MHC class 1-related chain A and B) are also expressed on endothelial cells. Antibodies against MICA and/or MICB can cause antibody-mediated rejection (AMR) and graft loss [10].

Other reported antibodies causing graft rejection include anti-angiotensin-2 receptor, anti-glutathione S-transferase T1, and anti-endothelial antibodies [11–13]. Anti-endothelial antibody can be detected by using donor monocytes for crossmatch [13]. Some minor transplant antigens may come from mitochondrial proteins and enzymes. As our knowledge in transplant immunology advances, there will likely be more alloreactive and autoreactive antibodies to be discovered in the future.

Allorecognition Pathways

Allorecognition can occur by one of the three mechanisms referred to as direct, indirect, and semi-direct pathways [14–16]. In the direct pathway, recipient T cells recognize intact allogeneic HLAs expressed by donor cells, while in the indirect pathway, T cells recognize peptides derived from donor HLAs presented by recipient APC. In the semi-direct pathway, recipient dendritic cells or other APC acquire intact HLAs from donor cells and present them to recipient T cells. The direct and indirect pathways are well understood in organ transplantation, the semi-direct pathway is not known of clinical importance. The direct pathway is very important in the immediate post transplant period. Without appropriate immunosuppression, a strong and effective alloresponse would follow, which is primarily due to the high number of recipient T cells that will recognize the graft antigens and cause acute cellular rejection (ACR). While the indirect pathway of allorecognition may also participate in acute rejection (AR), it usually dominates in the late onset of rejection, especially the chronic rejection [14–16]. As long as the allograft is present in the host, the recipient APCs can pick up the alloantigen shed from graft and start alloimmune response. Therefore, maintenance immunosuppression is required for the lifetime of allograft to prevent late rejection and chronic rejection.

Three-Signal Model of T-Cell Activation

T-cell activation is the key process of allograft rejection. T cells recognize alloantigen through T-cell receptor (TCR). The initiation of intracellular signaling requires additional peptides known as CD3 complex, and the antigen-specific signal (signal 1) is transduced through the TCR-CD3 complex [1–3]. Two signals are needed for T-cell full activation. The second co-stimulatory signal depends on the receptor–ligand interactions between T cells and APCs (signal 2). Numerous co-stimulatory pathways have been described and blockage of these pathways can lead to antigen-specific inactivation or death of T cells [17–19]. The best studied ones are the CD28-B7 and CD154-CD40 pathways. CD28 and CD154 are expressed on T cells, and their ligands B7 and CD40 are expressed on APCs. CD28 has two ligands, B7-1 (CD80) and B7-2 (CD86). T cells also express cytotoxic T-lymphocyte-associated antigen-4 (CTLA-4), which is homologous to CD28 and has a higher affinity than CD28 to bind B7. However, when CTLA-4 binds B7 (both CD80 and CD86), it produces an inhibitory signal to terminate T-cell response. This unique action leads to the clinical development of a fusion protein CTLA-4-Ig (belatacept) as a novel immunosuppressive medication [19]. CD154-CD40 blockages have also been shown to prevent allograft rejection in animal models, including anti-CD154 antibody and molecules that target CD40 [18].

The combination of signal 1 and 2 activates three downstream signal transduction pathways: the calcium-calcineurin pathway, the RAS-mitogen-activated protein (MAP) kinase pathway, and the IKK-nuclear factor kappa-beta (NF-kB) pathway. These three pathways further activate transcription factors including the nuclear factor of activated T cells (NFAT), activated protein-1 (AP-1), and NF-kB, respectively. Several new molecules and cytokines including CD25, CD154, IL-2, and IL-15 are subsequently expressed [1–3]. IL-2 and IL-15 deliver growth signals (signal 3) through the mammalian target-of-rapamycin (mTOR) pathway and phosphoinositide-3-kinase (PI-3K) pathway, which subsequently trigger the T-cell cycle and proliferation. The fully activated T cells undergo clonal expansion and produce a large number of cytokines and effector T cells, which eventually produce CD8+ T-cell mediated cytotoxicity, help macrophages-induced delayed type hypersensitivity (DTH) response (by CD4+ Th1), and help B cells for antibody production (by CD4+ Th2). A subset of activated T cells becomes the alloantigen-specific memory T cells [20, 21].

B Lymphocytes

B cells express clonally restricted antigen-specific receptors as immunoglobulins on their surfaces. When these receptors bind donor HLA antigen in the context of help from helper T cells (CD4+ Th2), B cells are activated. Then, they divide, differentiate, and become plasma cells to secret antibodies. Some activated B cells become memory B cells [22–24].

The helper T cells may help B-cell activation either through intimate membrane contact involving a variety of receptors and ligands (such as CD40:CD154) or through the secreted soluble cytokines (such as IL-4) [18, 23, 24]. These HLA antibodies bind antigens and can cause graft injury either by activating complement cascade (complement-dependent cytotoxicity, CDC), or via Fc receptor on NK cells, neutrophils, and eosinophils (antibody-dependent cellular cytotoxicity, ADCC) [1, 14]. In addition to antibody production, B cells are also APCs. B cells can present allograft-derived antigens to T cells for T cell activation through the indirect pathway of allorecognition [2–4].

Innate and Adaptive Immune Responses in Graft Rejection

Innate immunity refers to the nonspecific natural immune system that involves macrophages, neutrophils, NK cells, cytokines, toll-like receptors, and complement components [25]. Alloimmune is an adaptive immunity that involves recognition of alloantigen and confers antigen specificity and memory by T and B cells as discussed above. However, alloimmune response not only produces specific effector T cells and antibodies but also secretes chemokines and cytokines, which recruit components of the innate immune system, such as complement activation and leukocyte migration from the circulation into a site of inflammation [1–4]. On the other hand, ischemic injury of allograft initially activates the innate immune response, which leads to increased antigen presentation to T cells by up-regulating the expression of class II HLAs, adhesion molecules, and cytokines [2–4]. Therefore, the innate and adaptive immune responses are closely interrelated and both play important role in allograft rejection and rejection-associated tissue damage.

Sensitization and Panel Reactive Antibody

Human sensitization is defined by the presence of antibodies in the recipient's blood against a panel of selected HLA antigens representing donor population. It is reported as the percent panel reactive antibody (PRA). PRA estimates the likelihood of positive crossmatch to potential donors [1, 14]. The higher the PRA level, the lower the likelihood of receiving a compatible kidney, and the longer the waiting time on the kidney waitlist. Sensitization is caused by previous exposure to HLA antigens, usually through previous organ transplant, pregnancy, or blood transfusion. Particularly relevant is the exposure of women to their partner's HLA during pregnancy. This results in direct sensitization against the partner, potentially making the partner and/or their child an unsuitable donor. The percent PRA in an individual patient may vary from one testing date to another secondary to either a change in antibody titers, or a change in the usage of HLA antigens in the assay. The technology of PRA assay has been advanced from the initial CDC assay, then the enzyme-linked immunoabsorption (ELISA), to the current multiplexed particle-based flow cytometry (Luminex). Single antigen beads are increasingly used to characterize the preformed HLA antibodies before transplant as well as any de novo development of HLA antibodies (donor-specific antibodies, DSA) after transplant [1, 26].

Crossmatch and Donor-Specific Antibody

Solid phase-based ELISA or Luminex assay can detect and characterize the preformed HLA antibodies in an individual patient. The corresponding antigens are considered as unacceptable for that patient and are listed into the UNOS database. A patient will not be offered a kidney from the deceased donor who expresses an unacceptable HLA antigen (positive virtual crossmatch). Only those patients whose HLA antibodies are not donor directed will appear on the match run (negative virtual crossmatch). Such "virtual crossmatch" can improve efficiency of organ allocation by decreasing the risk of positive crossmatch before transplant [26]. When a potential donor is identified, a final crossmatch with fresh serum from recipient and lymphocytes from donor has to be performed to rule out any preformed DSA, which can produce hyperacute AMR. The final crossmatch must be negative to proceed with transplantation. The commonly used two tests are CDC crossmatch and flow cytometry crossmatch. The choice of crossmatch test remains a controversial issue. It is usually determined by individual transplant program according to center experience and availability.

T cells express HLA class I antigens only, while B cells express both HLA class I and class II antigens. Furthermore, B cells express HLA class I antigens at quantitatively greater level than on T cells. T-cell positive crossmatch is considered as true and significant sensitization with DSA against HLA class I antigens. T-cell negative/B-cell positive crossmatches may represent either HLA class II antibodies or low titers of HLA class I antibodies. T-cell positive/B-cell negative results are likely due to presence of non-HLA antibodies [1, 3].

Complement-dependent cytotoxicity (CDC) crossmatch. The donor lymphocytes (T cells, B cells, or mixed) are isolated from blood or lymph nodes, and placed in wells. The recipient serum is then added along with rabbit complement. The cytotoxicity is determined by counting the lyses of lymphocytes compared with a control. It is usually modified by addition of antihuman globulin to increase the sensitivity (AHG-CDC), as antihuman globulin can induce cross-linking of antibodies and increase the visual cytotoxicity. If the initial CDC crossmatch is positive, it will be repeated with the addition of dithiothreitol (DTT), which reduces the disulfide bonds of IgM if it is present. Initial positive and repeated DTT positive tests indicate the presence of DSA of IgG rather than IgM. IgM antibodies are generally not considered to be real sensitization. Transplantation should not proceed if there is evidence of a positive crossmatch secondary to a cytotoxic IgG anti-HLA antibody (DSA). However, there are various desensitization protocols that can be used to remove the preformed DSA to achieve negative final crossmatch for HLA incompatible transplants if a living donor is involved [27–31].

Flow cytometry crossmatch (FCXM). Donor T and B lymphocytes are isolated and mixed with recipient serum. A fluorescence-labeled antihuman IgG is then added. The cells bound any recipient antibodies are stained with fluorescence-labeled antihuman IgG, and cause the channel shifts (CS) in fluorescent intensity. FCXM is much more sensitive than CDC or AHG-CDC in detecting low level of antibodies. It does not depend on the complement activation of antibody; therefore, non-cytotoxic antibodies can also be detected. The significance of non-complement activating or non-cytotoxic antibodies in vivo is unclear. Single antigen bead (Luminex) can be used to further characterize any DSA presence and to determine if the DSA is responsible for the channel shift in the flow crossmatch [1–3].

Again, these two crossmatches differ in the degree of sensitivity. Conservative transplant program may choose sensitive FCXM, which will significantly reduce the incidence of post-transplant AMR. However, it may also be too sensitive in that clinically irrelevant antibodies are detected. Consequently, some viable transplant opportunities are potentially lost. Crossmatch test can also be performed with recipient's previous sera. The scenario of current sera negative, historical sera positive suggests previous antibodies may have waned in titer, but the specific memory B cells could rapidly expand and produce the antibodies when re-exposed to the specific alloantigen. Although this is not considered as a contraindication for transplantation, it does increase the risk of AMR after transplant. Close monitoring of DSA titer and more immunosuppression are usually recommended.

Immunosuppressive Therapy

Modern immunosuppressive protocol typically includes an induction therapy and a long-term maintenance. Antibody induction is recommended in patients with immunologic risk, but the choice of antibody remains controversial. In the USA, about 60 % of kidney transplant patients in the year of 2011 were given a T-cell depleting antibody induction, predominately the antithymocyte globulin (ATG). Other 40 % of patients received either IL-2 receptor antibody (IL-2R Ab) or no antibody induction [32]. Maintenance immunosuppression is required for the lifetime of functioning allograft to prevent rejection of transplanted kidney. It is generally accepted that more intensive immunosuppression is given initially and less immunosuppression is subsequently maintained to minimize the overall risk of infection and malignancy. A maintenance regimen typically consists of two of the four classes of drugs with or without glucocorticoids: (1) calcineurin inhibitor (CNI) (tacrolimus or cyclosporine), (2) antimetabolite (mycophenolate mofetil (MMF) or enteric-coated mycophenolate sodium), (3) mTOR inhibitor (sirolimus, or everolimus), and (4) costimulation blocker (belatacept). In the USA, the most popular maintenance either at beginning of transplant or at 1 year after transplant remains the combination of corticosteroid, mycophenolic acid (MFA), and tacrolimus [32].

Induction Antibody Preparations

OKT-3 is a murine monoclonal antibody against CD3 molecule. It binds to the TCR-associated CD3 glycoprotein, leading to initial activation and cytokine release, followed by blockade of function and T-cell depletion. It is associated with severe side effects, and ATG preparation was demonstrated to be superior than OKT-3 in decreasing the incidence of rejection and better tolerability [33–36]. The use of OKT-3 was subsequently decreased and led to cessation of its production in 2009.

Antithymocyte globulin (ATG). There are two forms of ATG that are polyclonal immunoglobulins from horses (ATGAM) or rabbits (thymoglobulin) immunized with human thymocytes. ATG binds to various cell surface markers, leads to complement-dependent lysis of lymphocytes. OKT-3, ATGAM, thymoglobulin, and alemtuzmab are often referred as lymphocyte-depleting antibodies, which are usually used in patients who have high immunological risk of rejection [33]. ATG use is associated with cytokine release syndrome, myelosuppression, and rarely anaphylactic reaction. Several studies found that thymoglobulin was more effective in preventing rejection and was associated with better graft survival than ATGAM [37–39]. The dose of thymoglobulin induction has ranged from 1 to 4 mg/kg/day for 3–10 days. Intraoperative administration of thymoglobulin was found to be associated with a lower incidence of delayed graft function (DGF) and shorter hospital stay [40]. Doses less than 3 mg/kg may not effectively prevent acute rejection (AR). Higher dose and longer duration of induction was associated with increased risk of infection and lymphoma. Therefore, the optimal dose of thymoglobulin induction might be a total of 6 mg/kg administered as 1.5 mg/kg/day in 3–5 days [41, 42].

IL-2 Receptor Antibody (*IL-2R Ab*). Daclizumab and basiliximab are the two IL-2R Abs. Daclizumab is a humanized antibody and basiliximab is a chimeric monoclonal antibody. Both bind to the alpha chain of IL-2 receptor (CD25) expressed on activated T lymphocytes. They prevent T cell proliferation without causing cell lysis and have minimal adverse effects. IL-2R Abs are also known as non-depleting antibodies, and frequently used in patients who have a low-to-moderate risk of rejection [43–46]. Basiliximab is administered as two doses within 4 days of transplantation, whereas daclizumab is administered as five doses over 8 weeks. This difference in convenience of administration led to more frequent use of basiliximab than daclizumab. Subsequently, Roche pharmaceuticals withdrew daclizumab from market in October 2008.

Alemtuzumab is a humanized anti-CD52 monoclonal antibody, which triggers antibody-dependent lysis of lymphocytes (both B and T cells), NK cells, and, to a lesser extent, of monocytes and macrophages. Alemtuzumab is FDA approved for treating B cell lymphomas. As an induction agent, it produces a profound depletion of lymphocytes and is associated with more frequent and severe adverse effects, such as neutropenia, thrombocytopenia, thyroid disease, autoimmune hemolytic anemia, and other autoimmune diseases [47–49]. It is hoped that alemtuzumab induction could permit patients to be maintained on unconventional strategy with less intensive immunosuppression, such as tacrolimus monotherapy [50], steroid-free [51], steroid- and CNI-free regimen [52].

Rituximab is a chimeric monoclonal Ab against CD20, which is expressed on the majority of B cells. It was first approved in 1997 for refractory B cell lymphomas and it is increasingly applied for autoimmune diseases. In the realm of kidney transplant, rituximab has been used in combination with plasmapheresis and IVIG to treat AMR, and to desensitize patients with preformed antibodies for ABO- and/or HLA incompatible kidney transplant [30, 53].

Considerations in Choosing Antibody Induction Therapy

Antibody selection should be guided by a comprehensive assessment of immunologic risk, patient comorbidities, financial burden, and the maintenance immunosuppressive regimen. Clinical trials comparing different antibody induction in various patient populations and with different maintenance immunosuppression are recently reviewed by the author [33]. The published data remain in line with the 2009 KDIGO guidelines [54]. Lymphocyte-depleting antibody is recommended for those with high immunologic risk as outlined in the 2009 KDIGO clinical practice guidelines (sensitized patient, presence of DSA, ABO incompatibility, high HLA mismatches, DGF, cold ischemia time >24 h, African American ethnicity, younger recipient age, older donor age), though it increases the risk of infection and malignancy [54]. For low or moderate risk patients, IL-2R Ab induction reduces the incidence of acute rejection and graft loss without much adverse effects, making its balance favorable in these patients [55–57]. IL-2R Ab induction should also be used in the high risk patients with other comorbidities (history of malignancy, viral infection with HIV, HBV, or HCV, hematological disorder of leucopenia or thrombocytopenia and elderly) that may preclude usage of lymphocyte-depleting antibody safely [58–60]. Many patients with very low risk (non-sensitized, Caucasian, Asian, well HLA-matched, living-related donor transplant) may be induced with intravenous steroids without using any antibody, as long as combined potent immunosuppressives are kept as maintenance. In these patients, benefits with antibody induction may be too small to outweigh its adverse effects and the financial cost [33, 54, 61]. Clinical comparison trials have not demonstrated any graft or patient survival benefit of using T-cell depleting Ab induction in patients with low immunological risk [33, 54]. Rituximab induction is useful in desensitization protocols for ABO and/or HLA incompatible transplants. Alemtuzumab induction might be more successful for adopting less intensive maintenance protocols. However, the long-term safety and efficacy of unconventional strategy remain to be determined.

Maintenance Immunosuppressive Drugs

Glucocorticoids have been used for preventing and treating graft rejection since the early 1960s. They have multiple actions. In addition to the nonspecific anti-inflammatory actions, glucocorticoids have critical immunosuppressive effect by blocking T-cell and APC-derived cytokine expression. Glucocorticoids bind to cytoplasmic receptor to form a complex, which translocates into the nucleus and binds to glucocorticoid response elements (GRE) in the promoter regions of cytokine genes. Glucocorticoids also inhibit the translocation of transcription factor AP-1 and NF-kB into the nucleus. Therefore, production of several cytokines (IL-1, 2, 3, 6, TNF-a, gamma-interferon) is inhibited [2, 62]. Large dose of glucocorticoids can be given in the perioperative period as induction therapy (methylprednisolone 250–500 mg IV), which is usually followed by oral prednisone 30–60 mg/day. The dose is tapered over 1–3 months to a typical maintenance dose of 5–10 mg/day. Side effects are well known, including weight gain, cataract, bone loss, fracture, avascular necrosis, glucose intolerance, hyperlipidemia, and hypertension [63, 64].

Calcineurin Inhibitors (*CNIs*). The introduction of *cyclosporine* into clinical usage in 1978 revolutionized solid organ transplant arena. It significantly decreased the incidence of acute rejection and improved early graft survival [65–68]. Cyclosporine is an 11-amino-acid cyclic peptide from *Tolypocladium inflatum*. It binds to intracellular cyclophilin to form a complex. This complex inhibits calcineurin phosphatase, blocks migration of NFAT from the cytoplasma into nucleus, therefore, inhibits cytokine (IL-2, IL-4, etc.) production [2, 62]. Microemulsion formulation (Neoral) is miscible in water and has better oral bioavailability than original preparation [66, 67]. Side effects of cyclosporine include acute and chronic nephrotoxicity, electrolyte disorders (hyperkalemia, hypomagnesemia, hyperuricemia), thrombotic microangiopathy (TMA), hypertension, neurotoxicity (tremor, dysesthesias, insomnia, headache), gingival hyperplasia, hypertrichosis, hirsutism, new onset diabetes after transplant (NODAT), hyperlipidemia, and bone pain syndrome. Clinical monitoring of trough level or peak level 2 h after administration is required to adjust cyclosporine dosage [69]. *Tacrolimus* (*FK506*) was approved by FDA in 1994 for liver transplant and in 1997 for kidney transplant. It is a macrolide antibiotic from *Streptomyces tsukubaensis*. It binds to FK506-binding protein (FKBP) to form a complex that inhibits calcineurin phosphatase with greater potency than cyclosporine. The use of tacrolimus has increased steadily, and it is now the dominant CNI, as it is associated with lower incidence of rejection [70–74]. Side effects are similar to cyclosporine in that it can cause acute and chronic nephrotoxicity, TMA, and electrolyte problems. But tacrolimus has a lower incidence of hypertension, hyperlipidemia, cosmetic skin changes, and gum hyperplasia, and a higher incidence of neurotoxicity and NODAT. The risk factor for NODAT includes African American ethnicity, older age, HCV infection, and obesity. Hirsutism is uncommon, but hair loss and even alopecia are associated with tacrolimus usage. Trough level monitoring is required to adjust its dosage. There is a new preparation of modified-release tacrolimus to permit once-daily dosing [75]. Both CNIs are metabolized by the cytochrome P-450 CYP3A4 enzyme. Any drug or nutrition supplement that induces or inhibits this enzyme may increase or decrease CNI level and need to adjust CNI dose respectively. Such common drug–drug interactions are summarized in Table 15.1.

Antimetabolites. There are several antimetabolites available. *Azathioprine* has been used as an immunosuppressive agent since early 1960s [76–78]. It is a prodrug of 6-mercaptopurine, which interferes with DNA synthesis by inhibiting metalloproteinase and synthesis of thioguanine nucleotides. It is metabolized by xanthine oxidase. Therefore, concurrent use of allopurinol, febuxostat, or any other xanthine oxidase inhibitor should be avoided as it can cause severe leucopenia. The usual maintenance dose is 2 mg/kg/day. Common side effects include bone marrow depression, leukopenia, macrocytosis, pancreatitis, and liver toxicity.

Mycophenolic acid (*MFA*) is from penicillium molds. It inhibits inosine monophosphate dehydrogenase, therefore, blocks the synthesis of guanosine monophosphate nucleotides and prevents the proliferation of T- and B cells [2, 77]. MMF is a prodrug that requires hydrolysis of the mofetil ester in acid environment to release MFA [79–82]. Thus, proton-pump inhibitor may reduce the exposure of MMF. Enteric-coated MFA is an active compound and its absorption is not affected by proton-pump inhibitor [83–86]. The typical dose is 1,000 mg of MMF or 720 mg of enteric-coated MFA twice daily when used in combination of cyclosporine, and cyclosporine can inhibit their absorption by 30–50 %. When used with tacrolimus, reduced dose of MMF or MFA may also be effective as tacrolimus does not reduce their absorption. MFA is superior to azathioprine in preventing acute rejection after kidney transplant [81, 82]. The combination of MFA and CNI has reduced graft rejection and improved graft survival. MFA has largely replaced azathioprine and is widely used in maintenance protocols [79–86]. The side effects include gastrointestinal symptoms and bone marrow suppression. The enteric-coated MFA is better tolerated due to less gastrointestinal symptoms [85–87]. MFA level can be measured as clinical monitoring, but it is usually unnecessary. MFA should be stopped 6 weeks before conception, as it increases the risk of fetal loss in the first trimester as well as fetus congenital malformations (cleft lip and palate, anomalies of external ear, distal limbs, heart, esophagus, and kidney).

Leflunomide is a synthetic isoxazole derivative and it inhibits pyrimidine synthesis by inhibiting dihydroorotate dehydrogenase. It is approved for rheumatoid arthritis, and it is sometimes used in transplant patients for BK virus nephropathy. However, its efficacy against BK virus remains controversial [88, 89]. Side effects include anemia, GI toxicity, and elevated liver enzymes.

Mammalian Target-of-Rapamycin (*mTOR*) *Inhibitors* *Sirolimus* (*rapamycin*) was approved by FDA in 1999 for prophylaxis of rejection in kidney transplant. It is a macrolide antibiotic derived from *S. hygroscopicus*. It binds to FKBP to form a complex, which inhibits mTOR. Inhibition of mTOR blocks the T-cell proliferation driven by IL-2 [90–92]. Everolimus is a derivative of sirolimus [93]. Both of them are metabolized by cytochrome P-450 CYP3A4. Therefore, they are subject to the similar drug–drug interaction as CNI in Table 15.1. The adverse effects of mTOR inhibitors include hyperlipidemia, leucopenia, thrombocytopenia, podocyte injury, proteinuria, focal and segmental glomerulosclerosis,

Table 15.1 Drugs that affect cytochrome P-450 enzyme and CNI metabolism

Induction of P-450 and reduction of CNI level
(1) Anticonvulsants: barbiturates, phenytoin, carbamazepine, and primidone
(2) Antimycobacterial drugs: rifampin, rifabutin, rifapentine, and isoniazid
(3) Herbal supplement: St. John's wort
Inhibition of P-450 and increase of CNI level
(1) Calcium channel blockers: verapamil, diltiazem, nicardipine, and amlodipine
(2) Antiarrhythmics: amiodarone, dronedarone, quinidine, and lidocaine
(3) Antifungal drugs: ketoconazole, itraconazole, clotrimazole, voriconazole, fluconazole, miconazole, and posaconazole
(4) Antibacterial agents: erythromycin, clarithromycin, telithromycin, and synercid
(5) Protease inhibitors: amprenavir, atazanavir, boceprevir, darunavir, delavirdine, fosamprenavir, ritonavir, indinavir, saquinavir, tipranavir, telaprevir, and nelfinavir
(6) Antidepressant: fluvoxamine
(7) Diet supplement: grapefruit juice

delayed recovery of ATN, delayed wound healing, lymphocele formation, oral ulcers, pneumonitis, pleural effusion, and ascites. The combination of mTOR inhibitor and CNI may increase the nephrotoxicity, TMA, and hypertension [91, 92, 94]. However, mTOR inhibitors may have antineoplastic and antiviral benefits and their usages are associated with lower incidence of malignancy and viral diseases (cytomegalovirus (CMV) and BKV infection) [90–94].

Belatacept is the first co-stimulatory pathway blockage approved as a maintenance immunosuppressive agent for kidney transplant. Belatacept is a fusion protein combining CTLA-4 with the Fc portion of IgG. It blocks the co-stimulatory pathway CD28–CD80/86 (signal 2) by binding to CD80/86 on T cells, therefore, inhibits T-cell activation [95]. In the clinical trials with basiliximab induction and MFA and glucocorticoid maintenance, belatacept group provides significantly better kidney function than cyclosporine control despite of higher incidence of acute rejection in the first year [95]. It is also associated with less chronic allograft nephropathy and better cardiovascular and metabolic profiles. Belatacept is given intravenously once monthly after the more frequent administration for the initial 2 months. The significant side effect is the increased risk of post-transplant lymphoproliferative disease (PTLD) primarily involving the CNS in patients without Epstein-Barr virus (EBV) immunity. Therefore, belatacept is contraindicated in patients who are EBV seronegative or with unknown EBV serostatus before transplant. Other risk factors for PTLD may include CMV infection and over immunosuppression [95–98].

Other Clinically Used Agents

IVIG is prepared from pooled donor plasma. It contains more than 90 % of intact IgG that can neutralize auto- and allo-antibodies. It blocks Fc receptor on effector cells, inhibits inflammatory cytokines, and attenuates complement-mediated injury. IVIG may also have a long-term immune modulate effect through inhibiting lymphocyte proliferation and antibody production [99]. IVIG is frequently used in treating AMR as well as in desensitization protocol for ABO and/or HLA incompatible transplants [100–102]. Commonly side effects include fever, chills, headache, chest tightness, sweating, and nausea. Occasionally, the IVIG forms containing high sucrose (such as sandoglobulin) can cause thrombotic event and AKI from sucrose nephropathy.

Bortezomib is a tripeptide that inhibits 26S proteasome. It prevents the degradation of pro-apoptotic factors and activates programmed cell death in immortal neoplastic cells, especially the plasma cells. Bortezomib is approved for the treatment of myeloma. It may be useful in desensitizing the patient with preformed DSA before transplant and for the treatment of AMR after transplant [103].

Eculizumab is a humanized antibody against complement C5. It inhibits the cleavage of C5 into C5a and C5b, therefore preventing formation of membrane attach complex C5b-9. Eculizumab is approved for paroxysmal nocturnal hemoglobinuria and atypical hemolytic uremia syndrome. It has been reported in treating AMR, especially the severe ones refractory to plasmapheresis and IVIG-based conventional therapy [104].

Considerations in Choosing a Maintenance Regimen

There are several important factors to consider when choosing a maintenance immunosuppressive regimen for a particular patient. The patient factor includes the immunologic risk, clinical characteristics, and comorbidities. The medication factor may include the drug efficacy, specific side effect, and financial cost. The ideal protocol should not only effectively prevent graft rejection (both acute and chronic) but also be affordable and tolerable, which can collectively provide better quality of life as well as superior graft and patient survival. In general, the risk for acute rejection is highest in the first several months after transplantation, while the risk of serious infection and malignancy as well as other adverse effects correlate with the total amount of immunosuppression. Therefore, the immunosuppression is usually tapered slowly to a maintenance level by 6–12 months after transplant in absence of rejection episode.

Steroid minimization (steroid-withdrawal or steroid-free) protocols have been tried as a strategy to avoid its adverse effects. The FREEDOM trial included three groups: steroid-free, steroid-withdrawal (after 7 days), and standard-steroids (tapering to 5–10 mg/day by 3 months). All groups received basiliximab induction, and enteric-coated MFA and cyclosporine maintenance. At 1 year, acute rejection rates were significantly higher in both steroid-free (31.5 %) and steroid-withdrawal (26.1 %) groups than standard-steroids group (14.7 %). There was no difference in renal function, graft, or patient survival [105]. Another trial compared long-term results of steroid withdrawal (after 7 days) with continuance of low-dose steroid. Enrolled patients received either thymoglobulin (68 %) or IL2R antibody (32 %) induction. All patients were treated with tacrolimus and MMF as the maintenance. At 5 years, early steroid-withdrawal group had significant increases in both biopsy-confirmed acute rejection (18 % vs. 11 %) and CAN (10 % vs. 4 %) without significant difference in steroid-associated adverse effects [106]. Therefore, continued steroid in the maintenance protocol is generally preferred, especially in high risk groups, such as African American patients or sensitized patients. Recent studies suggest steroid minimization might be achievable in selected low-risk patients when potent induction therapy with T-cell depleting antibody has been given and/or combination of tacrolimus and MFA is maintained [107–109].

Because of the acute and chronic nephrotoxicity, CNI-free or withdrawal protocols are desirable for renal graft benefit. The CAESAR study found that cyclosporine withdrawal at 4 months after transplant was associated with higher incidence of acute rejection than the group with either low-dose or standard-dose of cyclosporine. There was no difference in renal function among the three groups at 1 year of follow-up [110]. The SYMPHONY study compared four regimens: standard-dose cyclosporine/MMF/steriod, daclizumab/low-dose cyclosporine/MMF, daclizumab/MMF/steroid/low-dose tacrolimus, and daclizumab/MMF/steroid/sirolimus. The results clearly favored the group with daclizumab/MMF/steroid/low-dose tacrolimus. At the end of 1 year of follow-up, low-dose tacrolimus group (target trough levels of 3–7 ng/mL) had lowest rate of rejection (12.3 %, about half of other groups), superior graft function and significantly better graft survival, but higher incidence of NODAT than other groups. Interestingly, low-dose cyclosporine did not have a significant impact on any outcome than standard-dose cyclosporine [111]. At 3 years, low-dose tacrolimus group continued to provide the best results with highest renal function and best graft survival rate. Other three groups had similar outcomes to each other, but inferior to the low-dose tacrolimus group [112]. In another long-term study with a median follow-up of 8 years, patients were randomly assigned into tacrolimus/MMF, tacrolimus/sirolimus, or cyclosporine/sirolimus. All received IL2R antibody induction and maintenance steroid. Compared with other two groups, tacrolimus/MMF group had significantly lower incidence of acute rejection and better renal function at 1, 2, and 7 years. Tacrolimus/sirolimus group had higher incidence of death with functioning graft (DWFG) than other two groups [113].

Trials using mTOR inhibitor sirolimus to replace MMF or CNI in maintenance have not proved to be beneficial and are frequently associated with higher incidence of rejection and inferior graft survival [91, 92, 114–116]. Thus, low-dose tacrolimus combined with MFA and steroid seems to provide the most effective maintenance with good outcomes. The novel costimulation blockage belatacept is designed to provide effective immunosuppression while avoiding renal toxicity and metabolic adverse effects associated with CNI. Significantly better renal function and improved cardiovascular and metabolic profile have been demonstrated, which might be an important step towards ultimately better graft and/or patient survival [96–98].

Patient Selection and Transplant Surgery

Recipient Selection

As the waiting list for kidney transplantation continues to grow exponentially, the need for selecting appropriate candidates for transplant becomes paramount. To maximize the success rates of transplant, a careful review and evaluation of coexisting medical and psychosocial comorbidities should be performed to intervene if possible prior to the procedure. ESRD patients in the USA qualify for kidney transplant listing once they have a glomerular filtration rate (GFR) <20 ml/min or have initiated chronic dialysis. Preemptive transplantation prior to dialysis improves recipient survival [117]. A full review of recipient selection criteria is beyond the scope of this chapter; in addition, transplant centers and insurance companies may have specific criteria for their candidates. However, clinical guidelines from transplant societies have been published [118], and most centers adhere to these.

Transplant candidates are evaluated in a multidisciplinary setting, involving physicians and surgeons, psychologists and social workers, financial counselors and dieticians. This may take weeks, depending on the extent of testing that needs to be done for each patient. At the end of the evaluation, patients are presented at a multidisciplinary Selection Committee, where patients may be discussed in an unbiased setting and listed with unanimous voting. A brief summary of recipient criteria is described below.

Medical

Cardiovascular/pulmonary—Cardiopulmonary reserve should be tested to ensure that patients would be able to withstand major abdominal surgery. Patients with diabetes and other atherosclerotic diseases may need intervention prior to listing. Attention should be paid to the peripheral vascular system, especially in patients who have had previous hemodialysis catheters. Chronic thrombosis/atherosclerosis of iliac vessels may also preclude the possibility of transplant.

Infection—Recipients are typically tested serologically for presence of chronic infections such as CMV, EBV, hepatitis, syphilis, and HIV. Other infections may be tested for, based on endemic prevalence. These infections may not be contraindications by themselves, and some transplant centers around the country transplant HIV positive recipients as well [59].

Cancer—Candidates should undergo age-appropriate cancer screening. ESRD patients have a higher risk of native kidney cancers and these should be screened for. A recent history of cancer may require a period of waiting prior to listing, to avoid recurrence that may occur with transplant immunosuppression. This waiting period may vary by specific tumors and their pathology, but remote recurrences have been reported with aggressive cancers like breast cancers and melanomas [119].

HLA typing—Candidates will have HLA typing of their blood to be listed in the national database. In the current database, patients PRA (panel reactive antibody) level and unacceptable antigens (which the recipient cannot receive from a potential donor) must also be listed to minimize the risk of a positive crossmatch. Sensitizing history, such as previous transplants, pregnancies, and blood transfusions must be documented during the evaluation.

Psychosocial/Financial

A history of habitual noncompliance, especially with dialysis sessions and medications may indicate future risk of transplant failure. Patients with active substance abuse, recurrent criminal activity, mental illnesses, or other psychosocial situations that may impair the ability to understand or comply with a post-transplant regimen are also to be noted. Financial constraints are just as important for successful transplantation. Evaluation and discussion of specific coverage, copayments, and out of pocket expenses for the transplant procedure, immunosuppressive medications, lab testing, and clinical follow-up must be individualized for every patient.

Contraindications for Transplant

There are very few absolute contraindications to transplant, although most centers would not transplant candidates with

- Active untreated infection
- Current malignancy with short life expectancy
- Severe chronic comorbid diseases with shortened life expectancy or which would preclude safely undergoing major abdominal surgery
- Active substance abuse
- Reversible renal failure

Living Donor Selection

Living donation makes up a little less than 50 % of all kidney donations in the USA. While family members have usually been the predominant source of living donation, recently, unrelated donation from friends and coworkers has increased. Altruistic anonymous donation from strangers is also a phenomenon that is growing. A national UNOS sponsored swapping of incompatible donors for the purpose of facilitating multiple living donor transplants is currently underway.

The evaluation process of a potential living donor should be comprehensive and cautious, to minimize the risks in a healthy altruistic individual who is undergoing a major procedure simply to help another. To minimize a bias that a transplant program may have for recipients, current laws mandate that centers have an independent donor advocate that will not be involved in the care of the recipient, and acts only in the best interest of the donor, helping them through the whole process of donation.

The evaluation should determine the donors' understanding of this procedure, their motivation to donate and a review of any comorbid conditions. The short- and long-term risks of this procedure should be clearly described to candidates. Blood typing and crossmatching may be done initially to see if the donor is a match for the recipient. Incompatible blood and crossmatch transplants do currently occur, but is not the norm and will not be the focus of this chapter.

Sixty percent of transplant centers reported that they had no upper age limit for kidney donors [120], as long as they met all other criteria for donation. However, most transplant centers will not use donors aged <18, as they are not legally adults and hence cannot give informed consent. Most centers require donors to have a GFR of >80 mL/min. While this may be calculated from blood testing using the MDRD or CKD-EPI formulae, they are not always accurate and may underestimate true GFR. In equivocal cases, confirmatory testing with 24 h creatinine clearance or isotopic nuclear testing may be required.

Urine testing is typically performed as well for blood and protein. Most centers require <300 mg/day of protein loss in

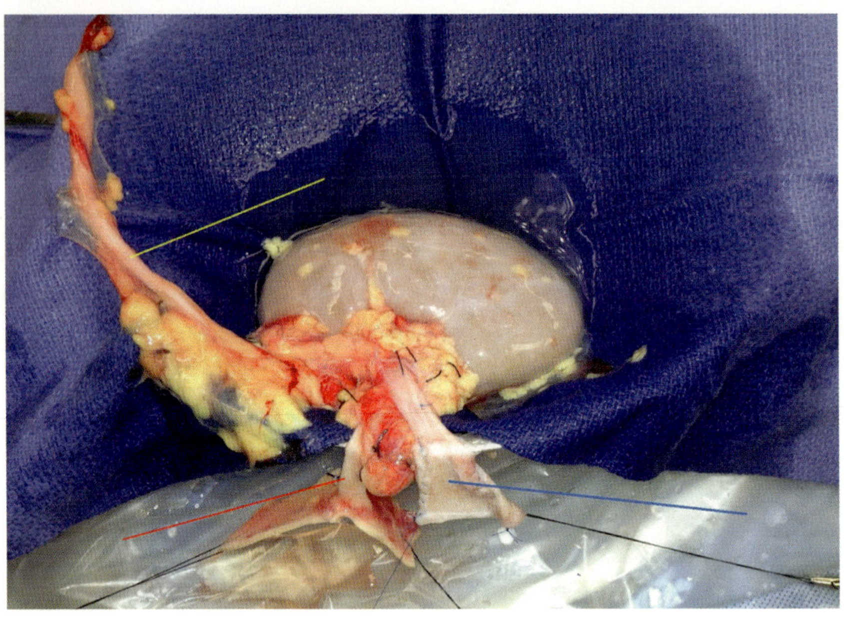

Fig. 15.1 Backtable reconstruction of deceased donor kidney. *Red line* indicates artery with attached aortic cuff; *blue line* indicates vein. Note the vein has been reconstructed by using donor vena cava to lengthen the vein. The *yellow line* indicates the ureter

the urine. Hematuria of >10 RBC/hpf should be further evaluated with urologic testing [120]. A history of nephrolithiasis should prompt a stone diathesis workup to ensure there is no metabolic predisposition to this. Hypertension in the donor needs to be worked up, possibly with ambulatory monitoring. Well-controlled hypertension with one or two medications may not be a contraindication to donation.

Other testing usually involves age-appropriate cancer screening, infectious screening, and other cardiopulmonary testing as required, similar to the recipient workup. Imaging of the donors' kidneys is done to determine anatomy and help decide if safe donation is feasible. Approximately 30 % of the population has abnormal vascular anatomy, which may factor in this decision [121].

Psycho/social testing is also paramount in the evaluation; it is illegal to be compensated for donating a kidney, and any evidence of coercion must be investigated. A confidential means of backing out of the surgery should be offered. The evaluation, surgery, and recovery period is paid by the recipients insurance; hence the donor is not required to have insurance to undergo this procedure. The transplant center is required to follow the donor for 2 years post donation. However, it is important to counsel donors on maintaining a healthy lifestyle to minimize the risk of any long-term complications.

Kidney Transplant Surgery Procedure

Although kidney transplantation is the most commonly performed solid organ transplant, recipients usually have multiple comorbidities that present individual challenges to each transplant. Also, there has a been a steady increase in the use of ECD kidneys and use of kidneys with anomalies, such as horseshoe kidneys, small pediatric kidneys, and kidneys with abnormal vascular anatomy, all of which increase the complexity of the operation.

Deceased Donor Procurement

In case of deceased donor organ procurement, the kidneys may be procured with other organs. The procedure involves cessation of blood flow and flushing the vascular system with organ preservative solution. The kidneys are separated, with an aortic cuff for each kidney. The vena cava is typically left attached to the right kidney due to the short length of the right renal vein. This allows for backtable reconstruction of the vein (see later). Each kidney is procured with adequate length of ureter, care being taken to preserve periureteral fat, which contains vasculature that supplies the ureter.

Living Donor Procurement

Living donor procurement has significantly increased over the past decade, especially with the advent of minimally invasive surgery. While most live donor procurements are performed laparoscopically, there have been reports of mini-incision removals and even robotic kidney removals. In most instances, the left kidney is procured, as the vein is much longer and easier to implant.

Backtable Preparation

Prior to implantation, backtable preparation is required to clean the kidney of perinephric fat and the adrenal gland, which may be adherent. The vessels are then dissected clean for a short length to make the anastomosis easier.

The veins may have branches that may need ligation. In the case of a cadaveric kidney right vein, which is short, the vein length may be extended by reconstructing the vena cava, which it is usually attached to (Fig. 15.1).

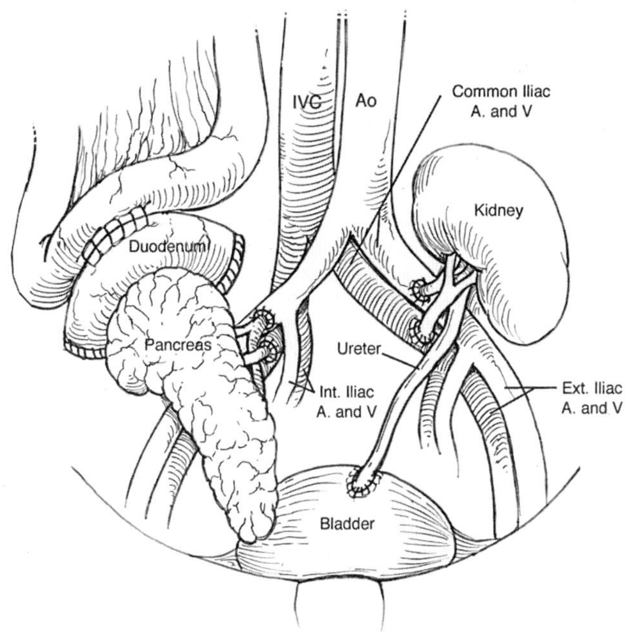

Fig. 15.2 Kidney and pancreas transplants. The donor renal artery and vein are anastomosed to the recipient left iliac artery and vein. The donor ureter is anastomosed to recipient bladder. The donor pancreas reconstructed artery and vein are anastomosed to the recipient right iliac artery and vein, while the donor duodenal segment is anastomosed to the recipient ileum

In cases of kidneys with multiple arteries, the arteries may require reconstruction by anastomosing a smaller artery to the side of a main artery, or by syndactylyzing the lumens of the arteries so that there is only one lumen for anastomosis. It is important to remember that each artery is typically and end artery with minimal collateralization. Hence it is important to preserve each of the arteries if possible.

Implantation

The implantation procedure usually lasts between 2 and 4 h. An incision is made in the iliac fossa. In smaller children a midline incision may sometimes be performed. A space is created in the retroperitoneum by sweeping the peritoneum upwards to expose the retroperitoneal iliac vessels.

The artery and vein are usually anastomosed in an end-to-side manner to the external iliac vessels. In cases of significant atherosclerotic disease of the external iliacs, the common iliacs may be explored and used if not as diseased. End-to-end anastomoses to the internal iliac vessels have also been described (Fig. 15.2). In cases of small children where the iliac vessels may be too small for anastomosis, they may need to be performed to the lower aorta and vena cave.

The ureter is anastomosed to the bladder using absorbable suture to minimize the risk of the retained suture acting as a nidus for future stone formation. In patients who have been anuric for years, the bladder may be very small and difficult to isolate. In such instances, anastomosing the transplant ureter to the native ureter may also be performed. Some surgeons may use ureteral stents within the ureteral anastomosis. There has been some literature suggesting this may reduce ureteral leaks, but may also increase the risk of a urinary tract infection. The stent is usually removed 4–6 weeks post-surgery [120].

Surgical Complications

A complex surgical procedure such as a kidney transplant is not without specific complications. For the purposes of this chapter, these complications may be divided into vascular, ureteral, and other occurrences.

Vascular

Intraoperative bleeding may occur postreperfusion if adequate attention has not been paid to backtable preparation or meticulous anastomotic technique. Immediate vasoconstriction of vessels may hide these bleeders until the postoperative period where a spike in blood pressure may open these up, so a careful inspection of all anastomoses and vessels is warranted prior to closure.

Thrombosis is probably the commonest cause of early graft loss. Thrombosis may occur in the artery or vein. Immediate vascular thrombosis that may occur with a hyperacute rejection due to an unrecognized positive crossmatch or incompatible blood typing is rare, but should be suspected in such instances.

Arterial thrombosis may occur due an unrecognized intimal flap that causes dissection along the vessel, causing obstruction. This may occur among patients with significant atherosclerotic disease of the iliac vessels.

Venous thrombosis usually occurs due to kinking of the vein. Being thin-walled, the vein is easily susceptible to this during the final positioning of the kidney at the end of the operation and this must be noted. The iliac veins themselves may be diseased from previous groin hemodialysis catheters, so it is often prudent to evaluate these preoperatively. Previous venous thrombosis of the iliac veins may predispose these patients to pulmonary embolus during the handling of this vein during the venous anastomosis.

Renal artery stenosis may occur with disease of the artery or with poor anastomotic technique and should be suspected with recalcitrant hypertension a few months after transplant. Reimplantation or balloon angioplasty has shown successful outcomes.

Ureteral

The ureter anastomosis may leak, causing urine to accumulate in the retroperitoneal space and creating an urinoma. Patients may present with a fluid collection around the kidney, which may be painful. It may be noted that the patients' serum creatinine levels may not fall, and may actually increase, as this urine is reabsorbed into the bloodstream. If the patient has a surgical drain in place, this condition may be suspected with increased drain output with drain fluid creatinine value being much higher than the serum creatinine value. Stenting of the ureter at surgery may reduce the incidence of leaks. Treatment of urine leaks is either surgical reimplantation if early (typically <2 weeks) or percutaneous drainage and anterograde stenting if diagnosed later.

Another complication of the ureteral anastomosis is stricturing. The ureter is very susceptible to ischemia due to its tenuous blood supply. Early strictures may be most likely to anastomotic surgical error or devascularization due to extensive dissection of the ureter. Late strictures may be due to chronic ischemia, although BK virus infection or a significant rejection episode may also do this. Patients may present with graft dysfunction or urinary infections with the presence of hydronephrosis. Treatment may require initial percutaneous drainage, with planned reconstruction once the kidney function has recovered. Short segment strictures may be treated with reanastomoses, although ballooning of such strictures has been described; long segment strictures may require a flap creation of the bladder (Boari flap) to bridge the resected segment.

Others

A lymphocele is a localized collection of lymphatic fluid draining from severed lymphatics around the iliac arteries during the surgical dissection. As the collection is extraperitoneal, this fluid collection cannot drain and thus may cause compression of the transplant kidney with dysfunction and may also get infected. Treatment is typically by creation of a peritoneal window, allowing this fluid to drain and be absorbed in the peritoneum. This procedure can typically be performed laparoscopically.

Kidney Allograft Dysfunction

The common causes of acute graft dysfunction are summarized in Table 15.2. The clinical workup is similar to AKI of native kidneys in both pre-renal and post-renal aspects. There are several types of rejection that can occur in transplanted kidney. In the era of potent immunosuppressive medicine, acute rejection rate is about 10 % within the first year after transplantation. However, it remains an important cause of graft loss if not diagnosed timely and treated properly [1, 14, 122, 123].

Hyperacute rejection occurs immediately after transplant. It is mediated by the preformed anti-donor antibodies, usually either anti-HLA (DSA), anti-ABO, or other non-HLA antibodies [123]. Hyperacute rejection results in an irreversible vascular rejection, intravascular thrombosis, and graft necrosis. The graft is tender and does not make much urine. Renal scan shows no or little uptake, which is different from ATN. Surgical exploration and graft nephrectomy is indicated. The routine pretransplant crossmatch and verification of ABO compatibility between donor and recipient should prevent the majority of hyperacute rejection episodes.

Table 15.2 Differential diagnosis of delayed graft function or acute graft dysfunction

1. Pre-renal azotemia
Volume depletion (diuretics, poor intake, vomiting, diarrhea)
Vascular constriction (CNI toxicity, NSAID)
2. Intrinsic renal diseases
Arterial or venous stenosis, thrombosis or compression
ATN
Acute or accelerated acute rejection (cellular, humoral, or both)
Pyelonephritis
Thrombotic microangiopathy (TMA)
Recurrent glomerular disease (FSGS, aHUS)
3. Post-renal obstruction
Foley catheter obstruction
Perinephris fluid collection (urine leak, hematoma, lymphocele)
Donor ureteral obstruction (kinking, stricture, blood clots)
Neurogenic bladder
Enlarged prostate (BPH, prostate cancer)

Accelerated acute rejection (or delayed hyperacute rejection) can occur within 24 h to several days after transplant. It represents an anamnestic response by memory B and T cells from prior sensitization events, and may involve both humoral and cellular components. Even a negative crossmatch before transplant may not prevent the development of accelerated acute rejection, as the preformed DSA (or non-HLA antibody) titer may be too low to be detected before kidney transplant [1, 123].

Acute rejection, either cellular, antibody-mediated or both, is more common and reversible than hyperacute rejection and accelerated acute rejection. The incidence of acute rejection has been steadily decreased over last two decades due to the wide use of antibody induction therapy and potent new immunosuppressive maintenance. Although the majority of acute rejection episodes occur in the first 3–6 months, it can happen anytime in the lifetime of an allograft kidney. It may develop in a graft already suffering from DGF after transplant surgery. This can be difficult to be recognized if the patient clinically is anuric or oliguric [124, 125]. Therefore, any new graft with DGF should have serial biopsies to detect the covert development of rejection and be treated properly. The classic signs and symptoms of acute rejection may include low grade of fever, malaise, decreased urine output, and graft tenderness. Urine analysis may show white blood cells and red blood cells. It is not uncommon for these patients to be misdiagnosed and treated as urinary tract infec-

Table 15.3 Banff 2007 classification of renal allograft pathology

1. Normal: a histologically normal biopsy
2. Antibody-mediated changes
(1) Acute AMR
• Type I: ATN-like histology (C4d positive), with minimal inflammation
• Type II: capillary-glomerulitis, with margination and/or thromboses (C4d positive)
• Type III: arterial-transmural inflammation/fibrinoid changes (C4d positive)
(2) Chronic active AMR: glomerular double counters and/or multilayering of the PTC basement membrane and/or IF/TA and/or fibrous intimal thickening in arteries and C4d positive.
3. Borderline changes: suspicious for acute T cell mediated rejection, tubulitis foci (t1, t2, or t3, with i0 or i1) without intimal arteritis.
4. T cell mediated rejection
(1) ACR
• Type IA: significant interstitial inflammation (>25 % of parenchyma affected, i2 or i3) and foci moderate tubulitis (t2).
• Type IB: significant interstitial inflammation (>25 % of parenchyma affected, i2 or i3) and severe tubulitis (t3)
• Type IIA: mild to moderate arteritis (v1)
• Type IIB: severe arteritis with greater than 25 % loss of the luminal area (v2)
• Type III: transmural arteritis, and/or arterial fibrinoid alterations, and necrosis of medial smooth muscle cells occurring in association with lymphocytic inflammation of the vessel (v3)
(2) Chronic active T cell mediated rejection: chronic arteriopathy involves arterial intimal fibrosis with mononuclear cell infiltration in fibrosis and formation of neo-intima.
5. Interstitial fibrosis and tubular atrophy (IF/TA) without evidence of any specific etiology
• Grade I: mild IF/TA (<25 % of cortical area)
• Grade II: moderate IF/TA (25–50 % of cortical area)
• Grade III: severe IF/TA (>50 % of cortical area)

tion at outside facility. However, the majority of patients do not have these classic signs and symptoms of acute rejection, instead, they only present as asymptomatic graft dysfunction as detected by laboratory monitoring. Kidney biopsy is necessary to make a definitive diagnosis of rejection. The use of noninvasive biomarkers in predicting and/or diagnosing acute rejection remains experimental. On the other hand, any patient presented with high grade fever, graft tenderness, and systemic symptoms should be worked up and treated for infectious process immediately, such as pyelonephritis, wound infection, abscess, or CMV disease.

Acute cellular rejection (ACR) is diagnosed by histologic finding of T-lymphocyte infiltration in tubular-interstitial parenchyma (tubulitis) and vascular wall (arteritis). The Banff classification (Table 15.3) provides standardized pathohistological definition of types and grades of rejection [122]. Pulse corticosteroid is the first-line therapy for ACR in most centers. Methylprednisolone, 3–5 mg/kg, is given intravenously for several (3–7) days. Mild or moderate ACR, such as Banff class borderline changes, 1A or 1B, usually responds well to steroid pulse therapy. After intravenous pulse steroids, oral steroids are given and then tapered rapidly to a maintenance dosage [126, 127].

Steroid-resistant ACR was traditionally defined as lack of improvement in renal function within 5–7 days of intravenous pulse steroids. We consider those with progressively decreasing urine output or worsening renal function despite of 2–3 days of pulse corticosteroids as steroid resistance. In these cases, we start polyclonal ATG early. Also, severe ACR with vascular involvement, such as Banff class 2A or above, often needs ATG therapy, as pulse steroids alone may not provide complete resolution of vascular rejection or recovery of renal function [128, 129]. There are two forms of ATG, either ATGAM or thymoglobulin. A direct comparison between thymoglobulin and ATGAM was performed in patients with ACR, and thymoglobulin resulted in a higher rate of reversal of rejection and a lower rate of recurrent ACR [128]. The typical dose of thymoglobulin is either 3 mg/kg per day for 3 days or 1.5 mg/kg per day for 5 days. The FDA-approved total dose of thymoglobulin for treatment of steroid-resistant acute rejection is 10 mg/kg. ATG is associated with severe side effects. The cytokine release syndrome can be prevented by concurrent administration of steroids, acetaminophen, and diphenhydramine. Antiviral and antimicrobial prophylaxis against CMV infection and pneumocystis carinii pneumonia (PCP) are recommended after ATG therapy [128, 129]. The risk of developing PTLD should be kept in mind, and patients should be monitored for this complication. Repeat kidney biopsy is indicated in ACR that is resistant to steroids and/or ATG to rule out other pathology, such as concurrent ATN, AMR, BKV nephropathy, or chronic irreversible fibrosis. The underline chronic fibrosis can be masked by interstitial inflammation of ACR, and it usually becomes more recognizable on repeat biopsy after the treatment of ACR.

Antibody-mediated rejection (AMR) was historically presumed when biopsy revealed severe vascular rejection or when the rejection was not responsive to the conventional treatment of ACR. The advent of C4d staining, sensitive assay to detect DSA, and the description of typical histologic findings of AMR has improved our recognition that rejection is often AMR either alone or in conjunction with ACR [1, 122, 130, 131]. Current diagnosis of AMR is based on three of the four criteria: (1) graft dysfunction; (2) detection of DSA; (3) the characteristic histologic findings; and (4) positive C4d staining in the peritubular capillaries (PTC). However, the risk of AMR is very high in pre-sensitized patients, such as HLA and/or ABO incompatible transplants after desensitization protocol, the husband to wife or the child to mother donation, and the patients with known preformed DSA. In such high risk patients, AMR should be considered with fewer (two of the four) diagnostic criteria in the absence of another identifiable cause of graft dysfunction, so the treatment may be initiated without delay.

DSA testing should be performed during the workup of graft dysfunction when AMR is concerned. Routine screening for the development of de novo DSA may permit early detection of AMR in high risk patients. C4d is a degradation product of the classic complement pathway. A unique feature of C4d is that it binds covalently to the endothelial basement membrane, thereby avoiding removal during tissue processing. C4d deposition in PTC serves as an immunologic footprint of AMR. It is in a linear pattern and best demonstrated by immunofluorescence in frozen tissue section [1, 130, 132]. But some patients with AMR may not have both positive DSA and C4d staining. Cases with positive DSA but negative C4d staining may result from either technique error (false negative), non-complement activating DSA, or low level of DSA detected by highly sensitive assay without clinical relevance [1, 131]. In addition, the production of DSA precedes C4d deposition in the course of AMR, and a biopsy performed too early may not find the typical C4d deposition. Also, AMR can be caused by non-HLA antibodies that result in C4d deposition without DSA; such non-HLA antibodies may include anti-MICA, anti-MICB, and anti-endothelial antibodies [10, 13].

Treatment of AMR is often refractory to the treatment used for ACR. The optimal therapy for AMR remains to be defined, but it usually consists of a combination of several modalities, such as plasmapheresis or immunoadsorption, IVIG, corticosteroids, rituximab, ATG, bortezomib, eculizumab, and occasionally splenectomy [27, 53, 100, 101, 103, 133, 134]. Plasmapheresis or immunoadsorption with protein A removes the circulating DSA, but neither can suppress antibody production [27, 101]. AMR associated with high circulating DSA titer usually justify plasmapheresis or immunoadsorption as a part of its treatment. IVIG is often administrated after plasmapheresis. Possible actions of IVIG include anti-idiotypic antibodies neutralizing DSA, inhibiting complement binding, or activation and suppressing DSA synthesis [100]. Rituximab depletes B cells and it has been used to treat AMR [53, 133]. Corticosteroids and ATG remain beneficial as they can control the B cell response by depleting or inhibiting the helper T cells. Bortezomib activates apoptosis of plasma cells, therefore directly decreases DSA production [103]. Eculizumab is now being reported in managing AMR, especially the severe ones refractory to the conventional therapy [104]. Splenectomy has also been reported as a rescue treatment in patients with severe AMR not responding to other treatments [134]. DSA should be quantified and the trends are monitored to guide clinical treatment. Repeat kidney biopsies are frequently needed to assess the success of treatment and to rule out other concurrent pathologic processes, especially in those not responding to a reasonable course of treatment.

Acute rejection is a predictor of developing CAN and/or transplant glomerulopathy [135]. An increase in proteinuria after rejection is associated with poor graft outcome. Early diagnosed and completely reversed rejection after treatment may not affect long-term graft survival [136]. Whenever a rejection is diagnosed and treated, it is important to address the possibility of noncompliance or inadequate immunosuppression. The failure to correct the contributing factor may increase the risk of recurrent rejection and/or development of chronic rejection. Patient noncompliance with medications may be caused by their inability to tolerate the side effects or by the financial difficulty to afford drugs. Inadequate immunosuppression may also be caused by adding new drug or herbal supplement (Table 15.1) that induces cytochrome P-450 enzyme and increases the metabolism of CNI and/or mTOR inhibitor, which leads to decline in the drug trough level. Rescue therapy for refractory rejection is commonly based upon the administration of tacrolimus and/or MFA to those not receiving them as maintenance prior to rejection episode [137, 138]. Other rescue modalities that may be considered include alemtuzumab [139, 140] and graft radiation [141].

Subclinical rejection is usually defined as histological evidence of acute rejection by protocol biopsies, but clinically patients have normal or stable graft function [142–144]. Untreated subclinical rejection may be a precursor to chronic rejection [144]. However, treatment of subclinical rejection may not consistently prevent chronic rejection and fibrosis lesions. It remains controversial whether protocol biopsy to diagnose subclinical rejection is necessary in all transplant patients. In many cases, it is difficult to separate a subclinical rejection from a normal graft accommodation. Therefore,

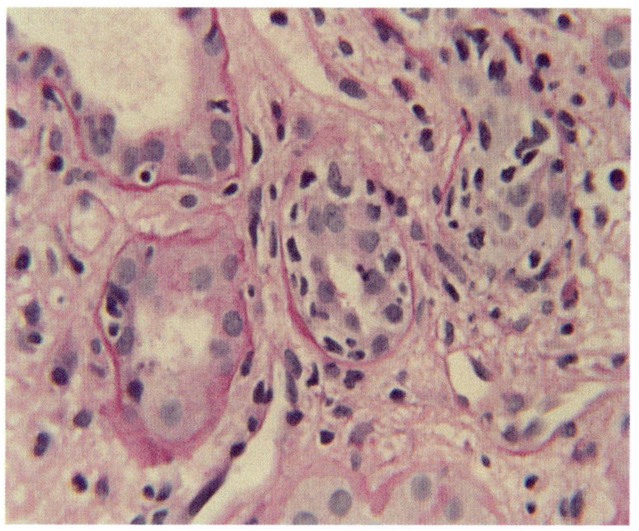

Fig. 15.3 Acute cellular rejection. There is infiltration of tubules (tubulitis) and interstitium with T cells (*courtesy of Suzanne Meleg-Smith, MD*)

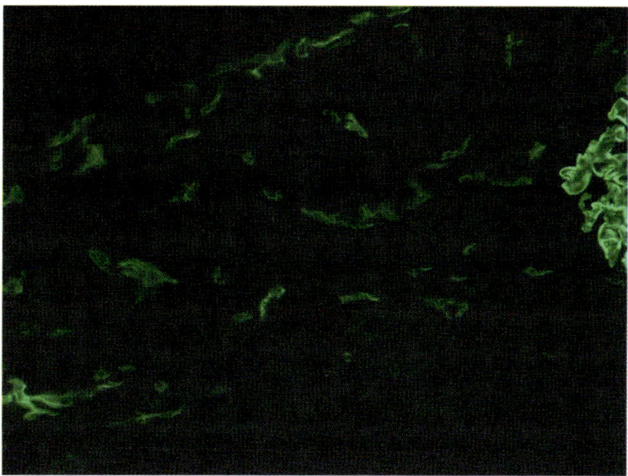

Fig. 15.5 Acute antibody-mediated rejection. There are positive C4d depositions in the peritubular capillaries (*courtesy of Suzanne Meleg-Smith, MD*)

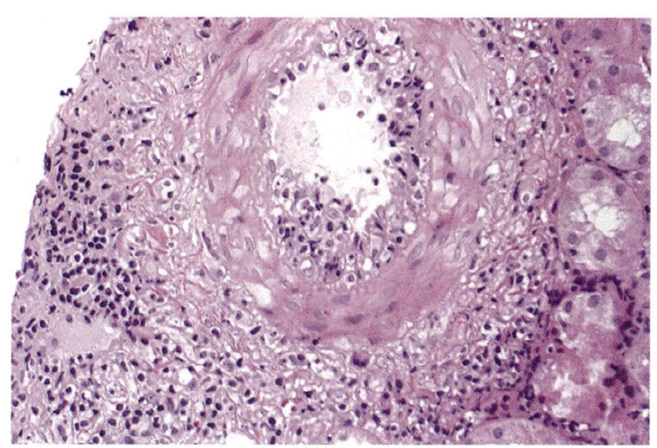

Fig. 15.4 Acute vascular rejection. In addition to the infiltration of tubules and interstitium, there is infiltration of arterial intima with T cells (*courtesy of Suzanne Meleg-Smith, MD*)

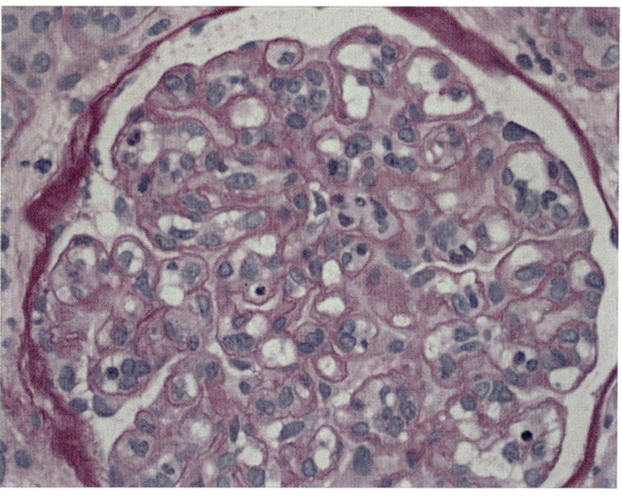

Fig. 15.6 Chronic rejection with transplant glomerulopathy. The glomerular capillary walls display "double contour" (*courtesy of Suzanne Meleg-Smith, MD*)

protocol biopsy probably should be limited to high risk patients at current clinical practice [142, 143].

Chronic active AMR is diagnosed by combination of the typical chronic changes from biopsy (glomerular double counters, multilayering of PTC basement membrane, IF/TA, fibrous intimal thickening in arteries) and ongoing humoral activity (positive DSA, C4d staining in PTC) [14, 122]. It is usually irreversible and there is no effective acute intervention for it. Empathetic treatment may include rituximab and/or IVIG to "control" the humoral activity. The maintenance immunosuppressive drugs may also be increased or adjusted with more potent ones wishfully to "stabilize" the graft function (Figs. 15.3, 15.4, 15.5, 15.6, 15.7, and 15.8).

Chronic allograft nephropathy (CAN) is a slow, progressive loss of renal function one or more years after kidney transplant, which is often referred as chronic rejection, transplant glomerulopathy, or IF/TA [14, 122]. Clinically, it is usually diagnosed by a slowly rising serum creatinine level, increasing proteinuria, and worsening hypertension. CAN represents a complex process culminating immunological and non-immunological injuries. It is the second most common cause of graft loss after the leading cause, death with a functioning graft. Optimal treatment of CAN remains unknown. Other causes of chronic allograft dysfunction are summarized in Table 15.4. When a specific cause of graft dysfunction is identified, then appropriate treatment may improve or stabilize the graft function.

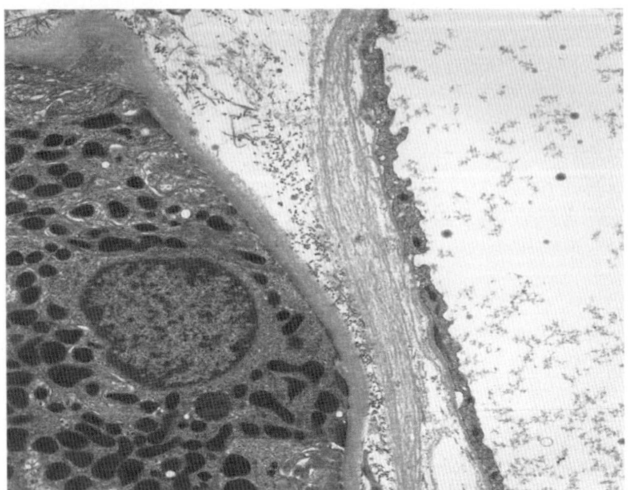

Fig. 15.7 Chronic transplant glomerulopathy. There is multilayering of glomerular basement membrane on electron microscopy (*courtesy of Suzanne Meleg-Smith, MD*)

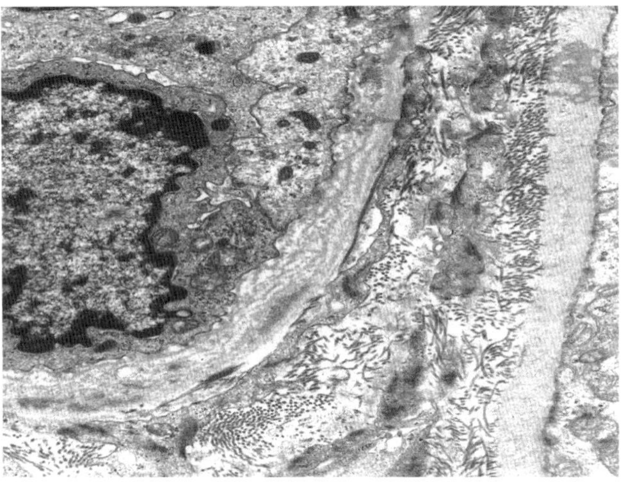

Fig. 15.8 Chronic antibody-mediated rejection. The peritubular capillary has laminated basement membrane on electron microscopy (*courtesy of Suzanne Meleg-Smith, MD*)

Table 15.4 Differential diagnosis of chronic allograft dysfunction

1. Immunological causes
Chronic active rejection (cellular, humoral, or both)
Chronic rejection (cellular, humoral, or both)
2. Non-immunological causes
Chronic CNI toxicity
Infection (BKV nephropathy, chronic pyeonephritis)
Chronic obstruction/hydronephrosis
Recurrent or de novo glomerular diseases
Recurrent or de novo diabetic nephropathy
Hypertensive nephrosclerosis
Renal artery stenosis

Long-Term Medical Complications

Obesity and Metabolic Syndrome (MS)

MS is a clustering of problems that include obesity, dyslipidemia, hypertension, and hyperglycemia. The key component of MS is obesity, especially abdominal obesity, which is associated with insulin-resistance as well as chronic inflammatory and pro-thrombotic status. Obesity/MS is increasingly recognized as an important cause of CKD. Each component of MS has been suggested to cause renal injury [145–147].

Obesity Paradox in ESRD Patients

Patients with ESRD have an exceptionally higher mortality rate compared to matched controls. Epidemiologic studies show that where obesity is concerned, there is a paradoxically inverse association between body mass index (BMI) and mortality in patients with ESRD. Higher BMI in dialysis patients has translated to a lower mortality, so called the "obesity paradox" or "dialysis paradox" [148, 149]. Recently, the mortality and BMI changes of dialysis patients during transplant waitlist period were studied, and it was found that lower BMI or muscle mass and/or unintentional weight loss or muscle loss was associated with a higher mortality [150]. Interestingly, there may be a "carry-over effect" of underweight after kidney transplant, as underweight status on dialysis was associated with higher mortality in the first year after kidney transplant [151]. Underweight or unintentional weight loss may reflect a poor health status and/or malnutrition, which is associated with high mortality in these patients. The impact of intentional weight loss among obese patients in preparation for kidney transplant remains unknown.

Kidney Transplantation in Obese Patients

There is no doubt obesity directly impacts transplant outcomes. Obesity is associated with higher surgical complication rate (wound infection, incision breakdown, and healing delay), longer hospital stay, and higher medical costs [152, 153]. Obesity also increases the risk for graft failure and patient death after kidney transplant [153]. Despite these relative poor outcomes, obese ESRD patients are routinely considered for kidney transplant because of the survival benefit as compared to dialysis therapy [154, 155]. One study demonstrated that kidney transplant was associated with a significantly lower risk of mortality of 61 % for deceased donor kidneys and 77 % for living donor kidneys [154]. This survival benefit of kidney transplant might drop off with a BMI >41 kg/m^2.

Obesity/MS After Kidney Transplantation

Successful kidney transplant not only prolongs patient life but also improves the quality of life [156]. Patients usually report a better appetite as the uremic syndrome has been resolved. Many patients develop new onset obesity/MS and the preexisting obesity/MS can get worse after kidney transplant [157]. Obesity/MS after kidney transplant is associated with cardiovascular morbidities and higher risk for patient death and graft failure [158]. The commonly used immunosuppressive drugs including corticosteroids, CNI (cyclosporine, tacrolimus), and mTOR inhibitor (sirolimus, zortress) have adverse metabolic effects and can cause or contribute to the development of obesity/MS as summarized in Table 15.5 [159, 160].

New Onset Diabetes After Transplant

NODAT is a serious complication in renal transplant patients as it is associated with CAN, CVD, graft failure, and patient death [161–163]. Risk factors for NODAT include African American or Hispanic ethnicity, family history of diabetes, pre-transplant glucose intolerance, hepatitis C infection, and immunosuppressive drugs. Obesity/MS is an independent predictor for developing NODAT [163, 164]. The commonly used immunosuppressive drugs (corticosteroids, cyclosporine, tacrolimus, sirolimus, and zortress) adversely affect insulin secretion and glucose metabolism and their usage can cause or contribute to NODAT (Table 15.5) [159, 160]. The new biologic agent belatacept is designed to provide effective immunosuppression while avoiding renal toxicity and metabolic adverse effects associated with CNI [165–167]. The BENEFIT and BEBEFIT-EXT studies have compared belatacept with cyclosporine-based regimens. There is significantly lower systolic and diastolic blood pressures and better lipid profile in the belatacept arm. Additionally there is a lower rate of NODAT after 12 months in the belatacept arm compared with cyclosporine arm [165, 166]. Although patient and graft survival are not significantly different in these trials, significant better renal function and improved cardiovascular profile might be an important step towards ultimately better graft and patient survival [166, 167]. The continuing research and innovation hopefully will lead to more biological agent lack of metabolic adverse effects to be developed, so that the full potential and benefit of kidney transplantation can be realized in all transplant patients.

Post-transplant Infection

The risk of infection is related to the cumulated overall immunosuppression and the epidemiologic exposure of transplant patients [168, 169]. Patients usually receive anti-bacterial and anti-PCP prophylaxis with TMP-SMX (either single strength daily or double strength every other day at bed time) for 1 year or longer. If patients cannot tolerate TMP-SMX, alternative regimen consisting of atovaquone with levofloxacin, pentamidine, or dapsone may be used [168–170]. Depending on the risk of CMV disease, patients should receive valganciclovir or acyclovir prophylaxis for

Table 15.5 The metabolic adverse effects of the commonly used immunosuppressive drugs in kidney transplant

Medications	Body weight	Blood pressure	Glucose	TG/LDL-C	HDL-C
Corticosteroids	Increase appetite	Overstimulation of mineralocorticoid receptor	Reduce insulin sensitivity	Decrease LDL degradation	Decrease hepatic HDL-C production
	Abnormal fat distribution (central obesity)	Sodium retention	Decrease insulin secretion	Stimulate hepatic VLDL production	
	Raise body weight	Increase blood pressure	Elevate blood glucose	Decrease VLDL removal	Low HDL-C
				Elevate LDL-C and TG	
Calcineurin inhibitors	Neutral effect	Increase sympathetic nerve activity	Inhibit glucokinase activity	Down-grade hepatic cholesterol 7a-hydroxylase and mitochondrial steroid 26-hydroxylase	Decrease cellular cholesterol and phospholipid efflux to apolipoprotein A-I
1. Cyclosporine		Stimulate renin-angiotensin system	Direct islet cell toxicity	Inhibit lipoprotein lipase	
2. Tacrolimus		Direct vasoconstriction	Suppress insulin release	Reduce bile acid synthesis	Lower HDL-C
		Elevate blood pressure	Increase glucose	Raise LDL-C and TG	
mTOR inhibitors	Neutral effect	Neutral effect	Prevent Akt activation	Increase lipase activity in adipose tissue	Neutral effect
1. Sirolimus			Inhibit glucose transporter expression	Decrease lipoprotein lipase activity	
2. Everolimus			Decrease glucose uptake and metabolism in skeletal muscle	Stimulate hepatic synthesis of TG and VLDL	
			Increase glucose	Increase TG and LDL-C	

herpes virus infection (see below in CMV disease). Anti-candida prophylaxis for mucocutaneous infection can be achieved with oral clotrimazole, nystatin, or fluconazole (in pancreas transplant recipients) for several weeks or months after transplant. Influenza vaccination should be given yearly. Due to safety concerns, live vaccines, such as nasal influenza, varicella, varicella zoster, MMR, smallpox, yellow fever, and oral typhoid, should be avoided after transplant surgery. Before transplant, patients should complete all necessary vaccines. Live vaccines should be given to patients not taking immunosuppressive drugs at least 1 month, preferably 3 months before transplant surgery [168].

BK Virus Nephropathy

BK virus is a "small, slow" polyoma virus, structurally similar to JC virus that causes progressive multifocal encephalopathy (PML) in immuocompromised patients. About 65–90 % of adults are infected with BK virus and it is latent in renal tubular cells [171, 172]. Reactivation occurs after kidney transplant presumptively due to the combination of immunosuppression and ischemia-reperfusion injury. Clinically, it can present as BK viruria, viremia, ureteral stenosis/hydronephrosis, hemorrhagic cystitis, sterile pyuria, or BK virus nephropathy. BK nephropathy has been reported in 3–10% of kidney transplant patients. Without recognition and treatment, BK nephropathy causes progressive deterioration of renal function and graft failure. BK nephropathy increases the risk of acute rejection, and it can also coexist with rejection [173, 174].

Kidney biopsy is necessary to diagnose BK nephropathy. Positive biopsy findings include viral inclusions in tubular cells, positive IF-antibody staining, positive in-situ hybridization for viral DNA, and/or viral particles on EM study. Negative kidney biopsy does not rule out BK nephropathy due to the nature of focal lesions initiated in deep medulla at early stage. Noninvasive tests suggesting possible BK nephropathy include high BK viremia ($>10^4$ copies/mL), viruria ($>10^7$ copies/mL), or presence of urine Decoy cells by cytology.

There is no FDA-approved antiviral agent for BKV. The cornerstone of treatment remains to be reduction of overall immunosuppression [168, 169, 171, 172]. This is frequently achieved by decreasing or discontinuing antimetabolite (such as MFA) and/or lower CNI trough level. Reduction of immunosuppression should control viral activation as reflected by reduction of viral load in plasma and urine. It may improve or stabilize renal function, and it also increases the risk of rejection. So, patient should be closely monitored for viral load as well as renal function. Other reported treatments include low-dose of cidofovir (0.25–0.5 mg/kg every other week), leflunomide (40 mg/day), quinolone, and IVIG [88, 89, 175–179]. The efficacies of these agents have not been well studied or approved, but they are frequently tried for patients with persistent high viral load and/or deteriorating graft function. Sirolimus may have antiviral effect for BKV proliferation [180]. After graft failure from BKV nephropathy, retransplant can be successfully performed [181].

Cytomegalovirus Disease

CMV disease is associated with high morbidity and mortality after kidney transplantation. It not only causes direct injury to the infected organs and tissues (such as CMV pneumonitis, colitis, hepatitis, encephalitis, nephropathy) but also has indirect effects on the allograft, including acute rejection and CAN [182–185]. It has been proposed that CMV may even play a role in the pathogenesis of CVD and other opportunistic infection. It is commonly recognized that donor-positive, recipient-negative serostatus (D+/R−) has the highest risk of developing CMV disease, while D+/R+ and D−/R+ have moderate risk, and D−/R− has the lowest risk. The patient who received T cell depleting antibody for induction or rejection is also at high risk for CMV disease [186–188].

There are two approaches for preventing CMV disease in high risk patients: universal chemoprophylaxis or preemptive treatment. Universal prophylaxis is to give oral ganciclovir or valganciclovir to patients at high risk immediately after transplant for a defined period, typically 3–6 months. Preemptive approach involves quantitative assays (CMV-PCRs) to monitor patients at predefined intervals, usually every 1–2 weeks for the first 3 months, and positive assays result in antiviral therapy. CMV prophylaxis has been shown to improve the graft survival [189, 190]. We use universal approach: patients at high risk (D+/R− mismatch or usage of T cell depleting antibody) are currently given 6-month prophylaxis and patients at moderate risk (D+/R+ or D−/R+) are given 3-month prophylaxis with valganciclovir. For those at low risk (D−/R−), we use acyclovir for herpes virus prophylaxis for 3 months.

CMV disease is usually diagnosed by clinical presentation with documentation of CMV involvement, such as CMV viral inclusions in biopsied tissues, positive antigenemia (early antigen pp65 in neutrophils), or DNA quantitative assays (CMV viral load). CMV culture is too slow and insensitive method, while CMV serology (IgG or IgM titers) is not reliable as patient may not produce any antibody to CMV due to immunosuppression. Our treatment of CMV disease includes 2–3 weeks of IV ganciclovir (5 mg/kg, twice daily, with dose adjustment for renal function) until clinical symptoms are resolved and viremia is cleared, then 3 months of oral ganciclovir (1 g three times daily) or valganciclovir

(900 mg once daily) with dose adjustment based on renal function. New data suggest that oral valganciclovir alone may be used to treat mild to moderate CMV disease [191]. When patients fail to response to treatment, CMV mutant assays should be sent to determine ganciclovir-resistance. Foscarnet is usually active against most ganciclovir-resistant strains of CMV and cidofovir may also be considered [168, 169, 182].

Epstein-Barr Virus Infection

EBV primarily infects B cells and plays a central role in the development of PTLD after organ transplant. PTLD spectrum ranges from benign polymorphic and polyclonal forms to monoclonal and highly malignant disease [192]. It may involve in kidney graft, lymph nodes, spleen, liver, and brain [192, 193]. Risk factors for PTLD include EBV serology mismatch with seropositive donor organ transplanted into seronegative recipients (D+/R−) and usage of T cell depleting antibody [36]. The new immunosuppressive drug belatacept has been noted to increase the risk of PTLD in patients without EBV immunity. Therefore, belatacept is contraindicated in patients who are EBV seronegative [165–167]. Although the majority of PTLD is of B-cell origin, T-cell, natural killer cell, and null cell tumors are also reported, and they are more often EBV negative and in late PTLD [194, 195]. PET scan is very sensitive imaging for localizing PTLD lesions and the clinical management usually depends on the stage of tumor [196]. Partial reduction or total withdrawal of immunosuppression is the first-line treatment, and it can cause PTLD to regress, especially in the early polyclonal forms. Antiviral agent, such as acyclovir, can be used to control EBV infection in cases of EBV-positive B-cell lymphomas. Cases with CD20-positive PTLD can be treated with rituximab [197, 198]. Radiation and/or chemotherapy with CHOP may be needed for diffuse lesions or incomplete response to other therapy. Sirolimus has been shown to have antiproliferative effect and is beneficial in managing PTLD [199, 200]. The trends of quantitative EBV viral loads should be closely monitored in high risk patients after kidney transplant (such as children) for timely adjusting immunosuppression and/or initiating antiviral therapy.

Other Malignancy

The incidence of malignancy has been rising in transplant recipients, and malignancy has become the second most common cause of death after CVD. The incidence of all types of cancer is higher for transplant recipients than the general population [201–203]. The most frequent cancers clinically observed are non-melanoma skin cancer, kidney cancer in native atrophic kidneys, PTLD, cervical, oral, and pharynx cancer. The increase in cancer risk may be associated with cumulative immunosuppression that inhibits the normal antitumor surveillance. Viral infections also contribute to several cancers, such as EBV in PTLD; HBV and HCV in liver cancer; HPV in cervical, vulva, oral, and anal cancer; and HHV-8 in Kaposi's sarcoma. Virus can be transmitted from donor organ to recipient and viral screening of organ donor may decrease the risk of viral infection [204, 205]. How to achieve a long-term balance between immunosuppression and risk of infection and malignancy is a challenging task. The routine cancer surveillance guidelines used in the general population are also the current care standard for transplant recipients. But high risk patients should have more frequent and specific screening based on individual's risk factor, such as annual imaging study of liver for hepatitis patients and native kidneys for positive cystic lesions, and regular skin examination by a dermatologist [206, 207]. mTOR inhibitor may have some anti-oncogenic effect, as mTOR inhibitor-based protocols are associated with lower rate of malignancy [199, 208, 209]. These lead clinician to choose mTOR inhibitor as maintenance for patients at risk for and/or suffering from cancer after kidney transplant.

Pancreas Transplantation

The first human pancreas transplant was performed in 1966 by Dr. Lillehei at the University of Minnesota [210]. The procedure was performed simultaneously with a kidney transplant in a young female with diabetic nephropathy. Unfortunately, the patient could only remain insulin-free for a few weeks. Although other pancreas transplants were performed over the next few years, the success rates did not improve much; by 1977, 1 year graft survival rates were only 5 % for 64 reported procedures, based on the International Pancreas Transplant Registry (IPTR) data.

But improvement in surgical techniques, immunosuppressive medications, and organ donor management has allowed pancreatic transplantation to become a well accepted and commonly performed procedure.

Indications for Pancreatic Transplants

The most common indication for a pancreatic transplant is insulin-dependant diabetes (IDDM). In most cases, patients have classic Type 1 DM, an autoimmune disease with the presence of anti-insulin or anti-islet cell antibodies. As these patients do not make insulin, they usually do not have measurable C-peptide levels. Such patients would also have a decreased stimulated insulin secretion test. Patients who develop IDDM from previous pancreatic resections or from chronic pancreatitis have also received pancreas transplants.

Many of these patients will have devastating complications of IDDM, including hypoglycemic unawareness, diabetic ketoacidosis as well as other organ sequelae such as nephropathy, retinopathy, and neuropathy.

Recently, there has been recognition of adult onset diabetes that is insulin responsive. So while these patients may previously have been characterized as Type 2 diabetics, they show features of Type 1 patients, in that they are not obese and they develop ketoacidosis and retinopathy. Some have even demonstrated late onset of insulin antibody development. Syndromes such as Latent Autoimmune Diabetes in Adults (LADA) [211] and Maturity Onset Diabetes of the Young (MODY) [212] have been described. Such patients had previously been classified as Type 1½ diabetics, but recognition of these syndromes would allow these patients to benefit from a pancreas transplant as well.

In most instances, pancreatic transplants are performed in conjunction with a kidney transplant. The presence of diabetic renal disease, resulting in a GFR of less than 20 cc/min or necessitating dialysis is an indication for a kidney transplant as well.

The workup for a transplant candidate is exhaustive and similar to that of the kidney transplant recipient (see previous). Recognition of the various sequelae of diabetics has to be described. In most centers, candidates are usually younger (<50 years of age) and non-obese (BMI <30). Results of pancreas transplants have not been as good in older or obese patients.

There are three scenarios in which pancreas transplants are performed:

(a) *Simultaneous pancreas kidney transplant* (*SPK*). In this scenario, a recipient receives both organs from the same cadaveric donor in a single surgical procedure. The advantages of this scenario are that the recipient only undergoes one surgical procedure and the organs are immunologically similar. Thus rejection will usually occur concomitantly in both organs and it is easier to diagnose. Also, in most parts of the USA, the kidney is allocated with the pancreas; thus the kidney may be allocated faster with the shorter pancreas waiting list, than with the much longer kidney list.

(b) *Pancreas after kidney transplant* (*PAK*). Here, the recipient receives a pancreas transplant after they have had a previous kidney transplant. This scenario has become more common with the popularity of living donor kidney transplants. So recipients may get on the list for a deceased donor pancreas after they receive a living donor kidney. The advantages of this are that the recipient will get a living donor kidney, which is typically better than a deceased donor one. Also, the living donor transplant may be timed so that the recipient may get their kidney transplant without needing to wait on the list or even before they start dialysis, which is also advantageous. The potential disadvantages are that the recipient has to undergo two surgical procedures. The two organs are not immunologically similar, and thus rejection could happen separately for each of these organs and this is difficult to monitor.

(c) *Pancreas transplants alone* (*PTA*). This transplant is done for patients that have IDDM without renal failure, and thus do not need a kidney transplant. This is perhaps the most controversial of pancreas transplant scenarios. The decision on how to manage complicated IDDM patients is not easy. Whether a brittle diabetic would be better off with an insulin pump, risking the sequelae of diabetes or choosing a major surgical procedure and immunosuppressant medications is difficult to answer. However, there are studies that have shown that in selected diabetics that are extremely brittle, with frequent attacks of hypoglycemic awareness and ketoacidosis despite intensive insulin regimen, pancreas transplants may be lifesaving. A PTA may also prevent the onset of renal failure in these patients, reducing the need for a future kidney transplant. The American Diabetic Association has supported PTA for these indications as well [213].

Surgical Procedure

The deceased donor organ is usually procured with a cuff of duodenum at the head and spleen attached to the tail. Preservation of the duodenum is necessary as it shares blood supply with the head of the pancreas and also serves as a repository of exocrine secretions for drainage. The preparation of the pancreas allograft requires removal of the spleen and vascular reconstruction of the arterial system. The pancreas has two arteries supplying it, the superior mesenteric artery for the head and the splenic artery for the body and tail. The two stumps of these vessels are sewn to a Y-graft of the donor common, internal and external iliac arteries to create a single arterial conduit for anastomosis.

The pancreas allograft is usually placed in the pelvis, with the arterial conduit and the portal vein (venous drainage of the pancreas) anastomosed to the iliac vessels in the recipient (Fig. 15.1). In some instances, the portal vein can be anastomosed to the superior mesenteric veins so the pancreas may have a portal rather than systemic drainage, and some consider this to be more physiologic.

The duodenum of the allograft is usually anastomosed to the recipients' intestine, so that the exocrine secretions of the allograft can be drained. Previous attempts at bladder drainage of the exocrine secretions resulted in high rates of hemorrhagic cystitis and metabolic acidosis, due to loss of exocrine bicarbonate in the urine.

Post-transplant Monitoring of Pancreas Transplants

With a successful transplant, serum glucose levels should normalize within hours after surgery. Serum amylase and lipase levels are very nonspecific, and may be elevated by rejection, infection, or other causes of pancreatitis, including some of the antirejection medications themselves. It is important to understand the development of hyperglycemia is a late finding and usually represents burnout of the pancreas. Measurement of C-peptide levels may confirm if the pancreas is still making insulin or not.

Rejection of the allograft is difficult to diagnose as biopsy of the pancreas is difficult. One of the benefits of an SPK as mentioned previously is that rejection tends to occur simultaneously in both organs; hence rejection in a pancreas allograft can be diagnosed by biopsy of the kidney allograft, which is much easier.

How Successful Are Pancreas Transplants?

Patients who receive pancreas transplants benefit from improved survival and quality of life. Secondary complications of diabetes may stop progressing, and may even reverse. The pancreas may also protect the kidney transplant from developing diabetic nephropathy. Long term US survival data from the Scientific Registry of Transplant Recipients (SRTR) [214] shows 1 and 5 year pancreas graft survival rates were 87 and 72 % for SPK recipients, 77.1 and 59 % PAK recipients, and 85 and 52 % for PTA recipients.

Pancreas Islet Transplantation

Islet transplantation via an injection would seem to be a better option than a major surgical procedure. However, long-term results of islet transplants have not yet shown good outcomes universally. In 2000, the University of Edmonton in Canada reported on seven patients that remained insulin-free 1 year after islet transplantation [215]. However, initial enthusiasm was dampened when in 2005, the same group reported that although 85 % of patients had measurable C-peptide levels, only 10 % of patients could remain insulin-free at 5 years [216]. Subsequent studies also showed that these patients also developed increased risk of renal failure [217] due to use of nephrotoxic immunosuppressants and many of them were now sensitized [218] due to the exposure of the foreign proteins, making it harder for them to receive kidney transplants. Due to these issues, further studies into pancreatic islet transplants are needed.

Other Advances in Pancreatic Transplantation

Living donor pancreas transplants utilizing the distal pancreas have been reported in several centers across the world. In one of the largest series, the University of Minnesota reported on 110 patients whose graft survival after living donor transplants was similar to cadaveric whole organ transplants [219]. Human bone marrow stem cells have been shown differentiation into pancreatic islet cells and glomerular cells, and potentially this could help treat diabetes and nephropathy as well [220].

References

1. Klein C, Brennan DC. HLA and ABO sensitization and desensitization in renal transplantation. UpToDate [Internet]. 2013. http://uptodate.medcity.net/. Accessed 16 March 2013.
2. Halloran PF. Immunosuppressive drugs for kidney transplantation. N Engl J Med. 2004;351(26):2715–29.
3. Danovitch GM. Handbook of kidney transplantation. 4th ed. Philadelphia: Lippincott Williams and Wilkins; 2005. p. 23–71.
4. Lakkis FG, Sayegh MH. Memory T cells: a hurdle to immunologic tolerance. J Am Soc Nephrol. 2003;14(9):2402–10.
5. Dinavahi R, George A, Tretin A, Akalin E, Ames S, Bromberg JS, Deboccardo G, Dipaola N, Lerner SM, Mehrotra A, Murphy BT, Nadasdy T, Paz-Artal E, Salomon DR, Schröppel B, Sehgal V, Sachidanandam R, Heeger PS. Antibodies reactive to non-HLA antigens in transplant glomerulopathy. J Am Soc Nephrol. 2011;22(6):1168–78.
6. Porcheray F, DeVito J, Yeap BY, Xue L, Dargon I, Paine R, Girouard TC, Saidman SL, Colvin RB, Wong W, Zorn E. Chronic humoral rejection of human kidney allografts associates with broad autoantibody responses. Transplantation. 2010;89(10):1239–46.
7. Montgomery RA. Renal transplantation across HLA and ABO antibody barriers: integrating paired donation into desensitization protocols. Am J Transplant. 2010;10:449–57.
8. Warren EH, Greenberg PD, Riddell SR. Cytotoxic T-lymphocyte-defined human minor histocompatibility antigens with a restricted tissue distribution. Blood. 1998;91(6):2197–207.
9. Scott DM, Ehrmann IE, Ellis PS, Chandler PR, Simpson E. Why do some females reject males? The molecular basis for male-specific graft rejection. J Mol Med (Berl). 1997;75(2):103–14.
10. Hankey KG, Drachenberg CB, Papadimitriou JC, Klassen DK, Philosophe B, Bartlett ST, Groh V, Spies T, Mann DL. MIC expression in renal and pancreatic allografts. Transplantation. 2002;73(2):304–6.
11. Dragun D, Müller DN, Bräsen JH, Fritsche L, Nieminen-Kelhä M, Dechend R, Kintscher U, Rudolph B, Hoebeke J, Eckert D, Mazak I, Plehm R, Schönemann C, Unger T, Budde K, Neumayer HH, Luft FC, Wallukat G. Angiotensin II type 1-receptor activating antibodies in renal-allograft rejection. N Engl J Med. 2005;352(6):558–69.
12. Aguilera I, Alvarez-Marquez A, Gentil MA, Fernandez-Alonso J, Fijo J, Saez C, Wichmann I, Nuñez-Roldan A. Anti-glutathione S-transferase T1 antibody-mediated rejection in C4d-positive renal allograft recipients. Nephrol Dial Transplant. 2008;23(7):2393–8.
13. Sun Q, Cheng Z, Cheng D, Chen J, Ji S, Wen J, et al. De novo development of circulating anti-endothelial cell antibodies rather than pre-existing antibodies is associated with post-transplant allograft rejection. Kidney Int. 2011;79(6):655–62.

14. Khan IE, Zhang R, Simon E, Hamm LL. The alloimmune injury in chronic allograft nephropathy. In: Göőz M, editor. Chronic kidney disease. Rijeka: InTech; 2012. p. 401–14.
15. Liu Z, Colovai AI, Tugulea S, Reed EF, Fisher PE, Mancini D, et al. Indirect recognition of donor HLA-DR peptides in organ allograft rejection. J Clin Invest. 1996;98(5):1150–7.
16. Vella JP, Spadafora-Ferreira M, Murphy B, Alexander SI, Harmon W, Carpenter CB, et al. Indirect allorecognition of major histocompatibility complex allopeptides in human renal transplant recipients with chronic graft dysfunction. Transplantation. 1997; 64(6):795–800.
17. Durrbach A, Francois H, Jacquet A, Beaudreuil S, Charpentier B. Co-signals in organ transplantation. Curr Opin Organ Transplant. 2010;15(4):474–80.
18. Denton MD, Reul RM, Dharnidharka VR, Fang JC, Ganz P, Briscoe DM. Central role for CD40/CD40 ligand (CD154) interactions in transplant rejection. Pediatr Transplant. 1998;2(1):6–15.
19. Larsen CP, Pearson TC, Adams AB, Tso P, Shirasugi N, Strobert E, et al. Rational development of LEA29Y (belatacept), a high-affinity variant of CTLA4-Ig with potent immunosuppressive properties. Am J Transplant. 2005;5(3):443–53.
20. Fiorentino DF, Bond MW, Mosmann TR. Two types of mouse T helper cell. IV. Th2 clones secrete a factor that inhibits cytokine production by Th1 clones. J Exp Med. 1989;170(6):2081–95.
21. Tsaur I, Gasser M, Aviles B, Lutz J, Lutz L, Grimm M, et al. Donor antigen-specific regulatory T-cell function affects outcome in kidney transplant recipients. Kidney Int. 2011;79(9):1005–12.
22. Mills DM, Cambier JC. B lymphocyte activation during cognate interactions with CD4+ T lymphocytes: molecular dynamics and immunologic consequences. Semin Immunol. 2003;15(6):325–9.
23. Richards S, Watanabe C, Santos L, Craxton A, Clark EA. Regulation of B-cell entry into the cell cycle. Immunol Rev. 2008;224:183–200.
24. Gatto D, Martin SW, Bessa J, Pellicioli E, Saudan P, Hinton HJ, et al. Regulation of memory antibody levels: the role of persisting antigen versus plasma cell life span. J Immunol. 2007;178(1):67–76.
25. Takeuchi O, Akira S. Pattern recognition receptors and inflammation. Cell. 2010;140(6):805–20.
26. Ren Q, Paramesh AS, Yau CL, Florman S, Killackey M, Slakey DP, Alper B, Simon E, Hamm LL, Zhang R. Kidney transplantation in highly sensitized African Americans. Transpl Int. 2011;24(3):259–65.
27. Lorenz M, Regele H, Schillinger M, Kletzmayr J, Haidbauer B, Derfler K, et al. Peritransplant immunoadsorption: a strategy enabling transplantation in highly sensitized crossmatch-positive cadaveric kidney allograft recipients. Transplantation. 2005;79(6):696–701.
28. Montgomery RA, Lonze BE, King KE, Kraus ES, Kucirka LM, Locke JE, et al. Desensitization in HLA-incompatible kidney recipients and survival. N Engl J Med. 2011;365(4):318–26.
29. Stegall MD, Gloor J, Winters JL, Moore SB, Degoey S. A comparison of plasmapheresis versus high-dose IVIG desensitization in renal allograft recipients with high levels of donor specific alloantibody. Am J Transplant. 2006;6(2):346–51.
30. Vo AA, Lukovsky M, Toyoda M, Wang J, Reinsmoen NL, Lai CH, et al. Rituximab and intravenous immune globulin for desensitization during renal transplantation. N Engl J Med. 2008;359(3):242–51.
31. Warren DS, Zachary AA, Sonnenday CJ, King KE, Cooper M, Ratner LE, et al. Successful renal transplantation across simultaneous ABO incompatible and positive crossmatch barriers. Am J Transplant. 2004;4(4):561–8.
32. US Department of Health and Human Services. 2011 Annual report of the organ procurement and transplantation network and the scientific registry of transplant recipients. Am J Transplant. 2013;13(S1):1–36.
33. Chouhan K, Zhang R. Editorial review: antibody induction therapy in adult kidney transplantation, a controversy continues. World J Transplant. 2012;2(2):19–26.
34. Hibberd PL, Tolkoff-Rubin NE, Cosimi AB, Schooley RT, Isaacson D, Doran M, Delvecchio A, Delmonico FL, Auchincloss Jr H, Rubin RH. Symptomatic cytomegalovirus disease in the cytomegalovirus antibody seropositive renal transplant recipient treated with OKT3. Transplantation. 1992;53(1):68–72.
35. Thistlethwaite Jr JR, Stuart JK, Mayes JT, Gaber AO, Woodle S, Buckingham MR, Stuart FP. Complications and monitoring of OKT3 therapy. Am J Kidney Dis. 1988;11(2):112–9.
36. Swinnen LJ, Costanzo-Nordin MR, Fisher SG, O'Sullivan EJ, Johnson MR, Heroux AL, Dizikes GJ, Pifarre R, Fisher RI. Increased incidence of lymphoproliferative disorder after immunosuppression with the monoclonal antibody OKT3 in cardiac-transplant recipients. N Engl J Med. 1990;323(25):1723–8.
37. Brennan DC, Flavin K, Lowell JA, Howard TK, Shenoy S, Burgess S, Dolan S, Kano JM, Mahon M, Schnitzler MA, Woodward R, Irish W, Singer GG. A randomized, double-blinded comparison of Thymoglobulin versus Atgam for induction immunosuppressive therapy in adult renal transplant recipients. Transplantation. 1999;67(7):1011–8.
38. Hardinger KL, Schnitzler MA, Miller B, Lowell JA, Shenoy S, Koch MJ, Enkvetchakul D, Ceriotti C, Brennan DC. Five-year follow up of thymoglobulin versus ATGAM induction in adult renal transplantation. Transplantation. 2004;78(1):136–41.
39. Hardinger KL, Rhee S, Buchanan P, Koch M, Miller B, Enkvetchakul D, Schuessler R, Schnitzler MA, Brennan DC. A prospective, randomized, double-blinded comparison of thymoglobulin versus Atgam for induction immunosuppressive therapy: 10-year results. Transplantation. 2008;86(7):947–52.
40. Goggins WC, Pascual MA, Powelson JA, Magee C, Tolkoff-Rubin N, Farrell ML, Ko DS, Williams WW, Chandraker A, Delmonico FL, Auchincloss H, Cosimi AB. A prospective, randomized, clinical trial of intraoperative versus postoperative thymoglobulin in adult cadaveric renal transplant recipients. Transplantation. 2003;76(5):798–802.
41. Wong W, Agrawal N, Pascual M, Anderson DC, Hirsch HH, Fujimoto K, Cardarelli F, Winkelmayer WC, Cosimi AB, Tolkoff-Rubin N. Comparison of two dosages of thymoglobulin used as a short-course for induction in kidney transplantation. Transpl Int. 2006;19(8):629–35.
42. Stevens RB, Mercer DF, Grant WJ, Freifeld AG, Lane JT, Groggel GC, Rigley TH, Nielsen KJ, Henning ME, Skorupa JY, Skorupa AJ, Christensen KA, Sandoz JP, Kellogg AM, Langnas AN, Wrenshall LE. Randomized trial of single-dose versus divided-dose rabbit anti-thymocyte globulin induction in renal transplantation: an interim report. Transplantation. 2008;85(10): 1391–9.
43. Vincenti F, Kirkman R, Light S, Bumgardner G, Pescovitz M, Halloran P, Neylan J, Wilkinson A, Ekberg H, Gaston R, Backman L, Burdick J. Interleukin-2-receptor blockade with daclizumab to prevent acute rejection in renal transplantation. Daclizumab Triple Therapy Study Group. N Engl J Med. 1998;338:161–5.
44. Kahan BD, Rajagopalan PR, Hall M. Reduction of the occurrence of acute cellular rejection among renal allograft recipients treated with basiliximab, a chimeric anti-interleukin-2-receptor monoclonal antibody. United States Simulect Renal Study Group. Transplantation. 1999;67:276–84.
45. Lawen JG, Davies EA, Mourad G, Oppenheimer F, Molina MG, Rostaing L, Wilkinson AH, Mulloy LL, Bourbigot BJ, Prestele H, Korn A, Girault D. Randomized double-blind study of immunoprophylaxis with basiliximab, a chimeric anti-interleukin-2 receptor monoclonal antibody, in combination with mycophenolate mofetil-containing triple therapy in renal transplantation. Transplantation. 2003;75:37–43.
46. Webster AC, Playford EG, Higgins G, Chapman JR, Craig JC. Interleukin 2 receptor antagonists for renal transplant recipients: a meta analysis of randomized trials. Transplantation. 2004;77: 166–76.

47. Kirk AD, Hale DA, Swanson SJ, Mannon RB. Autoimmune thyroid disease after renal transplantation using depletional induction with alemtuzumab. Am J Transplant. 2006;6(5 Pt 1):1084–5.
48. Pascual J, Mezrich JD, Djamali A, Leverson G, Chin LT, Torrealba J, Bloom D, Voss B, Becker BN, Knechtle SJ, Sollinger HW, Pirsch JD, Samaniego MD. Alemtuzumab induction and recurrence of glomerular disease after kidney transplantation. Transplantation. 2007;83(11):1429–34.
49. Hanaway MJ, Woodle ES, Mulgaonkar S, Peddi VR, Kaufman DB, First MR, Croy R, Holman J, for the INTAC Study Group. Alemtuzumab induction in renal transplantation. N Engl J Med. 2011;364(20):1909–19.
50. Tan HP, Donaldson J, Basu A, Unruh M, Randhawa P, Sharma V, Morgan C, McCauley J, Wu C, Shah N, Zeevi A, Shapiro R. Two hundred living donor kidney transplantations under alemtuzumab induction and tacrolimus monotherapy: 3-year follow-up. Am J Transplant. 2009;9(2):355–66.
51. Kaufman DB, Leventhal JR, Axelrod D, Gallon LG, Parker MA, Stuart FP. Alemtuzumab induction and prednisone-free maintenance immunotherapy in kidney transplantation: comparison with basiliximab induction—long-term results. Am J Transplant. 2005;5(10):2539–48.
52. Flechner SM, Friend PJ, Brockmann J, Ismail HR, Zilvetti M, Goldfarb D, Modlin C, Mastroianni B, Savas K, Devaney A, Simmonds M, Cook DJ. Alemtuzumab induction and sirolimus plus mycophenolate mofetil maintenance for CNI and steroid-free kidney transplant immunosuppression. Am J Transplant. 2005;5: 3009–14.
53. Mulley WR, Hudson FJ, Tait BD, Skene AM, Dowling JP, Kerr PG, et al. A single low-fixed dose of rituximab to salvage renal transplants from refractory antibody-mediated rejection. Transplantation. 2009;87(2):286–9.
54. Kidney Disease: Improving Global Outcomes (KDIGO) Transplant Work Group. KDIGO clinical practice guideline for the care of kidney transplant recipients. Am J Transplant. 2009;9 Suppl 3:S1–155.
55. Jindal RM, Das NP, Neff RT, Hurst FP, Falta EM, Elster EA, Abbott KC. Outcomes in African-Americans vs. Caucasians using thymoglobulin or interleukin-2 inhibitor induction: analysis of USRD database. Am J Nephrol. 2009;29:501–8.
56. Brennan DC, Daller JA, Lake KD, Cibrik D, Del Castillo D. Rabbit antithymocyte globulin versus basiliximab in renal transplantation. N Engl J Med. 2006;355:1967–77.
57. Patlolla V, Zhong X, Reed GW, Mandelbrot DA. Efficacy of anti IL2 receptor antibodies compared to no induction and to antilymphocyte antibodies in renal transplantation. Am J Transplant. 2007;7:832–1842.
58. Luan FL, Schaubel DE, Zhang H, Jia X, Pelletier SJ, Port FK, Magee JC, Sung RS. Impact of immunosuppressive regimen on survival of kidney transplant recipients with hepatitis C. Transplantation. 2008;85(11):1601–6.
59. Stock PG, Barin B, Murphy B, Hanto D, Diego JM, Light J, Davis C, Blumberg E, Simon D, Subramanian A, Millis JM, Lyon GM, Brayman K, Slakey D, Shapiro R, Melancon J, Jacobson JM, Stosor V, Olson JL, Stablein DM, Roland ME. Outcomes of kidney transplantation in HIV-infected recipients. N Engl J Med. 2010;363(21):2004–14.
60. Patel SJ, Knight RJ, Suki WN, Abdellatif A, Duhart Jr BT, Krauss AG, Mannan S, Nezakatgoo N, Osama GA. Rabbit antithymocyte induction and dosing in deceased donor renal transplant recipients over 60 yr of age. Clin Transplant. 2011;25(3):E250–6.
61. Morton RL, Howard K, Webster AC, Wong G, Craig JC. The cost effectiveness of induction immunosuppression in kidney transplantation. Nephrol Dial Transplant. 2009;24(7):2258–69.
62. Leichtman AB. Balancing efficacy and toxicity in kidney-transplant immunosuppression. N Engl J Med. 2007;357(25): 2625–7.
63. Hricik DE, Almawi WY, Strom TB. Trends in the use of glucocorticoids in renal transplantation. Transplantation. 1994;57(7):979–89.
64. Midtvedt K, Hjelmesaeth J, Hartmann A, Lund K, Paulsen D, Egeland T, et al. Insulin resistance after renal transplantation: the effect of steroid dose reduction and withdrawal. J Am Soc Nephrol. 2004;15(12):3233–9.
65. A randomized clinical trial of cyclosporine in cadaveric renal transplantation. Analysis at three years. The Canadian Multicentre Transplant Study Group. N Engl J Med. 1986;314(19):1219–25.
66. Mueller EA, Kovarik JM, van Bree JB, Lison AE, Kutz K. Pharmacokinetics and tolerability of a microemulsion formulation of cyclosporine in renal allograft recipients—a concentration-controlled comparison with the commercial formulation. Transplantation. 1994;57(8):1178–82.
67. Pescovitz MD, Barone G, Choc Jr MG, Hricik DE, Hwang DS, Jin JH, et al. Safety and tolerability of cyclosporine microemulsion versus cyclosporine: two-year data in primary renal allograft recipients: a report of the Neoral Study Group. Transplantation. 1997;63(5):778–80.
68. Ponticelli C, Minetti L, Di Palo FQ, Vegeto A, Belli L, Corbetta G, et al. The Milan clinical trial with cyclosporine in cadaveric renal transplantation. A three-year follow-up. Transplantation. 1988;45(5):908–13.
69. Knight SR, Morris PJ. The clinical benefits of cyclosporine C2-level monitoring: a systematic review. Transplantation. 2007;83(12):1525–35.
70. Knoll GA, Bell RC. Tacrolimus versus cyclosporin for immunosuppression in renal transplantation: meta-analysis of randomised trials. BMJ. 1999;318(7191):1104–7.
71. Hardinger KL, Bohl DL, Schnitzler MA, Lockwood M, Storch GA, Brennan DC. A randomized, prospective, pharmacoeconomic trial of tacrolimus versus cyclosporine in combination with thymoglobulin in renal transplant recipients. Transplantation. 2005;80(1):41–6.
72. Margreiter R, European Tacrolimus vs Ciclosporin Microemulsion Renal Transplantation Study Group. Efficacy and safety of tacrolimus compared with ciclosporin microemulsion in renal transplantation: a randomised multicentre study. Lancet. 2002; 359(9308):741–6.
73. Webster AC, Woodroffe RC, Taylor RS, Chapman JR, Craig JC. Tacrolimus versus ciclosporin as primary immunosuppression for kidney transplant recipients: meta-analysis and meta-regression of randomised trial data. BMJ. 2005;331(7520):810.
74. Krämer BK, Del Castillo D, Margreiter R, Sperschneider H, Olbricht CJ, Ortuño J, Sester U, Kunzendorf U, Dietl KH, Bonomini V, Rigotti P, Ronco C, Tabernero JM, Rivero M, Banas B, Mühlbacher F, Arias M, Montagnino G. Efficacy and safety of tacrolimus compared with ciclosporin A in renal transplantation: three-year observational results. Nephrol Dial Transplant. 2008;23(7):2386–92.
75. Silva Jr HT, Yang HC, Abouljoud M, Kuo PC, Wisemandle K, Bhattacharya P, et al. One-year results with extended-release tacrolimus/MMF, tacrolimus/MMF and cyclosporine/MMF in de novo kidney transplant recipients. Am J Transplant. 2007;7(3):595–608.
76. Bergan S, Rugstad HE, Bentdal O, Sodal G, Hartmann A, Leivestad T, et al. Monitored high-dose azathioprine treatment reduces acute rejection episodes after renal transplantation. Transplantation. 1998;66(3):334–9.
77. Remuzzi G, Cravedi P, Costantini M, Lesti M, Ganeva M, Gherardi G, et al. Mycophenolate mofetil versus azathioprine for prevention of chronic allograft dysfunction in renal transplantation: the MYSS follow-up randomized, controlled clinical trial. J Am Soc Nephrol. 2007;18(6):1973–85.
78. Kahan BD. Efficacy of sirolimus compared with azathioprine for reduction of acute renal allograft rejection: a randomised multicentre study. The Rapamune US Study Group. Lancet. 2000; 356(9225):194–202.

79. Meier-Kriesche HU, Steffen BJ, Hochberg AM, Gordon RD, Liebman MN, Morris JA, et al. Long-term use of mycophenolate mofetil is associated with a reduction in the incidence and risk of late rejection. Am J Transplant. 2003;3(1):68–73.
80. Neylan JF. Immunosuppressive therapy in high-risk transplant patients: dose-dependent efficacy of mycophenolate mofetil in African-American renal allograft recipients. U.S. Renal Transplant Mycophenolate Mofetil Study Group. Transplantation. 1997;64(9):1277–82.
81. Sollinger HW. Mycophenolate mofetil for the prevention of acute rejection in primary cadaveric renal allograft recipients. U.S. Renal Transplant Mycophenolate Mofetil Study Group. Transplantation. 1995;60(3):225–32.
82. The Tricontinental Mycophenolate Mofetil Renal Transplantation Study Group. A blinded, randomized clinical trial of mycophenolate mofetil for the prevention of acute rejection in cadaveric renal transplantation. Transplantation. 1996;61(7):1029–37.
83. Kofler S, Shvets N, Bigdeli AK, Konig MA, Kaczmarek P, Deutsch MA, et al. Proton pump inhibitors reduce mycophenolate exposure in heart transplant recipients—a prospective case-controlled study. Am J Transplant. 2009;9(7):1650–6.
84. Kiberd BA, Wrobel M, Dandavino R, Keown P, Gourishankar S. The role of proton pump inhibitors on early mycophenolic acid exposure in kidney transplantation: evidence from the CLEAR study. Ther Drug Monit. 2011;33(1):120–3.
85. Bolin P, Tanriover B, Zibari GB, Lynn ML, Pirsch JD, Chan L, et al. Improvement in 3-month patient-reported gastrointestinal symptoms after conversion from mycophenolate mofetil to enteric-coated mycophenolate sodium in renal transplant patients. Transplantation. 2007;84(11):1443–51.
86. Bunnapradist S, Lentine KL, Burroughs TE, Pinsky BW, Hardinger KL, Brennan DC, et al. Mycophenolate mofetil dose reductions and discontinuations after gastrointestinal complications are associated with renal transplant graft failure. Transplantation. 2006;82(1):102–7.
87. Langone AJ, Chan L, Bolin P, Cooper M. Enteric-coated mycophenolate sodium versus mycophenolate mofetil in renal transplant recipients experiencing gastrointestinal intolerance: a multicenter, double-blind, randomized study. Transplantation. 2011;91(4):470–8.
88. Chong AS, Zeng H, Knight DA, Shen J, Meister GT, Williams JW, et al. Concurrent antiviral and immunosuppressive activities of leflunomide in vivo. Am J Transplant. 2006;6(1):69–75.
89. Josephson MA, Gillen D, Javaid B, Kadambi P, Meehan S, Foster P, et al. Treatment of renal allograft polyoma BK virus infection with leflunomide. Transplantation. 2006;81(5):704–10.
90. Groth CG, Backman L, Morales JM, Calne R, Kreis H, Lang P, et al. Sirolimus (rapamycin)-based therapy in human renal transplantation: similar efficacy and different toxicity compared with cyclosporine. Sirolimus European Renal Transplant Study Group. Transplantation. 1999;67(7):1036–42.
91. Meier-Kriesche HU, Schold JD, Srinivas TR, Howard RJ, Fujita S, Kaplan B. Sirolimus in combination with tacrolimus is associated with worse renal allograft survival compared to mycophenolate mofetil combined with tacrolimus. Am J Transplant. 2005;5(9):2273–80.
92. Meier-Kriesche HU, Steffen BJ, Chu AH, Loveland JJ, Gordon RD, Morris JA, et al. Sirolimus with neoral versus mycophenolate mofetil with neoral is associated with decreased renal allograft survival. Am J Transplant. 2004;4(12):2058–66.
93. Budde K, Becker T, Arns W, Sommerer C, Reinke P, Eisenberger U, et al. Everolimus-based, calcineurin-inhibitor-free regimen in recipients of de-novo kidney transplants: an open-label, randomised, controlled trial. Lancet. 2011;377(9768):837–47.
94. Ciancio G, Burke GW, Gaynor JJ, Ruiz P, Roth D, Kupin W, et al. A randomized long-term trial of tacrolimus/sirolimus versus tacrolimums/mycophenolate versus cyclosporine/sirolimus in renal transplantation: three-year analysis. Transplantation. 2006;81(6):845–52.
95. Vincenti F, Larsen C, Durrbach A, Wekerle T, Nashan B, Blancho G, et al. Costimulation blockade with belatacept in renal transplantation. N Engl J Med. 2005;353(8):770–81.
96. Durrbach A, Pestana JM, Pearson T, Vincenti F, Garcia VD, Campistol J, et al. A phase III study of belatacept versus cyclosporine in kidney transplants from extended criteria donors (BENEFIT-EXT study). Am J Transplant. 2010;10(3):547–57.
97. Vincenti F, Charpentier B, Vanrenterghem Y, Rostaing L, Bresnahan B, Darji P, et al. A phase III study of belatacept-based immunosuppression regimens versus cyclosporine in renal transplant recipients (BENEFIT study). Am J Transplant. 2010;10(3):535–46.
98. Vincenti F, Blancho G, Durrbach A, Friend P, Grinyo J, Halloran PF, et al. Five-year safety and efficacy of belatacept in renal transplantation. J Am Soc Nephrol. 2010;21(9):1587–96.
99. Toyoda M, Pao A, Petrosian A, Jordan SC. Pooled human gammaglobulin modulates surface molecule expression and induces apoptosis in human B cells. Am J Transplant. 2003;3(2):156–66.
100. Luke PP, Scantlebury VP, Jordan ML, Vivas CA, Hakala TR, Jain A, et al. Reversal of steroid- and anti-lymphocyte antibody-resistant rejection using intravenous immunoglobulin (IVIG) in renal transplant recipients. Transplantation. 2001;72(3):419–22.
101. Rocha PN, Butterly DW, Greenberg A, Reddan DN, Tuttle-Newhall J, Collins BH, et al. Beneficial effect of plasmapheresis and intravenous immunoglobulin on renal allograft survival of patients with acute humoral rejection. Transplantation. 2003;75(9):1490–5.
102. Casadei DH, del C Rial M, Opelz G, Golberg JC, Argento JA, Greco G, et al. A randomized and prospective study comparing treatment with high-dose intravenous immunoglobulin with monoclonal antibodies for rescue of kidney grafts with steroid-resistant rejection. Transplantation 2001;71(1):53–8.
103. Everly MJ, Everly JJ, Susskind B, Brailey P, Arend LJ, Alloway RR, et al. Bortezomib provides effective therapy for antibody- and cell-mediated acute rejection. Transplantation. 2008;86(12):1754–61.
104. Locke JE, Magro CM, Singer AL, Segev DL, Haas M, Hillel AT, et al. The use of antibody to complement protein C5 for salvage treatment of severe antibody-mediated rejection. Am J Transplant. 2009;9(1):231–5.
105. Vincenti F, Schena FP, Paraskevas S, Hauser IA, Walker RG, Grinyo J, et al. A randomized, multicenter study of steroid avoidance, early steroid withdrawal or standard steroid therapy in kidney transplant recipients. Am J Transplant. 2008;8(2):307–16.
106. Woodle ES, First MR, Pirsch J, Shihab F, Gaber AO, Van Veldhuisen P, et al. A prospective, randomized, double-blind, placebo-controlled multicenter trial comparing early (7 day) corticosteroid cessation versus long-term, low-dose corticosteroid therapy. Ann Surg. 2008;248(4):564–77.
107. Hanaway MJ, Woodle ES, Mulgaonkar S, Peddi VR, Kaufman DB, First MR, Croy R, Holman J, INTAC Study Group. Alemtuzumab induction in renal transplantation. N Engl J Med. 2011;364(20):1909–19.
108. Chhabra D, Skaro AI, Leventhal JR, Dalal P, Shah G, Wang E, et al. Long-term kidney allograft function and survival in prednisone-free regimens: tacrolimus/mycophenolate mofetil versus tacrolimus/sirolimus. Clin J Am Soc Nephrol. 2012;7(3):504–12.
109. Heilman RL, Younan K, Wadei HM, Mai ML, Reddy KS, Chakkera HA, et al. Results of a prospective randomized trial of sirolimus conversion in kidney transplant recipients on early corticosteroid withdrawal. Transplantation. 2011;92(7):767–73.
110. Ekberg H, Grinyó J, Nashan B, Vanrenterghem Y, Vincenti F, Voulgari A, Truman M, Nasmyth-Miller C, Rashford M. Cyclosporine sparing with mycophenolate mofetil, daclizumab and corticosteroids in renal allograft recipients: the CAESAR Study. Am J Transplant. 2007;7(3):560–70.

111. Ekberg H, Tedesco-Silva H, Demirbas A, Vitko S, Nashan B, Gurkan A, et al. Reduced exposure to calcineurin inhibitors in renal transplantation. N Engl J Med. 2007;357(25):2562–75.
112. Ekberg H, Bernasconi C, Tedesco-Silva H, Vítko S, Hugo C, Demirbas A, Acevedo RR, Grinyó J, Frei U, Vanrenterghem Y, Daloze P, Halloran P. Calcineurin inhibitor minimization in the Symphony study: observational results 3 years after transplantation. Am J Transplant. 2009;9(8):1876–85.
113. Guerra G, Ciancio G, Gaynor JJ, Zarak A, Brown R, Hanson L, et al. Randomized trial of immunosuppressive regimens in renal transplantation. J Am Soc Nephrol. 2011;22(9):1758–68.
114. Srinivas TR, Schold JD, Guerra G, Eagan A, Bucci CM, Meier-Kriesche HU. Mycophenolate mofetil/sirolimus compared to other common immunosuppressive regimens in kidney transplantation. Am J Transplant. 2007;7(3):586–94.
115. Weir MR, Mulgaonkar S, Chan L, Shidban H, Waid TH, Preston D, et al. Mycophenolate mofetil-based immunosuppression with sirolimus in renal transplantation: a randomized, controlled Spare-the-Nephron trial. Kidney Int. 2011;79(8):897–907.
116. Flechner SM, Glyda M, Cockfield S, Grinyo J, Legendre C, Russ G, et al. The ORION study: comparison of two sirolimus-based regimens versus tacrolimus and mycophenolate mofetil in renal allograft recipients. Am J Transplant. 2011;11(8):1633–44.
117. Steinman TI, Becker BN, Frost AE, Olthoff KM, Smart FW, Suki WN, Wilkinson AH, Clinical Practice Committee, American Society of Transplantation. Guidelines for the referral and management of patients eligible for solid organ transplantation. Transplantation. 2001;71(9):1189–204.
118. Kasiske BL, Ramos EL, Gaston RS, Bia MJ, Danovitch GM, Bowen PA, Lundin PA, Murphy KJ. The evaluation of renal transplant candidates: clinical practice guidelines. Patient Care and Education Committee of the American Society of Transplant Physicians. J Am Soc Nephrol. 1995;6(1):1–34.
119. Penn I. The effect of immunosuppression on pre-existing cancers. Transplantation. 1993;55(4):742–7.
120. Tavakoli A, Surange RS, Pearson RC, Parrott NR, Augustine T, Riad HN. Impact of stents on urologic complications and health care expenditure in renal transplant recipients: results of a prospective, randomized clinical trial. J Urol. 2007;177(6):2260–4.
121. Mandelbrot DA, Pavlakis M, Danovitch GM, Johnson SR, Karp SJ, Khwaja K, Hanto DW, Rodrigue JR. The medical evaluation of living kidney donors: a survey of US transplant centers. Am J Transplant. 2007;7(10):2333–43.
122. Solez K, Colvin RB, Racusen LC, Haas M, Sis B, Mengel M, Halloran PF, Baldwin W, Banfi G, Collins AB, Cosio F, David DS, Drachenberg C, Einecke G, Fogo AB, Gibson IW, Glotz D, Iskandar SS, Kraus E, Lerut E, Mannon RB, Mihatsch M, Nankivell BJ, Nickeleit V, Papadimitriou JC, Randhawa P, Regele H, Renaudin K, Roberts I, Seron D, Smith RN, Valente M. Banff 07 classification of renal allograft pathology: updates and future directions. Am J Transplant. 2008;8(4):753–60.
123. Mauiyyedi S, Crespo M, Collins AB, Schneeberger EE, Pascual MA, Saidman SL. Acute humoral rejection in kidney transplantation: II. Morphology, immunopathology, and pathologic classification. J Am Soc Nephrol. 2002;13(3):779–87.
124. Saidi RF, Elias N, Kawai T, Hertl M, Farrell ML, Goes N. Outcome of kidney transplantation using expanded criteria donors and donation after cardiac death kidneys: realities and costs. Am J Transplant. 2007;7(12):2769–74.
125. Humar A, Matas AJ. Surgical complications after kidney transplantation. Semin Dial. 2005;18(6):505–10.
126. Shinn C, Malhotra D, Chan L, Cosby RL, Shapiro JI. Time course of response to pulse methylprednisolone therapy in renal transplant recipients with acute allograft rejection. Am J Kidney Dis. 1999;34(2):304–7.
127. Gray D, Shepherd H, Daar A, Oliver DO, Morris PJ. Oral versus intravenous high-dose steroid treatment of renal allograft rejection. The big shot or not? Lancet. 1978;1(8056):117–8.
128. Gaber AO, First MR, Tesi RJ, Gaston RS, Mendez R, Mulloy LL, et al. Results of the double-blind, randomized, multicenter, phase III clinical trial of Thymoglobulin versus Atgam in the treatment of acute graft rejection episodes after renal transplantation. Transplantation. 1998;66(1):29–37.
129. Webster AC, Pankhurst T, Rinaldi F, Chapman JR, Craig JC. Monoclonal and polyclonal antibody therapy for treating acute rejection in kidney transplant recipients: a systematic review of randomized trial data. Transplantation. 2006;81(7):953–65.
130. Worthington JE, McEwen A, McWilliam LJ, Picton ML, Martin S. Association between C4d staining in renal transplant biopsies, production of donor-specific HLA antibodies, and graft outcome. Transplantation. 2007;83(4):398–403.
131. Mengel M, Sis B, Haas M, Colvin RB, Halloran PF, Racusen LC, et al. Banff 2011 meeting report: new concepts in antibody-mediated rejection. Am J Transplant. 2012;12(3):563–70.
132. Troxell ML, Weintraub LA, Higgins JP, Kambham N. Comparison of C4d immunostaining methods in renal allograft biopsies. Clin J Am Soc Nephrol. 2006;1(3):583–91.
133. Becker YT, Becker BN, Pirsch JD, Sollinger HW. Rituximab as treatment for refractory kidney transplant rejection. Am J Transplant. 2004;4(6):996–1001.
134. Locke JE, Zachary AA, Haas M, Melancon JK, Warren DS, Simpkins CE, et al. The utility of splenectomy as rescue treatment for severe acute antibody mediated rejection. Am J Transplant. 2007;7(4):842–6.
135. Opelz G, Dohler B, Collaborative Transplant Study Report. Influence of time of rejection on long-term graft survival in renal transplantation. Transplantation. 2008;85(5):661–6.
136. Madden RL, Mulhern JG, Benedetto BJ, O'Shea MH, Germain MJ, Braden GL, et al. Completely reversed acute rejection is not a significant risk factor for the development of chronic rejection in renal allograft recipients. Transpl Int. 2000;13(5):344–50.
137. Woodle ES, Thistlethwaite JR, Gordon JH, Laskow D, Deierhoi MH, Burdick J, et al. A multicenter trial of FK506 (tacrolimus) therapy in refractory acute renal allograft rejection. A report of the Tacrolimus Kidney Transplantation Rescue Study Group. Transplantation. 1996;62(5):594–9.
138. Briggs D, Dudley C, Pattison J, Pfeffer P, Salmela K, Rowe P, et al. Effects of immediate switch from cyclosporine microemulsion to tacrolimus at first acute rejection in renal allograft recipients. Transplantation. 2003;75(12):2058–63.
139. Clatworthy MR, Friend PJ, Calne RY, Rebello PR, Hale G, Waldmann H, et al. Alemtuzumab (CAMPATH-1H) for the treatment of acute rejection in kidney transplant recipients: long-term follow-up. Transplantation. 2009;87(7):1092–5.
140. Csapo Z, Benavides-Viveros C, Podder H, Pollard V, Kahan BD. Campath-1H as rescue therapy for the treatment of acute rejection in kidney transplant patients. Transplant Proc. 2005;37(5):2032–6.
141. Wahl AO, Small Jr W, Dixler I, Strom S, Rademaker A, Leventhal J, et al. Radiotherapy for rejection of renal transplant allografts refractory to medical immunosuppression. Am J Clin Oncol. 2006;29(6):551–4.
142. Rush D, Arlen D, Boucher A, Busque S, Cockfield SM, Girardin C, et al. Lack of benefit of early protocol biopsies in renal transplant patients receiving TAC and MMF: a randomized study. Am J Transplant. 2007;7(11):2538–45.
143. Nemeth D, Ovens J, Opelz G, Sommerer C, Dohler B, Becker LE, et al. Does borderline kidney allograft rejection always require treatment? Transplantation. 2010;90(4):427–32.
144. Seron D, Moreso F. Protocol biopsies in renal transplantation: prognostic value of structural monitoring. Kidney Int. 2007;72(6):690–7.
145. Zhang R, Lia J, Morse S, Donelon S, Reisin E. Kidney disease in the metabolic syndrome. Am J Med Sci. 2005;330(6):319–25.
146. Zhang R, Thakur V, Morse S, Reisin E. Renal and cardiovascular considerations for the non pharmacological and pharmacological therapies of obesity-hypertension. J Hum Hypertens. 2002;16(12):819–27.

147. Chen J, Muntner P, Hamm LL, Jones DW, Batuman V, Fonseca V, Whelton PK, He J. The metabolic syndrome and chronic kidney disease in U.S. adults. Ann Intern Med. 2004;140(3):167–74.
148. Kalantar-Zadeh K, Block G, Humphreys MH, Kopple JD. Reverse epidemiology of cardiovascular risk factors in maintenance dialysis patients. Kidney Int. 2003;63:793–808.
149. Leavey SF, McCullough K, Hecking E, Goodkin D, Port FK, Young EW. Body mass index and mortality in 'healthier' as compared with 'sicker' haemodialysis patients: results from the Dialysis Outcomes and Practice Patterns Study (DOPPS). Nephrol Dial Transplant. 2001;16:2386–94.
150. Molnar MZ, Streja E, Kovesday CP, Bunnapradist S, Sampaio MS, Jing J, Krishnan M, Nissenson AR, Danovitch GM, Kalantar-Zadeh K. Associations of body mass index and weight loss with mortality in transplant waitlisted maintenance of hemodialysis patients. Am J Transplant. 2011;11:725–36.
151. Chang SH, Coates PT, McDonald SP. Effects of body mass index at transplant on outcomes of kidney transplantation. Transplantation. 2007;84:981–7.
152. Molnar MZ, Kovesdy CP, Musci I, Bunnapradist S, Streja E, Krishnan M, Kalantar-Zadeh K. Higher recipient body mass index is associated with post-transplant delayed kidney graft function. Kidney Int. 2011;80:218–24.
153. Meier-Kriesche H, Arndorfer J, Kaplan B. The impact of body mass index on renal transplant outcomes: a significant independent risk factor for graft failure and patient death. Transplantation. 2002;73:70–4.
154. Friedman AN, Miskulin DC, Rosenberg IH. Demographics and trends in overweight and obesity in patients at time of kidney transplantation. Am J Kidney Dis. 2003;41:480–7.
155. Glanton C, Kao T, Cruess D, Agodoa LY, Abbott KC. Impact of renal transplantation on survival in end-stage renal disease with elevated body mass index. Kidney Int. 2003;63:647–53.
156. Kovas AZ, Molnar MZ, Szeifert L. Sleep disorders, depressive symptoms and health related quality of life—a cross sectional comparison between kidney transplant recipients and waitlisted patients on maintenance dialysis. Nephrol Dial Transplant. 2011;26(3):1058–65.
157. Johnson CP, Gallagher-Lepak S, Zhu YR, et al. Factors influencing weight gain after renal transplantation. Transplantation. 1993;56:822–7.
158. Hoogeveen EK, Aalten J, Rothman KJ, Roodnat JI, et al. Effect of obesity on the outcome of kidney transplantation: a 20 year follow up. Transplantation. 2011;91:869–74.
159. Marcén R. Immunosuppressive drugs in kidney transplantation: impact on patient survival, and incidence of cardiovascular disease, malignancy and infection. Drugs. 2009;69:2227–43.
160. Miller L. Cardiovascular toxicities of immunosuppressive agents. Am J Transplant. 2002;1:807–18.
161. Ducloux D, Kazory A, Chalopin JM. Post transplant diabetes mellitus and atherosclerotic events in renal transplant recipients: A prospective study. Transplantation. 2005;79:438–43.
162. Kasiske B, Snyder JJ, Gilbertson D, et al. Diabetes mellitus after kidney transplantation in the United States. Am J Transplant. 2003;3:178–85.
163. Nathaniel B, Cochetti P, Mysore S, et al. Association of metabolic syndrome with development of new-onset diabetes after transplant. Transplantation. 2010;90:861–6.
164. Ajay I, Snyder J, Skeans M, et al. Clinical diagnosis of metabolic syndrome: predicting new-onset diabetes, coronary heart disease, and allograft failure late after kidney transplant. Transpl Int. 2012;25:748–75.
165. Larsen CP, et al. Belatacept-based regimens versus a cyclosporine A-based regimen in kidney transplant recipients: 2-year results from the BENEFIT and BENEFIT-EXT studies. Transplantation. 2010;90:1528–35.
166. Pestana JO, Grinyo JM, Vanrenterghem Y, et al. Three year outcomes from BENEFIT-EXT: a phase III study of belatacept versus cyclosporine in recipients of extended criteria donor kidneys. Am J Transplant. 2012;12(3):630–9.
167. Vanrenterghem Y, Bresnahan B, Campistol J, et al. Belatacept-based regimens are associated with improved cardiovascular and metabolic risk factors compared with cyclosporine in kidney transplant recipients. Transplantation. 2011;91(9):976–83.
168. The AST infectious disease community of practice, American Society of Transplantation, infectious disease guidelines 3rd edition. Am J Transplant. 2013;13 Suppl 4:3–336.
169. Fishman JA. Infection in solid-organ transplant recipients. N Engl J Med. 2007;357(25):2601–14.
170. Fishman JA. Prevention of infection due to Pneumocystis carinii. Antimicrob Agents Chemother. 1998;42(5):995–1004.
171. Hirsch HH, Knowles W, Dickenmann M, Passweg J, Klimkait T, Mihatsch MJ, et al. Prospective study of polyomavirus type BK replication and nephropathy in renal-transplant recipients. N Engl J Med. 2002;347(7):488–96.
172. Schold JD, Rehman S, Kayle LK, Magliocca J, Srinivas TR, Meier-Kriesche HU. Treatment for BK virus: incidence, risk factors and outcomes for kidney transplant recipients in the United States. Transpl Int. 2009;22(6):626–34.
173. Nickeleit V, Hirsch HH, Zeiler M, Gudat F, Prince O, Thiel G, et al. BK-virus nephropathy in renal transplants-tubular necrosis, MHC-class II expression and rejection in a puzzling game. Nephrol Dial Transplant. 2000;15(3):324–32.
174. McGilvray ID, Lajoie G, Humar A, Cattral MS. Polyomavirus infection and acute vascular rejection in a kidney allograft: coincidence or mimicry? Am J Transplant. 2003;3(4):501–4.
175. Kuypers DR, Vandooren AK, Lerut E, Evenepoel P, Claes K, Snoeck R, et al. Adjuvant low-dose cidofovir therapy for BK polyomavirus interstitial nephritis in renal transplant recipients. Am J Transplant. 2005;5(8):1997–2004.
176. Vats A, Shapiro R, Singh Randhawa P, Scantlebury V, Tuzuner A, Saxena M, et al. Quantitative viral load monitoring and cidofovir therapy for the management of BK virus-associated nephropathy in children and adults. Transplantation. 2003;75(1):105–12.
177. Gabardi S, Waikar SS, Martin S, Roberts K, Chen J, Borgi L, et al. Evaluation of fluoroquinolones for the prevention of BK viremia after renal transplantation. Clin J Am Soc Nephrol. 2010;5(7):1298–304.
178. Leung AY, Chan MT, Yuen KY, Cheng VC, Chan KH, Wong CL, et al. Ciprofloxacin decreased polyoma BK virus load in patients who underwent allogeneic hematopoietic stem cell transplantation. Clin Infect Dis. 2005;40(4):528–37.
179. Sener A, House AA, Jevnikar AM, Boudville N, McAlister VC, Muirhead N, et al. Intravenous immunoglobulin as a treatment for BK virus associated nephropathy: one-year follow-up of renal allograft recipients. Transplantation. 2006;81(1):117–20.
180. Wali RK, Drachenberg C, Hirsch HH, Papadimitriou J, Nahar A, Mohanlal V, et al. BK virus-associated nephropathy in renal allograft recipients: rescue therapy by sirolimus-based immunosuppression. Transplantation. 2004;78(7):1069–73.
181. Dharnidharka VR, Cherikh WS, Neff R, Cheng Y, Abbott KC. Retransplantation after BK virus nephropathy in prior kidney transplant: an OPTN database analysis. Am J Transplant. 2010;10(5):1312–5.
182. Brennan DC. Cytomegalovirus in renal transplantation. J Am Soc Nephrol. 2001;12(4):848–55.
183. Reinke P, Fietze E, Ode-Hakim S, Prosch S, Lippert J, Ewert R, et al. Late-acute renal allograft rejection and symptomless cytomegalovirus infection. Lancet 1994;344(8939–8940):1737–8.
184. Paya CV. Indirect effects of CMV in the solid organ transplant patient. Transpl Infect Dis. 1999;1(S1):8–12.
185. Kotton CN, Kumar D, Caliendo AM. International consensus guidelines on the management of cytomegalovirus infection in solid organ transplantation. Transplantation. 2010;89:775–95.
186. Issa NC, Fishman JA. Infectious complications of antilymphocyte therapies in solid organ transplantation. Clin Infect Dis. 2009;48(6):772–86.

187. Reischig T, Jindra P, Hes O, Svecova M, Klaboch J, Treska V. Valacyclovir prophylaxis versus preemptive valganciclovir therapy to prevent cytomegalovirus disease after renal transplantation. Am J Transplant. 2008;8(1):69–77.
188. Kliem V, Fricke L, Wollbrink T, Burg M, Radermacher J, Rohde F. Improvement in long-term renal graft survival due to CMV prophylaxis with oral ganciclovir: results of a randomized clinical trial. Am J Transplant. 2008;8(5):975–83.
189. Humar A, Lebranchu Y, Vincenti F, Blumberg EA, Punch JD, Limaye AP, et al. The efficacy and safety of 200 days valganciclovir cytomegalovirus prophylaxis in high-risk kidney transplant recipients. Am J Transplant. 2010;10(5):1228–37.
190. Reischig T, Hribova P, Jindra P, Hes O, Bouda M, Treska V, et al. Long-term outcomes of pre-emptive valganciclovir compared with valacyclovir prophylaxis for prevention of cytomegalovirus in renal transplantation. J Am Soc Nephrol. 2012;23(9):1588–97.
191. Asberg A, Humar A, Jardine AG, Rollag H, Pescovitz MD, Mouas H, et al. Long-term outcomes of CMV disease treatment with valganciclovir versus IV ganciclovir in solid organ transplant recipients. Am J Transplant. 2009;9(5):1205–13.
192. Hanto DW, Frizzera G, Gajl-Peczalska KJ, Sakamoto K, Purtilo DT, Balfour Jr HH, et al. Epstein-Barr virus-induced B-cell lymphoma after renal transplantation: acyclovir therapy and transition from polyclonal to monoclonal B-cell proliferation. N Engl J Med. 1982;306(15):913–8.
193. Cavaliere R, Petroni G, Lopes MB, Schiff D, International Primary Central Nervous System Lymphoma Collaborative Group. Primary central nervous system post-transplantation lymphoproliferative disorder: an International Primary Central Nervous System Lymphoma Collaborative Group Report. Cancer. 2010;116(4):863–70.
194. Leblond V, Davi F, Charlotte F, Dorent R, Bitker MO, Sutton L, et al. Posttransplant lymphoproliferative disorders not associated with Epstein-Barr virus: a distinct entity? J Clin Oncol. 1998;16(6):2052–9.
195. Rajakariar R, Bhattacharyya M, Norton A, Sheaff M, Cavenagh J, Raftery MJ, et al. Post transplant T-cell lymphoma: a case series of four patients from a single unit and review of the literature. Am J Transplant. 2004;4(9):1534–8.
196. Bakker NA, Pruim J, de Graaf W, van Son WJ, van der Jagt EJ, van Imhoff GW. PTLD visualization by FDG-PET: improved detection of extranodal localizations. Am J Transplant. 2006;6(8):1984–5.
197. Elstrom RL, Andreadis C, Aqui NA, Ahya VN, Bloom RD, Brozena SC, Olthoff KM, Schuster SJ, Nasta SD, Stadtmauer EA, Tsai DE. Treatment of PTLD with rituximab or chemotherapy. Am J Transplant. 2006;6(3):569–76.
198. Trappe R, Oertel S, Leblond V, Mollee P, Sender M, Reinke P, Neuhaus R, Lehmkuhl H, Horst HA, Salles G, Morschhauser F, Jaccard A, Lamy T, Leithäuser M, Zimmermann H, Anagnostopoulos I, Raphael M, Riess H, Choquet S, German PTLD Study Group, European PTLD Network. Sequential treatment with rituximab followed by CHOP chemotherapy in adult B-cell post-transplant lymphoproliferative disorder (PTLD): the prospective international multicentre phase 2 PTLD-1 trial. Lancet Oncol. 2012;13(2):196–206.
199. Salgo R, Gossmann J, Schofer H, Kachel HG, Kuck J, Geiger H, et al. Switch to a sirolimus-based immunosuppression in long-term renal transplant recipients: reduced rate of (pre-)malignancies and nonmelanoma skin cancer in a prospective, randomized, assessor-blinded, controlled clinical trial. Am J Transplant. 2010;10(6):1385–93.
200. Vaysberg M, Balatoni CE, Nepomuceno RR, Krams SM, Martinez OM. Rapamycin inhibits proliferation of Epstein-Barr virus-positive B-cell lymphomas through modulation of cell-cycle protein expression. Transplantation. 2007;83(8):1114–21.
201. Dantal J, Soulillou JP. Immunosuppressive drugs and the risk of cancer after organ transplantation. N Engl J Med. 2005;352(13):1371–3.
202. Buell JF, Gross TG, Woodle ES. Malignancy after transplantation. Transplantation. 2005;80(2 Suppl):S254–64.
203. Engels EA, Pfeiffer RM, Fraumeni Jr JF, Kasiske BL, Israni AK, Snyder JJ, et al. Spectrum of cancer risk among US solid organ transplant recipients. JAMA. 2011;306(17):1891–901.
204. Zou S, Dodd RY, Stramer SL, Strong DM, Tissue Safety Study Group. Probability of viremia with HBV, HCV, HIV, and HTLV among tissue donors in the United States. N Engl J Med. 2004;351(8):751–9.
205. Fishman JA, Greenwald MA, Grossi PA. Transmission of infection with human allografts: essential considerations in donor screening. Clin Infect Dis. 2012;55(5):720–7.
206. Euvrard S, Kanitakis J, Claudy A. Skin cancers after organ transplantation. N Engl J Med. 2003;348(17):1681–91.
207. Schwarz A, Vatandaslar S, Merkel S, Haller H. Renal cell carcinoma in transplant recipients with acquired cystic kidney disease. Clin J Am Soc Nephrol. 2007;2(4):750–6.
208. Euvrard S, Morelon E, Rostaing L, Goffin E, Brocard A, Tromme I, et al. Sirolimus and secondary skin-cancer prevention in kidney transplantation. N Engl J Med. 2012;367(4):329–39.
209. Campistol JM, Eris J, Oberbauer R, Friend P, Hutchison B, Morales JM, et al. Sirolimus therapy after early cyclosporine withdrawal reduces the risk for cancer in adult renal transplantation. J Am Soc Nephrol. 2006;17(2):581–9.
210. Kelly WD, Lillehei RC, Merkel FK, Idezuki Y, Goetz FC. Allotransplantation of the pancreas and duodenum along with the kidney in diabetic nephropathy. Surgery. 1967;61(6):827–37.
211. Zimmet PZ, Tuomi T, Mackay IR, Rowley MJ, Knowles W, Cohen M, Lang DA. Latent autoimmune diabetes mellitus in adults (LADA): the role of antibodies to glutamic acid decarboxylase in diagnosis and prediction of insulin dependency. Diabet Med. 1994;11(3):299–303.
212. Saudek F, Průhová S, Boucek P, Lebl J, Adamec M, Ek J, Pedersen O, Hansen T. Maturity onset diabetes of the young with end stage nephropathy: a new indication for simultaneous pancreas and kidney transplantation? Transplantation. 2004;77(8):1298–301.
213. Robertson RP, Davis C, Larsen J, Stratta R, Sutherland DER. Pancreas and islet transplantation in type I diabetes. Diabetes Care. 2006;29(4):935.
214. www.srtr.org. Accessed 15 April 2013.
215. Shapiro AM, Lakey JR, Ryan EA, Korbutt GS, Toth E, Warnock GL, Kneteman NM, Rajotte RV. Islet transplantation in seven patients with type 1 diabetes using a glucocorticoid-free immunosuppressive regimen. N Engl J Med. 2000;343:230–8.
216. Ryan EA, Paty BW, Senior PA, Bigam D, Alfadhli E, Kneteman NM, Lakey JR, Shapiro AM. Five year follow-up after clinical islet transplantation. Diabetes. 2005;54(7):2060–9.
217. Senior PA, Zeman M, Paty BW, Ryan EA, Shapiro AM. Changes in renal function after clinical islet transplantation: four-year observational study. Am J Transplant. 2007;7(1):91–8.
218. Campbell PM, Senior PA, Salam A, LaBranche K, Bigam DL, Kneteman NM, Imes S, Halpin A, Ryan EA, Shapiro AM. High risk of sensitization after failed islet transplantation. Am J Transplant. 2007;7(10):2311–7.
219. Sutherland DE, Gruessner R, Dunn D, Moudry-Munns K, Gruessner A, Najarian JS. Pancreas transplants from living-related donors. Transplant Proc. 1994;26(2):443–5.
220. Lee RH, Seo MJ, Reger RL, Spees JL, Pulin AA, Olson SD, Prockop DJ. Multipotent stromal cells from human marrow home to and promote repair of pancreatic islets and renal glomeruli in diabetic NOD/scid mice. Proc Natl Acad Sci U S A. 2006;103(46):17438–43.

Part III

Treatment and Prognosis

16 Glycemic Control

Allison J. Hahr and Mark E. Molitch

Introduction

Glycemic control in diabetes mellitus (DM) can be challenging to every physician. Management of blood sugars is the hallmark by which we measure our success (and failure), and it is critical in the prevention of complications related to diabetes including kidney disease. Glycemic control in those with chronic kidney disease (CKD) brings another level of challenge to care of the patient with diabetes. It requires detailed knowledge of which medications can be safely used and how kidney disease affects metabolism of these medications. In addition, the glycemic target needs to be individualized for each patient and our ability to interpret the data can be altered in the setting of kidney disease.

Medications

Medical therapy for diabetes is continually advancing with new therapies available for use and updates to our current understanding and the safety profile of medications already in use. Please refer to Table 16.1 for adjustments in dosing for diabetes medications used in CKD.

Insulin

All available types of insulin can be used in CKD. However, the insulin type, dose, and pattern of administration must be adjusted to each individual patient to achieve target glycemia while limiting hypoglycemia. There are multiple forms of insulin available (Table 16.2).

A.J. Hahr, M.D. • M.E. Molitch, M.D. (✉)
Division of Endocrinology, Metabolism and Molecular Medicine, Medicine Department, Northwestern University Feinberg School of Medicine, 645 N. Michigan Avenue, Suite 530, Chicago, IL, USA
e-mail: molitch@northwestern.edu

Rapid-Acting Insulins

There are three rapid-acting insulin analogs available, aspart (Novolog), lispro (Humalog), and glulisine (Apidra). They have the most rapid onset of action with peak concentrations at about 30–90 min and overall short duration, estimated to be about 5 h. However, the duration of action of glulisine may be slightly longer than that of aspart or lispro.

Because of their rapid peak and relatively short duration, these insulin analogs most resemble physiologic insulin secretion making their use ideal for mealtime administration and when rapid correction of high blood sugars is needed. They can be given immediately before or up to 15 min prior to eating which is convenient for patients. They are used as part of the regimen in "basal–bolus therapy," also known as multiple daily injections (MDI).

In patients with gastroparesis, giving these insulin analogs after meals can be beneficial resulting in better matching of the peak insulin levels with the glucose absorption from the meal. In addition, in patients with poor appetites, sometimes the insulin can be given after meals to allow for adjustment of the insulin dose in proportion to how much food was actually consumed. These insulin analogs are also used in continuous subcutaneous insulin infusions (CSII), also known as insulin pumps.

Short-Acting Insulin

Regular crystalline insulin has an onset of action at 30–60 min, peak concentration at 2–3 h, and a total duration of about 5–8 h after administration. It is recommended that regular insulin be given about 30 min before eating. The only advantage of regular insulin is substantially lower cost compared to the rapid-acting insulin analogs.

Intermediate-Acting Insulin

Isophane insulin or NPH (neutral protamine Hagedorn) is the only available intermediate-acting insulin. It has an onset of action at 2–4 h, peak concentration at 4–10 h, and duration anywhere from 10 to 18 h. Therefore, to achieve 24 h coverage as a basal insulin, it usually has to be given twice daily. It can have

E.V. Lerma and V. Batuman (eds.), *Diabetes and Kidney Disease*,
DOI 10.1007/978-1-4939-0793-9_16, © Springer Science+Business Media New York 2014

Table 16.1 Dose adjustment for insulin compounds and medications for diabetes in CKD

Medication class	CKD stages 3 and 4 and predialysis stage 5
Insulin	
Glargine	No advised dose adjustment[a]
Detemir	No advised dose adjustment[a]
NPH	No advised dose adjustment[a]
Regular	No advised dose adjustment[a]
Aspart	No advised dose adjustment[a]
Lispro	No advised dose adjustment[a]
Glulisine	No advised dose adjustment[a]
First-generation sulfonylureas	
Acetohexamide[b]	Avoid use
Chlorpropamide	eGFR 50–80: reduce dose by 50 %
	eGFR <50: avoid use
Tolazamide	Avoid use
Tolbutamide	Avoid use
Second-generation sulfonylureas	
Glipizide	eGFR <30: use with caution
Glimepiride	eGFR <60: use with caution
	eGFR <30: avoid use
Glyburide	eGFR <60: avoid use
Gliclazide[b]	No dose adjustment
Meglitinides	
Repaglinide	No dose adjustment but may wish to use caution with eGFR <30
Nateglinide	eGFR <60: avoid use (but may consider use if patient is on hemodialysis)
Biguanides	
Metformin[c]	Per FDA, do not use if serum Cr ≥1.5 mg/dL in men
	≥1.4 mg/dL in women
	Consider
	eGFR ≥45–59: use caution with dose and follow renal function closely (every 3–6 months)
	eGFR ≥30–44: max dose 1,000 mg/day or use 50 % dose reduction. Follow renal function every 3 months. Do not start as new therapy
	eGFR <30: avoid use
Thiazolidinediones	
Pioglitazone	No dose adjustment
Rosiglitazone	No dose adjustment
Alpha-glucosidase inhibitors	
Acarbose	Serum Cr >2 mg/dL: avoid use
Miglitol	eGFR <25 or serum Cr >2 mg/dL: avoid use
DPP-4 inhibitor	
Sitagliptin	eGFR ≥50: 100 mg daily
	eGFR 30–49: 50 mg daily
	eGFR<30: 25 mg daily
Saxagliptin	eGFR>50: 2.5 or 5 mg daily
	GFR≤50: 2.5 mg daily
Linagliptin	No dose adjustment
Alogliptin	eGFR >60: 25 mg daily
	eGFR 30–59: 12.5 mg daily
	eGFR <30: 6.25 mg daily
Incretin mimetic	
Exenatide	eGFR 30–50: use caution
	eGFR <30: avoid use
Liraglutide	No dose adjustment but use caution when starting or titrating the dose
Amylin analog	
Pramlintide	No dose adjustment known but not studied in ESRD
Dopamine receptor agonist	
Bromocriptine mesylate	No dose adjustment known but not studied: use with caution
Bile acid sequestrant	
Colesevelam	No dose adjustment known but limited data
SGLT2 inhibitor	
Canagliflozin	eGFR 45 to <60: max dose 100 mg once daily
	eGFR <45: avoid use
Dapagliflozin	eGFR <60: avoid use

[a]Adjust doses based on patient response
[b]Not available in the United States
[c]Recommendations are controversial

Table 16.2 Pharmacokinetic properties of insulin

Insulin	Onset	Peak	Duration
Long-acting			
Glargine (Lantus)	2–4 h	None	20–24 h
Detemir (Levemir)	1–3 h	6–8 h	18–20 h
Intermediate-acting			
NPH	2–4 h	4–10 h	10–18 h
Short-acting			
Regular	0.5–1 h	2–3 h	5–8 h
Rapid-acting			
Aspart (Novolog)	5–15 min	0.5–2 h	3–5 h
Lispro (Humalog)	5–15 min	0.5–2 h	3–5 h
Glulisine (Apidra)	5–15 min	0.5–2 h	3–5 h
Premixed			
70 % NPH/30 % regular	0.5–1 h	3–12 h (dual)	10–16 h
50 % NPH/50 % regular	0.5–1 h	2–12 h (dual)	10–16 h
75 % NPL/25 % lispro	5–15 min	1–4 h (dual)	10–16 h
50 % NPL/50 % lispro	5–15 min	1–4 h (dual)	10–16 h
70 % NPA/30 % aspart	5–15 min	1–4 h (dual)	10–16 h

NPH neutral protamine Hagedorn, *NPL* neutral protamine lispro, *NPA* neutral protamine aspart

unpredictable absorption and high variability even within the same patient, making its use sometimes problematic.

Long-Acting Insulins

Glargine insulin (Lantus) was the first long-acting insulin analog that was developed. Glargine is soluble at an acidic pH but less soluble at a physiologic pH. Subcutaneous injection leads to precipitation which results in slower absorption. A unique property of glargine is that it does not have a clear peak concentration; it lasts approximately 22 h after injection and usually only has to be given once daily.

Detemir insulin (Levemir) was the second long-acting insulin analog developed. After injection, detemir binds to albumin thus giving its prolonged action. It has a slight peak about 6–8 h after injection and lasts about 18–20 h. For patients with type 1 diabetes, it usually is given twice daily; for those with type 2 diabetes, once daily administration sometimes suffices.

Premixed Insulin

There are multiple premixed preparations of insulin that contain a fixed percentage of two different types of insulin. The most commonly used form is insulin "70/30" which consists of 70 % NPH and 30 % regular insulin mixed together and is injected twice daily. There are also other mixtures of NPH with rapid-acting insulins in a 75/25 % ratio. Because two different insulin types are present, there are two different peaks in insulin concentration. These combinations, though simpler for the patient to administer, greatly restrict adjustment of the insulin and require fixed dosing and mealtimes. In a patient who has stopped eating or has a decreased appetite, the risk of hypoglycemia is high.

Insulin U-500

All insulin is U-100, which is defined as 100 units of insulin per 1 mL. The exception is U-500 which is 500 units of insulin per 1 mL and is only available as regular insulin. However, the high concentration of U-500 insulin alters the properties of regular insulin and its pharmacokinetics is instead more like those of NPH. It is generally used in patients who are severely insulin resistant and require very high doses of insulin. Although generally given as a subcutaneous injection, it may also be administered via an insulin pump.

Use in Kidney Disease

Approximately one-third of insulin degradation is by the kidney, and a decrease in kidney function is associated with prolongation of the insulin half-life, so less insulin is needed as GFR declines [1]. The kidney is responsible for approximately 30–80 % of insulin breakdown. Patients with kidney disease are at higher risk of hypoglycemia due to decreased clearance of insulin but also a decline in renal gluconeogenesis from lower kidney mass. The presence of anorexia and weight loss in nephropathy can contribute to increased insulin sensitivity as well. There are no limitations on which insulin can be used in kidney disease; however, the doses may need to be adjusted; there are no specific guidelines for this. The insulin type chosen and the dose must be individualized for each patient. As with all therapy in diabetes, doses should be used to attain goal glycemic control with a minimum of hypoglycemic events. An inpatient study randomizing weight-based basal and bolus insulin in patients with an eGFR <45 mL/min/1.73 m^2 to 0.5 units/kg body weight vs. 0.25 units/kg showed similar glycemic control but significantly less hypoglycemia in the group with the lower weight-based dose [2]. All patients on insulin need to have an individualized regimen based on their level of glucose control and level of CKD, and these patients need to be extra vigilant in monitoring glucose levels and adjusting insulin doses.

Patients with more advanced kidney disease (stage 4–5) and on dialysis may have delayed gastric emptying. Thus, use of rapid-acting insulin after the meal, similar to patients with gastroparesis, can be helpful. Patients on dialysis have additional factors to consider. Those on hemodialysis can have different clearance rates of insulin that correlate with the timing of dialysis. However, glucose control in patients on dialysis tends to be highly variable and even unpredictable, making glycemic control in this population challenging. Patients who are on peritoneal dialysis will have exposure to large amounts of glucose in the dialysate which can cause problematic hyperglycemia. In those who cycle peritoneal dialysis overnight, the use of NPH or a premixed insulin such as 70/30 can be useful to address the glucose absorption from the dialysis fluid.

Oral Medications

Sulfonylureas

Sulfonylureas represent the oldest oral medications available for treatment of diabetes. They bind to the sulfonylurea receptor on the pancreatic beta-cells and lead to an increase in insulin secretion. The first-generation sulfonylureas (acetohexamide, chlorpropamide, tolazamide, tolbutamide) are rarely prescribed. The second-generation sulfonylureas which include glipizide, glimepiride, glyburide, and gliclazide (the latter is not available in the United States) are commonly prescribed. They are typically taken once to twice daily and are also available in long-acting preparations. Sulfonylureas typically lower hemoglobin A1c (A1c) by 1.5–2 % and can cause hypoglycemia.

Sulfonylureas and their metabolites are cleared by the kidney which leads to an increased risk of hypoglycemia as GFR declines. The first-generation sulfonylureas should be avoided in CKD stage 3 or worse since these medications and their metabolites are dependent on the kidney for clearance. With the second-generation sulfonylureas, the risk of hypoglycemia is greatly increased with glimepiride and glyburide if the eGFR is <60 mL/min/1.73 m^2 due to decreased clearance of glyburide and two active metabolites of glimepiride [3]. The use of glyburide should be avoided with eGFR <60 mL/min/1.73 m^2 [4]. Glimepiride should be used cautiously if the eGFR is <60 mL/min/1.73 m^2 and not be used with eGFR <30 mL/min/1.73 m^2 [3]. Less than 10 % of glipizide is cleared renally but it should still be used with caution with an eGFR <30 mL/min/1.73 m^2 due to the risk of hypoglycemia [5, 6].

Meglitinides

Nateglinide and repaglinide, like sulfonylureas, increase insulin secretion by closing an ATP-dependent potassium channel on the beta-cells of the pancreas. They require the presence of glucose and result in a rapid and short duration of insulin release. Because of this, they should be taken prior to meals. They also can cause hypoglycemia.

The active metabolite of nateglinide accumulates in CKD and can cause hypoglycemia; nateglinide should not be used with an eGFR <60 mL/min/1.73 m^2. However, this active metabolite is cleared by hemodialysis, so nateglinide can be used in these individuals [7]. Conversely, repaglinide appears safe to use in individuals with CKD [8]. However, it is reasonable to exercise caution in those with more severe renal dysfunction, such as an eGFR <30 mL/min/1.73 m^2, and start at the lowest dose (0.5 mg) with slow titration upwards.

Biguanides (Metformin)

Metformin reduces hepatic gluconeogenesis and increases insulin sensitivity. On average, metformin reduces A1c by 1.0–2.0 %. It does not cause hypoglycemia and it may lead to weight loss in some patients. The most common side effects are gastrointestinal and include diarrhea, bloating, and cramping. Vitamin B12 deficiency has also been reported with extended use [9].

The FDA recommends that metformin should not be used with serum creatinine levels ≥1.5 mg/dL in men and ≥1.4 mg/dL in women or with decreased creatinine clearance in people over age 80. Because metformin is renally cleared [10], this recommendation is in place to reduce the risk of lactic acidosis in individuals with even modest renal impairment. The overall incidence of lactic acidosis with metformin use, however, appears to be rare. A Cochrane database review of 347 prospective trials and observational cohort studies showed no cases of fatal or nonfatal lactic acidosis in 70,490 patient-years of metformin users or in 55,451 patient-years of users of other antihyperglycemic agents [11]. In a study evaluating metformin-associated lactic acidosis in 14 patients, other causes of lactic acidosis (including clinical shock or tissue hypoxia) seemed to be the driving cause and not specifically metformin; 10 of these patients did have metformin accumulation related to elevated serum creatinine (range 3.05–11.8 mg/dL) whereas 4 patients, all with lower creatinine levels though still reduced GFR, had no evidence of metformin accumulation [12]. It is reasonable to consider use of a GFR-based guideline such as outlined here rather than one based on creatinine alone. Metformin can be used without dose reduction with eGFR >60 mL/min/1.73 m^2. Given the very rare occurrence of lactic acidosis even with reduced GFR and the excellent efficacy of metformin, there is a general consensus now that metformin can be used even in patients with stage 3 CKD [13, 14]. If the eGFR is ≥45–59 mL/min/1.73 m^2, it may be prudent to continue use of metformin but caution with dosing should be taken and the renal function followed more closely, such as every 3–6 months. If the eGFR is ≥30–44 mL/min/1.73 m^2, the dose should be limited to a maximum of 1,000 mg daily and renal function followed every 3 months. Metformin should be avoided with eGFR <30 mL/min/1.73 m^2. It is recommended that metformin be stopped in the presence of situations that are associated with hypoxia or an acute decline in kidney function such as sepsis/shock, hypotension, acute myocardial infarction, and use of radiographic contrast or other nephrotoxic agents [13, 14].

Thiazolidinediones

Thiazolidinediones are peroxisome-proliferator-activated receptor γ (PPARγ) agonists that increase peripheral insulin sensitivity. The average reduction in A1c is 0.5–1.5 %. The major side effects are weight gain and fluid retention. They do not cause hypoglycemia. Pioglitazone is the only thiazolidinedione commonly prescribed.

The Rosiglitazone Evaluated for Cardiovascular Outcomes and Regulation of Glycemia in Diabetes (RECORD) study and additional data were reviewed by the FDA and in 2010, due to its association with adverse cardiovascular events, use of rosiglitazone was restricted to those unable to control their diabetes with other medications [15]. Physician must document a patient's eligibility for the medication, and patients are required to review safety information regarding the cardiovascular side effects and acknowledge the risks associated with use. Recently, the FDA has reviewed the restrictions and removed them.

No dose adjustment is indicated with pioglitazone or rosiglitazone in CKD since they are cleared by the liver. However, since the thiazolidinediones are associated with fluid retention, this may be problematic in patients with more advanced CKD. Pioglitazone has been associated with an adverse effect on bones, and this should be taken into consideration in those with or at risk of developing renal osteodystrophy.

Dipeptidyl Peptidase Inhibitors

The dipeptidyl peptidase (DPP)-4 inhibitors (sitagliptin, saxagliptin, linagliptin, alogliptin) decrease the breakdown of the incretin hormones, such as glucagon-like peptide 1 (GLP-1). GLP-1 is secreted by the GI tract in response to food and leads to insulin secretion in a glucose-dependent mechanism while also decreasing glucagon release. GLP-1 also slows gastric emptying.

Sitagliptin was the first available DPP-4 inhibitor. Approximately 80 % of sitagliptin is cleared by the kidney; a reduction in the standard dose of 100 mg daily is advised with declines in GFR. With an eGFR of ≥30 to <50 mL/

min/1.73 m^2, 50 mg once daily should be used and with an eGFR <30 mL/min/1.73 m^2, a dose of 25 mg once daily is advised [16]. Saxagliptin also needs a dose reduction with eGFR ≤ 50 mL/min/1.73 m^2 to 2.5 mg daily; otherwise, the standard dose with eGFR >50 mL/min is 2.5 or 5 mg daily. Only a small amount of linagliptin is cleared renally; thus, no dose adjustment is indicated with a reduced GFR [17]. Alogliptin similarly needs a dose reduction from 25 to 12.5 mg daily with an eGFR < 60 mL/min/1.73 m^2 and then to 6.25 mg daily with an eGFR < 30 mL/min/1.73 m^2.

Alpha-Glucosidase Inhibitors

Alpha-glucosidase inhibitors (acarbose, miglitol) decrease the breakdown of oligo- and disaccharides in the small intestine. The ingestion of carbohydrates is delayed and slows the absorption of glucose after a meal. The major side effects are bloating, flatulence, and abdominal cramping. They typically lower A1c by 0.5–1.0 %.

Acarbose is minimally absorbed, with <2 % of the drug and active metabolites present in the urine. However, with reduced renal function, serum levels of acarbose and metabolites are significantly higher. Miglitol has greater systemic absorption with >95 % renal excretion. It is recommended that use of miglitol be avoided if the GFR is <25 mL/min/1.73 m^2 [18]. Additionally, neither medication has been studied long term in patients with a creatinine >2 mg/dL; their use should be avoided in this population.

Other Oral Agents

The use of bromocriptine, a dopamine receptor agonist, has not been adequately studied in patients with CKD.

Colesevelam (bile acid sequestrant) shows no difference in efficacy or safety in those with an eGFR <50 but the data are limited. It has not been adequately studied in more advanced CKD.

Canagliflozin reduces renal glucose absorption by inhibiting the sodium-glucose co-transporter 2 (SGLT2) which is found in the proximal tubule. This leads to a reduction in the reabsorption of glucose and therefore increases the excretion of glucose in the urine. The increase in urine glucose results in a weight loss of up to 5 kg over 1 year. Because of an increase in adverse events, no more than 100 mg once daily should be used in patients with an eGFR of 45 to <60 mL/min/1.73 m^2, and it should not be used at all if the eGFR is <45 mL/min/1.73 m^2. Dapagliflozin, a second SGLT2 inhibitor, should not be used if the eGFR is <60 ml/min/1.73m^2.

Other Subcutaneous Medications

GLP-1 Receptor Agonists

Exenatide (Byetta) and liraglutide (Victoza) are injectable incretin mimetics. They are FDA approved for use with metformin and/or sulfonylureas. However, in practice, they are also used in conjunction with insulin therapy. They contribute to central satiety leading to a reduction in appetite and therefore weight loss. They also promote insulin release, delay glucagon release, and slow gastric emptying. Some studies have shown an association with an increased risk of pancreatitis.

Clearance of exenatide decreases with declines in GFR [19]. Additionally, in a case report of a patient with renal impairment and CKD, use of exenatide led to a rise in serum creatinine that resolved when the medication was stopped [20]. The FDA reported cases of acute renal failure associated with exenatide use and recommends it be used with caution in those with a GFR of 30–50 mL/min and not be used if the GFR is <30 mL/min [21]. Liraglutide is not metabolized primarily by the kidney and no dose adjustment is indicated in those with renal impairment, including ESRD, though data in this population are limited [22]. The manufacturer has reported cases of renal failure and worsening of chronic renal impairment with liraglutide and advises caution with initiating or increasing the dose in those with nephropathy.

Amylin Analog

Pramlintide (Symlin) is the only available amylin analog; it is given as an injection along with insulin therapy at meals. Amylin is co-secreted by beta-cells of the pancreas and endogenous levels tend to be low in those with diabetes. Pramlintide decreases glucagon secretion, slows gastric emptying, and can decrease appetite.

Dose adjustments for pramlintide are not indicated in the presence of mild–moderate renal disease; its use has not been studied in ESRD.

Strategy for Glycemic Control

Insulin therapy for patients with type 1 and type 2 DM differs greatly. However, the primary goal of optimizing glycemic control to reduce the development of microvascular and macrovascular complications is the same. Those with type 1 diabetes have an absolute need, of course, for insulin. On occasion, additional therapies are used in conjunction with insulin. Those with type 2 diabetes have a wide array of therapies available for use, ranging from a single oral medication to insulin.

Type 1 Diabetes

In type 1 diabetes, the ideal method for insulin dosing is to reproduce physiologic secretion by the pancreas. For best success in achieving target glycemic control, patients with type 1 diabetes should use a regimen that mimics endogenous insulin secretion. This is best achieved with combination therapy through use of a long-acting basal insulin and MDI of a rapid-acting insulin with meals.

Prior to the availability of insulin analogs, a combination of twice daily NPH and regular insulin was used in attempt to mimic physiologic insulin secretion. Typically, the two were given together before breakfast and before dinner. Since both types of insulin serve to treat fasting and postprandial glucose levels, it can be a difficult regimen to use to achieve target glycemic control. This regimen requires that patients maintain similar mealtimes and meal sizes each day, and it also does not truly imitate normal physiologic insulin secretion. Thus, the use of insulin analogs has greatly advanced our care for type 1 diabetes.

Glargine insulin does not have a distinct peak, is superior to twice daily NPH in reducing fasting glucose levels with less hypoglycemia [23], and results in more stable fasting values [24]. Long-term reductions in A1c and number of hypoglycemic events, with improvement in hypoglycemic awareness, were seen in individuals receiving glargine for 1 year who had at baseline an A1c of 7.1 % [25]. Compared to NPH, glargine has been shown to have less intra- and interindividual variability with greater predictability and reproducibility.

Detemir is another option as a basal insulin for patients with type 1 diabetes and may offer less variability than NPH. In comparisons of twice daily detemir and NPH, those receiving detemir had less variability in fasting glucose levels and overnight plasma glucose profiles as well as less hypoglycemia [26]. Whereas glargine can be given once daily, detemir should be dosed twice daily due to its shorter duration of action.

Use of a rapid-acting insulin analog such as lispro, aspart, or glulisine as the bolus insulin is superior to regular insulin with respect to better postprandial glucose control and less hypoglycemia [27–29].

Which regimen to use is based on the comfort of the patient and physician; the insulin regimen should be tailored for each person. For basal therapy, once daily glargine would be an optimal first choice, followed by twice daily detemir, then NPH, with any of the rapid-acting insulin analogs as prandial insulin.

The closest approximation of physiologic insulin secretion can be achieved by using a pump that delivers insulin by continuous subcutaneous infusion. A single type of insulin is used in the pump such as a rapid-acting analog. This insulin serves as the basal, bolus, and correction insulin. The pump is programmed to deliver different basal rates throughout the day, which is an advantage over the use of a long-acting insulin such as glargine or detemir. As an example, often basal rates are lower overnight but need to increase in the early morning to address the "dawn phenomenon." As another example, different basal rates can be programmed to take into account exercise patterns or dialysis patterns. Insulin pumps can be used in all stages of CKD. Insulin pumps require vigilance on the part of the patient and their use should be overseen by endocrinologists and diabetes educators with experience in their use.

External devices known as continuous glucose monitoring systems (CGMS) are now available that can continually measure glucose levels. A small plastic catheter is inserted subcutaneously and measures glucose every 5 min. Patients can view this in real time and detect upward and downward trends in glucose. Also helpful is that alarms for high and low readings can be set. We recommend these systems also be supervised by experienced endocrinologists and diabetes educators.

Type 2 Diabetes

There are multiple treatment options for type 2 diabetes. When medical therapy is initiated in type 2 diabetes, if the diabetes is mild, starting with an oral agent is preferred because of ease of administration. If kidney function permits, metformin is an ideal first choice given the lack of associated hypoglycemia and its potential benefits on weight; it is also inexpensive and readily available. As noted above, CKD can be a limiting factor in its use. A DPP-4 inhibitor can also be considered as there is no associated hypoglycemia, though reduction in A1c tends to be modest. Sulfonylureas are inexpensive and effective; however, as they carry a risk of hypoglycemia they require vigilant monitoring on the part of the physician and patient; the initial starting dose should be low and titrated with caution. It is possible that they may also contribute to premature beta-cell failure as they "squeeze" insulin production from the pancreas. Pioglitazone can be a reasonable choice since it decreases insulin resistance and is safe in CKD. However, weight gain and fluid retention are undesirable side effects. The recently approved SGLT2 inhibitors, canagliflozin and dapagliflozin, are also reasonable choices as second agents, although they will have limited use when the eGFR dips below 60 mL/min/1.73 m^2.

GLP-1 receptor agonists can be added to oral agents such as sulfonylureas (but not DPP-4 inhibitors); in CKD, liraglutide is the preferred choice. Since they are injections, they may not be desirable to patients but the potential for reduction in hyperglycemia along with weight loss is appealing. They can also be used as single agents.

In type 2 diabetes, there is a combination of a defect in insulin action leading to insulin resistance combined with progressive beta-cell failure. In patients with severe insulin resistance, beta-cell failure, or uncontrolled A1c despite use of other medications, insulin therapy should be initiated. There is no clear consensus on which regimen to use in which patient. The insulin regimen needs to be customized to the patient and time of day when hyperglycemia is occurring in an effort to minimize hypoglycemia while providing adequate control.

Often a long-acting insuin is added to oral hypoglycemic agnets or a GLP-1 agonist. A typical regimen includes adding basal insulin at bedtime to treat suboptimal fasting blood glucose levels due to hepatic gluconeogenesis that is inadequately treated with the oral agent [30]. In the Treat-to-Target trial, glargine or NPH was added at bedtime in patients already taking one or two oral hypoglycemic agents and titrated to a target fasting glucose of ≤100 mg/dL. The starting insulin dose was 10 U and the dose was titrated weekly with an increase of 2 U for every 20 mg/dL glucose level above target. Nearly 60 % of participants attained an A1c ≤7 % after 14 weeks. Study end A1c and fasting glucose levels were similar; however, those taking NPH experienced more hypoglycemic events [31]. A basal insulin such as glargine, detemir, or NPH, therefore, can be initiated at a dose of 10–15 U at bedtime. Subsequently, every 3 days, the insulin dose can be increased by 1–2 U to reach a target fasting blood sugar of 100–140 mg/dL [32]. The risk of nocturnal hypoglycemia may be higher with NPH. Basal insulin can also be used in the morning and titrated to normalize daytime hyperglycemia.

If goal glycemic control cannot be attained with basal insulin alone, or there is concurrent hypo- and hyperglycemia, then prandial insulin may need to be added. This is typically found in individuals who are hyperglycemic during the day but have controlled fasting blood sugar levels. Postprandial hyperglycemia has been associated with increased risk of cardiovascular disease (CVD) [33, 34], and is an equally important target for glycemic control. The addition of lispro to failing sulfonylurea therapy was studied in 25 patients with baseline poor glycemic control. The use of lispro plus sulfonylureas compared to sulfonylureas alone significantly reduced postprandial glucose levels, decreased A1c levels by 1.9 %, and also decreased fasting glucose levels [35].

Glycemic Target

Uncontrolled hyperglycemia is the prime cause of vascular complications including kidney disease. Glycemic control is necessary to delay the progression of diabetes-related kidney disease, and multiple factors must be taken into consideration when determining the appropriate level of glycemic control.

Glycemic Goal to Attain A1c ~7.0 %

In general, the recommended target A1c in diabetes has been less than or around 7 % by the ADA [36]; the ADA also recommends stricter (<6.5 %) or looser (<8 %) goals for certain individuals. AACE endorses a goal A1c of ≤6.5 % in healthy patients at low risk of hypoglycemia but it acknowledges that the goals should be individualized [37]. The 2007 Kidney Disease Outcomes Quality Initiative (KDOQI) guidelines for diabetes and CKD endorse a target A1c of <7.0 % [38]. However, their updated guidelines from 2012 instead recommend a target A1c of ~7.0 % [39].

In type 1 diabetes, a number of studies have shown that the development of microalbuminuria is associated with worse glycemic control. The Diabetes Control and Complications Trial (DCCT) showed that intensive therapy in patients with type 1 diabetes (mean A1c 9.1 % vs. 7.2 %) reduced the occurrence of microalbuminuria by 34 % in the primary prevention group and by 43 % in the secondary intervention group who had known early complications at baseline. Similarly, risk reduction in progression to clinical albuminuria was noted [40, 41]. To assess whether risk reduction of diabetic nephropathy persists long term, the Epidemiology of Diabetes Interventions and Complications (EDIC) Study demonstrated there were fewer cases of new microalbuminuria and progression to albuminuria in the original intensive group [42]. In the long-term follow-up study of the original DCCT treatment groups, it was found that intensive treatment also resulted in a significant decrease in the development of estimated GFR levels of <60 mL/min/1.73 m^2.

In patients with type 2 diabetes, the UK Prospective Diabetes Study (UKPDS) demonstrated a reduction in development of microalbuminuria by 24 % in subjects in the intensive management group (A1c 7.0 % vs. 7.9 %). These subjects also had significantly reduced rates of rises in creatinine. Similar findings were shown in the Veteran Affairs Cooperative Study on Glycemic Control and Complications in Type 2 Diabetes Feasibility Trial, where subjects had significantly lower rates of microalbuminuria and albuminuria. Similar results were also found in the Kumamoto study and ADVANCE trial [43–46]. A systematic review and meta-analysis of seven trials evaluating the impact of intensive glucose control on kidney-related end points in patients with type 2 diabetes showed reduced risk of developing microalbuminuria and macroalbuminuria. However, they also found there was no benefit in regard to doubling of serum creatinine, development of ESRD, or death related to kidney disease [47].

The ACCORD study showed higher risks of hypoglycemia and mortality in patients with type 2 diabetes treated with intensive glucose control (mean A1c 6.4 % vs. 7.5 %) without any risk reduction on CVD. The increased mortality could not be attributed to hypoglycemia [48]. In the ADVANCE trial more intensive glycemic control (A1c 6.5 % vs. 7.3 %) showed no reduction in CVD but a 21 % reduction in nephropathy [46]. The VADT study (intensive group with A1c 6.9 % vs. 8.4 %) also showed no benefit on CVD risk with stricter glucose control [49]. The data clearly show that lowering A1c leads to benefit in regard to microvascular complications including nephropathy. Benefits in A1c reduction are also clearly seen on rates of retinopathy and neuropathy. However, the positive effect of lowering A1c is much less in regard to macrovascular disease. Thus, it is reasonable that a target A1c ~7.0 % offers an optimal risk-to-benefit ratio rather than a target that is considerably lower. Additionally, any improvement in glycemic control even to A1c levels above 7 % results in improvement in nephropathy, as well as retinopathy and neuropathy, when compared to a higher A1c. This supports that the best A1c attainable should be achieved when possible, even if it cannot be 7 %.

Patients on chronic dialysis no longer need to achieve good glycemic control to prevent deterioration of kidney function. However, good control can still have benefits in delaying the progression of retinopathy and neuropathy. Whether improved glucose control reduces mortality in those undergoing dialysis is unclear. Some analyses suggest that there is no clear correlation, indicating the need to individualize glucose control without routinely recommending intensive control for all patients on dialysis [50, 51]. Conversely, there are a number of studies demonstrating improved survival with lower A1c levels [52–55]. The Dialysis Outcomes and Practice Patterns Study (DOPPS) concluded the optimal target A1c is 7–7.9 % as mortality was found to be increased with A1c levels that were both higher and lower than this range [56].

Hypoglycemia Risk

As expected, lower A1c levels are associated with higher risk of hypoglycemia, necessitating tailored A1c targets for different individuals. The risk of hypoglycemia, which in turn can cause injury, myocardial infarction, seizure, stroke, or death, is greatest in those who are frail and elderly, with erratic eating habits, on insulin and sulfonylureas, and with CKD. In patients at risk of hypoglycemia, a higher target A1c should be strongly considered. Higher A1c targets should also be considered for children, those with shortened life expectancies, those with a known history of severe hypoglycemia or hypoglycemia unawareness, the presence of comorbidities such as seizures, or a long (>25 years) history of diabetes with development of only minimal complications.

As noted previously, patients with progressing kidney disease with substantial decreases in GFR have increased risks for hypoglycemia for multiple reasons: decreased clearance of insulin, decreased clearance of oral agents, and impaired renal gluconeogenesis. This decline in gluconeogenesis may reduce the ability of a patient to defend against hypoglycemia in the face of excessive insulin, excess oral agents, or lack of food intake.

Monitoring Glycemic Control

Hemoglobin A1c should be measured every 3 months if therapy is changed or if the A1c is not at goal; it can otherwise be followed every 6 months if at goal and glucose control is stable. Patients should be encouraged to check their blood sugars frequently with a calibrated, validated glucose meter. The intensity of blood glucose monitoring is dependent on the severity of diabetes and intensity of treatment. For example, a patient taking insulin injections four times daily should check blood glucose levels four times per day or more. Conversely, a patient with mild diabetes controlled with lifestyle management may only need to check blood sugars a few times per week. Goal fasting and premeal blood sugars are <130 mg/dL and goal postprandial blood sugars are <180 mg/dL [36].

Accuracy of A1c in Chronic Kidney Disease

The measurement of hemoglobin A1c can be inaccurate in some patients with progressive kidney disease. Contributing factors include anemia from reduced life-span of the red blood cell, hemolysis, and iron deficiency, which may result in falsely low values, but falsely increased levels can occur from carbamylation of hemoglobin and the presence of acidosis. Fructosamine and glycated albumin are alternative measures available to estimate glycemic control. Fructosamine reflects the glycation of multiple serum proteins whereas glycated albumin reflects glycation of only albumin; both provide an estimate of control over the past 2 weeks. It is unclear if they offer superior measures of glucose control compared to A1c in patients with CKD. Studies suggest glycated albumin is superior to A1c in dialysis patients since A1c tends to underestimate glycemic control in those with ESRD [57]; however, the differences are rather small.

Conclusion

Caring for diabetes in patients with CKD demands detailed attention to multiple aspects of their care. At the center of this is glycemic control. Control should be optimized for the patient, taking measures to reduce complications while minimizing adverse events. Adequate treatment often necessitates a multifactorial approach through the use of an endocrinologist, nephrologist, dietician, diabetes educator, and additional specialists experienced in the complications of diabetes to provide a comprehensive care program to reduce progression of disease.

References

1. Rabkin R, Ryan MP, Duckworth WC. The renal metabolism of insulin. Diabetologia. 1984;27(3):351–7.
2. Baldwin D, Zander J, Munoz C, Raghu P, DeLange-Hudec S, Lee H, et al. A randomized trial of two weight-based doses of insulin glargine and glulisine in hospitalized subjects with type 2 diabetes and renal insufficiency. Diabetes Care. 2012;35(10):1970–4.
3. Holstein A, Plaschke A, Hammer C, Ptak M, Kuhn J, Kratzsch C, et al. Hormonal counterregulation and consecutive glimepiride serum concentrations during severe hypoglycaemia associated with glimepiride therapy. Eur J Clin Pharmacol. 2003;59(10):747–54.
4. Holstein A, Beil W. Oral antidiabetic drug metabolism: pharmacogenomics and drug interactions. Expert Opin Drug Metab Toxicol. 2009;5(3):225–41.
5. Balant L, Zahnd G, Gorgia A, Schwarz R, Fabre J. Pharmacokinetics of glipizide in man: influence of renal insufficiency. Diabetologia. 1973;331–8.
6. Arjona Ferreira JC, Marre M, Barzilai N, Guo H, Golm GT, Sisk CM, et al. Efficacy and safety of sitagliptin versus glipizide in patients with type 2 diabetes and moderate-to-severe chronic renal insufficiency. Diabetes Care. 2013;36:1067–73.
7. Inoue T, Shibahara N, Miyagawa K, Itahana R, Izumi M, Nakanishi T, et al. Pharmacokinetics of nateglinide and its metabolites in subjects with type 2 diabetes mellitus and renal failure. Clin Nephrol. 2003;60(2):90–5.
8. Hasslacher C. Safety and efficacy of repaglinide in type 2 diabetic patients with and without impaired renal function. Diabetes Care. 2003;26(3):886–91.
9. Wile DJ, Toth C. Association of metformin, elevated homocysteine, and methylmalonic acid levels and clinically worsened diabetic peripheral neuropathy. Diabetes Care. 2010;33(1):156–61.
10. Sambol NC, Chiang J, Lin ET, Goodman AM, Liu CY, Benet LZ, et al. Kidney function and age are both predictors of pharmacokinetics of metformin. J Clin Pharmacol. 1995;35(11):1094–102.
11. Salpeter SR, Greyber E, Pasternak GA, Salpeter EE. Risk of fatal and nonfatal lactic acidosis with metformin use in type 2 diabetes mellitus. Cochrane Database Syst Rev. 2010;(4):CD002967.
12. Lalau JD, Lacroix C, Compagnon P, de Cagny B, Rigaud JP, Bleichner G, et al. Role of metformin accumulation in metformin-associated lactic acidosis. Diabetes Care. 1995;18(6):779–84.
13. Lipska KJ, Bailey CJ, Inzucchi SE. Use of metformin in the setting of mild-to-moderate renal insufficiency. Diabetes Care. 2011; 34(6):1431–7.
14. Herrington WG, Levy JB. Metformin: effective and safe in renal disease? Int Urol Nephrol. 2008;40(2):411–7.
15. U.S. Food and Drug Administration. FDA significantly restricts access to the diabetes drug Avandia. http://www.fda.gov/Drugs/DrugSafety/PostmarketDrugSafetyInformation for patients and providers/ucm226956htm, 9-23-10.
16. Bergman AJ, Cote J, Yi B, Marbury T, Swan SK, Smith W, et al. Effect of renal insufficiency on the pharmacokinetics of sitagliptin, a dipeptidyl peptidase-4 inhibitor. Diabetes Care. 2007;30(7):1862–4.
17. Graefe-Mody U, Friedrich C, Port A, Ring A, Retlich S, Heise T, et al. Effect of renal impairment on the pharmacokinetics of the dipeptidyl peptidase-4 inhibitor linagliptin(*). Diabetes Obes Metab. 2011;13(10):939–46.
18. Snyder RW, Berns JS. Use of insulin and oral hypoglycemic medications in patients with diabetes mellitus and advanced kidney disease. Semin Dial. 2004;17(5):365–70.
19. Linnebjerg H, Kothare PA, Park S, Mace K, Reddy S, Mitchell M, et al. Effect of renal impairment on the pharmacokinetics of exenatide. Br J Clin Pharmacol. 2007;64(3):317–27.
20. Johansen OE, Whitfield R. Exenatide may aggravate moderate diabetic renal impairment: a case report. Br J Clin Pharmacol. 2008;66:568–9.
21. U.S. Food and Drug Administration. Information for Healthcare Professionals: reports of altered kidney function in patients using Exenatide (Marketed as Byetta). http://www.fda.gov/Drugs/DrugSafety/PostmarketDrugSafetyInformation for Patients and Providers/DrugSafetyInformation for Healthcare Professionals/ucm188656.htm, 11-02-2009.
22. Davidson JA, Brett J, Falahati A, Scott D. Mild renal impairment and the efficacy and safety of liraglutide. Endocr Pract. 2011;17(3):345–55.
23. Ratner RE, Hirsch IB, Neifing JL, Garg SK, Mecca TE, Wilson CA. Less hypoglycemia with insulin glargine in intensive insulin therapy for type 1 diabetes. U.S. Study Group of Insulin Glargine in Type 1 Diabetes. Diabetes Care. 2000;23(5):639–43.
24. Rosenstock J, Park G, Zimmerman J. Basal insulin glargine (HOE 901) versus NPH insulin in patients with type 1 diabetes on multiple daily insulin regimens. U.S. Insulin Glargine (HOE 901) Type 1 Diabetes Investigator Group. Diabetes Care. 2000;23(8):1137–42.
25. Porcellati F, Rossetti P, Pampanelli S, Fanelli CG, Torlone E, Scionti L, et al. Better long-term glycaemic control with the basal insulin glargine as compared with NPH in patients with Type 1 diabetes mellitus given meal-time lispro insulin. Diabet Med. 2004;21(11):1213–20.
26. Vague P, Selam JL, Skeie S, De Leeuw I, Elte JW, Haahr H, et al. Insulin detemir is associated with more predictable glycemic control and reduced risk of hypoglycemia than NPH insulin in patients with type 1 diabetes on a basal-bolus regimen with premeal insulin aspart. Diabetes Care. 2003;26(3):590–6.
27. Torlone E, Pampanelli S, Lalli C, Del Sindaco P, Di Vincenzo A, Rambotti AM, et al. Effects of the short-acting insulin analog [Lys(B28), Pro(B29)] on postprandial blood glucose control in IDDM. Diabetes Care. 1996;19(9):945–52.
28. Raskin P, Guthrie RA, Leiter L, Riis A, Jovanovic L. Use of insulin aspart, a fast-acting insulin analog, as the mealtime insulin in the management of patients with type 1 diabetes. Diabetes Care. 2000;23(5):583–8.
29. Garg SK, Rosenstock J, Ways K. Optimized Basal-bolus insulin regimens in type 1 diabetes: insulin glulisine versus regular human insulin in combination with Basal insulin glargine. Endocr Pract. 2005;11(1):11–7.
30. DeFronzo RA. Pharmacologic therapy for type 2 diabetes mellitus. Ann Intern Med. 1999;131(4):281–303.
31. Riddle MC, Rosenstock J, Gerich J. The treat-to-target trial: randomized addition of glargine or human NPH insulin to oral therapy of type 2 diabetic patients. Diabetes Care. 2003;26(11):3080–6.
32. Mooradian AD, Bernbaum M, Albert SG. Narrative review: a rational approach to starting insulin therapy. Ann Intern Med. 2006;145(2):125–34.
33. Gerstein HC, Yusuf S. Dysglycaemia and risk of cardiovascular disease. Lancet. 1996;347(9006):949–50.
34. Goldberg RJ, Burchfiel CM, Benfante R, Chiu D, Reed DM, Yano K. Lifestyle and biologic factors associated with atherosclerotic disease in middle-aged men. 20-year findings from the Honolulu Heart Program. Arch Intern Med. 1995;155(7):686–94.
35. Feinglos MN, Thacker CH, English J, Bethel MA, Lane JD. Modification of postprandial hyperglycemia with insulin lispro improves glucose control in patients with type 2 diabetes. Diabetes Care. 1997;20(10):1539–42.
36. American Diabetes Association. Standards of medical care in diabetes—2013. Diabetes Care. 2013;36 Suppl 1:S11–66.
37. Garber AJ, Abrahamson MJ, Barzilay JI, Blonde L, Bloomgarden ZT, Bush MA, et al. AACE comprehensive diabetes management algorithm 2013. Endocr Pract. 2013;19(2):327–36.

38. KDOQI. KDOQI clinical practice guidelines and clinical practice recommendations for diabetes and chronic kidney disease. Am J Kidney Dis. 2007;49(2 Suppl 2):S12–154.
39. KDOQI. KDOQI Clinical Practice Guideline for Diabetes and CKD: 2012 Update. Am J Kidney Dis. 2012;60(5):850–86.
40. DCCT. The effect of intensive treatment of diabetes on the development and progression of long-term complications in insulin-dependent diabetes mellitus. The Diabetes Control and Complications Trial Research Group. N Engl J Med. 1993;329(14):977–86.
41. DCCT. Effect of intensive therapy on the development and progression of diabetic nephropathy in the Diabetes Control and Complications Trial. The Diabetes Control and Complications (DCCT) Research Group. Kidney Int. 1995;47(6):1703–20.
42. EDIC. Sustained effect of intensive treatment of type 1 diabetes mellitus on development and progression of diabetic nephropathy: the Epidemiology of Diabetes Interventions and Complications (EDIC) study. JAMA. 2003;290(16):2159–67.
43. Levin SR, Coburn JW, Abraira C, Henderson WG, Colwell JA, Emanuele NV, et al. Effect of intensive glycemic control on microalbuminuria in type 2 diabetes. Veterans Affairs Cooperative Study on Glycemic Control and Complications in Type 2 Diabetes Feasibility Trial Investigators. Diabetes Care. 2000;23(10):1478–85.
44. Ohkubo Y, Kishikawa H, Araki E, Miyata T, Isami S, Motoyoshi S, et al. Intensive insulin therapy prevents the progression of diabetic microvascular complications in Japanese patients with non-insulin-dependent diabetes mellitus: a randomized prospective 6-year study. Diabetes Res Clin Pract. 1995;28(2):103–17.
45. UKPDS. Intensive blood-glucose control with sulphonylureas or insulin compared with conventional treatment and risk of complications in patients with type 2 diabetes (UKPDS 33). UK Prospective Diabetes Study (UKPDS) Group. Lancet. 1998;352(9131):837–53.
46. Patel A, MacMahon S, Chalmers J, Neal B, Billot L, Woodward M, et al. Intensive blood glucose control and vascular outcomes in patients with type 2 diabetes. N Engl J Med. 2008;358(24):2560–72.
47. Coca SG, Ismail-Beigi F, Haq N, Krumholz HM, Parikh CR. Role of intensive glucose control in development of renal end points in type 2 diabetes mellitus: systematic review and meta-analysis intensive glucose control in type 2 diabetes. Arch Intern Med. 2012;172(10):761–9.
48. Gerstein HC, Miller ME, Byington RP, Goff Jr DC, Bigger JT, Buse JB, et al. Effects of intensive glucose lowering in type 2 diabetes. N Engl J Med. 2008;358(24):2545–59.
49. Duckworth W, Abraira C, Moritz T, Reda D, Emanuele N, Reaven PD, et al. Glucose control and vascular complications in veterans with type 2 diabetes. N Engl J Med. 2009;360(2):129–39.
50. Shurraw S, Majumdar SR, Thadhani R, Wiebe N, Tonelli M. Glycemic control and the risk of death in 1,484 patients receiving maintenance hemodialysis. Am J Kidney Dis. 2010;55(5):875–84.
51. Williams ME, Lacson Jr E, Wang W, Lazarus JM, Hakim R. Glycemic control and extended hemodialysis survival in patients with diabetes mellitus: comparative results of traditional and time-dependent Cox model analyses. Clin J Am Soc Nephrol. 2010; 5(9):1595–601.
52. Oomichi T, Emoto M, Tabata T, Morioka T, Tsujimoto Y, Tahara H, et al. Impact of glycemic control on survival of diabetic patients on chronic regular hemodialysis: a 7-year observational study. Diabetes Care. 2006;29(7):1496–500.
53. Duong U, Mehrotra R, Molnar MZ, Noori N, Kovesdy CP, Nissenson AR, et al. Glycemic control and survival in peritoneal dialysis patients with diabetes mellitus. Clin J Am Soc Nephrol. 2011;6(5):1041–8.
54. Kalantar-Zadeh K, Kopple JD, Regidor DL, Jing J, Shinaberger CS, Aronovitz J, et al. A1C and survival in maintenance hemodialysis patients. Diabetes Care. 2007;30(5):1049–55.
55. Drechsler C, Krane V, Ritz E, Marz W, Wanner C. Glycemic control and cardiovascular events in diabetic hemodialysis patients. Circulation. 2009;120(24):2421–8.
56. Ramirez SP, McCullough KP, Thumma JR, Nelson RG, Morgenstern H, Gillespie BW, et al. Hemoglobin A(1c) levels and mortality in the diabetic hemodialysis population: findings from the Dialysis Outcomes and Practice Patterns Study (DOPPS). Diabetes Care. 2012;35(12):2527–32.
57. Freedman BI, Shenoy RN, Planer JA, Clay KD, Shihabi ZK, Burkart JM, et al. Comparison of glycated albumin and hemoglobin A1c concentrations in diabetic subjects on peritoneal and hemodialysis. Perit Dial Int. 2010;30(1):72–9.

17 Computerized Clinical Decision Support for Patients with Diabetes and Chronic Kidney Disease

Shayan Shirazian, John K. Maesaka, Louis J. Imbriano, and Joseph Mattana

Scope of the Problem

Epidemiology

Diabetes mellitus (DM) is the most common cause of chronic kidney disease (CKD) and end stage renal disease (ESRD) in the United States [1]. Diabetes affects approximately 40 % of the over 20 million Americans with CKD and 45 % of the approximately 413,725 Americans on dialysis [1, 2]. Patients with diabetes and CKD are at increased risk of cardiovascular and all-cause mortality [3, 4]. This mortality risk increases as kidney function deteriorates. The mortality for patients with ESRD and diabetes is estimated to be greater than 70 % at 5 years [1]. In addition to these substantial health risks, Medicare spends nearly 36 billion dollars treating ESRD annually, a number that has increased by approximately 15 billion dollars in the past 10 years [1].

Early Recognition

The problem of CKD in patients with diabetes is expected to worsen in the next two decades, as the incidence of diabetes increases. It has been estimated that by the year 2030, diabetes will reach pandemic proportions worldwide with over 366 million adults afflicted [5]. In order to slow the growing epidemic of kidney disease in patients with diabetes and improve outcomes in this population, the National Kidney Foundation (NKF) and National Institute of Health (NIH) have established programs that promote the early recognition and treatment of patients with diabetes and CKD [6, 7]. One example of such a program is the Kidney Early Evaluation Program (KEEP) [7, 8]. Established by the NKF in 1997, KEEP is a free community-screening program for adults at high risk for CKD. High-risk status is defined as a personal history of diabetes or hypertension, or a first-degree relative with diabetes, hypertension, or kidney disease. The KEEP program was designed to increase awareness of CKD among high-risk individuals, to provide free testing for kidney disease, to recommend a CKD treatment plan with educational information and to provide referrals and ongoing support for follow-up. Since its establishment, the KEEP program has screened approximately 170,000 people in the United States [9]. Although the full impact of the KEEP program is not yet known, the hope is that early detection will facilitate early treatment and slow the growing prevalence of ESRD and CKD-related mortality.

Proven Interventions

Multiple interventions have been proven to decrease cardiovascular risk and slow the progression of kidney disease in patients with diabetes and CKD. These interventions include the use of angiotensin inhibitors and strict control of blood pressure and blood glucose. Although not as rigorously supported, additional treatments such as cholesterol control, smoking cessation, dietary interventions, and weight reduction may also slow the progression of CKD. When implemented together, these interventions have additive risk reduction benefits.

Angiotensin Inhibition

The clinical benefits of angiotensin inhibition in the treatment of patients with diabetes and albuminuria have been shown in multiple large randomized controlled trials [10–15]. These benefits have included improved blood pressure control, regression of proteinuria, slower rates of renal function decline, decreased rates of ESRD,

S. Shirazian, M.D. (✉) • J.K. Maesaka, M.D. • L.J. Imbriano, M.D. • J. Mattana, M.D.
Department of Medicine, Winthrop-University Hospital, 200 Old Country Road, Suite 135, Mineola, NY 11501, USA

Division of Nephrology and Hypertension, Department of Medicine, Winthrop-University Hospital, 200 Old Country Road, Suite 135, Mineola, NY 11501, USA
e-mail: sshirazian@winthrop.org

E.V. Lerma and V. Batuman (eds.), *Diabetes and Kidney Disease*, DOI 10.1007/978-1-4939-0793-9_17, © Springer Science+Business Media New York 2014 and decreased mortality [16]. Due to these benefits, NKF has issued guidelines recommending the use of either an angiotensin-converting enzyme (ACE) inhibitor or an angiotensin receptor blocker (ARB) for the treatment of patients with diabetes and either microalbuminuria, macroalbuminuria, or CKD [17].

Blood Glucose Control

Tight glucose control has been shown to prevent the development and progression of albuminuria [18–22]. Furthermore, large randomized controlled trials have shown that intensive glucose control slows decline in renal function [19, 23]. Determining the optimal blood glucose to target for treatment has been more difficult, as controlling hemoglobin A1c (HgBA1c) to a target of 6 % or less has been associated with a higher risk of all-cause mortality [22]. It is currently recommended by the American Diabetes Association (ADA) and NKF to control HgBA1c to a target level of approximately 7.0 % in patients with diabetes with or without CKD [17, 24].

Blood Pressure Control

Strict blood pressure control has been shown to slow the decline of kidney function in patients with diabetes and CKD in multiple prospective trials [25, 26]. The optimal level of blood pressure to minimize risk remains uncertain. The Kidney Disease: Improving Global Outcomes (KDIGO) clinical practice guidelines currently recommends targeting a blood pressure lower than 140/90 in nonalbuminuric patients with diabetes and CKD and targeting a blood pressure of less than 130/80 in albuminuric patients with diabetes and CKD [27].

Additional Therapies

Additional interventions have shown limited benefit in the treatment of patients with diabetes and CKD. Salt restriction to ≤70 mEq/day has been shown to enhance the anti-proteinuric effects of angiotensin inhibition [28]. Weight loss has been shown to decrease proteinuria in overweight patients with diabetes [29]. Cholesterol lowering with statins or fibrates may slow the rate of renal function decline and progression of albuminuria [30, 31]. Smoking has been associated with the progression of kidney disease in patients with type 2 diabetes [32] and its cessation has been associated with a decreased risk of CKD progression [33]. Finally, decreasing dietary protein may mitigate the risk of ESRD and death in patients with diabetes and CKD [34].

Combined Therapy

The potential additive benefits of intensive intervention in patients with diabetes and CKD has been shown in a prospective study of 160 white Danish patients, the Steno 2-trial [35]. In this study, patients were randomly assigned to multifactorial intensive therapy or standard therapy. Multifactorial intervention included dietary counseling, exercise, smoking cessation, targeting blood glucose to HgBA1C <6.5 %, targeting blood pressure to <140/85 and <130/80 mmHg for the last 2 years, ACE inhibitor therapy, targeting total cholesterol <190 and <175 mg/dL for the last 2 years, targeting triglycerides <150 mg/dL, aspirin, and vitamin therapy. After 7.8 years of follow-up, the intensive therapy group had a significant reduction in the primary composite cardiac end point, which included cardiac death, as well as a significant reduction in albuminuria [35]. At 13.3 years, including 5.5 years of observational follow-up, the intensive therapy group has a significantly decreased risk of all-cause mortality when compared to the control group [36].

Under-Recognition of CKD

CKD has been shown to be under-recognized in the general population, in populations at high risk for CKD and in patients with diabetes [37, 38]. Cross-sectional analysis of the National Health and Nutrition Examination Survey (NHANES) from 1999 to 2000 revealed awareness rates of 40.5 %, 29.3 %, 22 %, and 44.5 % in patients with stage 1, 2, 3, and 4 kidney disease, respectively [38]. Of the 274 patients with CKD who were unaware of their diagnosis, 68.8 % were also noted to have a history of diabetes. In a more recent analysis of the KEEP database, which includes patients at high risk for CKD, awareness rates were found to be similarly low; 4.36 %, 4.86 %, 5.39 %, 32.08 %, 44.87 % in patients with stage 1, 2, 3, 4, and 5 kidney disease, respectively [37]. When patients from the KEEP database with diabetes were examined only 9.4 % of patients were aware of their CKD diagnosis [39].

Low rates of CKD documentation and coding have also been reported among primary care physicians [40–42]. Retrospective and cross-sectional chart reviews have revealed documentation rates between 4 and 38 % in patients with moderate CKD [40, 41]. These low documentation and coding rates may be related to a lack of CKD knowledge. In a recent analysis by Navaneethan et al., only 36.5 % of primary care physicians were aware of NKF guidelines for nephrology referral [42]. Furthermore analysis of the KEEP database has revealed that only 12.3 % of patients with CKD who met NKF nephrology referral criteria were actually seen by a nephrologist [43]. This is an important finding given the known benefits of early referral in patients with CKD [44, 45]. These benefits include cost savings and decreased morbidity and mortality rates [44]. In a retrospective study of the Veterans Health Administration clinic records, including 39,031 patients, consistent nephrology care was independently associated with a lower risk of death in patients with moderately severe to severe CKD [46].

Undertreatment of CKD

As outlined above, several key interventions have been proven to slow the progression of CKD in patients with diabetes. Despite the proven benefit of these interventions, the majority of patients with diabetes and CKD are not receiving appropriate treatment. Analysis of the KEEP database, using data from 2005 to 2010, has revealed that target levels of blood pressure, blood glucose, and cholesterol were achieved concurrently in only 8.4 % of patients. In patients with stage 1 and stage 2 CKD, 6.0 % achieved these target levels, in patients with stage 3 CKD 8.5 % achieved these target levels and in patients with stage 4 and stage 5 CKD 9.0 % achieved these target levels [43]. Interestingly, only 9.9 % of patients with CKD co-managed by a nephrologist achieved target level control. Similar studies have shown that rates of uncontrolled blood pressure exceed 50 % in patients with CKD [47]. In a retrospective study of the NHANES database from 2003 to 2008, in which CKD awareness rates were only 7.4 % among patients with stage 1 through 4 disease, awareness of CKD was not associated with improvements in BP control, ACEI/ARB use, or blood glucose control [48].

Given the importance of early diagnosis and treatment of CKD in patients with diabetes and the known benefits of interventions, it is imperative that health care professionals increase their rates of guideline adherence. This includes improved rates of blood pressure, blood glucose, and cholesterol control and the employment of multifactorial lifestyle interventions including dietary and weight-loss counseling and smoking cessation. Novel strategies to improve the treatment of patients with diabetes and patients with CKD have been employed but with only limited success. These strategies have included educational programs, multidisciplinary programs, behavioral interventions, telephone interventions, close follow-up by mid-level providers, and risk-communication interventions [49–54]. One potential strategy for increasing the adherence of patients and physicians to treatment guidelines is through the use of information technology interventions built into the electronic medical record (EMR) including the use of computerized clinical decision support (CCDS). The rest of this chapter will focus on the use of CCDS to improve the care of patients with diabetes and CKD. We will first define CCDS, we will then review existing CCDS systems that have been used to facilitate the treatment of patients with diabetes and CKD and we will finish by discussing the characteristics of an optimal CCDS system to help manage patients with diabetes and CKD.

Introduction to CCDS

Clinical decision-making is part of the art of medicine. Deciding what diagnostic tests to order, when to initiate treatment, and how to treat is learned through countless hours of study and experience in medical school, training, and practice. Despite our best efforts, health care professionals make medical errors on a daily basis and adherence to guideline-appropriate treatment is poor. The Institute of Medicine has estimated that approximately 98,000 US residents die each year due to preventable medical errors [55]. Although health care professionals are often extremely bright, talented, and dedicated individuals, there are too many decisions to be made during a finite medical encounter. In addition, the growing body of medical literature makes it is near impossible for health care professionals to stay completely up-to-date on studies that should be guiding their decisions. CCDS strives to improve the decision-making process of physicians.

CCDS has been defined as the application of health information technology to aid clinical decision-making through the use of patient-specific electronic health information [56]. The most common features of these CCDS systems are a clinical knowledge base, an integration of that clinical knowledge base with patient-specific information stored in the EMR, and a system by which recommendations are presented back to the clinician [57]. A recent systematic review by Bright et al. identified 148 randomized controlled trials done between January 1976 and January 2011 that implemented CCDS at the point of care to aid decision-making [58]. The identified trials varied greatly with regard to the population studied, the clinical problem, the design and features of the CCDS system used, and the outcomes measured. Besides underscoring the breadth of CCDS systems studied over the past 25 years, this review also highlights the current problems with CCDS research. In order to simplify the classification of CCDS systems, we will only focus on clinically relevant aspects of CCDS for the rest of this chapter.

Clinically Relevant CCDS

CCDS has been most commonly used to address clinical needs. The four most commonly described clinically relevant aspects of CCDS systems include: (1) the primary clinical problem for which CCDS is being implemented, (2) the target audience for which recommendations are presented, (3) when recommendations are presented, (4) how recommendations are presented and the control given to users in accessing or manipulating the recommendations [57].

Primary Clinical Problem

CCDS systems have been used to improve the quality of care across multiple target areas. These areas have included preventive care, diagnosis, treatment, efficiency, and cost containment [57]. With regard to preventive care, CCDS tools have been studied as a means to improve immunization rates, cancer-screening rates, and adherence to disease management guidelines for secondary prevention of cardiovascular disease [59–62]. In a systematic review by Souza et al. of existing randomized CCDS systems for primary preventive care, 41 trials were identified [62]. These CCDS systems improved the screening and treatment of dyslipidemia in primary care, but were less rigorously supported for use in cancer screening, vaccinations, and other preventive care. They also did not improve patient outcomes, safety, cost, or provider satisfaction.

CCDS systems have been used to aid physician diagnosis. In radiology, CCDS systems have improved image interpretation for a multitude of diseases including breast and lung cancer [63, 64]. In internal medicine, CCDS systems have been used to aid in the diagnosis of pneumonia through self-auscultation [65], diabetic proliferative retinopathy [66], tuberculosis [67], and acute coronary syndrome [68]. There are also many popular online diagnostic websites for both physicians and patients including webMD® and DxExplain®.

CCDS systems have been most extensively used to improve medical treatment. CCDS systems have been used to alert physicians to drug–drug interactions, drug dosing errors, and nonadherence to treatment guidelines [68–70]. These systems have also been used to improve adherence to disease management guidelines in multiple chronic conditions including asthma, HIV, neonatal care, diabetes, and hypertension [71–75]. For the most part, CCDS has improved the process of care in chronic conditions, but have not significantly improved patient outcomes [58].

In addition to screening, diagnosis, and treatment, interventions implemented by CCDS have been used to improve the efficiency of delivered care [76]. Examples of these interventions include care plans, order set guides, and drug formulary alerts [57]. These interventions have been designed to prevent duplicate testing and maximize cost savings. Few studies have examined the impact of these systems on efficiency and cost. Although difficult to implement and initially costly, CCDS systems may eventually result in significant cost savings by decreasing hospitalizations, shortening length of stay, decreasing the frequency of drug adverse events, and eliminating duplicate or excessive tests [71, 77].

Target Audience

CCDS systems have been designed for use by physician, nurses, nurse-practitioners, physician-assistants, pharmacists, and health care professionals in training [56, 77]. The majority of existing systems are targeted for physician use [56].

When to Present Recommendations

There has been considerable variation in when recommendations are presented to CCDS users. Information has been presented prior to patient encounters, in real-time during patient encounters or after patient encounters. It appears CCDS recommendations are most often followed when they are presented in real-time; however, patient summaries or lists of high-risk patients may be useful before or after patient encounters [78, 79].

How to Present Alerts and User Control of Alerts

An area of extensive study in CCDS implementation has been how to present recommendations or alerts to providers and the degree of provider control over these alerts. Considerations have included the format of alerts, how intrusive alerts and recommendations are to workflow, and how health care professional access and dismiss alerts [78–80].

The format of recommendations and alerts and their intrusiveness to workflow has varied greatly among CCDS trials. CCDS output has been presented as automatic pop-ups during a patient encounter that alert of incorrect prescribing or inadequate treatment, a list of patients not meeting appropriate screening or treatment goals, or as passive guidelines that can assist providers with treatment. The format of alert presentation often varies according to the importance of information presented with pop-up alerts that interrupt workflow presenting urgent information and passive lists conveying less urgent information.

The ease with which providers access and dismiss alerts has been described as its user control. CCDS can vary with regard to user control from interruptive alerts that physicians cannot clear until the problem is noted and corrected to completely passive alerts that health care professionals access on demand [57]. Furthermore, the degree of user control can be matched to the intention of the alert. Alerts indicating severe drug–drug interactions are often interruptive alerts that must be addressed prior to completing an order, while alerts that guide optimal care of chronic illness are often passive reminders that physicians can choose to address. The degree of user control of CCDS can dramatically impact a health care professional's impression of the CCDS system and the resultant actions which they may take. Interruptive reminders may disrupt workflow and frustrate physicians, while passive reminders have a tendency to be ignored. Furthermore, important interruptive reminders may start to be ignored if they appear too frequently or if CCDS users deem them inaccurate or unnecessary, a phenomenon known as "alert fatigue."

"Alert fatigue" has the potential to prevent changes in provider practice [79]. The overall frequency of over-ridden alerts has been estimated to be approximately 96 % [79]. Interruptive alerts have fared better than non-interruptive alerts. The frequency of provider over-riding drug interaction alerts has been found to 88 % and providers over-riding drug allergy alerts has been found to be 69 % [81], while the frequency with which providers have been found to ignore non-interruptive alerts has been found to be 98.6 % [82]. In designing future CCDS systems, an integral component will be to how to optimally configure user control of CCDS output to the importance of the alert. In order to prevent "alert fatigue" it may become necessary to configure alert presentation and to control an individual provider's tendencies. For example, for a provider that regularly dismisses or ignores alerts, CCDS systems could only present messages that are deemed urgent and make these messages difficult to dismiss or ignore [80].

Future Directions with CCDS

In this brief overview of clinically relevant aspects of CCDS interventions, we have introduced a variety of terms used to describe existing designs of CCDS. For the most part, although varied, current CCDS systems have successfully improved provider practice. In a systematic review by Kawamoto et al. characteristics of CCDS that successfully improved provider practice were described, and included computer-based recommendations/alerts, automated alerts that did not disrupt workflow, and action-oriented recommendations [81].

Despite improvements in provider practice, consistent improvements in clinical outcomes with CCDS implementation have not yet been realized. As described in a recent systemic review by Roshanov et al., CCDS systems improved the process of medical care in 52–64 % of studies, but only 15–31 % of those studies led to an improvement in patient outcomes [79]. Furthermore, initial studies have shown significant costs associated with CCDS implementation. In order to validate their adoption by health care systems, future CCDS studies need to show improvements in patient outcomes as well as prove their efficiency and cost-effectiveness.

Existing CCDS Systems for Diabetes, Hypertension, and CKD

There have been many studies addressing the effect of CCDS systems on the care of patients with diabetes, hypertension, and CKD. These interventions have addressed nephrologic care along different content areas with dramatically different CCDS designs. Content areas have included preventive care, treatment, efficiency, and cost. We will now introduce the existing studies of CCDS systems in patients with diabetes, hypertension, and CKD and end with a discussion of the optimal CCDS system for patients with diabetes and CKD.

Preventing Adverse Drug Events in CKD

CCDS systems have been used to check drug–drug interactions, drug allergies, and drug dosing in patients with kidney disease [77, 83]. These systems have been used in both acute and chronic kidney failure and in both outpatient and acute care settings [77, 83]. The ultimate goal of these systems is to reduce adverse drug events (ADEs), defined as drug-related patient injuries [69], though results thus far have been mixed.

Acute Kidney Injury

CCDS has successfully improved medication dosing during episodes of acute kidney injury (AKI). In a study by McCoy et al., 1598 adult inpatients with an episode of AKI were randomized to a CCDS system which consisted of a passive alert or an interruptive alert if one of at least 122 known nephrotoxic or renally cleared medications were dosed [84]. The interruptive alert but not the passive alert significantly improved the frequency with which providers modified or discontinued nephrotoxic or renally cleared medications during episodes of AKI.

CKD

In a study by Chertow et al., the effect of CCDS on prescriber practices and patient outcomes in hospitalized patients with CKD was evaluated [85]. The intervention consisted of real-time recommendations for drug selection, drug dosing, and drug frequency which appeared as alerts in the EMR. This intervention was compared to controls, in which drug dosing information was available online but not incorporated real-time into the ordering process, over four consecutive 2-month intervals (intervention—alternating with control) in a sample of 7,490 patients with a creatinine clearance <80 mL/min. CCDS was found to significantly increase the frequency of appropriate medication prescribing in patients with CKD to 51 % compared to 30 % in the control group. This included appropriate orders for dose changes (67 % vs. 54 %) and frequency changes (59 % vs. 35 %). There was also found to be a significant difference in length of stay in the intervention group vs. control (4.3 vs. 4.5) days, but no difference in hospital costs or episodes of AKI with the intervention [85].

In a review by Tawadrous et al., the effect of CCDS systems on prescribing practices in patients with AKI and CKD was examined [77]. The review yielded 17 prospective studies of CCDS. Of these 17 studies, 12 studies recommended drug dosing relative to the level of kidney function and the remaining five recommended dosing in response to clinical parameters of serum drug levels. The majority of these studies improved clinician-prescribing outcomes by improving rates of appropriate dosing and/or frequency of medication as well as the time to modify inappropriate drugs. Overall in this review, CCDS was found to decrease the rate at which patients developed AKI. However, other patient-important outcomes, such as rates of ADEs and length of hospital stay, were not shown to improve.

The above studies demonstrate a clear role for CCDS in improving clinician prescribing in terms of avoiding contraindicated medications and properly dosing medications in patients with kidney disease. Further research is needed to determine whether CCDS improves clinical outcomes such as decreasing the frequency of drug adverse events and whether CCDS can ultimately decrease costs.

CCDS to Prompt Recognition of CKD

Despite mandatory estimated glomerular filtration rate (eGFR) reporting only modest increases in CKD awareness among primary care providers has been realized [86, 87]. CCDS systems have been integrated into outpatient primary care EMRs to prompt recognition of CKD in an effort to improve clinical outcomes. Two of these CCDS systems were designed to provide comprehensive CKD care and will be discussed in an upcoming section, with only one study concentrated primarily on increasing recognition of CKD in a primary care [88, 89].

In a study by Abdel-Khader et al., the effect of a CCDS plus an educational session for primary care providers versus an educational session alone on nephrology referral and proteinuria quantification was tested in primary care clinics throughout Canada [86]. The study was designed as a cluster randomized trial. The CDSS consisted of a passive alert in the EMR that would be activated for patients who had an eGFR <45 mL/min/1.73 m^2 within 12 months of the patient's office visit and had not been seen by a university nephrologist. The first alert suggested a nephrology referral and provided the option to enter an order set containing an order for the referral. The second alert suggested ordering a spot urine albumin–creatinine ratio for patients who had not had a quantitative albuminuria/proteinuria assessment within the last year. The educational session and CCDS prompt did not improve nephrology referrals or proteinuria quantifications between the intervention and control group [86]. Although this study was an excellent example of a randomized controlled trial of a CCDS system for patients with CKD, it had several limitations on its generalizability to all CCDS systems for CKD. It was relatively small and underpowered, it was performed in university-based primary care clinics and finally and most importantly the CCDS was designed with a passive, non-interruptive alert [87]. Given the high frequency with which providers ignore passive alerts, future trials of CCDS to improve provider recognition of CKD should probably be designed with interruptive alerts that force provider recognition.

CCDS Systems to Improve Blood Pressure Control

The effect of decision support systems on blood pressure control has been reviewed by Anchala et al. [90]. This review identified four cluster-randomized controlled trials that measured differences in systolic blood pressure from the beginning to the end of the study. Three of these studies used computer-based clinical decision support systems that provided recommendations for medication management if a patient was not at goal blood pressure [75, 91, 92], while one study utilized a CCDS system that provided only a real-time patient-specific cardiovascular risk assessment with no hypertension management recommendations [93]. Based on results from the existing four studies, the authors of the review concluded that CCDS did not result in a significant reduction in systolic blood pressure. Limitations of this review included the exclusion of studies that did not report outcomes, the heterogeneity in the included studies and a large percentage of patients that were lost to follow-up (>25 %). The most notable limitation of their study was that not all of the included studies provided recommendations to providers regarding how to treat and specifically what medications and dosages to use.

An example of a good study in this review that included treatment recommendations as part of the CCDS treatment algorithm was done by Hicks et al. [92]. In this cluster randomized trial performed in 14 primary clinics affiliated with a large academic medical center in Boston, practices were randomized to a CCDS intervention designed to remind physicians of blood pressure treatment guidelines versus standard of care. Guidelines for blood pressure control were developed emphasizing disease-specific medication use. Patients were eligible for inclusion in the trial if they had a least one outpatient visit for hypertension in the preceding year to one of the clinics participating in the trial. The CCDS consisted of a reminder to start an appropriate antihypertensive medication in patients with a diagnosis of hypertension in the problem list or with three blood pressure readings ≥140/90 who were not on an appropriate guideline recommended medication for their disease class. The reminder was generated by an algorithm that was run in the EMR which searched vitals, medications, allergies, and problem lists and cross-checked these patient-specific problems with a disease-specific algorithm. If the patient was not on a disease-appropriate medication, a reminder was given to the provider in the EMR. Paper print outs of the reminders were also given to providers prior to a patient encounter. Of 2,027 eligible patients 1,048 were randomized to usual care, 786 to the CCDS intervention, 120 to care with a nurse practitioner, and 73 to care with NP and CCDS. Analysis of results revealed no significant improvement in blood pressure control between the CCDS group and the control group; however, CCDS use did result in a significant increase in recommended medication prescribing. The lack of improvement in blood pressure was thought to be due to the fact that the CCDS was designed to remind physicians to prescribe an appropriate class of medication and not to intensify therapy.

In fact 90 % of patients in both groups were taking a guideline-appropriate medication at the start of the study. The authors suggested that future CCDS designs for hypertension management focus on intensification of therapy.

In summary, existing studies of CCDS in hypertension have shown an improvement in processes of care such as medication prescribing, without an improvement in blood pressure control. To accomplish this, future studies should ideally focus on treatment recommendations built into the EMR with appropriate recommendations for intensification of therapy.

CCDS Systems to Improve Diabetes Management

The largest percentage of CCDS systems designed to treat chronic disease have been used to treat diabetes mellitus [79]. These CCDS systems have added many advantageous elements to diabetes care including a standardized care process for providers with emphasis on multifaceted risk reduction, improved continuity among providers due to a shared multidisciplinary EMR, and the ability to involve and empower patients in the care process through patient portals with accessible personalized health information [79]. Two examples of diabetes CCDS studies with effective interventions include the TRANSLATE trial and the COMPETE II trial.

The TRANSLATE trial was a group randomized trial that tested the effect of a multicomponent diabetes intervention on diabetes care in 24 single specialty community primary care practices without an existing EMR system [94]. In practices randomized to the intervention, a site coordinator and local physician advocate was assigned, an electronic diabetes registry was established and a site coordinator was trained in its use. The electronic registry, based on coordinator and clinic staff input as well as a laboratory interface, generated reminders for unscheduled appointments (for foot exams, eye exams, etc.), and reminders that graphed HgBA1c, SBP, and LDL values over time and indicated whether a patient was at target. These reminders were given to patients at every visit. In addition, high-risk patients were contacted by study coordinators. Site coordinators updated physicians on their progress monthly. In this study of 7,101 randomized patients, intervention practices resulted in significant improvements in SBP, HgBA1c, LDL cholesterol from baseline to 12 months when compared to control. This study found that at 12 months, 15 more targets for SBP, HgBA1c, or LDL were achieved by the intervention compared to the control for every 100 individuals randomized.

In the COMPETE II randomized trial, Holbrook et al. tested the effect of a web-based diabetes tracker shared by both patient and provider on 13 diabetes risk markers [95]. Patients with diabetes were assigned to the intervention arm consisting of an electronic, web-based, color-coded, diabetes tracker that interfaced with the patient's EMR and with a telephone reminder system or to standard care. The tracker monitored 13 diabetes-related quality variables for patients giving them targets for each variable as well as advice to help them reach these targets. In addition to the intervention patients received monthly mailings of the tracker coder page with instructions to bring this page to their physician appointments as well as receiving monthly automated telephone reminders for medications, laboratory, and physician visits. A total of 511 patients were randomized into the trial and these patients were followed for an average of 5.9 months. The primary outcome for this study was an "improvement of process," defined as the difference between intervention and control with regard to a composite outcome of quality that was calculated based on achieved values of HgBA1c, blood pressure, LDL cholesterol, body mass index, albuminuria, foot check frequency, smoking and physical activity index compared to targets. The process composite score increased significantly more in the intervention group than the control group. The authors also noted a small but statistically significant improvement in SBP control and HgBA1c between the intervention and control groups, but at the end of the 6-month study only 19 patients or 7.5 % of patients in the intervention group had SBP, HgBA1c, and LDL in target. The authors concluded that they achieved only modest improvements in outcome, attributing this to short follow-up and their focus on process outcomes.

Ali et al. reviewed published studies from the Medline database looking at the effect of an EMR equipped with CCDS on clinical diabetes care [96]. The result was 33 individual studies of which 21 reported on quantitative clinical care process indicators with pre- and post-intervention measures. There were 13 reported randomized or cluster randomized trials and 23 of 26 trials were set in primary health care clinics. There were no studies that reported on hard clinical end points such as cardiovascular events or mortality. Major findings from this review were that CDSS incorporated into EMR led to a decrease in the variability of clinical care received between clinics and between providers at the same clinic. It was also noted that multifaceted interventions, for example those that also involved implementation of clinical case managers, improved outcomes to a greater degree than single interventions and that CCDS tools that were interactive with patient portals and a greater number of features were associated with better outcomes. The majority of the studies received good reviews from patients who reported an increased sense of empowerment with CCDS. This review was limited by the heterogeneity of reviewed studies and a lack of reporting on hard clinical end points like cardiovascular events or mortality. In conclusion CCDS systems for diabetes have been shown to improve the clinical care process with multifaceted interventions and patient accessible options predicting the greatest success. Future studies should utilize a standard evaluation metric and include evaluation of hard clinical end points.

CCDS to Treat CKD

There have been only two prospective studies examining the effect of CDS in patients with CKD. Both trials identified patients with CKD from the EMR and then recommended treatment based on this designation; however, only one study gave computerized real-time recommendations to the provider.

In the first study by Fox et al., the effect of quality improvement measures implemented at two urban minority practice sites, one with an EMR and one with paper-based charting, were measured [88]. These quality improvement measures included the use of practice enhancement assistants, CCDS and academic detailing. A CCDS tool was designed based on NKF guidelines. This tool extracted laboratory elements from the EMR including eGFR, HgBA1c, medications related to CKD as well as calcium, phosphorous, intact parathyroid hormone, and 25-OH vitamin D levels. Based on these current laboratory parameters, a recommendation reminder sheet was created for each patient with CKD seen by a specific provider. This reminder sheet included current laboratory parameters for the patient and recommendations for quality improvement to help the patient achieve NKF-defined CKD treatment goals. In the practice with EMR, the reminder sheet was placed in a physician "to do" section as a passive task reminder, once approved reminder notes were placed into the EMR to improve CKD care including notes to diagnose CKD, discontinue harmful medications and to order appropriate diagnostic tests. In the paper-based clinic, the initial reminder sheet and reminder notes were placed in the paper-based chart. In addition to the CCDS tools, the quality improvement intervention included the implementation of two practice enhancement assistants who would review charts and check for guideline implementation approximately every 3 months and make suggestions for meeting CKD guidelines. Inclusion criteria for CDSS implementation into the EMR included age older than 18 and estimated GFR (eGFR) <60 mL/min, and 180 patients from both clinics met this criteria. The quality improvement project with CCDS improved rates of CKD and anemia diagnosis and decreased the use of potentially harmful medications in CKD including metformin and NSAIDs. The authors also noted a small but significant improvement in eGFR at 1 year post-intervention.

In the second study by Manns et al., the effect of an enhanced eGFR laboratory prompt was evaluated at 93 primary care clinics in Canada in patients older than 66 with an eGFR <60 mL/min and diabetes or proteinuria [89]. The enhanced prompt included education about the significance of CKD and management suggestions including recommendations to measure urine albumin/creatinine ratio (UACR), prescribe an ACEi or ARB in patients with diabetes with UACR >35 mg/mmol, reduce BP to <130/80 mmHg, reduce LDL cholesterol to <2.5 mmol/L, and target hemoglobin A1c to <7 %. These recommendations were mailed to the provider. Primary care clinics were cluster randomized to receive a paper-based standard eGFR prompt which consisted of a statement defining CKD and indications for nephrology referral or the enhanced prompt as described. The primary outcome was the proportion of patients who filled a prescription for an ACEi or ARB within 1 year of the first prompt being received by the physician. The authors found that the enhanced prompt did not improve ACEi or ARB prescribing practices in 5,444 elderly CKD patients with diabetes or proteinuria. There was also no difference in the proportion of patients receiving a prescription for new a cholesterol-lowering drug or an additional antihypertensive medication from a different therapeutic class between groups for the year after the prompt was instituted. Although this was a large randomized trial, the design of the study and the intervention limit the generalizability of these findings. Treatment recommendations were not incorporated into the EMR and were not given at the time and place of the physician visit. Furthermore 77 % of patient had achieved the primary outcome, were on an ACEi or ARB, prior to intervention suggesting minimal room for improvement [97]. Future studies of CDS in CKD should be designed with computerized systems that incorporate real-time recommendations into the EMR and be powered to detect improvements in clinical outcomes.

Optimal CCDS for Diabetes and CKD

Caring for patients with diabetes mellitus requires attention to detail, close follow-up, and a multidisciplinary approach. Moreover patients with diabetes and CKD represent a very high-risk subgroup that requires even more diligence. Physicians must remain up-to-date on the latest treatments for these patients, manage complex comorbidities including psychiatric illness and deal with challenging social problems. As we have previously documented, physicians are falling short in the care of patients with diabetes and CKD. Furthermore, the growing epidemic of patients with diabetes and CKD makes the future care of a large number of these patients daunting. It is obvious that physicians need help. We believe that the addition of CCDS tools into the EMR can greatly augment the care of patients with diabetes and CKD. In the previous section we introduced studies examining the effect of CCDS on diabetes, hypertension, and CKD care. In this section we will describe what we believe are characteristics of an optimal CCDS system for patients with diabetes and CKD, characteristics we hope will improve patient outcomes.

Based on the successes and failures of the previously described CCDS systems [78], we feel that the optimal CCDS for diabetes and CKD should have several key systematic characteristics. These characteristics include integration into the existing EMR, real-time recommendations with minimal disruption to workflow, recommendations rather than assessments whenever appropriate, and customized alert messages with situation-specific user control. Furthermore we believe the optimal CCDS for diabetes and CKD should address five key functions: (1) identify patients with CKD and those at high risk for progression to ESRD; (2) prevent drug adverse events; (3) identify patients who are not meeting diabetes, hypertension, or hyperlipidemia treatment goals; (4) make recommendations to help providers and patients reach treatment goals; and (5) engage the patient with the help of tools to help them better understand their condition and the rationale for their therapeutic plan. In the rest of this chapter we will review how a CCDS for patients with diabetes and CKD could be designed to optimally address these five functions.

Identify Patients with CKD and Those at High Risk for Progression

The optimal CCDS system would automatically identify patients with diabetes as having CKD if their eGFR is less than 60 mL/min or if they have proteinuria, an abnormal urine sediment or structural renal abnormalities regardless of their eGFR. A message would appear passively in the EMR (accessed by clicking an icon) only if a patient is determined to have CKD without clear documentation of this diagnosis. This alert could also include a link to standard NKF classifications of CKD or other educational material for providers and patients.

This alert would be the first step in classifying patients with CKD who are at increased cardiovascular and renal risk. Given the high prevalence of CKD in patients with diabetes, it will also be important to subclassify patients in the highest risk category and alert providers and patients to this. A more sophisticated risk stratification algorithm (described below) could be utilized to identify these patients. The charts of these patients would then be flagged with their high-risk status, possibly with an interruptive alert to prevent it from being overlooked. If a nephrologist or cardiologist is not seeing these patients, a recommendation for referral would be made by the system. Furthermore, more intensive care could be recommended for high-risk patients including protein restriction, bicarbonate or phosphate binder therapy, depression screening, insomnia screening, health psychology referral, CKD education referral, and renal replacement planning.

Risk Prediction Using CCDS

Risk prediction is a potentially valuable tool in patients with diabetes and CKD, enabling physicians to stratify patients as low risk or as high risk for cardiovascular events and or progression to ESRD. Determining which patients with diabetes and CKD are at high risk for progression to ESRD would enable either early preparation for dialysis, preparation for renal transplant, or if the patient chooses, end of life planning. Conversely, identifying patients at high risk for cardiovascular events rather than progression to ESRD could prompt cardiology referral or end-of-life discussions and conserve valuable health resources that would otherwise be used preparing a patient for dialysis or transplant.

CCDS has the potential to enable easier risk stratification of patients with diabetes and CKD by applying well-validated risk stratification equations to patient-specific health information in real-time [54, 98]. Risk presentations could be expressed in the EMR as either a numeric percentage, a risk category (high, medium, or low) or as a graphical alert. This risk presentation could then be linked to other CCDS interventions that recommend strategies for reducing cardiovascular and renal risk and for preparing for ESRD.

Risk presentation built into the EMR could also have beneficial effects for patients. Risk output could be printed out from the EMR or displayed through a patient-accessible portal and given to patients. These risk assessments could help patients make informed decisions regarding their care including renal replacement planning and could motivate patients to improve their blood pressure, hemoglobin A1c, and cholesterol control through diet and exercise. These risk presentations would ideally be presented through simple risk graphics, which focus on frequencies and which are tailored to a population with low numeracy [99–101]. A comparable risk, such as the decrease in risk with appropriate treatment, could be displayed next to current risk, and strategies to decrease risk could also be provided for patients [99].

Preventing Drug Adverse Events

We have described previous CCDS systems to decrease drug adverse events in patients with kidney disease [77]. The optimal CCDS system for patients with diabetes and CKD would provide alerts for drug–drug interactions and drug dosing errors. For serious alerts, severe drug–drug interactions or drug dosing errors, alerts would be interruptive and difficult to ignore. This format of alert has been shown to be more effective than passive alerts in modifying physician behavior [81]. In addition, interruptive alerts would appear when nephrotoxic medications such as aminoglycosides, NSAIDs, and intravenous contrast dye are ordered in patients with diabetes and CKD. The CCDS system could also generate a printable list of nephrotoxic medications that could be given to high-risk patients.

For less severe drug interactions or dose recommendations, a passive alert would appear in the EMR. The user control of these alerts could be customized based on an ongoing review of the CCDS system. Commonly ignored alerts could be made more passive with little to no interruption of workflow and ultimately could be removed from the CCDS system. This would prevent "alert fatigue" and ensure continued support of the CCDS by physician users.

Identify Patients Not Meeting DM, Hypertension, or Hyperlipidemia Treatment Goals

With the recent promotion of EMR by the federal government, it is believed the majority of patients with diabetes and CKD will have an electronic chart by the year 2014 [102]. From this electronic chart, it is imperative that key diabetes and CKD treatment parameters be easily searchable including, at minimum, HgBA1c, blood pressure, and LDL cholesterol. The ideal CCDS system would be able to identify patients who are not meeting targets for these three variables. A provider would be flagged through a passive alert in real-time that their patient is not meeting the target and would also get an email list of patients not meeting specific targets. If a patient with diabetes and CKD has not had the appropriate diagnostic work-up, recommendations for subsequent testing would be generated. These recommendations would ideally be linked to the guidelines that support them.

Recommendations to Help Providers Reach Treatment Goals

The most complicated part of implementing CCDS for patients with diabetes and CKD will be the generation of patient-specific recommendations for blood pressure, blood glucose, and cholesterol control. An additional level of sophistication would allow the provider and patient to set goals that might in some instances differ from the standard target, such as a higher blood pressure goal for a patient intolerant to attempts to lower blood pressure below 130/80 mmHg or a patient who has developed symptomatic hypoglycemia with attempts at achieving a HbA1c at the recommended level. These patient-specific goals would remain as part of the record and would be used as the parameters for treatment recommendations.

Blood Pressure

The optimal CCDS system for patients with diabetes, CKD, and hypertension would provide recommendations for medication initiation and titration until blood pressure is at goal. In order to improve provider acceptance, recommendations would be based on up-to-date clinical knowledge and would be guided by patient-specific information.

The knowledge base would be generated from clinician review of recent randomized trials and would be continually updated. This knowledge base would also be supplemented by patient-specific information. For example, rather than recommending an angiotensin inhibitor for all patients, the CCDS system would suggest an alternative medication or medication dosing in patients with an allergy to ACE inhibitors and would recognize the patient previously treated with an ACEI or ARB who did not tolerate it for other reasons. This patient-specific feedback would be an integral component of such a CCDS system. All medication recommendations would flow through a step-wise algorithm, which would be cross-checked with current medications and contraindicated medications until a specific medication or a dose increase is suggested. This would continue at each subsequent visit until the patient reaches a goal blood pressure of 130/80 (or other goal determined by provider and patient as discussed above).

HgBA1c

The optimal CCDS system for patients with CKD and diabetes would identify high-risk patients who are not at goal HgBA1c and would then provide therapeutic recommendations for providers. As described above, goal HgBA1c would be set based on patient-specific information; HgBA1c goals higher than 7.0 would be set for older patients and patients with multiple prior episodes of symptomatic hypoglycemia. Alerts would recommend increasing or altering insulin therapy or recommend nutrition referral or a specific diet plan for patients not at goal HgBA1c.

In order to optimize the diabetes treatment portion of such a CCDS system, one would build on successful attributes of previous systems [96]. These attributes include multifactorial and multidisciplinary CCDS recommendations, and patient portals [96]. Such a CCDS system would be used by a multidisciplinary team of providers including nephrologists, endocrinologists, cardiologists, nutritionists, and health psychologists. Patient-specific portals would allow patients and providers to jointly track patient-specific diabetes information. This portal would protect health care information and would ideally include the recommendations of providers. Furthermore care coordinators could jointly tract patient information and help navigate patients to different appointments.

Cholesterol Management

Previous studies have used CCDS to successfully improve cholesterol management [90]. One can envision a CCDS system that would alert physicians when the LDL level of their patient with diabetes and CKD is over goal. The CCDS would then recommend a multifactorial patient-specific plan to improve cholesterol levels. Again patients would be able to track their cholesterol management along with the physician using a patient portal with specific health information and recommendations.

Other Interventions

An ideal CCDS system would also suggest additional health management strategies for high-risk patients. This would include protein restriction for patients with advanced kidney disease, renal replacement options for patients at high risk of progressing to ESRD, and referral to weight loss or smoking cessation clinic for obese patients and smokers. In addition, recommendations could be made by the CCDS system to promote psychiatric and social health. These recommendations could include insomnia or depression screens, referral to educational interventions, which stress patient empowerment, or substance abuse rehabilitation. The goal through the implementation of these recommendations would be to improve the patient's quality of health by keeping them active and employed members of society.

Ensuring Success

Part of ensuring the success of a CCDS system requires building on the success of previous systems. As mentioned, such an intervention would be computerized with real-time recommendations and would utilize customized alert messages with situation-specific user control. As advocated by the Agency for Healthcare Research and Quality and Sirajuddin et al., the goal would be to provide the right alert, for the right patient, in the right format at the right time [103]. In addition, the CCDS system would have several unique features that address the shortcomings of previous systems. The CDS would be multicomponent and multidisciplinary and would be able to be used and shared by all providers for a particular patient. Care would be comprehensive across a range conditions that afflict patients with diabetes and CKD. The CCDS would deliver recommendations for both providers and patients and would include patient portals where patients would be able to access their health information including treatment targets and recommendations for reaching these targets. All recommendations would be accompanied by links to supporting literature. Finally, such a CCDS system would include pathways for accessing additional resources that augment recommendations whenever possible such as involvement of nurse educators, care coordinators, and patient navigators in the patient's care.

Monitoring Outcomes

The success of a novel CCDS system such as that outlined here will need to be documented by the results of studies that demonstrate its efficacy in not only improving patient and provider practice, but also in improving clinical outcomes and quality of life. Studies of such a CCDS system will need to demonstrate improvements in hard clinical end points like progression to ESRD and all-cause and cardiovascular mortality. Other important clinical end points that should be measured include the percentage of patients being transplanted rather than receiving dialysis as well as the graft survival rates of transplanted patients. In addition to these clinical end points, important quality of life and user satisfaction markers should be measured.

The ideal CCDS system will also need to demonstrate cost-effectiveness. Initial studies of CCDS systems have shown that start-up can be costly, with the majority of the cost coming from clinician review and maintenance of the CCDS knowledge base [104]. Future studies will need to demonstrate cost savings over time. Ideally if given enough time, optimal CCDS systems would be self-sustaining with a decreased need for intensive clinical input. Ultimately they could deliver care to multiple patients with minimal provider input, and could become a viable option for care in low income and resource challenged settings. It is plausible that health care costs could be reduced by preventing the major morbidity and mortality associated with CKD and its progression to ESRD and the resultant need for renal replacement therapy.

In conclusion CCDS is a potentially valuable tool to improve the management of patients with diabetes and CKD. CCDS can be used to identify patients with diabetes and CKD from the EMR, prevent drug adverse events and make specific recommendations to help providers and patients reach treatment goals. Key features of optimal CCDS will be computerized, real-time, patient-specific recommendations that are integrated into workflow, multidisciplinary provider use, and patient portals. Ultimately the success of these systems will be defined by whether they improve ESRD and mortality rates as well as quality of life.

References

1. Collins AJ, Foley RN, Herzog C, Chavers B, Gilbertson D, Ishani A, et al. US renal data system 2012 annual data report. Am J Kidney Dis. 2013;61(1 Suppl 1):A7, e1–476.
2. Coresh J, Selvin E, Stevens LA, Manzi J, Kusek JW, Eggers P, et al. Prevalence of chronic kidney disease in the United States. JAMA. 2007;298(17):2038–47.
3. Go AS, Chertow GM, Fan D, McCulloch CE, Hsu CY. Chronic kidney disease and the risks of death, cardiovascular events, and hospitalization. N Engl J Med. 2004;351(13):1296–305.

4. Stamler J, Vaccaro O, Neaton JD, Wentworth D. Diabetes, other risk factors, and 12-yr cardiovascular mortality for men screened in the Multiple Risk Factor Intervention Trial. Diabetes Care. 1993;16(2):434–44.
5. Hossain P, Kawar B, El Nahas M. Obesity and diabetes in the developing world—a growing challenge. N Engl J Med. 2007;356(3):213–5.
6. Khwaja A, Throssell D. A critique of the UK NICE guidance for the detection and management of individuals with chronic kidney disease. Nephron Clin Pract. 2009;113(3):c207–13.
7. Brown WW, Peters RM, Ohmit SE, Keane WF, Collins A, Chen SC, et al. Early detection of kidney disease in community settings: the Kidney Early Evaluation Program (KEEP). Am J Kidney Dis. 2003;42(1):22–35.
8. McGill JB, Brown WW, Chen SC, Collins AJ, Gannon MR. Kidney Early Evaluation Program (KEEP). Findings from a community screening program. Diabetes Educ. 2004;30(2):196–8, 200–2, 206.
9. Whaley-Connell A, Kurella Tamura M, McCullough PA. A decade after the KDOQI CKD guidelines: impact on the National Kidney Foundation's Kidney Early Evaluation Program (KEEP). Am J Kidney Dis. 2012;60(5):692–3.
10. Captopril reduces the risk of nephropathy in IDDM patients with microalbuminuria. The Microalbuminuria Captopril Study Group. Diabetologia. 1996;39(5):587–93.
11. Lewis EJ, Hunsicker LG, Bain RP, Rohde RD. The effect of angiotensin-converting-enzyme inhibition on diabetic nephropathy. The Collaborative Study Group. N Engl J Med. 1993; 329(20):1456–62.
12. Hovind P, Rossing P, Tarnow L, Smidt UM, Parving HH. Remission and regression in the nephropathy of type 1 diabetes when blood pressure is controlled aggressively. Kidney Int. 2001;60(1):277–83.
13. Lewis EJ, Hunsicker LG, Clarke WR, Berl T, Pohl MA, Lewis JB, et al. Renoprotective effect of the angiotensin-receptor antagonist irbesartan in patients with nephropathy due to type 2 diabetes. N Engl J Med. 2001;345(12):851–60.
14. Brenner BM, Cooper ME, de Zeeuw D, Keane WF, Mitch WE, Parving HH, et al. Effects of losartan on renal and cardiovascular outcomes in patients with type 2 diabetes and nephropathy. N Engl J Med. 2001;345(12):861–9.
15. Keane WF, Brenner BM, de Zeeuw D, Grunfeld JP, McGill J, Mitch WE, et al. The risk of developing end-stage renal disease in patients with type 2 diabetes and nephropathy: the RENAAL study. Kidney Int. 2003;63(4):1499–507.
16. Ruggenenti P, Cravedi P, Remuzzi G. The RAAS in the pathogenesis and treatment of diabetic nephropathy. Nat Rev Nephrol. 2010;6(6):319–30.
17. KDOQI. KDOQI Clinical Practice Guideline for Diabetes and CKD: 2012 Update. Am J Kidney Dis. 2012;60(5):850–86.
18. The effect of intensive treatment of diabetes on the development and progression of long-term complications in insulin-dependent diabetes mellitus. The Diabetes Control and Complications Trial Research Group. N Engl J Med. 1993;329(14):977–86.
19. Intensive blood-glucose control with sulphonylureas or insulin compared with conventional treatment and risk of complications in patients with type 2 diabetes (UKPDS 33). UK Prospective Diabetes Study (UKPDS) Group. Lancet. 1998;352(9131):837–53.
20. Fioretto P, Steffes MW, Sutherland DE, Goetz FC, Mauer M. Reversal of lesions of diabetic nephropathy after pancreas transplantation. N Engl J Med. 1998;339(2):69–75.
21. Duckworth W, Abraira C, Moritz T, Reda D, Emanuele N, Reaven PD, et al. Glucose control and vascular complications in veterans with type 2 diabetes. N Engl J Med. 2009;360(2):129–39.
22. Ismail-Beigi F, Craven T, Banerji MA, Basile J, Calles J, Cohen RM, et al. Effect of intensive treatment of hyperglycaemia on microvascular outcomes in type 2 diabetes: an analysis of the ACCORD randomised trial. Lancet. 2010;376(9739):419–30.
23. de Boer IH, Rue TC, Cleary PA, Lachin JM, Molitch ME, Steffes MW, et al. Long-term renal outcomes of patients with type 1 diabetes mellitus and microalbuminuria: an analysis of the Diabetes Control and Complications Trial/Epidemiology of Diabetes Interventions and Complications cohort. Arch Intern Med. 2011;171(5):412–20.
24. Inzucchi SE, Bergenstal RM, Buse JB, Diamant M, Ferrannini E, Nauck M, et al. Management of hyperglycemia in type 2 diabetes: a patient-centered approach: position statement of the American Diabetes Association (ADA) and the European Association for the Study of Diabetes (EASD). Diabetes Care. 2012;35(6):1364–79.
25. Adler AI, Stratton IM, Neil HA, Yudkin JS, Matthews DR, Cull CA, et al. Association of systolic blood pressure with macrovascular and microvascular complications of type 2 diabetes (UKPDS 36): prospective observational study. BMJ. 2000;321(7258):412–9.
26. Berl T, Hunsicker LG, Lewis JB, Pfeffer MA, Porush JG, Rouleau JL, et al. Impact of achieved blood pressure on cardiovascular outcomes in the Irbesartan Diabetic Nephropathy Trial. J Am Soc Nephrol. 2005;16(7):2170–9.
27. Wheeler DC, Becker GJ. Summary of KDIGO guideline. What do we really know about management of blood pressure in patients with chronic kidney disease? Kidney Int. 2013;83(3):377–83.
28. Houlihan CA, Allen TJ, Baxter AL, Panangiotopoulos S, Casley DJ, Cooper ME, et al. A low-sodium diet potentiates the effects of losartan in type 2 diabetes. Diabetes Care. 2002;25(4):663–71.
29. Morales E, Valero MA, Leon M, Hernandez E, Praga M. Beneficial effects of weight loss in overweight patients with chronic proteinuric nephropathies. Am J Kidney Dis. 2003;41(2):319–27.
30. Ansquer JC, Foucher C, Rattier S, Taskinen MR, Steiner G. Fenofibrate reduces progression to microalbuminuria over 3 years in a placebo-controlled study in type 2 diabetes: results from the Diabetes Atherosclerosis Intervention Study (DAIS). Am J Kidney Dis. 2005;45(3):485–93.
31. Tonolo G, Velussi M, Brocco E, Abaterusso C, Carraro A, Morgia G, et al. Simvastatin maintains steady patterns of GFR and improves AER and expression of slit diaphragm proteins in type II diabetes. Kidney Int. 2006;70(1):177–86.
32. Chuahirun T, Khanna A, Kimball K, Wesson DE. Cigarette smoking and increased urine albumin excretion are interrelated predictors of nephropathy progression in type 2 diabetes. Am J Kidney Dis. 2003;41(1):13–21.
33. Orth SR. Effects of smoking on systemic and intrarenal hemodynamics: influence on renal function. J Am Soc Nephrol. 2004;15 Suppl 1:S58–63.
34. Hansen HP, Tauber-Lassen E, Jensen BR, Parving HH. Effect of dietary protein restriction on prognosis in patients with diabetic nephropathy. Kidney Int. 2002;62(1):220–8.
35. Gaede P, Vedel P, Parving HH, Pedersen O. Intensified multifactorial intervention in patients with type 2 diabetes mellitus and microalbuminuria: the Steno type 2 randomised study. Lancet. 1999;353(9153):617–22.
36. Gaede P, Lund-Andersen H, Parving HH, Pedersen O. Effect of a multifactorial intervention on mortality in type 2 diabetes. N Engl J Med. 2008;358(6):580–91.
37. Saab G, Whaley-Connell AT, McCullough PA, Bakris GL. CKD awareness in the United States: the Kidney Early Evaluation Program (KEEP). Am J Kidney Dis. 2008;52(2):382–3.
38. Nickolas TL, Frisch GD, Opotowsky AR, Arons R, Radhakrishnan J. Awareness of kidney disease in the US population: findings from the National Health and Nutrition Examination Survey (NHANES) 1999 to 2000. Am J Kidney Dis. 2004;44(2):185–97.
39. Whaley-Connell A, Sowers JR, McCullough PA, Roberts T, McFarlane SI, Chen SC, et al. Diabetes mellitus and CKD aware-

ness: the Kidney Early Evaluation Program (KEEP) and National Health and Nutrition Examination Survey (NHANES). Am J Kidney Dis. 2009;53(4 Suppl 4):S11–21.
40. Rothberg MB, Kehoe ED, Courtemanche AL, Kenosi T, Pekow PS, Brennan MJ, et al. Recognition and management of chronic kidney disease in an elderly ambulatory population. J Gen Intern Med. 2008;23(8):1125–30.
41. Chase HS, Radhakrishnan J, Shirazian S, Rao MK, Vawdrey DK. Under-documentation of chronic kidney disease in the electronic health record in outpatients. J Am Med Inform Assoc. 2010;17(5):588–94.
42. Navaneethan SD, Kandula P, Jeevanantham V, Nally Jr JV, Liebman SE. Referral patterns of primary care physicians for chronic kidney disease in general population and geriatric patients. Clin Nephrol. 2010;73(4):260–7.
43. Jurkovitz CT, Elliott D, Li S, Saab G, Bomback AS, Norris KC, et al. Physician utilization, risk-factor control, and CKD progression among participants in the Kidney Early Evaluation Program (KEEP). Am J Kidney Dis. 2012;59(3 Suppl 2):S24–33.
44. Kinchen KS, Sadler J, Fink N, Brookmeyer R, Klag MJ, Levey AS, et al. The timing of specialist evaluation in chronic kidney disease and mortality. Ann Intern Med. 2002;137(6):479–86.
45. Levinsky NG. Specialist evaluation in chronic kidney disease: too little, too late. Ann Intern Med. 2002;137(6):542–3.
46. Tseng CL, Kern EF, Miller DR, Tiwari A, Maney M, Rajan M, et al. Survival benefit of nephrologic care in patients with diabetes mellitus and chronic kidney disease. Arch Intern Med. 2008;168(1):55–62.
47. Peralta CA, Hicks LS, Chertow GM, Ayanian JZ, Vittinghoff E, Lin F, et al. Control of hypertension in adults with chronic kidney disease in the United States. Hypertension. 2005;45(6):1119–24.
48. Tuot DS, Plantinga LC, Hsu CY, Powe NR. Is awareness of chronic kidney disease associated with evidence-based guideline-concordant outcomes? Am J Nephrol. 2012;35(2):191–7.
49. Thompson DM, Kozak SE, Sheps S. Insulin adjustment by a diabetes nurse educator improves glucose control in insulin-requiring diabetic patients: a randomized trial. CMAJ. 1999;161(8):959–62.
50. Rothman RL, Malone R, Bryant B, Shintani AK, Crigler B, Dewalt DA, et al. A randomized trial of a primary care-based disease management program to improve cardiovascular risk factors and glycated hemoglobin levels in patients with diabetes. Am J Med. 2005;118(3):276–84.
51. Frosch DL, Uy V, Ochoa S, Mangione CM. Evaluation of a behavior support intervention for patients with poorly controlled diabetes. Arch Intern Med. 2011;171(22):2011–7.
52. Sperl-Hillen J, Beaton S, Fernandes O, Von Worley A, Vazquez-Benitez G, Parker E, et al. Comparative effectiveness of patient education methods for type 2 diabetes: a randomized controlled trial. Arch Intern Med. 2011;171(22):2001–10.
53. Weinger K, Beverly EA, Lee Y, Sitnokov L, Ganda OP, Caballero AE. The effect of a structured behavioral intervention on poorly controlled diabetes: a randomized controlled trial. Arch Intern Med. 2011;171(22):1990–9.
54. Edwards AG, Naik G, Ahmed H, Elwyn GJ, Pickles T, Hood K, et al. Personalised risk communication for informed decision making about taking screening tests. Cochrane Database Syst Rev. 2013;(2):CD001865.
55. Dunsford J. Structured communication: improving patient safety with SBAR. Nurs Womens Health. 2009;13(5):384–90.
56. Garg AX, Adhikari NK, McDonald H, Rosas-Arellano MP, Devereaux PJ, Beyene J, et al. Effects of computerized clinical decision support systems on practitioner performance and patient outcomes: a systematic review. JAMA. 2005;293(10):1223–38.
57. Berner ES. Clinical decision support systems: state of the art. AHRQ publication no. 09-0060-EF. Rockville, MD: Agency for Healthcare Research and Quality; 2009.
58. Bright TJ, Wong A, Dhurjati R, Bristow E, Bastian L, Coeytaux RR, et al. Effect of clinical decision-support systems: a systematic review. Ann Intern Med. 2012;157(1):29–43.
59. Burack RC, Gimotty PA, George J, Stengle W, Warbasse L, Moncrease A. Promoting screening mammography in inner-city settings: a randomized controlled trial of computerized reminders as a component of a program to facilitate mammography. Med Care. 1994;32(6):609–24.
60. Flanagan JR, Doebbeling BN, Dawson J, Beekmann S. Randomized study of online vaccine reminders in adult primary care. Proc AMIA Symp. 1999:755–9.
61. Bertoni AG, Bonds DE, Chen H, Hogan P, Crago L, Rosenberger E, et al. Impact of a multifaceted intervention on cholesterol management in primary care practices: guideline adherence for heart health randomized trial. Arch Intern Med. 2009;169(7):678–86.
62. Souza NM, Sebaldt RJ, Mackay JA, Prorok JC, Weise-Kelly L, Navarro T, et al. Computerized clinical decision support systems for primary preventive care: a decision-maker-researcher partnership systematic review of effects on process of care and patient outcomes. Implement Sci. 2011;6:87.
63. Chen JJ, White CS. Use of CAD to evaluate lung cancer on chest radiography. J Thorac Imaging. 2008;23(2):93–6.
64. Shiraishi J, Li Q, Appelbaum D, Doi K. Computer-aided diagnosis and artificial intelligence in clinical imaging. Semin Nucl Med. 2011;41(6):449–62.
65. Morillo DS, Leon Jimenez A, Moreno SA. Computer-aided diagnosis of pneumonia in patients with chronic obstructive pulmonary disease. J Am Med Inform Assoc. 2013;20:e111–7.
66. Oloumi F, Rangayyan RM, Ells AL. Computer-aided diagnosis of proliferative diabetic retinopathy. Conf Proc IEEE Eng Med Biol Soc. 2012;2012:1438–41.
67. Marcelo A, Fatmi Z, Firaza PN, Shaikh S, Dandan AJ, Irfan M, et al. An online method for diagnosis of difficult TB cases for developing countries. Stud Health Technol Inform. 2011;164:168–73.
68. Milani RV, Lavie CJ, Dornelles AC. The impact of achieving perfect care in acute coronary syndrome: the role of computer assisted decision support. Am Heart J. 2012;164(1):29–34.
69. Wolfstadt JI, Gurwitz JH, Field TS, Lee M, Kalkar S, Wu W, et al. The effect of computerized physician order entry with clinical decision support on the rates of adverse drug events: a systematic review. J Gen Intern Med. 2008;23(4):451–8.
70. Haynes RB, Wilczynski NL. Effects of computerized clinical decision support systems on practitioner performance and patient outcomes: methods of a decision-maker-researcher partnership systematic review. Implement Sci. 2010;5:12.
71. Roshanov PS, Misra S, Gerstein HC, Garg AX, Sebaldt RJ, Mackay JA, et al. Computerized clinical decision support systems for chronic disease management: a decision-maker-researcher partnership systematic review. Implement Sci. 2011;6:92.
72. Lomotan EA, Hoeksema LJ, Edmonds DE, Ramirez-Garnica G, Shiffman RN, Horwitz LI. Evaluating the use of a computerized clinical decision support system for asthma by pediatric pulmonologists. Int J Med Inform. 2012;81(3):157–65.
73. Oluoch T, Santas X, Kwaro D, Were M, Biondich P, Bailey C, et al. The effect of electronic medical record-based clinical decision support on HIV care in resource-constrained settings: a systematic review. Int J Med Inform. 2012;81(10):e83–92.
74. Balas EA, Krishna S, Kretschmer RA, Cheek TR, Lobach DF, Boren SA. Computerized knowledge management in diabetes care. Med Care. 2004;42(6):610–21.
75. Bosworth HB, Olsen MK, Dudley T, Orr M, Goldstein MK, Datta SK, et al. Patient education and provider decision support to control blood pressure in primary care: a cluster randomized trial. Am Heart J. 2009;157(3):450–6.
76. Main C, Moxham T, Wyatt JC, Kay J, Anderson R, Stein K. Computerised decision support systems in order communication

for diagnostic, screening or monitoring test ordering: systematic reviews of the effects and cost-effectiveness of systems. Health Technol Assess. 2010;14(48):1–227.
77. Tawadrous D, Shariff SZ, Haynes RB, Iansavichus AV, Jain AK, Garg AX. Use of clinical decision support systems for kidney-related drug prescribing: a systematic review. Am J Kidney Dis. 2011;58(6):903–14.
78. Kawamoto K, Houlihan CA, Balas EA, Lobach DF. Improving clinical practice using clinical decision support systems: a systematic review of trials to identify features critical to success. BMJ. 2005;330(7494):765.
79. Roshanov PS, Fernandes N, Wilczynski JM, Hemens BJ, You JJ, Handler SM, et al. Features of effective computerised clinical decision support systems: meta-regression of 162 randomised trials. BMJ. 2013;346:f657.
80. Ash JS, Sittig DF, Campbell EM, Guappone KP, Dykstra RH. Some unintended consequences of clinical decision support systems. AMIA Annu Symp Proc. 2007:26–30.
81. Payne TH, Nichol WP, Hoey P, Savarino J. Characteristics and override rates of order checks in a practitioner order entry system. Proc AMIA Symp. 2002:602–6.
82. Seidling HM, Phansalkar S, Seger DL, Paterno MD, Shaykevich S, Haefeli WE, et al. Factors influencing alert acceptance: a novel approach for predicting the success of clinical decision support. J Am Med Inform Assoc. 2011;18(4):479–84.
83. Chang J, Ronco C, Rosner MH. Computerized decision support systems: improving patient safety in nephrology. Nat Rev Nephrol. 2011;7(6):348–55.
84. McCoy AB, Waitman LR, Gadd CS, Danciu I, Smith JP, Lewis JB, et al. A computerized provider order entry intervention for medication safety during acute kidney injury: a quality improvement report. Am J Kidney Dis. 2010;56(5):832–41.
85. Chertow GM, Lee J, Kuperman GJ, Burdick E, Horsky J, Seger DL, et al. Guided medication dosing for inpatients with renal insufficiency. JAMA. 2001;286(22):2839–44.
86. Abdel-Kader K, Fischer GS, Li J, Moore CG, Hess R, Unruh ML. Automated clinical reminders for primary care providers in the care of CKD: a small cluster-randomized controlled trial. Am J Kidney Dis. 2011;58(6):894–902.
87. Reynolds CJ, O'Donoghue DJ. Clinical decision support systems and the management of CKD by primary care physicians. Am J Kidney Dis. 2011;58(6):868–9.
88. Fox CH, Swanson A, Kahn LS, Glaser K, Murray BM. Improving chronic kidney disease care in primary care practices: an upstate New York practice-based research network (UNYNET) study. J Am Board Fam Med. 2008;21(6):522–30.
89. Manns B, Tonelli M, Culleton B, Faris P, McLaughlin K, Chin R, et al. A cluster randomized trial of an enhanced eGFR prompt in chronic kidney disease. Clin J Am Soc Nephrol. 2012;7(4): 565–72.
90. Anchala R, Pinto MP, Shroufi A, Chowdhury R, Sanderson J, Johnson L, et al. The role of Decision Support System (DSS) in prevention of cardiovascular disease: a systematic review and meta-analysis. PLoS One. 2012;7(10):e47064.
91. Roumie CL, Elasy TA, Greevy R, Griffin MR, Liu X, Stone WJ, et al. Improving blood pressure control through provider education, provider alerts, and patient education: a cluster randomized trial. Ann Intern Med. 2006;145(3):165–75.
92. Hicks LS, Sequist TD, Ayanian JZ, Shaykevich S, Fairchild DG, Orav EJ, et al. Impact of computerized decision support on blood pressure management and control: a randomized controlled trial. J Gen Intern Med. 2008;23(4):429–41.
93. Montgomery AA, Fahey T, Peters TJ, MacIntosh C, Sharp DJ. Evaluation of computer based clinical decision support system and risk chart for management of hypertension in primary care: randomised controlled trial. BMJ. 2000;320(7236):686–90.
94. Peterson KA, Radosevich DM, O'Connor PJ, Nyman JA, Prineas RJ, Smith SA, et al. Improving Diabetes Care in Practice: findings from the TRANSLATE trial. Diabetes Care. 2008;31(12): 2238–43.
95. Holbrook A, Thabane L, Keshavjee K, Dolovich L, Bernstein B, Chan D, et al. Individualized electronic decision support and reminders to improve diabetes care in the community: COMPETE II randomized trial. CMAJ. 2009;181(1–2):37–44.
96. Ali MK, Shah S, Tandon N. Review of electronic decision-support tools for diabetes care: a viable option for low- and middle-income countries? J Diabetes Sci Technol. 2011;5(3):553–70.
97. Narva AS. Decision support and CKD: not there yet. Clin J Am Soc Nephrol. 2012;7(4):525–6.
98. Echouffo-Tcheugui JB, Kengne AP. Risk models to predict chronic kidney disease and its progression: a systematic review. PLoS Med. 2012;9(11):e1001344.
99. Fagerlin A, Zikmund-Fisher BJ, Ubel PA. Helping patients decide: ten steps to better risk communication. J Natl Cancer Inst. 2011;103(19):1436–43.
100. Abdel-Kader K, Dew MA, Bhatnagar M, Argyropoulos C, Karpov I, Switzer G, et al. Numeracy skills in CKD: correlates and outcomes. Clin J Am Soc Nephrol. 2010;5(9):1566–73.
101. Zikmund-Fisher BJ, Fagerlin A, Ubel PA. A demonstration of "less can be more" in risk graphics. Med Decis Making. 2010;30(6):661–71.
102. Ahmad FS, Tsang T. Diabetes prevention, health information technology, and meaningful use: challenges and opportunities. Am J Prev Med. 2013;44(4 Suppl 4):S357–63.
103. Sirajuddin AM, Osheroff JA, Sittig DF, Chuo J, Velasco F, Collins DA. Implementation pearls from a new guidebook on improving medication use and outcomes with clinical decision support. Effective CDS is essential for addressing healthcare performance improvement imperatives. J Healthc Inf Manag. 2009;23(4):38–45.
104. Field TS, Rochon P, Lee M, Gavendo L, Subramanian S, Hoover S, et al. Costs associated with developing and implementing a computerized clinical decision support system for medication dosing for patients with renal insufficiency in the long-term care setting. J Am Med Inform Assoc. 2008;15(4):466–72.

Antihypertensive and Other Treatments in Early Stages of Diabetic Nephropathy

18

William J. Elliott

Introduction

Prevention of progression of diabetic nephropathy is a multi-faceted task, and has proven to be a "moving target" over the last several decades. Although the lifetime risk of developing end-stage renal disease is now quite similar for type 1 and type 2 diabetics (perhaps due to reducing death rates from cardiovascular diseases) [1, 2], the earlier (and usually more easily identified) age of onset of type 1 diabetics suggests they have a lower time-dependent risk of nephropathy. This had been reasonably well characterized in the decades before preventive measures were envisioned or widely available, and has been discussed in Part I of this book. From a clinical perspective, 5–10 years after diagnosis of type 1 diabetes, about 40 % of individuals reproducibly excreted abnormal amounts of protein (especially albumin) in the urine (see Table 18.1 for the historical and new ranges and nomenclature [3, 4]). These were typically small enough amounts to escape detection by the traditional dipstick urinalysis, although special techniques were later developed to quantitate them. The new terminology for this level of urinary albumin excretion is "moderately increased" albuminuria [3, 4], as many people were apparently confused by the older term (now relegated to the dustbin of history), and thought it represented much smaller molecules of albumin that were cleared into the urine. Classically, this amount of urinary albumin did not yet meet the diagnostic criterion for "diabetic nephropathy" (which was >300 mg/day of albumin), and therefore many research projects were launched to determine if various therapeutic interventions could reduce the incidence of progression to the defined threshold for urinary albumin excretion (which varied somewhat geographically, according to the units of common measurement at the time: μg/min or mg/day). In type 1 diabetics, about 50 % of those who produced 30–299 mg/day of albuminuria went on, over the next 10 years, to excrete >300 mg/day of albumin (producing a "positive dipstick test for proteinuria"). Several investigators have reported that individuals who cross this diagnostic threshold were more likely to have had an early detection of "moderately increased albuminuria" (or 30–299 mg/day) in the preceding decade. Detection of clinical proteinuria typically preceded a steady decline in glomerular filtration rate, with about 50 % of these progressing to end-stage renal disease over the next 7–10 years. Interestingly, but not well understood, was the fact that *regression* of (usually short-term) moderately elevated albuminuria (30–299 mg/day) occurred in a substantial proportion of type 1 diabetic patients (range over the literature: 15–65 %) [7]. However, once a patient developed >300 mg/day of albuminuria, regression back to <30 mg/day was not observed. The situation in type 2 diabetics is generally somewhat more complex, because the age of onset of diabetes is less certain, and type 2 diabetics are generally older (and therefore at higher risk for many other complications, including death). Despite all this, the degree of albuminuria at baseline was a significant, strong, and graded predictor of both cardiovascular events and mortality [5], as well as renal outcomes [6] in meta-analyses of large cohorts.

It is now recognized, however, that urinary albumin excretion rates can be confounded by many parameters, including recent exercise, blood pressure control, urinary flow rate, urinary dilution, intravascular volume status, and dietary sodium intake. The intrinsic variability of albuminuria (even day-to-day) is such a major issue that the US Food and Drug Administration (FDA) has never recognized it as an appropriate surrogate endpoint for clinical trials, despite wide acceptance in the diabetes and kidney disease community [1–3]. Many improvements to methodology for specimen collection and analysis have resulted in the early morning

The writing of this manuscript was not supported by any specific entity. For a list of the author's "Real or Potential Conflicts of Interest," See the attached "Standard Financial Disclosure Form."

W.J. Elliott, M.D., Ph.D. (✉)
Division of Pharmacology, Pacific Northwest University of Health Sciences, 200 University Parkway, Yakima, WA 98901, USA
e-mail: wj.elliott@yahoo.com

E.V. Lerma and V. Batuman (eds.), *Diabetes and Kidney Disease*,
DOI 10.1007/978-1-4939-0793-9_18, © Springer Science+Business Media New York 2014

Table 18.1 Historical comparison of important levels of urinary albumin excretion

Albumin excretion rate (mg/day)	Historical descriptor	Albumin/creatinine ratio (mg/g)	"New" classification (before "albuminuria")
<30	"Normal"	<30	"Normal to mildly increased"
30–300	"Microalbuminuria"	30–300	"Moderately increased"
>300	"Macroalbuminuria"	>300	"Severely increased"

Adapted from [3, 4]

first-voided urine as the currently recommended technique for estimating urinary albumin excretion [1–3]. Most clinical trial endpoints that use this technique also require two successive determinations about the diagnostic threshold, in an attempt to minimize the intrinsic variability of the test.

Once the diabetic patient has reached the threshold of >300 mg/day of albuminuria (or albumin/creatinine ratio ≥300 mg/g), some authorities claim that the diagnosis of diabetic nephropathy is met; for example, Canadian health authorities reimburse physicians more for office visits for such diabetic patients, which is presumably why this diagnostic threshold was chosen by the Heart Outcomes Prevention Evaluation investigators [8]. Yet, even after this diagnosis, there are several useful interventions to prevent an inexorable decline to end-stage renal disease in diabetics with nephropathy (see below, and Chap. 10). Although some might characterize these as "late interventions" for diabetic nephropathy, they are still worthwhile, as delay of dialysis or transplantation carries a large human and economic cost.

Interventions for Early Diabetic Nephropathy

Glycemic Control

The most impressive results for control of blood glucose were seen in the Diabetes Control and Complications Trial (DCCT) [9], and its long-term follow-up, Epidemiology of Diabetes Interventions and Complications (EDIC) study [10]. This trial originally enrolled 1,441 type 1 diabetics with no retinopathy at baseline (1,365 of whom had normal albumin excretion rates), and randomized them to an intensive vs. standard insulin regimen. After the first 6.5 years, the intensive therapy group (average A1c = 7.2 %) had a significant, 39 % reduction in incident "albuminuria >40 mg/day," as well as a significant 54 % reduction in incident "albuminuria >300 mg/day," compared to the standard therapy group (average A1c = 9.1 %) [11]. Longitudinal follow-up showed the significantly increased risk of cardiovascular events in those who developed albuminuria, with a significant difference observed across randomized treatment groups [10]. In addition, those originally randomized to intensive glucose control were significantly less likely to develop incident "albuminuria >40 mg/day" (7 % vs. 16 %), "albuminuria >300 mg/day" (1.4 % vs. 9 %), or hypertension (30 % vs. 40 %). Follow-up 22 years after randomization showed a persistent benefit on development of impaired renal function (estimated glomerular filtration rate <60 mL/min/1.73 m^2, 3.9 % vs. 7.6 %) [12]. Similar benefits were seen in a prospective, 7.5-year, Swedish trial that enrolled 102 type 1 diabetic patients: only 1 of 48 treated to an average A1c of 7.1 % developed urinary albumin excretion >200 μg/min, compared to 9 of 54 treated to an average A1c of 8.5 % [13], as well as a meta-analysis of smaller trials reported through 1993 [14]. Perhaps the most impressive report of the efficacy of glycemic control in type 1 diabetes comes from a series of 8 patients who received pancreatic transplants, which led not only to persistent euglycemia, but also striking reductions in albuminuria, 5 and 10 years later, with reversal of much of the glomerular pathology seen on biopsy during the transplant [15].

The clinical trial data about improved glycemic control and early renal endpoints in type 2 diabetes are consistent with those in type 1 diabetes, but are somewhat less impressive, perhaps because of smaller numbers of enrolled patients, a relatively short duration of follow-up, or small differences in achieved A1c levels across randomized groups. Many of these individual trials are discussed in detail in Chap. 16. It is perhaps more efficient to summarize the data from seven trials involving 28,065 type 2 diabetics, as combined in meta-analyses. Subjects who received the more intensive glucose control experienced a significantly reduced risk of developing albuminuria >30 mg/day (risk ratio: 0.86, 95 % confidence interval [CI]: 0.76–0.96), albuminuria >300 mg/day (risk ratio: 0.74, 95 % CI: 0.65–0.85), but *not* of doubling serum creatinine, end-stage renal disease, or death [16]. Meta-regression analysis showed, as have many earlier observational studies, that greater differences in achieved A1c levels across randomized groups were associated with greater benefits on albuminuria (at both thresholds). It is likely that, since the publication of the Action to Control Cardiovascular Risk in Diabetes-Glucose trial results [17], which showed significant harm (including death), associated with more intensive lowering of A1c, no further trials exploring aggressive lowering of A1c levels will be performed in type 2 diabetics.

Inhibitors of the Renin-Angiotensin System

Although the first FDA-approved angiotensin converting-enzyme (ACE)-inhibitor initially caused an increase in the incidence of dipstick-detectable proteinuria, essentially all subsequent studies have shown a strong antiproteinuric effect of all ACE-inhibitors, angiotensin receptor blockers (ARBs), and aliskiren, a direct renin inhibitor. These effects on protein and albumin excretion appear to be independent of their blood pressure-lowering efficacy. As a result, they have been widely studied, and are now often recommended for diabetic patients with persistent albuminuria, although this indication is not formally sanctioned by the US FDA.

Normotensive Type 1 Diabetics (with "Normal to Mildly Increased Albuminuria")

Five trials have randomized normotensive type 1 diabetics with "normal to mildly increased albuminuria" to placebo or an inhibitor of the renin-angiotensin system; none have shown significant benefits in this earliest possible stage of diabetic nephropathy (often called "primary prevention" by nephrologists). The largest was the Diabetic Retinopathy Candesartan Trials (DIRECT) Program, which enrolled 3,326 normotensive type 1 diabetics with a median urinary albumin excretion rate of 5.0 μg/min, and randomized them to placebo or 16 mg/day of candesartan (with a dose increase to 32 mg/day after 1 month) [18]. Although the trial was primarily designed to compare retinopathy rates, over 4.7 years of median follow-up, there were no significant differences across randomized groups in either the primary renal endpoint (urinary albumin excretion ≥20 μg/min in timed, overnight urine collections), or the rate of change in urinary albumin excretion compared to randomization. Although understandably disappointed, the investigators cited their subjects' low burden of vasculopathy, young age, normotensive status, and very low baseline albumin excretion rate as possible reasons why candesartan showed no significant prevention of "moderately increased albuminuria." An earlier trial enrolled 530 normotensive insulin-dependent diabetics aged 20–59 years, 83 % of whom had "normal to mildly increased albuminuria" (i.e., <20 μg/min), and randomized them to lisinopril 10 mg/day (initially) or placebo [19]. After 2 years of median follow-up, diastolic blood pressures were lower in the lisinopril-treated subjects, but the albumin excretion rate was only 12.7 % lower (95 % CI: −2.9–26.0 %, $P=0.10$), and the numbers of subjects who crossed threshold levels of albuminuria were not significantly different ($P=0.50$) across randomized groups. Many supplemental analyses were undertaken, but all showed very little, if any, benefit in the group of subjects who had the lowest amounts of albuminuria at baseline. A third trial compared losartan, enalapril, and placebo in 285 normotensive type 1 diabetics with "normal" baseline albumin excretion rates [20]. There were no significant differences across the groups with respect to the primary outcome (mesangial fractional volume per glomerulus, on biopsy), but the albumin excretion rate increased significantly in those randomized to losartan, but not enalapril, each compared to placebo. Similarly, the 5-year cumulative incidence rate of developing "moderately increased albuminuria" was 17 % for losartan ($P=0.01$), 6 % for placebo, and 4 % for enalapril ($P=0.96$).

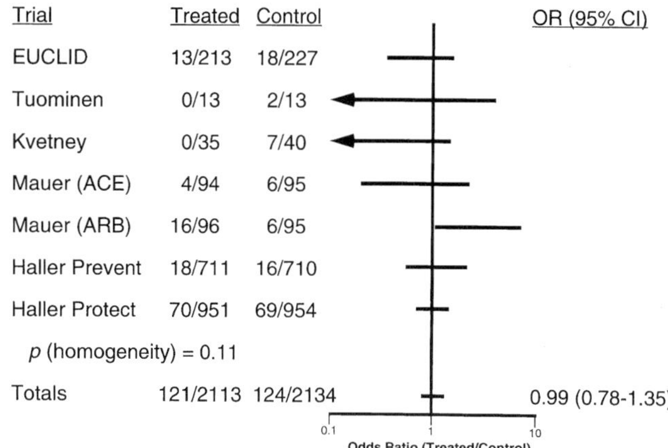

Fig. 18.1 Results of a Mantel–Haenszel meta-analysis of trials comparing an angiotensin converting-enzyme inhibitor (ACE-I) or angiotensin receptor blocker (ARB) with another "control" treatment, on the transition of normotensive type 1 diabetics with "normal to mildly increased albuminuria" (traditionally <30 mg/day or 20 μg/min) past the lower threshold for "moderately increased albuminuria" (traditionally 30 mg/day or 20 μg/min). *OR* odds ratio; *95 % CI* 95 % confidence interval, *EUCLID* EUrodiab Controlled trial of Lisinopril in Insulin-dependent Diabetes [19], Tuomenin = Diabetes Care. 1998;21:1345–1348, Kvetney = Q J Med. 2001;94:89–94, Mauer (ACE) = ACE-inhibitor arm [20], Mauer (ARB) = ARB arm [20], Haller Prevent = Prevention arm of [18], Haller Protect = Protection arm of [18]

Taken together (Fig. 18.1), these data indicate that there is little reason to recommend "prophylactic" administration of either an ACE-inhibitor or ARB to a type 1 diabetic with an albumin/creatinine ratio <30 mg/g [21]. This strategy fits well with other data, especially if "regression" of albumin/creatinine ratios in the 30–299 mg/g range is as frequent now as in early studies (15–65 %). Most authors, and recent guidelines [1, 3, 4], recommend instead annual screening of type 1 diabetics with a first morning voided urinary albumin/creatinine ratio (after the fifth year of diabetes), and potential treatment (with an ACE-inhibitor or ARB) of only those who show persistent albumin/creatinine ratios >30 mg/g.

Normotensive Type 1 Diabetics (with "Moderately Increased Albuminuria")

Several ACE-inhibitors have significantly reduced urinary albumin excretion rates in multiple randomized trials in normotensive type 1 diabetics with what would now be called "moderately increased albuminuria" (at baseline) [21]. In one of the larger European trials, 92 normotensive type 1 diabetics with persistent urinary albumin excretion rates between 20 and 200 μg/min were randomized to captopril 50 mg twice daily, or placebo, and followed for 2 years [22]. The primary outcome was a persistent increase in urinary albumin excretion to ≥200 μg/min, and at least 30 % higher than baseline, which was seen in 12 placebo-treated, vs. four captopril-treated subjects ($P=0.05$). The time course of progression to

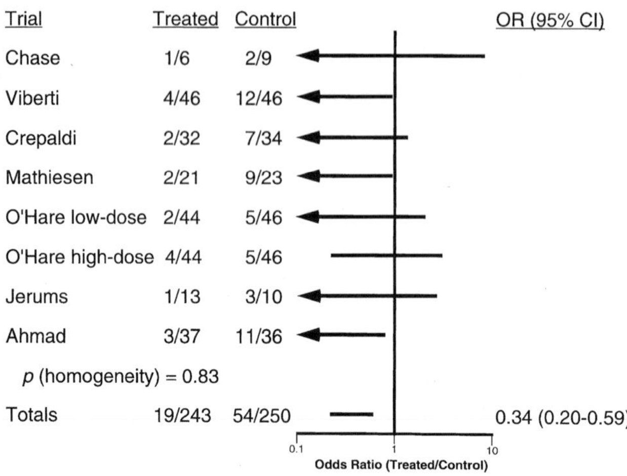

Fig. 18.2 Results of a Mantel–Haenszel meta-analysis of trials comparing an ACE-I or ARB with another "control" treatment, on the transition of normotensive type 1 diabetics with "moderately increased albuminuria" (traditionally 30–299 mg/day or 20–199 µg/min) past the threshold for "severely increased albuminuria" (traditionally 300 mg/day or 200 µg/min). *OR* odds ratio, *95% CI* 95 % confidence interval, Chase=Ann Ophthalmol. 1993;25:284–289, Viberti=JAMA. 1994;271:275–279, Crepaldi=Diabetes Care. 1998;21:104–110, Mathiesen=BMJ. 1999;319:24–25, O'Hare=Diabetes Care. 2000;23:1823–1829, Ahmad=Diabetes Res Clin Pract. 2003;60:131–138

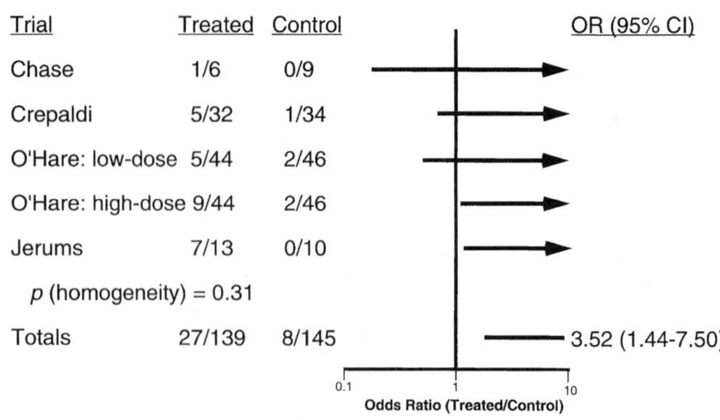

Fig. 18.3 Results of a Mantel–Haenszel meta-analysis of trials comparing an ACE-I or an ARB, with another "control treatment," on regression of moderately increased albuminuria (traditionally 30–299 mg/day or 20–200 µg/min) back to normal to mildly increased albuminuria (traditionally <30 mg/day or <20 µg/min). *OR* odds ratio, *95% CI* 95 % confidence interval, Chase=Ann Ophthalmol. 1993;25:284–289, Crepaldi=Diabetes Care. 1998;21:104–110, O'Hare=Diabetes Care. 2000;23:1823–1829, Jerums=Am J Kidney Dis. 2001;37:890–899

the primary endpoint was significantly delayed by captopril ($P=0.03$), as was the geometric mean of the albumin excretion rate ($P<0.01$). Analysis of two similar trials that randomized 235 normotensive type 1 diabetics with baseline urinary albumin excretion between 20 and 199 µg/min to either placebo or captopril 50 mg twice daily, also showed a significant reduction in progression to ≥200 µg/min of albuminuria (25 of 114 placebo-treated, vs. 8 of 111 captopril-treated, $P=0.004$), as well as an overall reduction in albuminuria only in the captopril-treated group, which was statistically independent of the hypotensive effect of captopril [23]. Lisinopril was compared with placebo for 2 years in 79 normotensive type 1 diabetics with "moderately increased albuminuria" in a subgroup of the EUCLID study [19]. Although an intention-to-treat analysis of this subgroup failed to show a significant difference (despite a 50 % difference in albumin excretion rates), the rates *fell* (compared to baseline) in the lisinopril-treated subjects, and *rose* in the placebo-treated subjects. Other analyses, including a per-protocol analysis and adjustment for numerous covariates (including blood pressure at 1 month), did show a significant effect of lisinopril on albumin excretion rates. A 2005 meta-analysis that included data from 11 randomized clinical trials concluded that an ACE-inhibitor reduced the risk of normotensive type 1 diabetics with "moderately increased albuminuria" developing clinical proteinuria (relative risk: 0.36, 95 % CI: 0.22–0.58), and regression to "normal or mildly elevated albuminuria" (relative risk: 5.3, 95 % CI: 2.5–11.5) [24]. These estimates were little changed in subsequent meta-analyses [21] (Fig. 18.2). Figure 18.3 summarizes the effects of inhibitors of the renin-angiotensin system on the regression of moderately increased albuminuria back to normal to mildly increased albuminuria in type 1 diabetics.

Hypertensive Type 1 Diabetics with Overt Nephropathy (and Proteinuria)

Although some would not classify such patients as having "early diabetic nephropathy," the only trial in type 1 diabetic nephropathy with "hard renal endpoints" was the Captopril Cooperative Study Group's comparison of captopril and placebo in 409 subjects [25], discussed in detail in Chap. 10. The clear, major benefits of the ACE-inhibitor are not only reducing the risk of doubling serum creatinine (the primary endpoint), but also in the clinically important endpoint of death, dialysis, or renal transplantation, as well as proteinuria (with 8 captopril-treated patients experiencing a complete, long-term remission of proteinuria! [26]). This also made it ethically difficult for others to evaluate the effects of other (newer) antihypertensive agents against placebo in type 1 diabetic nephropathy patients. This historical situation left the door open to investigation of newer agents in type 2 diabetics.

Trials in Type 2 Diabetics

Although a 2012 meta-analysis from the Cochrane Collaboration concluded that ACE-inhibitors prevented both new onset diabetic kidney disease and death in diabetics with albuminuria <30 mg/day [27], no distinction was made in these meta-analyses between types 1 and 2 diabetes. Furthermore, this conclusion was largely driven by the HOPE trial [8], which included both hypertensive and non-hypertensive type 2 diabetics. This review recognized that some ARBs may have similar benefits [28], as discussed below, in addition to their significant, and very important, benefits on reducing the risk of doubling serum creatinine, end-stage renal disease, or death in type 2 diabetics with overt nephropathy [29, 30], as discussed briefly below, and in detail in Chap. 10.

Normotensive Type 2 Diabetics

Perhaps because type 2 diabetics are older and more likely to have hypertension, the number of trials in normotensive subjects is much smaller in type 2 than type 1 diabetes. The first trial that compared enalapril and placebo in normotensive type 2 diabetics was performed in Israel, but is thought to be generalizable to most other populations [31]. The trial successfully followed 94 of the original 156 normotensive type 2 diabetics with serum creatinine levels <1.4 mg/dL and 24-h urinary albumin excretion between 30 and 300 mg/day. After 7 years of treatment, albuminuria was stable in those given enalapril, but increased significantly in those given placebo; the relative risk reduction was 42 % for development of "moderately increased albuminuria" with enalapril compared to placebo. Similarly, serum creatinine increased in those given placebo, but stabilized in the enalapril-treated group.

The Appropriate Blood pressure Control in Diabetes trial randomized 480 normotensive type 2 diabetics to either placebo ($n=243$, but 48 % required antihypertensive medication during the 5.3 years of follow-up), or nisoldipine ($n=118$) or enalapril ($n=119$) [32]. Subjects randomized to antihypertensive therapy had significantly lower blood pressures (128/75 vs. 137/81 mmHg, on average), but no significant difference in creatinine clearance ($P=0.43$), compared to those originally given placebo. However, active antihypertensive therapy significantly reduced the time to transitions from "normal to mildly increased albuminuria" to "moderately increased albuminuria" ($P=0.04$) or from the latter to "severely increased albuminuria" ($P=0.02$), with no significant difference between enalapril and nisoldipine. During follow-up, 15 subjects given antihypertensive drugs reverted from "moderately increased albuminuria" to "normal to mildly increased albuminuria," as compared to 8 in those originally assigned to placebo. There was no significant change over the 5.3 years of follow-up in the 11 % of subjects who had severely increased albuminuria at randomization. The authors therefore concluded that lowering blood pressure, rather than ACE-inhibitor therapy per se, was associated with a reduction in progression of albuminuria.

The most recent results come from 725 type 2 diabetics in the normotensive subgroup in the DIRECT study [18], all of whom had <20 (median = 8) μg/min of albuminuria at randomization. As with the pooled results (in both normotensive type 1, and normotensive and hypertensive type 2 diabetics) after 4.7 years, there was no significant difference in either incident "moderately increased albuminuria," or the annual rate of change of albuminuria, between candesartan or placebo. These results carry the same *caveats* as those from this trial pertaining to normotensive type 1 diabetics

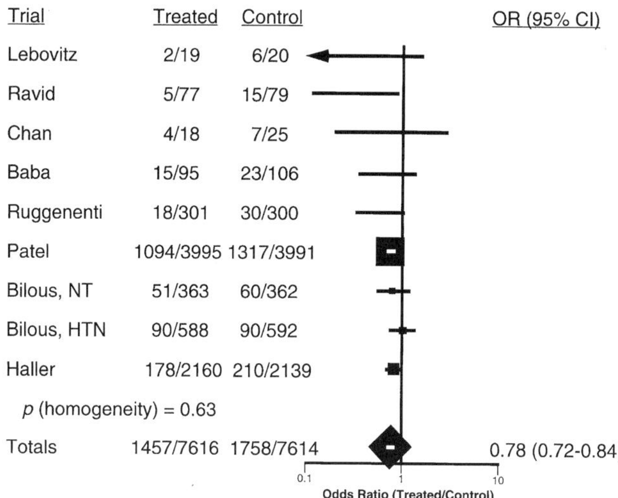

Fig. 18.4 Results of a Mantel–Haenszel meta-analysis of trials comparing an ACE-I or an ARB with another "control" treatment, on progression of normal to mildly increased albuminuria (traditionally <30 mg/day or <20 μg/min) to moderately increased albuminuria (traditionally 30–299 mg/day or 20–199 μg/min) in type 2 diabetics. *OR* odds ratio, *95 % CI* 95 % confidence interval, Lebovitz = Kidney Int. 1994;45 (Suppl. 45):S150–S155, Chan = Kidney Int. 2000;57:590–600, Baba = Diabetes Res Clin Pract. 2001;54:191–201, Ruggenenti [35], Patel = [40] and J Am Soc Nephrol. 2009;20:883–92, Bilous, NT = normotensive group in [18], Bilous, HTN = hypertensive group in [18], Haller = [46]

(discussed above), and may simply reflect the very low albumin excretion rates and low burden of vasculopathy in the enrolled subjects.

A set of 2012 meta-analyses that included 49 trials found a smaller, yet still significant, effect of renin-angiotensin system inhibitors in type 2 diabetics (normotensive or hypertensive) with albuminuria <30 mg/day (~12 % reduction in seven trials), compared to individuals with 30–299 mg/day (~23 % reduction in 21 trials) [21]. Similar conclusions can be derived from Figs. 18.4 and 18.5, which include a somewhat different set of trials. In the 2012 meta-analyses [21], the reduction in progression from the former to the latter was significant for type 2, but not type 1 diabetics. The authors therefore suggested that *all* type 2 diabetics might benefit from such therapy, which was deemed cost-effective, as far back as 1999 [33]. Similarly, two random-effects meta-analyses ([21] and Fig. 18.6) have shown significant regression of moderately increased albuminuria to normal or mildly increased albuminuria with either an ACE-inhibitor or an ARB; the significant inhomogeneity across the included trials is likely due to a smaller effect of the ARB (see below).

Hypertensive Type 2 Diabetics with Moderately Increased Albuminuria

A wider variety of agents has been tested in hypertensive type 2 diabetics, consistent with the greater prevalence of this condition than normotensive type 2 diabetes. In the United Kingdom Prospective Diabetes Study, there were no

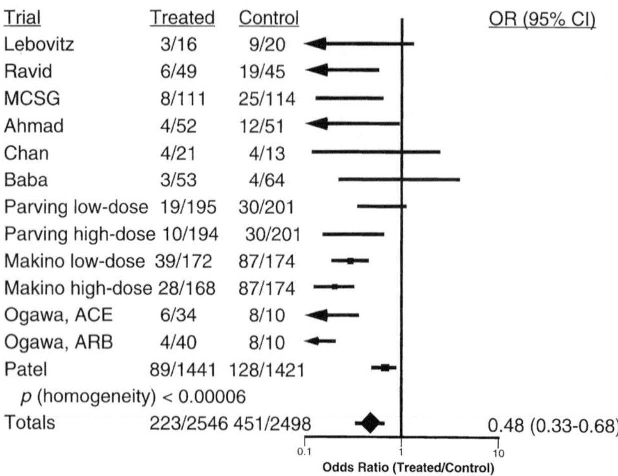

Fig. 18.5 Results of a random-effects meta-analysis of trials comparing an ACE-I or an ARB with another "control" treatment on progression of moderately increased albuminuria (traditionally 30–299 mg/day, or 20–199 μg/min) to severely increased albuminuria (traditionally ≥ 300 mg/day or ≥200 μg/min) in type 2 diabetics. *OR* odds ratio, *95 % CI* 95 % confidence interval, Lebovitz = Kidney Int. 1994;45 (Suppl. 45):S150–S155, Ravid = [31], CMSG = Captopril Microalbuminuria Study Group [23], Ahmad = Diabetes Care. 1997;20:1576–1581, Chan = Kidney Int. 2000;57:590–600, Baba = Diabetes Res Clin Pract. 2001;54:191–201, Parving = [41], Makino = Diabetes Care. 2007;30:1577–1578, Ogawa = Hypertens Res. 2007;30:325–334, Patel = [40]. Note that the fixed-effects meta-analysis shows significant inhomogeneity, likely due to a smaller effect of the low doses of an ARB

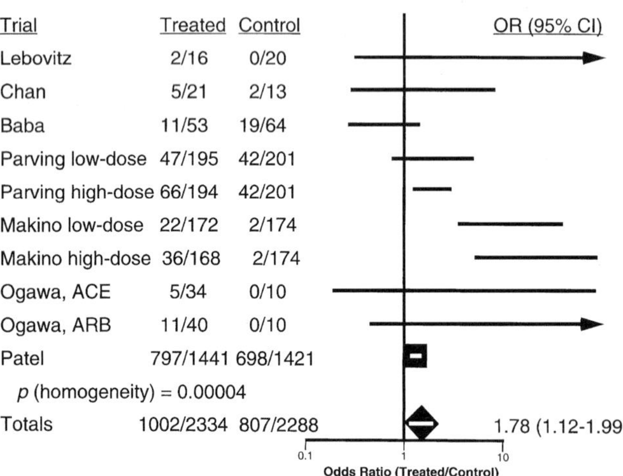

Fig. 18.6 Results of a random-effects meta-analysis of trials comparing an ACE-I or an ARB with another "control" treatment on regression of moderately increased albuminuria (traditionally 30–299 mg/day or 20–199 μg/min) back to normal to mildly increased albuminuria (traditionally <30 mg/day or <20 μg/min) in type 2 diabetics. *OR* odds ratio, *95 % CI* 95 % confidence interval, Lebovitz = Kidney Int. 1994;45 (Suppl. 45):S150–S155, Chan = Kidney Int. 2000;57:590–600, Baba = Diabetes Res Clin Pract. 2001;54:191–201, Parving = [41], Makino = Diabetes Care. 2007;30:1577–1578, Ogawa = Hypertens Res. 2007;30:325–334, Patel = [40]. Note that the fixed-effects meta-analysis shows significant inhomogeneity, likely due to a smaller effect of the low doses of an ARB

significant differences between atenolol and captopril in doubling serum creatinine, average serum creatinine concentrations, or urinary albumin concentration ≥50 mg/L [34]. However, the numbers of subjects developing urinary albumin concentrations >300 mg/L were higher in the atenolol group (14/146 vs. 7/153, $P = 0.09$). These findings may be confounded by the use of urinary concentrations of albumin, lower adherence to atenolol, and other factors. In another trial, half-maximal doses of trandolapril were studied, alone and in combination with 180 mg/day of verapamil-sustained release, compared to placebo or verapamil 240 mg/day, in 1,204 hypertensive diabetics with baseline albumin excretion <20 μg/min, with the primary endpoint being time to two consecutive determinations of overnight albumin excretion ≥20 μg/min [35]. After a median of 3.6 years, those given trandolapril (alone: 18/301, or in combination: 17/300) had a significantly lower risk of the primary endpoint, compared to placebo (30/300), with verapamil monotherapy not significant (36/303, $P = 0.54$). The authors believed these results were independent of blood pressure changes. Similarly, half-maximal doses of candesartan and lisinopril, or their combination, were given to 199 hypertensive type 2 diabetics who had moderately increased albuminuria at randomization [36]. Over 12 weeks, both monotherapies reduced blood pressure (12/10 and 16/10 mmHg, for candesartan and lisinopril, respectively), and albumin excretion rates compared to baseline (30 and 46 %, both $P < 0.001$), and even more so in those given the combination (25/16 mmHg, and 50 %). In contrast, full doses of an ACE-inhibitor + ARB were associated with renal harm (and an increase in albuminuria) in the overall Ongoing Telmisartan Alone or in combination with Ramipril Global Endpoints Trial (ONTARGET) cohort [37]. When these results were combined in a meta-analysis of 85 trials involving 21,708 subjects, progression of albuminuria from moderately increased to severely increased was significantly reduced by an ACE-inhibitor vs. placebo, an ARB vs. placebo, but not the combination vs. monotherapy [38]. Only one trial has been performed comparing the long-term renal effects of an ARB vs. an ACE-inhibitor in hypertensive type 2 diabetics; it enrolled only 250 subjects and was designed as a non-inferiority study [39]. Although the dropout rate was a concern (see Chap. 10), the change in isotopically measured glomerular filtration rate was not significantly different after 5 years of treatment with either enalapril or telmisartan.

Two "mega-trials" have reported changes in albuminuria after randomizing type 2 diabetics (with or without hypertension) to an ACE-inhibitor [8] or an ACE-inhibitor + diuretic combination [40]. The Heart Outcomes Prevention Evaluation trial analyzed a subset of 3,677 diabetics who were not well treated for other cardiovascular risk factors, but nonetheless observed, in the group given ramipril, instead of placebo, a significant 24 % reduction in the incidence of albuminuria >300 mg/day (or equivalent, $P = 0.027$) [8].

The Action in Diabetes and Vascular disease: preterAx® and diamicroN®-MR Controlled Evaluation (ADVANCE) trial enrolled 11,140 hypertensive type 2 diabetics, randomized them to either placebo or perindopril + indapamide, and followed them for a median of 4.3 years [44]. In the entire recruited cohort, the combination of the ACE-inhibitor + diuretic reduced the incidence of "moderately increased albuminuria" by 21 % (95 % CI: 14–27 %, $P<0.0001$), although the rates of significantly new or worsening nephropathy did not quite meet statistical thresholds (3.3 % vs. 3.9 %, $P=0.055$). In each study, there was no evidence that the antihypertensive effects of the ACE-inhibitor (or combination) were significantly related to the improvement in these renal outcomes. Many subsequent meta-analyses have therefore concluded that an ACE-inhibitor should be part of the antihypertensive regimen for hypertensive type 2 diabetics, regardless of the baseline urinary protein excretion rate.

Several trials have investigated the role of an ARB in reducing albuminuria in hypertensive type 2 diabetics. Perhaps the clearest was the Irbesartan Microalbuminuria Trial #2 [41], which randomized 590 subjects to placebo or irbesartan (150 or 300 mg/day), and followed them for 2 years for the development of albumin excretion rates >200 μg/min, and a 30 % increment from baseline. This endpoint was significantly prevented only by the 300 mg/day dose, although a trend was present for the 150 mg/day dose, compared to placebo. A similar, significant response of albumin excretion to the dose of an ARB has been detected in a meta-analysis of this and similar studies [42]. In a substudy of 133 subjects in this trial, a month after withdrawal of antihypertensive agents, blood pressure was unchanged in those originally taking placebo, but returned nearly to baseline in the irbesartan-treated groups [43]. Perhaps more importantly, the urinary albumin excretion rate increased in the placebo and low-dose irbesartan groups, but remained 47 % below baseline in the high-dose irbesartan group, which suggested that the high-dose ARB had persistent long-term benefits, even after it was discontinued for a month. Even more interesting was the 2-year follow-up after the study's completion, which showed that individuals who experienced the greatest degree of reduction in urinary albumin excretion had the slowest rates of decline in glomerular function [44]. This is therefore one of the few trials in diabetics with initially normal to mildly increased albuminuria that has been able to link progression to moderately increased albuminuria, and then to a decline in renal function, both independent of blood pressure changes. A 24-week comparison of valsartan with amlodipine in 332 type 2 diabetics (with or without hypertension) with moderately increased albuminuria showed valsartan (with a 44 % reduction) more effective than amlodipine (with a 8 % reduction) [45], despite similar reductions in blood pressure. A much larger, 3.2-year-long, trial compared olmesartan vs. placebo in 4,447 type 2 diabetics with normal to mildly increased albuminuria at baseline [46]. The blood pressure target of <130/80 mmHg was achieved in 80 % of those given olmesartan and 71 % of those given placebo, but the time to onset of an albumin/creatinine ratio of ≥35 (for women) or ≥25 (for men) mg/g was significantly delayed in the olmesartan-treated group (8.2 % of the eligible patients, compared to 9.8 % of placebo-treated subjects). This "benefit" was perhaps balanced by no significant differences in doubling of serum creatinine and a larger number of fatal cardiovascular events (15 vs. 3) in the olmesartan-treated subjects.

More recently, the direct renin inhibitor has been used in clinical trials, but because of the prior proven efficacy of an ARB in preventing renal endpoints in hypertensive type 2 diabetics, the study design involved adding aliskiren (or placebo) to an ARB (or ACE-inhibitor). The 6-month trial, in which all subjects received losartan, used urinary albumin excretion as the endpoint, and was positive (showing a 20 % reduction with aliskiren vs. placebo, $P<0.001$), with only a small difference in blood pressures between the groups [47]. However, the long-term study, which layered aliskiren or placebo on either an ARB or an ACE-inhibitor was stopped prematurely at 2.7 years, because of excess hyperkalemia and hypotension in the aliskiren-treated group [48], despite a significant 14 % reduction in the urinary albumin/creatinine ratio.

Hypertensive Type 2 Diabetics with Overt Nephropathy

In addition to the DETAIL trial that found "non-inferiority" of an ACE-inhibitor with an ARB in preventing the time-dependent decline in glomerular filtration rate in 250 hypertensive type 2 diabetics with nephropathy [39], three trials have randomized hypertensive type 2 diabetics with overt nephropathy to placebo, an ARB, or amlodipine, in the Irbesartan Diabetic Nephropathy Trial (IDNT) [29]. As mentioned briefly above (and discussed in detail in Chap. 10), the IDNT and the Reduction of Endpoints in Non-Insulin Dependent Diabetes Mellitus with the Angiotensin II Antagonist Losartan (RENAAL) study [30] showed a significant 20 or 16 % reduction, respectively, in the incidence of doubling serum creatinine, end-stage renal disease, or death, compared to placebo. In both trials, reductions in this endpoint were preceded by, and associated with, a significant decline in urinary albumin excretion. Elaborate statistical analyses suggested that the reduction in the primary renal endpoint in each trial was independent of blood pressure-lowering. This was perhaps easier to demonstrate in IDNT, which included the amlodipine arm as a sort of "positive control" for its hypotensive effects, which were quite similar to those of irbesartan (141/77 vs. 140/77 mmHg, respectively), yet irbesartan was better than amlodipine (by 23 %, $P=0.006$) in prevention of the primary renal endpoint.

A more recent trial, the Olmesartan Reducing Incidence of End-stage Renal Disease in Diabetic Nephropathy Trial (ORIENT), randomized 577 hypertensive Japanese or Chinese type 2 diabetics with overt nephropathy (morning albumin/creatinine ratio >300 mg/g) to olmesartan or placebo for an average of 3.2 years [49]. The primary endpoint was the same as that of IDNT and RENAAL, but the major difference was that ~73 % of subjects in both randomized groups continued therapy with an ACE-inhibitor (although dose changes were prohibited by protocol). During follow-up, the olmesartan-treated group had significantly lower blood pressure (by 2.8/1.6 mmHg, on average), a highly significant reduction in urinary albumin excretion (−24.9 % at 144 weeks compared to baseline, vs. −3.1 % compared to baseline in the placebo-group, $P=0.005$), but a non-significant reduction in the primary renal endpoint (41.1 % vs. 45.4 %, $P=0.79$). Cardiovascular death was more common (10 vs. 3) in the olmesartan-treated group, which was attributed to an imbalanced randomization: 21.3 % of those randomized to olmesartan had cardiovascular disease at baseline, compared to only 11.6 % given placebo. Further subgroup analyses of the ORIENT trial are underway, but the simple message may be (as with combinations of ramipril+telmisartan [37] or aliskiren+an ACE-inhibitor or ARB [48]), that combining two inhibitors of the renin-angiotensin system increases the risk of hypotension and hypokalemia, and does not improve renal outcomes in type 2 diabetics.

Blood Pressure Lowering

Although often overlooked in the vigorous debate about the importance of having an inhibitor of the renin-angiotensin system in the treatment regimen of many type 1 and all type 2 diabetics, simply lowering blood pressure both reduces albuminuria (particularly in the higher categories), and delays the loss of renal function. During the last millennium, this was hotly debated, and frequently cited as "the reason" that early trials of ACE-inhibitors showed renal benefits in diabetic nephropathy. The clearest early demonstration of the role of strict blood pressure control was a series of 11 type 1 diabetics with baseline blood pressure of 143/96 mmHg, albumin excretion rate of 1,038 μg/min, and decline in glomerular filtration rate of 0.89 mL/min/month [50]. After 72 months of intensive antihypertensive treatment (usually with a diuretic, beta-blocker, and hydralazine), blood pressure fell to 129/84 mmHg, albumin excretion rate was only 504 μg/min, and the decline in renal function was 0.22 mL/min/month. These observations have been validated by subsequent analyses of on-treatment blood pressures in both IDNT [51] and RENAAL [52].

Calcium antagonists appear to be heterogeneous with respect to reducing urinary albumin excretion in diabetic subjects, particularly in short-term trials. Dihydropyridine compounds, notably nifedipine, have been associated with increases in urinary protein excretion, whereas the non-dihydropyridine compounds, verapamil and diltiazem, tend to reduce it [53]. These effects were more easily discerned in patients who were not treated with an inhibitor of the renin-angiotensin system (which is now commonly recommended). It appears that combining even a dihydropyridine calcium antagonist with an inhibitor of the renin-angiotensin system reduces not only albuminuria, but also the longer-term risk of renal deterioration, as demonstrated in RENAAL [52]. Verapamil did not reduce the long-term risk of severely increased albuminuria, either as monotherapy (compared to placebo), or when added to trandolapril (compared to trandolapril monotherapy) [35].

Several recent trials have demonstrated that aldosterone antagonists have an antiproteinuric effect, even when added to ACE-inhibitors in either type 1 or type 2 diabetics [54]. However, experience with the combination in patients with impaired renal excretory function (e.g., >Stage 2 chronic kidney disease) indicates that serum potassium, creatinine, and non-steroidal anti-inflammatory drugs must be carefully monitored in such patients who are given spironolactone or eplerenone.

Dietary Protein Restriction

There is currently much less enthusiasm for dietary protein restriction as a means of preventing the progression of diabetic nephropathy, although two trials done in the last millennium were positive. These two trials enrolled 19 and 35 type 1 diabetics, and showed that daily consumption of only 0.6 g of protein per kg of ideal body weight reduced the rate of decline in glomerular filtration rate by 60–75 %, and urinary albumin excretion [55, 56]. A subsequent trial in Denmark, however, showed no differences in the decline in renal function, but instead a higher risk of both end-stage renal disease or death, and mortality alone [57]. While some would argue that these trials were done in patients with late diabetic nephropathy, there are general concerns about the wisdom of restricting dietary protein in diabetics with nephropathy, who are already at risk for protein-calorie malnutrition, and must follow strict dietary regimens that limit carbohydrate, fat, and potassium consumption.

Dietary Sodium Restriction

Dietary sodium intake (or diuretic therapy) has a direct effect on proteinuria in patients with non-diabetic chronic kidney disease who are treated with inhibitors of the renin-angiotensin system. Several small studies in patients with diabetic nephropathy suggest a similar antiproteinuric effect of low-sodium diets [58–60], but it is not clear whether this phenomenon is mediated or otherwise influenced by concomitant blood pressure changes. It is likely that a low-sodium diet will lower blood pressure and reduce the need for diuretic therapy; both outcomes would presumably be beneficial for diabetics with early or late nephropathy.

Summary

To summarize, commonly recommended interventions for diabetics with early stages of nephropathy include: strict glycemic control, one inhibitor (but *not* two inhibitors) of the renin-angiotensin system to prevent progression (and possibly enhance the chance of regression) of albuminuria, adequate (but probably not intensive) lowering of blood pressure, and dietary sodium restriction. An exception is the type 1 diabetic with normal to mildly elevated albuminuria, in whom trials of inhibitors of the renin-angiotensin system have not proven significant prevention of progression to moderately increased albuminuria. Otherwise, these recommendations hold for all stages of diabetic nephropathy, although outcomes data are better in type 1 diabetics with ACE-inhibitors than ARBs, with the reverse being true for type 2 diabetics.

References

1. American Diabetes Association. Executive summary: standards of medical care in diabetes—2013. Diabetes Care. 2013;36 Suppl 1:S11–66.
2. Hassalacher C, Ritz E, Wahl P, Michale C. Similar risk of nephropathy in patients with type I or type II diabetes mellitus. Nephrol Dial Transplant. 1989;4:859–63.
3. Kidney Disease: Improving Global Outcomes (KDIGO) CKD Work Group. KDIGO clinical practice guideline for the evaluation and management of chronic kidney disease. Kidney Int Suppl. 2013;3:1–150.
4. Stevens PE, Levin A, for the Kidney Disease: Improving Global Outcomes Chronic Kidney Disease Guideline Development Work Group Members. Evaluation and management of chronic kidney disease: synopsis of the kidney disease: improving global outcomes 2012 clinical practice guideline. Ann Intern Med. 2013;158:825–30.
5. Matsushita K, van der Velde M, Astor BC, Woodward M, Levey AS, de Jong PE, Coresh J, Gansevoort RT, for the Chronic Kidney Disease Prognosis Consortium. Association of estimated glomerular filtration rate and albuminuria with all-cause and cardiovascular mortality in general population cohorts: a collaborative meta-analysis. Lancet. 2010;375:2073–81.
6. Gansevoort RT, Matsushita K, van der Velde M, Astor BC, Woodward M, Levey AS, Jong PE, Coresh J, for the Chronic Kidney Disease Prognosis Consortium. Lower estimated glomerular filtration rate and higher albuminuria are associated with adverse kidney outcomes. A collaborative meta-analysis of general and high-risk population cohorts. Kidney Int. 2011;80:93–104.
7. Perkins BA, Ficociello LH, Silva KN, Finklestein DM, Warram JH, Krolewski AS. Regression of microalbuminuria in type 1 diabetes. N Engl J Med. 2003;348:2285–93.
8. Effects of ramipril on cardiovascular and microvascular outcomes in people with diabetes mellitus: the HOPE study and MICRO-HOPE substudy. Heart Outcomes Prevention Evaluation (HOPE) Study Investigators. Lancet. 2000;355:253–9.
9. The effect of intensive treatment of diabetes on the development and progression of long-term complications in insulin-dependent diabetes mellitus. The Diabetes Control and Complications Trial Research Group. N Engl J Med. 1993;329:977–86.
10. Nathan DM, Cleary PA, Backlund JY, Genuth SM, Lachin JM, Orchard TJ, Raskin P, Zinman B, Diabetes Control and Complication Trial/Epidemiology of Diabetes Interventions and Complications (DCCT/EDIC) Study Research Group. Intensive diabetes treatment and cardiovascular disease in patients with type 1 diabetes. N Engl J Med. 2005;353:2643–53.
11. Effect of intensive therapy on the development and progression of diabetic nephropathy in the Diabetes Control and Complications Trial. The Diabetes Control and Complications (DCCT) Research Group. Kidney Int. 1995;47:1703–20.
12. de Boer IH, Sun W, Cleary PA, Lachin JM, Molitch ME, Steffes MW, Zinman B, for the DCCT/EDIC Research Group. Intensive diabetes therapy and glomerular filtration rate in type 1 diabetes. N Engl J Med. 2011;365:2366–76.
13. Reichard P, Nilsson BY, Rosengvist U. The effect of long-term intensified insulin treatment on the development of microvascular complications of diabetes mellitus. N Engl J Med. 1993;329:304–9.
14. Wang PH, Lau J, Chalmers TC. Meta-analysis of effects of intensive blood-glucose control on late complications of type 1 diabetes. Lancet. 1993;341:1306–9.
15. Fioretto P, Steffes MW, Sutherland DE, Goetz FC, Mauer M. Reversal of lesions of diabetic nephropathy after pancreas transplantation. N Engl J Med. 1998;339:69–75.
16. Coca SG, Ismail-Beigi F, Haq N, Krumholz HM, Parikh CR. Role of intensive glucose control in development of renal end points in type 2 diabetes mellitus: systematic review and meta-analysis intensive glucose control in type 2 diabetes. Arch Intern Med. 2012;172:761–9.
17. Gerstein HC, Miller ME, Byington RP, Goff Jr DC, Bigger JT, Buse JB, Cushman WC, Genuth S, Ismail-Beigi F, Grimm Jr RH, Probstfield JL, Simons-Morton DG, Friedewald WT, for the Action to Control Cardiovascular Risk in type 2 Diabetes Study Group. Effects of intensive glucose lowering in type 2 diabetes. N Engl J Med. 2008;358:2545–59.
18. Bilous R, Chaturvedi N, Sjølle AK, Fuller J, Klein R, Orchard T, Porta M, Parving H-H. Effect of candesartan on microalbuminuria and albumin excretion rates in diabetes: three randomized trials. Ann Intern Med. 2009;151:11–20.
19. Randomised placebo-controlled trial of lisinopril in normotensive patients with insulin-dependent diabetes and normoalbuminuria or microalbuminuria. The EUCLID Study Group. Lancet. 1997;349:1787–92.
20. Mauer M, Zinman B, Gardiner R, Suissa S, Sinaiko A, Strand T, Drummond K, Donnelly S, Goodyer P, Gubler MC, Klein R. Renal and retinal effects of enalapril and losartan in type 1 diabetes. N Engl J Med. 2009;361:40–51.
21. Hirst JA, Taylor KS, Stevens RJ, Blacklock CL, Roberts NW, Pugh CW, Farmer AJ. The impact of renin-angiotensin-aldosterone system inhibitors on type 1 and type 2 diabetic patients with and without early diabetic nephropathy. Kidney Int. 2012;81:674–83.
22. Viberti G, Mogensen CE, Groop LC, Pauls JF, Boner G, van Dyk J, Lucas A, Romero R, Salinas I, Sanmarti A, Blomqvist AC, Ekstrand A, Kirsi VL, Koivisto VA, Groop PH, Escobar F, Jimenez FE, Campos-Pastor MM, Muñoz M, Gomez M, Mangili R, Pozza G, Spotti D, Wurgler Hansen K, Sandahl Christiansen J, Klein F, Mogensen CE, van Doorn LG, Spooren PFMJ, Cruickshank JK, Jervell J, Paus PN, Collins A, Viberti G, Williams G. Effect of captopril on progression to clinical proteinuria in patients with insulin-

dependent diabetes mellitus and microalbuminuria. European Microalbuminuria Captopril Study Group. JAMA. 1994;271: 275–9.
23. Captopril reduces the risk of nephropathy in IDDM patients with microalbuminuria. The Microalbuminuria Captopril Study Group. Diabetologia. 1996;39:587–93.
24. Newman DJ, Mattock MG, Dawnay ABS, Kerry S, McGuire A, Yaqoob M, Hitman GA, Hawke C. Systemic review on urine albumin testing for early detection of diabetic complications. Health Technol Assess. 2005;9:III–vi, xiii–163.
25. Lewis EJ, Hunsicker LG, Bain RP, Rohde RD. The effect of angiotensin-converting-enzyme inhibition on diabetic nephropathy. The Captopril Collaborative Study Group. N Engl J Med. 1993;329:1456–62.
26. Wilmer WA, Hebert LA, Lewis EJ, Rohde RD, Whittier F, Cattran D, Levey AS, Lewis JB, Spitalewitz S, Blumenthal S, Bain RP. Remission of nephrotic syndrome in type 1 diabetes: long-term follow-up of patients in the Captopril Study. Am J Kidney Dis. 1999;34:308–14.
27. Lv J, Perkovic V, Foote CV, Craig ME, Craig JC, Strippoli GF. Antihypertensive agents for preventing diabetic kidney disease. Cochrane Database Syst Rev. 2012;(12):CD004136. doi: 10.1002/14651858.CD004136.pub3.
28. Kunz R, Friedrich C, Wolbers M, Mann JF. Meta-analysis: effect of monotherapy and combination therapy with inhibitors of the renin angiotensin system on proteinuria in renal disease. Ann Intern Med. 2008;148:30–48.
29. Lewis EJ, Hunsicker LG, Clarke WR, Berl T, Pohl MA, Lewis JB, Ritz E, Atkins RC, Rohde R, Raz I. Renoprotective effect of the angiotensin-receptor antagonist irbesartan in patients with nephropathy due to type 2 diabetes. Collaborative Study Group. N Engl J Med. 2001;345:851–60.
30. Brenner BM, Cooper ME, de Zeeuw D, Keane WF, Mitch WE, Parving HH, Remuzzi G, Snapinn SM, Zhang G, Shahinfar S. Effects of losartan on renal and cardiovascular outcomes in patients with type 2 diabetes and nephropathy. Reduction of Endpoints in Non-Insulin Dependent Diabetes Mellitus with the Angiotensin II Antagonist Losartan (RENAAL) Study Group. N Engl J Med. 2001;345:861–9.
31. Ravid M, Savin H, Jutrin I, Bental T, Lang R, Lishner M. Long-term effect of ACE inhibition on development of nephropathy in diabetes mellitus type II. Kidney Int. 1994;45 Suppl 45:S161–4.
32. Schrier RW, Estacio RO, Esler A, Mehler P. Effects of aggressive blood pressure control in normotensive type 2 diabetic patients on albuminuria, retinopathy, and strokes. Kidney Int. 2002;61: 1086–97.
33. Golan L, Birkmeyer JD, Welch HG. The cost-effectiveness of treating all patients with type 2 diabetes with angiotensin-converting enzyme inhibitors. Ann Intern Med. 1999;131:660–7.
34. Efficacy of atenolol and captopril in reducing the risk of macrovascular and microvascular complications in type 2 diabetes: UKPDS 39. UK Prospective Diabetes Study Group. BMJ. 1998;317: 713–20.
35. Ruggenenti P, Fassi A, Ilieva AP, Bruno S, Iliev IP, Brusegan V, Rubis N, Gherardi G, Arnoldi F, Ganeva M, Ene-Iordache B, Gaspari F, Perna A, Bossi A, Trevisan R, Dodesini AR, Remuzzi G, Preventing microalbuminuria in type 2 diabetes. N Engl J Med. 2004;351:1941–51.
36. Mogensen CE, Neldam S, Tikkanen I, Oren S, Viskoper R, Watts RW, Cooper ME. Randomised controlled trial of dual blockade of renin-angiotensin system in patients with hypertension, microalbuminuria, and non-insulin dependent diabetes: the candesartan and lisinopril microalbuminuria (CALM) study. BMJ. 2000;321: 1440–4.
37. Mann JFE, Schmieder RE, McQueen M, Dyal L, Schumacher M, Pogue J, Wang X, Maggioni A, Budaj A, Chaithiraphan S, Dickstein K, Keltai M, Metsärinne K, Oto A, Parkhomenko A, Piegas LS, Svendsen TL, Teo KK, Yusuf S, on behalf of the ONTARGET Investigators. Renal outcomes with telmisartan, ramipril, or both, in people at high vascular risk (the ONTARGET study): a multicentre, randomised, double-blind, controlled trial. Lancet. 2008;372: 547–53.
38. Maione A, Navaneethan SD, Graziano G, Mitchell R, Johnson D, Mann JFE, Gao P, Craig JC, Tognoni G, Perkovic V, Nicolucci A, De Cosmo S, Sasso A, Lamacchia O, Cignarelli M, Manfreda VM, Gentile G, Strippoli GFM. Angiotensin-converting enzyme inhibitor, angiotensin receptor blockers, and combined therapy in patients with micro- and macroalbuminuria and other cardiovascular risk factors: a systematic review of randomized controlled trials. Nephrol Dial Transplant. 2011;26:2827–47.
39. Barnett AH, Bain SC, Bouter P, Karlberg B, Madsbad S, Jervell J, Mustonen J, for the Diabetics Exposed to Telmisartan and Enalapril Study Group. Angiotensin-receptor blockade versus converting-enzyme inhibition in type 2 diabetes and nephropathy. N Engl J Med. 2004;351:1952–61.
40. Patel A, MacMahon S, Chalmers J, Neal B, Woodward M, Billot L, Harrap S, Poulter N, Marre M, Cooper M, Glasziou P, Grobbee DE, Hamet P, Heller S, Liu LS, Mancia G, Mogensen CE, Pan CY, Rodgers A, Williams B. Effects of a fixed combination of perindopril and indapamide on macrovascular and microvascular outcomes in patients with type 2 diabetes mellitus (the ADVANCE trial): a randomised controlled trial. Lancet. 2007;370:829–40.
41. Parving H-H, Lehnert H, Bröchner-Mortensen J, Gomis R, Andersen S, Arner P. The effect of irbesartan on the development of diabetic nephropathy in patients with type 2 diabetes. The Irbesartan in Patients with Type 2 Diabetes and Microalbuminuria Study Group. N Engl J Med. 2001;345:870–8.
42. Andersen S, Bröchner-Mortensen J, Parving H-H, for the Irbesartan in Patients with Type 2 Diabetes and Microalbuminuria Study Group. Kidney function during and after withdrawal of long-term irbesartan treatment in patients with type 2 diabetes and microalbuminuria. Diabetes Care. 2003;26:3296–302.
43. Hellemons ME, Persson F, Bakker SJL, Rossing P, Parving H-H, de Zeeuw D, Lambers Heerspink HJ. Initial angiotensin receptor-blockade-induced decrease in albuminuria is associated with long-term renal outcome in type 2 diabetic patients with microalbuminuria: a post-hoc analysis of the IRMA-2 trial. Diabetes Care. 2011; 34:2078–83.
44. Blacklock CL, Hirst JA, Taylor KS, Stevens RJ, Roberts NW, Farmer AJ. Evidence for a dose effect of renin-angiotensin system inhibition on progression of microalbuminuria in type 2 diabetes: a meta-analysis. Diabet Med. 2011;28:1182–7.
45. Viberti G, Wheeldon NM, for the MicroAlbuminuria Reduction with VALsartan (MARVAL) Study Investigators. Microalbuminuria reduction with valsartan in patients with type 2 diabetes mellitus: a blood pressure-independent effect. Circulation. 2002;106:672–8.
46. Haller H, Ito S, Izzo Jr JL, Januszewicz A, Katayama S, Menne J, Mimran A, Rabelinki TJ, Ritz E, Ruilope LM, Rump LC, Viberti G, for the ROADMAP Trial Investigators. Olmesartan for the delay or prevention of microalbuminuria in type 2 diabetes. N Engl J Med. 2011;364:907–17.
47. Parving H-H, Persson F, Lewis JB, Lewis EJ, Hollenberg NK, for the AVOID Study Investigators. Aliskiren combined with losartan in type 2 diabetes and nephropathy. N Engl J Med. 2008;358: 2433–46.
48. Parving H-H, Brenner BM, McMurray JJV, de Zeeuw D, Haffner SM, Solomon SD, Chaturvedi N, Persson F, Desai AS, Nicolaides M, Richard A, Xiang Z, Brunel P, Pfeffer MA, for the ALTITUDE Investigators. Cardiorenal end points in a trial of aliskiren for type 2 diabetes. N Engl J Med. 2012;367:2204–13.
49. Imai E, Chan CN, Ito S, Yamasaki T, Kobayashi F, Haneda M, Makino H, for the ORIENT Study Investigators. Effects of olmesartan

on renal and cardiovascular outcomes in type 2 diabetics with overt nephropathy: a multicentre, randomised, placebo-controlled study. Diabetologia. 2011;54:2978–86.
50. Parving H-H, Andersen AR, Smidt UM, Hommel E, Mathiesen ER, Svendsen PA. Effect of antihypertensive treatment on kidney function in diabetic nephropathy. Br Med J (Clin Res). 1987; 294:1443–7.
51. Pohl MA, Blumenthal S, Cordonnier DJ, De Alvaro F, Deferrar G, Eisner G, Esmatjes E, Gilbert RE, Hunsicker LG, de Faria JB, Mangilli R, Moor Jr J, Reisin E, Ritz E, Schernthanaer G, Spitalewitz S, Tindall H, Rodby RA, Lewis EJ. Independent and additive impact of blood pressure control and angiotensin II receptor blockade on renal outcomes in the Irbesartan Diabetic Nephropathy Trial: clinical implications and limitations. J Am Soc Nephrol. 2005;16:3027–37.
52. Bakris GL, Weir MR, Shanifar S, Zhang Z, Douglas J, van Dijk DJ, Brenner BM, for the RENAAL Study Group. Effects of blood pressure level on progression of diabetic nephropathy: results from the RENAAL study. Arch Intern Med. 2003; 163:1555–65.
53. Böhlen L, de Courten M, Wiedmann P. Comparative study of the effect of ACE-inhibitors and other antihypertensive agents on proteinuria in diabetic patients. Am J Hypertens. 1994;7 Suppl 2: 84S–92.
54. Epstein M, Williams GH, Weinberger M, Lewin A, Krause S, Mukherjee R, Patni R, Beckerman B. Selective aldosterone blockade with eplerenone reduces albuminuria in patients with type 2 diabetes. Clin J Am Soc Nephrol. 2006;1:940–51.
55. Walker JD, Bending JJ, Dodds RA, Mattock MB, Murrells TJ, Keen H, Viberti GC. Restriction of dietary protein and progression of renal failure in diabetic nephropathy. Lancet. 1989;2:1411–5.
56. Zeller K, Whittaker E, Sullivan L, Raskin P, Jacobson HR. Effect of restricting dietary protein on the progression of renal failure in patients with insulin-dependent diabetes mellitus. N Engl J Med. 1991;324:78–84.
57. Hansen HP, Tauber-Lassen E, Jensen BR, Parving H-H. Effect of dietary protein restriction on prognosis in patients with diabetic nephropathy. Kidney Int. 2002;62:220–8.
58. Bakris GL, Smith A. Effects of sodium intake on albumin excretion in patients with diabetic nephropathy treated with long-acting calcium antagonists. Ann Intern Med. 1996;125:201–4.
59. Houlihan CA, Allen TJ, Baxter AL, Panangiotopoulos S, Casley DJ, Cooper ME, Jerums G. A low-sodium diet potentiates the effects of losartan in type 2 diabetes. Diabetes Care. 2002;25:663–71.
60. Esnault VL, Ekhias A, Decroix C, Moutel MG, Nguyen JM. Diuretic and enhanced sodium restriction results in improved antiproteinuric response to RAS blocking agents. J Am Soc Nephrol. 2005;16:474–81.

Novel Treatments and the Future of Diabetic Nephropathy: What Is on the Horizon?

19

Vecihi Batuman

Introduction

Since the emergence of diabetic kidney disease as a major public health issue in the 1970s, the scope and the extent of the problem have continued to grow. Worldwide intense research continues. There has been much new insight gained in the last quarter century, still however short of a cure. In this chapter we will briefly review the future frontiers of diabetes research focused mostly as relates to diabetic kidney disease.

During the past decade new types of medications that counter glucose dysregulation through different mechanisms have been introduced to clinical practice. Currently many studies are in progress to evaluate how these new types of blood glucose regulating drugs will influence the natural course of diabetes and target organ damage caused by diabetes especially diabetic nephropathy. These new drugs that are currently approved by the FDA and available for use in the US are discussed in detail in Chap. 16, and elsewhere in the published literature [1–4]. Included among these newer therapeutics are: (1) the dipeptidyl peptidase (DPP) 4 inhibitors (sitagliptin, saxagliptin, linagliptin, aloglitpin), which decrease the breakdown of the incretin hormones, such as glucagon-like peptide 1 (GLP-1), (2) the alpha-glucosidase inhibitors (acarbose, miglitol) which decrease the breakdown of oligo- and disaccharides in the small intestine, (3) the *GLP-1 Receptor Agonists* (*incretin mimetics*), exenatide (Byetta) and liraglutide (Victoza), and (4) the sodium-glucose co-transporter 2 inhibitors that include the recently approved canagliflozin (and several others under development) [5].

These new drugs have opened a new frontier in the treatment of diabetes, as they work through mechanisms other than stimulating insulin secretion. Among these novel classes of drugs, SGLT2 inhibitors, which block renal tubular reabsorption of glucose and lead to a caloric deficit as well as increased sodium excretion in the kidney may have weight losing and blood pressure lowering effects and may be uniquely helpful in preventing diabetic nephropathy [5–7]. In a recent study a newer SGLT2 inhibitor, empagliflozin, was shown to attenuate GFR measured by inulin clearance measured under clamped hyperglycemia in hyperfiltering type 1 diabetics by as much as 33 mL/min/1.73 m^2 from a baseline of 172 ± 23 to 139 ± 25 mL/min/1.73 m^2 [8]. As hyperfiltration is an early change in diabetic nephropathy, this favorable effect raises the expectation that SGLT2 inhibitors may prevent or delay the onset of nephropathy if initiated early during the course of diabetes. Additional clinical trials are needed to determine if this modality reduces kidney complications.

Despite the recent progress, there is need for further groundbreaking research to reduce the burden of disease as well as the target organ damage caused by diabetes.

The Role of Immune System and Prospects of Immunotherapy in Diabetes

An exciting front has opened exploring the role of immune system, especially the innate immunity in the pathogenesis of diabetes. Pointing to the relation between the recent obesity epidemic and the rapidly rising prevalence of both type 1 and type 2 diabetes, research has revealed evidence that chronic low-level inflammation predominantly mediated through innate immunity as a primary determinant of obesity-related pathology including the full spectrum of diabetic disease [9].

Since the first demonstration in 1974 of islet cell antibodies [10], type 1 diabetes was believed to be autoimmune in nature. Although initially these antibodies were believed to be responsible for β-cell destruction, later research has shown that these antibodies (representing the humoral arm of the immune system) are not necessarily responsible for the β-cell destruction but they are rather markers of islet cell destruction, and that the cellular arm of the immune system,

V. Batuman, M.D. (✉)
Tulane University Medical Center, Nephrology Section, 1430 Tulane Avenue, New Orleans, LA 70112, USA
e-mail: vbatuma@tulane.edu

E.V. Lerma and V. Batuman (eds.), *Diabetes and Kidney Disease*,
DOI 10.1007/978-1-4939-0793-9_19, © Springer Science+Business Media New York 2014

specifically T-lymphocytes, mediate the β-cell destruction [11]. Studies have further shown that the T-lymphocytes do not act alone. They initiate the response after interaction with antigen-presenting cells such as dendritic cells and macrophages, and appear to receive help also from B-lymphocytes involving a complex array of interactions between the innate and adaptive immunity systems. The initial immune response triggers and propagates secondary and tertiary responses that result in impairment of β-cell function, progressive destruction of β-cells, and consequent development of type 1 diabetes. The process may be insidious and may evolve at different speeds, over many years in older individuals and much more rapidly in young children, with the overt expression of clinical symptoms becoming apparent only when most β-cells have been destroyed. Initially it has been thought that this process results in complete β-cell destruction, but several studies have now demonstrated some degree of residual β-cell function or existence (at autopsy) in long-standing type 1 diabetes. This has inspired studies aimed at the preservation and even regeneration of the β-cells as well as β-cell function, with the hope that restoring endogenous insulin secretion will yield better glycemic control, and slow the development of the dreaded complications of diabetes, such as retinopathy and nephropathy [11].

Glycemic control reflects the balance between dietary intake and gluconeogenesis (rate of appearance of glucose in circulation) and tissue uptake or utilization through storage as glycogen or fat and oxidation (rate of glucose disappearance from circulation). This is coordinated primarily by insulin production in the pancreas from the β-cells along with interplay of other glucoregulatory hormones including glucagon, amylin, the incretins GLP-1 and glucose-dependent insulinotropic peptide (GIP), epinephrine, cortisol, growth hormone, etc. [12]. Insulin regulates serum glucose through its actions on liver, skeletal muscle, and fat tissue. When there is insulin resistance, insulin cannot suppress hepatic gluconeogenesis, which leads to hyperglycemia. On the other hand, insulin resistance in the adipose tissue and skeletal muscle leads to increased lipolysis causing hyperlipidemia in addition to hyperglycemia, and compensatory hyperglycemia. Evidence suggests that when there is insulin resistance the pancreas is forced to increase its insulin output, which stresses the β-cells eventually resulting in β-cell exhaustion. The high blood glucose levels and high levels of saturated fatty acids create an inflammatory environment resulting in activation of the innate immune cells in metabolic tissues, which result in activation of the nuclear transcription factors-kappa B (NF-κB), and release of inflammatory mediators, including, interleukin-1β (IL-1β), and tumor necrosis factor-alpha (TNFα), promoting systemic insulin resistance and β-cell damage as a result of autoimmune insulitis [9]. The consequent insulin resistance further leads to high glucose levels, along with high serum levels of free fatty acids, as well as IL-1, leading to glucotoxicity, lipotoxicity, and IL-1 toxicity resulting in apoptotic β-cell death. These studies have revealed that, in obesity, adipose tissue is an immunologically active site for both MHC class I and MHC class II-mediated antigen presentation by macrophages to CD8+ and CD4+ T cells, which contribute to adipose tissue inflammation and peripheral insulin resistance. This line of research has revealed an important role of regulatory T cells (Treg) in the pathogenesis of diabetes and has led to studies exploring specific sequences on T cells responsible for mediating immune destruction of islet cells, and potential strategies to neutralize these cells [13]. Importantly, investigations into immunopathogenesis of diabetes suggest that the traditional dualistic concept of type 1 and type 2 may no longer be valid, and may inspire in the future therapies that may pre-empt diabetic pathophysiology in both young and older individuals [9].

This line of research has already identified potential novel therapy interventions [14–16]. A recent 2-year trial has demonstrated that selective depletion of B-lymphocytes with rituximab, an anti-CD20 monoclonal antibody, slowed decline of β-cell function in recent-onset type 1 diabetes mellitus (T1DM), although it did not appear to fundamentally alter the underlying pathophysiology of the disease [16]. Interestingly, however, therapeutic approaches originally believed to be applicable to type 2 diabetes, i.e., exercise, weight loss, and insulin sensitizing agents have been found effective in slowing or even preventing type 1 diabetes [9, 17].

Also on the horizon are therapies aimed at countering the progressive destruction of β-cells, and attempting to exploit the inherent regenerative capacity of the β-cell mass. Based on the recent insight that revealed a pivotal role for IL-1β in β-cell destruction, therapy attempts utilizing a novel IL-1β neutralizing antibody, XOMA 052, have shown promise in animal models [18, 19]. Clinical trials to explore feasibility of anti-IL-β approach using either monoclonal neutralizing antibodies, such as, canakinumab, or IL-1 receptor antagonist (IL-Ra) anakinra, have been initiated [14, 20, 21].

In a preliminary clinical trial in children with newly diagnosed type 1 diabetes, the effects of a short course (28 days) treatment with recombinant IL-1R antagonist protein, anakinra, were evaluated. Anakinra-treated patients had similar HbA1c and mixed-meal tolerance testing (MMTT) responses, but insulin requirements were lower at 1 and 4 months after diagnosis compared to controls. Children treated with anakinra had lower insulin-dose-adjusted HbA1c 1 month after diagnosis. Although anakinra did not prevent the development of diabetes in these children with newly diagnosed type 1 diabetes, it was well tolerated and appeared promising justifying additional studies perhaps with different protocols to explore clinical efficacy [21].

Currently, there are also ongoing trials exploring primary prevention in genetically susceptible infants by maneuvers, such as, using infant formulas free of either cow's milk or of bovine insulin, infant formula supplemented with the omega-3-fatty acid docosahexaenoic acid, delayed introduction of gluten-containing foods, and vitamin D supplementation [22].

Renal Fibrosis and Epithelial-to-Mesenchymal Transition: Potential for Reversibility?

Regardless of the etiology, kidney disease progresses predominantly through tubulointerstitial fibrosis, which is another major consequence of the heightened immune environment present in the diabetic kidney. The inflammatory milieu that leads to the activation of both the innate and adaptive immune systems that results in the production of IL-1β, activation of NF-κB and increased transcription, and release to medium of a cascade of cytokines. These cytokines include TNF-α, MCP-1, interleukins 6, 8, etc., but most prominently TGF-β1, which has been recognized as a major mediator of kidney fibrosis in both diabetic and non-diabetic kidney diseases [23–25]. In a recent study, the expression levels of TGF-β1, p53, and microRNA-192 (miR-192) were shown increased in the renal cortex of diabetic mice, and these changes were associated with glomerular expansion and fibrosis [26]. Detailed studies showed that the inflammatory setting responsible for these events include recruitment of monocytes from the circulation and $CD14^+$ fibrocytes from the bone marrow. The monocytes differentiate into both M1 and M2 macrophages, contribute more cytokines in the medium perpetuating the cycle of inflammatory events [27]. A major component of fibrosis has now been shown to be due to the resident macrophages, kidney tissue fibroblasts, and epithelial-to-mesenchymal transformation (EMT) and endothelial-to-mesenchymal proliferation (EndEMT) driven through the effects of TGF-βs. The residential fibroblasts proliferate, the renal epithelia and endothelia acquire myofibroblast phenotype, and with increased synthesis and decreased degradation of matrix proteins resulting in increased collagen and matrix deposition especially in the tubulointerstitial space the kidney is progressively destroyed [26–29]. Evidence suggests that intrarenal renin-angiotensin system may have a key role in this process, which may be independent of circulating angiotensin, and measurement of urinary angiotensinogen levels has been proposed as a marker of intrarenal renin-angiotensin system [30–33]. Urinary angiotensinogen levels may have a particular value in identifying patients at risk of diabetic kidney disease and suggest that renal renin-angiotensin system plays a key role in the pathogenesis of diabetic nephropathy [32, 34].

Our improved understanding of the process of fibrosis has identified some exciting potential therapeutic opportunities that can halt the process, but also, conceivably, that can even reverse established fibrosis. First, antagonizing pro-fibrotic cytokines, especially TGF-βs, and other growth factors including PDGF, VEGF may slow progression of kidney disease. Of interest is the relation between angiotensin II and TGF-β1, and the well-known role of renin-angiotensin-aldosterone system (RAAS) antagonists in slowing progression of kidney disease [27, 28, 35]. Clearly, these interventions although found helpful in slowing progression, have not reduced the incidence of diabetic nephropathy. Strategies that can reverse renal and other tissue fibrosis are now imaginable through use of agents that can reverse EMT in the opposite direction towards restoring original phenotypes of the epithelia or endothelia through agents, such as BMP-7 [27]. The BMP7 receptor Alk3 plays a key role in opposing fibrogenesis, and Alk3 agonists also appear as an attractive therapeutic approach in diabetic nephropathy [27].

Another promising therapeutic target in diabetic nephropathy is the nuclear factor erythroid 2-related factor 2 (Nrf2), a master regulator of oxidative stress, which has an anti-EMT effect through its interaction with hemeoxygenase-1. In addition, it was recently shown that BMP7 receptor Alk3 in renal tubules is essential for anti-fibrogenesis and tissue repair in the kidneys. Alk3-agonistic compounds showed renoprotection in experimental kidney fibrosis models, including models of diabetic nephropathy; this renal protection was associated with the inhibition of EMT, inflammation, and apoptosis [27]. Strategies to prevent or reverse EMT are likely to be part of the future therapies in diabetic kidney disease as well as other complications associated with diabetes.

It has been recognized for some time that the kidneys may have intrinsic ability for self-regeneration. An earlier 10-year follow-up study of eight type 1 diabetes patients who received pancreas transplants and who had varying degrees of diabetic nephropathy before reaching end-stage demonstrated reversal of all the kidney lesions after 10 years of normoglycemia [36]. In experimental models as well as in humans with diabetic and non-diabetic kidney disease, reversal of kidney lesions and functional restoration was observed. Research since then has confirmed the existence of a "renopoietic" renal stem cell/progenitor system that can replace tubular cells as well as podocytes, which are neuron-like cells with limited ability to regenerate and which are the principal drivers of the characteristic glomerular sclerosis in diabetic nephropathy [37]. There are indications that these podocyte- and tubule-committed progenitor cells can be pharmacologically manipulated to promote kidney regeneration, or also isolated, clonally expanded, directed to injury site by molecular manipulations and transplanted into injured kidney to reverse kidney damage [37]. Further research into understanding the molecular mechanisms of activating progenitor cells is likely to contribute to regenerative nephrology and be part of future strategies for the treatment of diabetic and non-diabetic kidney disease.

Vascular changes seen in diabetes are largely responsible for not only kidney disease, but also are the main cause of cardiovascular morbidity as well as retinopathy. Accelerated atherosclerosis is a main feature of diabetes, and multiple factors along with hyperglycemia, including advanced glycation end products (AGE), increased free fatty acids and LDL cholesterol, reactive oxygen species, angiotensin II, activation of NF-κB and production of inflammatory cytokines, etc., contribute to vascular injury [38]. The effects of insulin receptors beyond glucose regulation have been shown to promote the integrity of both the vascular endothelial cells as well as podocytes, thus identifying another mechanism through which vasculopathy, and podocytopathy, which aggravate both atherosclerosis and glomerulosclerosis is mediated as a result of insulin resistance [27, 38]. Ongoing research suggests that enhancing the protective effects of insulin-regulated genes on vascular endothelial cells, and delivery of non-diabetic endothelial progenitor cells can prevent or even reverse the vascular disease in diabetes [38, 40]. Countering accelerated atherosclerosis through the use of statins and renin-angiotensin system antagonists is already an established therapy in diabetes. These newer insights are likely to generate more effective treatments through gene manipulations that can lead to induction of antioxidant and anti-inflammatory factors that promote vascular survival and preserve vascular integrity, which in turn would be expected to help prevent both diabetic kidney disease and retinopathy [38].

The Promise of Metabolomics and Proteomics

A significant constraint in the approach against treatment of diabetic nephropathy is the limited availability of biomarkers. Microalbuminuria has its limitations and is not always predictable (see the chapters 8 and 9 in this book. Some investigators have suggested that increased urinary excretion of polyclonal immune globulin light chains, particularly kappa light chains, as a reflection of early tubular dysfunction, i.e., decreased endocytosis through the endocytic receptors megalin and cubilin [41], may be a more reliable marker [42–44]. A more comprehensive search for biomarkers through metabolomics studies using gas chromatography–mass spectrometry to screen for large numbers of metabolites in the urine of patients with diabetic nephropathy are under way, and have yielded promising clues [45]. In a recent pilot study Sharma et al. observed that urine from subjects with diabetic kidney disease showed reduced levels of metabolites, many were soluble organic anions related to mitochondrial function and reflecting globally suppressed mitochondrial function in diabetic nephropathy patients. The authors also found that exosomes from patients with diabetes and kidney disease had less mitochondrial DNA, and kidney tissues from patients with diabetic kidney disease had lower gene expression of PGC1a (a master regulator of mitochondrial biogenesis). These observations suggest that urine metabolomics may be a promising strategy to identify early biomarkers of kidney disease in diabetic patients, and that organic anion transporters and mitochondrial function maybe dysregulated in diabetic kidney disease [45].

The field is likely to expand as studies on urinary exosomes are more closely investigated. Exosomes are 40–100 nm vesicles that contain proteins, mRNA, and microRNAs (miRNA) that have the potential to serve as biomarkers of renal dysfunction. Newer methodologies including various ultracentrifugation techniques are now allowing more efficient exosome isolation enabling proteomics analysis and RNA and miRNA analysis. Such techniques are likely to lead to identification of newer biomarkers of kidney involvement in diabetics, as well as newer insight into mechanisms of kidney disease [46].

Proteomic analyses from diabetic kidneys and other organs, such as liver and skin, are relatively new and appear to identify differential expression of various proteins in affected organs compared to healthy organs. These studies have identified accumulation of protein aggregates due to impaired proteasomal activity, novel oxidative and glycolytic mechanisms, and novel regulators of TGF-β signaling, tight junction maintenance, oxidative stress, etc. [47–50]. These investigations have started to point to potential novel therapeutic approaches awaiting pre-translational and translational studies.

Genes, Epigenetics, and microRNAs

The genetic determinants of kidney disease in diabetes are still not fully defined. Although nearly half the diabetics will develop kidney disease, the other half will not suggesting a genetic basis of vulnerability independent of hyperglycemia, hypertension, or albuminuria. Earlier studies have focused on angiotensin converting enzyme insertion/deletion polymorphism as a determinant of susceptibility to kidney disease in both type 1 and type 2 diabetes and suggested that the D allele or DD homozygous might be associated with increased risk of nephropathy [51–55]. It has also been suggested that the DD genotype may respond better to angiotensin converting enzyme inhibitors or angiotensin receptor blockers prompting investigators to suggest a pharmacogenomics approach to treatment in diabetic populations [56]. However, most of the studies were not definitive, suggested a much more complex gene–environment interaction and pointed to the need for further investigations [55].

Nearly two decades of use of converting enzyme inhibitors and angiotensin receptor blockers may have helped to slow the progression of diabetic nephropathy in many people, but the incidence of diabetic nephropathy continues to increase.

More recent genetic research has broadened our understanding of the role of genetics and epigenetics in the pathogenesis of diabetic nephropathy and suggested novel directions of therapeutic interventions. Genome wide association scans (GWAS) for single nucleotide polymorphisms (SNPs) have pointed to previously unidentified pathways that may be responsible for susceptibility to diabetic nephropathy [57–59]. Multiple chromosomal loci including 3q, 7q, 10p, 14q, and 18q have been identified as possible determinants of susceptibility to diabetic nephropathy in both type 1 and type 2 diabetes, however, the specific roles of these loci in the pathogenesis of diabetic nephropathy have not been fully established [60].

Gene–environment interactions and the role of epigenetics appear to be closely involved in the pathobiology of diabetes, obesity, and diabetic nephropathy [61, 62]. Some of these studies have focused on the intrauterine environment and alterations in DNA methylation and histone post-translational modifications that result in disease in adult life and some even persist across generations [61]. Dysregulation of post-transcriptional modifications of histones in chromatin that include histone methylation can result in aberrant gene behavior that favors development of diabetes and its complications. Genome-wide studies have revealed cell-type specific changes in histone methylation patterns in diabetic populations. Experimental studies in vitro have shown long lasting epigenetic alterations of inflammatory gene promoters after prior exposure to diabetic conditions implying a possible mechanism for metabolic memory [62].

Histone deacetylases, especially sirtuins, which deacetylate histones and various transcription factors, are also being explored as epigenetic therapeutic targets in many acute and chronic diseases. A recent study observed that sirtuin 1 was down-regulated in the kidneys of diabetic mice before the onset of albuminuria, and overexpression of sirtuin in the proximal tubules of mice prevented diabetic nephropathy [63].

In addition to histone methylation, DNA methylation miRNAs have also been implicated in diabetic nephropathy [64, 65]. miRNAs are small (19–23 nucleotide long) non-coding RNA molecules that play important roles in the transcriptional and post-transcriptional gene expression through either mRNA degradation or translational repression [66]. Studies have demonstrated that a long non-coding RNA, the plasmacytoma variant translocation 1 (PVT1), increases plasminogen activator inhibitor 1 (PAI-1) and TGF-β1 in mesangial cells, the two main contributors to ECM accumulation in the glomeruli under hyperglycemic conditions, as well as fibronectin 1 (FN1), a major ECM component, and miR-1207-5p, a PVT derived miRNA plays a key role in this process [67, 68]. Recent studies in diabetic mice have suggested that cross talk between mRNAs, TGF-β1, and p53 may play an important role in the pathogenesis of diabetic nephropathy. Among many miRNAs, this study has suggested that miR-192 is increased in the kidneys of diabetic mice along with p53, TGF-β1, and blocking miR-192 reversed increased expression of p53 and TGF-β1. This intervention reduced and reversed renal fibrosis, suggesting an important role for miRNAs in the pathogenesis of diabetic nephropathy and identified miRNA targeting as a novel therapeutic strategy [26].

In a streptozotocin model of diabetes, high concentrations of miR-375 appeared as a marker of beta cell death and a potential predictor of diabetes in mice [69]. Other investigators showed similar associations with miR-21, i.e., increased expression in the kidney as a potential marker for diabetic nephropathy, and as a therapeutic target as miR-21 knockdown plasmid delivery, similar to opposing miR-192, also reduced TGF-β1 expression, suppressed NF-κB activation and helped reverse proteinuria and renal inflammation in db/db diabetic mice, a model for type 2 diabetes [70]. To date miRNAs that have been identified as contributing to diabetic kidney disease include miR-192, miR-216a, miR-217; miR-377, miR-21, miR-29c, as well as miR-1207-5p, and miRNA targeted therapies are being explored as a possible strategy to treat diabetes and diabetic kidney disease [67, 68].

Thus, genetics, search for loci and SNPs in GWAS studies, along with exciting new insight revealed through better understanding of epigenetics, and the role of miRNAs have opened up new areas of research in the pathobiology of diabetes. This research is identifying new mechanisms and new therapy approaches that are on the verge of translational studies that may enable us to not only treat diabetes and its serious complications including diabetic nephropathy, but, more importantly, identify susceptible populations and possibly prevent diabetes through pre-emptive strategies.

In Pursuit of Futuristic Therapies

During the past few years, significant progress has been made with gene-based therapies in animal models, and we can expect that some translational studies will be initiated in humans in the near future. Gene therapy aimed at protection and regeneration of β-cells is one area that has attracted attention. A broad array of strategies is being explored with gene therapy approaches, including insulin gene, various growth factors, and modulators of the inflammatory pathways involved in the pathogenesis of islet cell failure [48, 71, 72]. Some studies have shown that the serine-threonine kinase Akt1, encoded by the Akt1-gene, can promote β-cell survival and regeneration. Using an enhanced adenoviral vector delivery of constitutively active Akt1 targeted to islet cells was shown to promote β-cell survival and proliferation in a streptozotocin-induced model of diabetes in mice [73, 74].

Innovative strategies are currently being explored to exploit the transdifferentiation of the pluripotential cells in the pancreas to regenerate into β-cells. Attempts are underway to reconstruct pancreas development, including islet β-cell and α-cell differentiation, from fetal progenitor cells [75].

Plasmid DNAs targeted to the pancreas in vivo using ultrasound-targeted microbubble destruction (UTMD) appears promising to achieve islet regeneration. In this technique intravenous microbubbles carrying plasmids are destroyed within the pancreatic microcirculation by ultrasound, achieving local gene expression that is further targeted to β-cells by a rat insulin promoter (RIP3.1). In one study, a series of genes involved in the development of endocrine pancreas were delivered to rats after streptozotocin-induced diabetes. RIP3.1-NeuroD1 promoted islet cell regeneration from surviving β-cells, with normalization of glucose, insulin, and C-peptide levels at 30 days; however the improvement was transient. Nevertheless, this proof-of-concept study demonstrated the feasibility of selective gene delivery to the pancreas without using viral vectors, opening up further possibilities for successful gene therapy [76].

Other techniques that appear effective in rodent models of diabetes include delivery of bone marrow-derived mesenchymal stem cells (BM-MSCs). BM-MSCs transplantation decreased blood glucose concentrations and attenuated β-cell injury, prevented renal damage, and decreased proteinuria by inhibiting TGF-β1 expression and upregulating synaptopodin and IL-10 expression in rats with diabetic nephropathy [77].

At a time when pancreatic islet cell transplantation appeared to have limited potential because of limited donor availability and rejection (discussed elsewhere in the book), novel strategies are emerging to improve the chances of transplanted cells' survival and proliferation to achieve sufficient mass, and prevent rejection. There are multiple different approaches to preserve β-cell viability and functionality both in situ and in islet cell transplantation. One promising line of research is exploring the role of estrogen and estrogen receptors in the preservation of β-cells, demonstrating that estrogen receptor modulation can be helpful in preventing islet cell failure [78–80].

In another line of research, various methodologies are being pursued to encapsulate cultured human islet cells before implantation to improve the chances of engraftment and reduce the risk of rejection. In one study alginate-encapsulated islet cells yielded superior outcomes in a mouse model of diabetes as well as a single type 1 diabetes patient [81], while another study used coating by biosilicification to improve survival and function of islet cells in culture [82]. Other strategies include directing engraftment to other sites, such as, the small intestine rather than the portal vein, which seems to yield better control of diabetes in an animal model [83]. Investigators have also attempted to differentiate human endometrial stromal stem cells (ESSC) into insulin secreting cells and found in a mouse model of diabetes that when injected into the renal capsule these cells secreted insulin in response to high glucose levels and achieved normoglycemia [84].

Novel immunosuppression protocols are also being explored to improve the success rate in single donor islet cell transplants and in one study the use of antithymoglobulin plus anti-inflammatory agents of anakinra and etanercept for induction and tacrolimus plus mycophenolate mofetil for maintenance was shown to result in successful single-donor islet cell transplantation in eight patients [85]. Obviously larger scale clinical trials are needed to demonstrate the efficacy of such protocols, however, in the upcoming years, it is likely that we will see more effective immune suppression protocols that will improve the success rate in single donor islet cells. Clearly, during the recent years, multiple strategies have emerged that promise successful engraftment or differentiation of islet cells.

Xenotransplantation

Cross-species transplantation of organs from animals into humans was attempted since as early as the seventeenth century. An early example in the twentieth century was when Dr Keith Reethma transplanted chimpanzee kidneys to 13 patients at Tulane between 1963 and 1964. Although the patients lived only 9–60 days, one patient survived for 9 months and even returned to work, indicating potential feasibility [86, 87]. Attempts to cross-species transplantation of organs including kidney, liver, neuronal cells, pancreas, and islet cells continued through the 2000s. Zoonotic infections and rejection were the main causes of failure, and as of today these difficulties inherent in xenotransplantation have not been overcome [87, 88]. However, xenotransplantation still appears to be a promising but difficult frontier, which could potentially provide reliably an endless source of insulin producing cells, although severe rejection continues to be an insurmountable challenge.

If a xenograft from an animal could be genetically modified to express human genes and avoid rejection by the human body, then we would have an endless supply of spare organs for patients with organ failure including diabetes with pancreas failure. Genetic manipulations are now being attempted to counter rejection along with experiments with biologicals that selectively target costimulatory molecules, or suppression of immunity locally and by encapsulating xenografts in immunologically inert scaffolds, some designed and fabricated by three-dimensional printing are strategies that are being explored [78, 89–91]. Although this technology is not ready for translational studies yet, animal experiments suggest that they could be introduced to clinical trials in the near future.

Regenerative Medicine and Nanotechnology

Imagining the future of diabetes and diabetic nephropathy must include the exciting developments in regenerative medicine and nanotechnology. There is work on newer implantable devices that can sense blood glucose concentration and deliver appropriate doses of insulin continuously. Recent advances in nanotechnology and biosensors raise the expectation that biochips can be designed that can continuously monitor blood glucose as well as other disease biomarkers. Such devices would need to be fully integrated closed loop systems and implantable via minimally invasive methods, possibly subcutaneously. Issues such as long-term biocompatibility, reliability, and high-degree of integration need to be overcome before such technology can be introduced clinically [92, 93].

A major breakthrough in biotechnology that can help diabetic patients with kidney disease can be imagined in the field of regenerative medicine and three-dimensional printing [94–96]. Significant strides have been made in this field during the past decade, and the feasibility of fabricating viable and potentially transplantable tissues has been demonstrated [97, 98]. Using this technology, recently scientists from Massachusetts General Hospital successfully constructed a kidney that produced rudimentary urine in vitro when perfused through their intrinsic vascular bed. When transplanted orthotopically and perfused by the recipient's circulation, the grafts produced urine through the ureteral conduit in vivo. The technological advances in the field of three-dimensional printing are likely to find broad applications including creation of biocompatible scaffolds encapsulating functional islet cells to facilitate successful engraftment, or creating functional sheets of cells to replace injured parts of organs [99, 100].

Thus, emerging technologies and interdisciplinary efforts are likely to produce increasingly sophisticated solutions for not only diabetic patients with kidney disease but also for other organ failures. But can we prevent diabetes before it presents as full-blown clinical disease?

Strategies to Prevent Diabetes and Diabetic Nephropathy

The recent insights into the immunopathogenesis and immunogenetics of diabetes have yielded a large number of promising biomarkers, which can identify diabetics in the earliest phases of the disease, and may even help identify patients at risk. This, in turn would allow preventive interventions, taking advantage of our increased understanding of pathophysiology. Studies evaluating the effect of various immunotherapies aimed at preventing β-cell destruction in type 1 diabetics with residual C-peptide or patients developing diabetes are under way. Clinical trial networks such as TrialNet and the Immune Tolerance Network in the U.S. and similar networks in Europe have been have started exploring such pre-emptive strategies [101, 102]. It is now in the realm of possibility that with early biomarkers, such as miRNAs pre-emptive interventions to avert clinical diabetes will become available. These pre-emptive therapies are likely to include new therapies that involve epigenetic manipulations and biologicals that will halt β-cell destruction and perhaps even help regenerate residual β-cells to sufficient mass. There will likely be advanced technologies that may help with the replenishment of islet cells, or interventions to regenerate islet cells, and new drugs that help correct the metabolic disorders associated with diabetes beyond glucose control, which in turn would help prevent diabetic nephropathy and other crippling organ damage associated with diabetes, such as retinopathy, limb loss, etc. It looks as though thanks to new insight into the molecular biology and immunopathogenesis of diabetes along with the advances in space age technologies, we are on the verge of an explosion in new treatment options for diabetes and diabetic kidney disease. However, we should not lose sight of the fact that the increase in the diabetes epidemics and the associated organ damage that wreaks havoc on lives and the societies across the globe is above all a consequence of the modern life style that involves unhealthy diet as well as decreased physical activity and the rising epidemic in the closely associated metabolic disorder, obesity [102–105].

Without doubt, there is a need for more effective medical and perhaps technological treatments for particularly the "true" type 1 diabetes, as our ability to intervene pre-emptively before full-blown disease develops. Clearly there is impressive progress in this area and we can expect novel therapies and technologies in the near future. Yet, there is little question that the many more hundreds of millions of patients can be helped much more cost effectively through an internationally coordinated program that can help reduce obesity, increase physical activity, and educate populations on healthy diet. Studies have shown that people at high risk for type 2 diabetes, i.e., individuals with impaired glucose tolerance without overt diabetes, could sharply lower their chances of developing the disorder through diet and exercise [102, 106, 107]. The future strategies must therefore include coordinated efforts globally to implement lifestyle changes that will likely have the greatest impact on lowering the burden of diabetes and diabetic kidney disease.

References

1. Tonjes A, Kovacs P. SGLT2: a potential target for the pharmacogenetics of type 2 diabetes? Pharmacogenomics. 2013;14(7):825–33.
2. Raskin P. Sodium-glucose cotransporter inhibition: therapeutic potential for the treatment of type 2 diabetes mellitus. Diabetes Metab Res Rev. 2013;29(5):347–56.

3. Panchapakesan U, Pegg K, Gross S, Komala MG, Mudaliar H, Forbes J, et al. Effects of SGLT2 inhibition in human kidney proximal tubular cells–renoprotection in diabetic nephropathy? PLoS One. 2013;8(2):e54442.
4. Mikhail N. Use of dipeptidyl peptidase-4 inhibitors for the treatment of patients with type 2 diabetes mellitus and chronic kidney disease. Postgrad Med. 2012;124(4):138–44.
5. Andrianesis V, Doupis J. The role of kidney in glucose homeostasis—SGLT2 inhibitors, a new approach in diabetes treatment. Expert Rev Clin Pharmacol. 2013;6:519–39.
6. Komala MG, Panchapakesan U, Pollock C, Mather A. Sodium glucose cotransporter 2 and the diabetic kidney. Curr Opin Nephrol Hypertens. 2013;22(1):113–9.
7. Whaley JM, Tirmenstein M, Reilly TP, Poucher SM, Saye J, Parikh S, et al. Targeting the kidney and glucose excretion with dapagliflozin: preclinical and clinical evidence for SGLT2 inhibition as a new option for treatment of type 2 diabetes mellitus. Diabetes Metab Syndr Obes. 2012;5:135–48.
8. Cherney DZ, Perkins BA, Soleymanlou N, Maione M, Lai V, Lee A, et al. The renal hemodynamic effect of SGLT2 inhibition in patients with type 1 diabetes. Circulation. 2014;129:587–97.
9. Odegaard JI, Chawla A. Connecting type 1 and type 2 diabetes through innate immunity. Cold Spring Harb Perspect Med. 2012;2(3):a007724.
10. Bottazzo GF, Florin-Christensen A, Doniach D. Islet-cell antibodies in diabetes mellitus with autoimmune polyendocrine deficiencies. Lancet. 1974;2(7892):1279–83.
11. Skyler JS. Immune intervention for type 1 diabetes mellitus. Int J Clin Pract Suppl. 2011;170:61–70.
12. Marini MA, Succurro E, Frontoni S, Mastroianni S, Arturi F, Sciacqua A, et al. Insulin sensitivity, beta-cell function, and incretin effect in individuals with elevated 1-hour postload plasma glucose levels. Diabetes Care. 2012;35(4):868–72.
13. Nakayama M, Eisenbarth GS. Paradigm shift or shifting paradigm for type 1 diabetes. Diabetes. 2012;61(5):976–8.
14. Moran A, Bundy B, Becker DJ, DiMeglio LA, Gitelman SE, Goland R, et al. Interleukin-1 antagonism in type 1 diabetes of recent onset: two multicentre, randomised, double-blind, placebo-controlled trials. Lancet. 2013;381(9881):1905–15.
15. Skyler JS. The year in immune intervention for type 1 diabetes. Diabetes Technol Ther. 2013;15 Suppl 1:S88–95.
16. Pescovitz MD, Greenbaum CJ, Bundy B, Becker DJ, Gitelman SE, Goland R, et al. B-lymphocyte depletion with rituximab and beta-cell function: two-year results. Diabetes Care. 2014;37:453–9.
17. Pozzilli P, Guglielmi C. Double diabetes: a mixture of type 1 and type 2 diabetes in youth. Endocr Dev. 2009;14:151–66.
18. Roell MK, Issafras H, Bauer RJ, Michelson KS, Mendoza N, Vanegas SI, et al. Kinetic approach to pathway attenuation using XOMA 052, a regulatory therapeutic antibody that modulates interleukin-1beta activity. J Biol Chem. 2010;285(27):20607–14.
19. Owyang AM, Maedler K, Gross L, Yin J, Esposito L, Shu L, et al. XOMA 052, an anti-IL-1{beta} monoclonal antibody, improves glucose control and {beta}-cell function in the diet-induced obesity mouse model. Endocrinology. 2010;151(6):2515–27.
20. Ridker PM, Howard CP, Walter V, Everett B, Libby P, Hensen J, et al. Effects of interleukin-1beta inhibition with canakinumab on hemoglobin A1c, lipids, C-reactive protein, interleukin-6, and fibrinogen: a phase IIb randomized, placebo-controlled trial. Circulation. 2012;126(23):2739–48.
21. Sumpter KM, Adhikari S, Grishman EK, White PC. Preliminary studies related to anti-interleukin-1beta therapy in children with newly diagnosed type 1 diabetes. Pediatr Diabetes. 2011;12(7):656–67.
22. Skyler JS. Primary and secondary prevention of type 1 diabetes. Diabet Med. 2013;30(2):161–9.
23. Kalluri R, Neilson EG. Epithelial-mesenchymal transition and its implications for fibrosis. J Clin Invest. 2003;112(12):1776–84.
24. Liu Y. Renal fibrosis: new insights into the pathogenesis and therapeutics. Kidney Int. 2006;69(2):213–7.
25. Ziyadeh FN. Mediators of diabetic renal disease: the case for tgf-Beta as the major mediator. J Am Soc Nephrol. 2004;15 Suppl 1:S55–7.
26. Deshpande SD, Putta S, Wang M, Lai JY, Bitzer M, Nelson RG, et al. Transforming growth factor-beta-induced cross talk between p53 and a microRNA in the pathogenesis of diabetic nephropathy. Diabetes. 2013;62(9):3151–62.
27. Kanasaki K, Taduri G, Koya D. Diabetic nephropathy: the role of inflammation in fibroblast activation and kidney fibrosis. Front Endocrinol. 2013;4:7.
28. Ziyadeh FN, Wolf G. Pathogenesis of the podocytopathy and proteinuria in diabetic glomerulopathy. Curr Diabetes Rev. 2008;4(1):39–45.
29. Cheng X, Gao W, Dang Y, Liu X, Li Y, Peng X, et al. Both ERK/MAPK and TGF-Beta/Smad signaling pathways play a role in the kidney fibrosis of diabetic mice accelerated by blood glucose fluctuation. J Diabetes Res. 2013;2013:463740.
30. Jang HR, Lee YJ, Kim SR, Kim SG, Jang EH, Lee JE, et al. Potential role of urinary angiotensinogen in predicting antiproteinuric effects of angiotensin receptor blocker in non-diabetic chronic kidney disease patients: a preliminary report. Postgrad Med J. 2012;88(1038):210–6.
31. Mills KT, Kobori H, Hamm LL, Alper AB, Khan IE, Rahman M, et al. Increased urinary excretion of angiotensinogen is associated with risk of chronic kidney disease. Nephrol Dial Transplant. 2012;27(8):3176–81.
32. Park S, Bivona BJ, Kobori H, Seth DM, Chappell MC, Lazartigues E, et al. Major role for ACE-independent intrarenal ANG II formation in type II diabetes. Am J Physiol Renal Physiol. 2010; 298(1):F37–48.
33. Thethi T, Kamiyama M, Kobori H. The link between the renin-angiotensin-aldosterone system and renal injury in obesity and the metabolic syndrome. Curr Hypertens Rep. 2012;14(2):160–9.
34. Kobori H, Kamiyama M, Harrison-Bernard LM, Navar LG. Cardinal role of the intrarenal renin-angiotensin system in the pathogenesis of diabetic nephropathy. J Investig Med. 2013; 61(2):256–64.
35. Ritz E. Limitations and future treatment options in type 2 diabetes with renal impairment. Diabetes Care. 2011;34 Suppl 2:S330–4.
36. Fioretto P, Steffes MW, Sutherland DE, Goetz FC, Mauer M. Reversal of lesions of diabetic nephropathy after pancreas transplantation. N Engl J Med. 1998;339(2):69–75.
37. Romagnani P, Remuzzi G. Renal progenitors in non-diabetic and diabetic nephropathies. Trends Endocrinol Metab. 2013;24(1): 13–20.
38. Rask-Madsen C, King GL. Vascular complications of diabetes: mechanisms of injury and protective factors. Cell Metab. 2013; 17(1):20–33.
39. Oh BJ, Oh SH, Jin SM, Suh S, Bae JC, Park CG, et al. Co-transplantation of bone marrow-derived endothelial progenitor cells improves revascularization and organization in islet grafts. Am J Transplant. 2013;13(6):1429–40.
40. Steiner S, Winkelmayer WC, Kleinert J, Grisar J, Seidinger D, Kopp CW, et al. Endothelial progenitor cells in kidney transplant recipients. Transplantation. 2006;81(4):599–606.
41. Nakhoul N, Batuman V. Role of proximal tubules in the pathogenesis of kidney disease. Contribut Nephrol. 2011;169:37–50.
42. Hassan SB, Hanna MO. Urinary kappa and lambda immunoglobulin light chains in normoalbuminuric type 2 diabetes mellitus patients. J Clin Lab Anal. 2011;25(4):229–32.
43. Hutchison CA, Cockwell P, Harding S, Mead GP, Bradwell AR, Barnett AH. Quantitative assessment of serum and urinary polyclonal free light chains in patients with type II diabetes: an early marker of diabetic kidney disease? Expert Opin Ther Targets. 2008;12(6):667–76.

44. Groop L, Makipernaa A, Stenman S, DeFronzo RA, Teppo AM. Urinary excretion of kappa light chains in patients with diabetes mellitus. Kidney Int. 1990;37(4):1120–5.
45. Sharma K, Karl B, Mathew AV, Gangoiti JA, Wassel CL, Saito R, et al. Metabolomics reveals signature of mitochondrial dysfunction in diabetic kidney disease. J Am Soc Nephrol. 2013;24(11):1901–12.
46. Alvarez ML, Khosroheidari M, Kanchi Ravi R, DiStefano JK. Comparison of protein, microRNA, and mRNA yields using different methods of urinary exosome isolation for the discovery of kidney disease biomarkers. Kidney Int. 2012;82(9):1024–32.
47. Cummins TD, Barati MT, Coventry SC, Salyer SA, Klein JB, Powell DW. Quantitative mass spectrometry of diabetic kidney tubules identifies GRAP as a novel regulator of TGF-beta signaling. Biochim Biophys Acta. 2010;1804(4):653–61.
48. Diao WF, Chen WQ, Wu Y, Liu P, Xie XL, Li S, et al. Serum, liver, and kidney proteomic analysis for the alloxan-induced type I diabetic mice after insulin gene transfer of naked plasmid through electroporation. Proteomics. 2006;6(21):5837–45.
49. Folli F, Guzzi V, Perego L, Coletta DK, Finzi G, Placidi C, et al. Proteomics reveals novel oxidative and glycolytic mechanisms in type 1 diabetic patients' skin which are normalized by kidney-pancreas transplantation. PLoS One. 2010;5(3):e9923.
50. Manwaring V, Heywood WE, Clayton R, Lachmann RH, Keutzer J, Hindmarsh P, et al. The identification of new biomarkers for identifying and monitoring kidney disease and their translation into a rapid mass spectrometry-based test: evidence of presymptomatic kidney disease in pediatric Fabry and type-I diabetic patients. J Proteome Res. 2013;12(5):2013–21.
51. Bouhanick B, Gallois Y, Hadjadj S, Boux de Casson F, Limal JM, Marre M. Relationship between glomerular hyperfiltration and ACE insertion/deletion polymorphism in type 1 diabetic children and adolescents. Diabetes Care. 1999;22(4):618–22.
52. Kimura H, Gejyo F, Suzuki Y, Suzuki S, Miyazaki R, Arakawa M. Polymorphisms of angiotensin converting enzyme and plasminogen activator inhibitor-1 genes in diabetes and macroangiopathy1. Kidney Int. 1998;54(5):1659–69.
53. Marre M, Bouhanick B, Berrut G, Gallois Y, Le Jeune JJ, Chatellier G, et al. Renal changes on hyperglycemia and angiotensin-converting enzyme in type 1 diabetes. Hypertension. 1999;33(3):775–80.
54. Weekers L, Bouhanick B, Hadjadj S, Gallois Y, Roussel R, Pean F, et al. Modulation of the renal response to ACE inhibition by ACE insertion/deletion polymorphism during hyperglycemia in normotensive, normoalbuminuric type 1 diabetic patients. Diabetes. 2005;54(10):2961–7.
55. Yu ZY, Chen LS, Zhang LC, Zhou TB. Meta-analysis of the relationship between ACE I/D gene polymorphism and end-stage renal disease in patients with diabetic nephropathy. Nephrology (Carlton). 2012;17(5):480–7.
56. Ruggenenti P, Bettinaglio P, Pinares F, Remuzzi G. Angiotensin converting enzyme insertion/deletion polymorphism and renoprotection in diabetic and nondiabetic nephropathies. Clin J Am Soc Nephrol. 2008;3(5):1511–25.
57. Krolewski AS, Poznik GD, Placha G, Canani L, Dunn J, Walker W, et al. A genome-wide linkage scan for genes controlling variation in urinary albumin excretion in type II diabetes. Kidney Int. 2006;69(1):129–36.
58. Ng DP, Krolewski AS. Molecular genetic approaches for studying the etiology of diabetic nephropathy. Curr Mol Med. 2005;5(5):509–25.
59. Pezzolesi MG, Poznik GD, Mychaleckyj JC, Paterson AD, Barati MT, Klein JB, et al. Genome-wide association scan for diabetic nephropathy susceptibility genes in type 1 diabetes. Diabetes. 2009;58(6):1403–10.
60. Thomas MC, Groop PH, Tryggvason K. Towards understanding the inherited susceptibility for nephropathy in diabetes. Curr Opin Nephrol Hypertens. 2012;21(2):195–202.
61. Seki Y, Williams L, Vuguin PM, Charron MJ. Minireview: epigenetic programming of diabetes and obesity: animal models. Endocrinology. 2012;153(3):1031–8.
62. Reddy MA, Natarajan R. Epigenetics in diabetic kidney disease. J Am Soc Nephrol. 2011;22(12):2182–5.
63. Hasegawa K, Wakino S, Simic P, Sakamaki Y, Minakuchi H, Fujimura K, et al. Renal tubular Sirt1 attenuates diabetic albuminuria by epigenetically suppressing Claudin-1 overexpression in podocytes. Nat Med. 2013;19(11):1496–504.
64. Villeneuve LM, Reddy MA, Natarajan R. Epigenetics: deciphering its role in diabetes and its chronic complications. Clin Exp Pharmacol Physiol. 2011;38(7):451–9.
65. Villeneuve LM, Natarajan R. The role of epigenetics in the pathology of diabetic complications. Am J Physiol Renal Physiol. 2010;299(1):F14–25.
66. Tyagi AC, Sen U, Mishra PK. Synergy of microRNA and stem cell: a novel therapeutic approach for diabetes mellitus and cardiovascular diseases. Curr Diabetes Rev. 2011;7(6):367–76.
67. Alvarez ML, DiStefano JK. Towards microRNA-based therapeutics for diabetic nephropathy. Diabetologia. 2013;56(3):444–56.
68. Alvarez ML, Khosroheidari M, Eddy E, Kiefer J. Role of microRNA 1207-5P and its host gene, the long non-coding RNA Pvt1, as mediators of extracellular matrix accumulation in the kidney: implications for diabetic nephropathy. PLoS One. 2013; 8(10):e77468.
69. Erener S, Mojibian M, Fox JK, Denroche HC, Kieffer TJ. Circulating miR-375 as a biomarker of beta-cell death and diabetes in mice. Endocrinology. 2013;154(2):603–8.
70. Zhong X, Chung AC, Chen HY, Dong Y, Meng XM, Li R, et al. miR-21 is a key therapeutic target for renal injury in a mouse model of type 2 diabetes. Diabetologia. 2013;56(3):663–74.
71. Lin X, Tao L, Tang D. Gene therapy, a targeted treatment for diabetic nephropathy. Curr Med Chem. 2013;20(30):3774–84.
72. Flaquer M, Franquesa M, Vidal A, Bolanos N, Torras J, Lloberas N, et al. Hepatocyte growth factor gene therapy enhances infiltration of macrophages and may induce kidney repair in db/db mice as a model of diabetes. Diabetologia. 2012;55(7):2059–68.
73. Zhang Y, Zhang Y, Bone RN, Cui W, Peng JB, Siegal GP, et al. Regeneration of pancreatic non-beta endocrine cells in adult mice following a single diabetes-inducing dose of streptozotocin. PLoS One. 2012;7(5):e36675.
74. Bone RN, Icyuz M, Zhang Y, Zhang Y, Cui W, Wang H, et al. Gene transfer of active Akt1 by an infectivity-enhanced adenovirus impacts beta-cell survival and proliferation differentially in vitro and in vivo. Islets. 2012;4(6):366–78.
75. Sugiyama T, Benitez CM, Ghodasara A, Liu L, McLean GW, Lee J, et al. Reconstituting pancreas development from purified progenitor cells reveals genes essential for islet differentiation. Proc Natl Acad Sci U S A. 2013;110(31):12691–6.
76. Chen S, Shimoda M, Wang MY, Ding J, Noguchi H, Matsumoto S, et al. Regeneration of pancreatic islets in vivo by ultrasound-targeted gene therapy. Gene Ther. 2010;17(11):1411–20.
77. Zhang Y, Ye C, Wang G, Gao Y, Tan K, Zhuo Z, et al. Kidney-targeted transplantation of mesenchymal stem cells by ultrasound-targeted microbubble destruction promotes kidney repair in diabetic nephropathy rats. Biomed Res Int. 2013;2013:526367.
78. Liu S, Kilic G, Meyers MS, Navarro G, Wang Y, Oberholzer J, et al. Oestrogens improve human pancreatic islet transplantation in a mouse model of insulin deficient diabetes. Diabetologia. 2013;56(2):370–81.
79. Tiano J, Mauvais-Jarvis F. Selective estrogen receptor modulation in pancreatic beta-cells and the prevention of type 2 diabetes. Islets. 2012;4(2):173–6.
80. Tiano JP, Delghingaro-Augusto V, Le May C, Liu S, Kaw MK, Khuder SS, et al. Estrogen receptor activation reduces lipid synthesis in pancreatic islets and prevents beta cell failure in rodent models of type 2 diabetes. J Clin Invest. 2011;121(8):3331–42.

81. Jacobs-Tulleneers-Thevissen D, Chintinne M, Ling Z, Gillard P, Schoonjans L, Delvaux G, et al. Sustained function of alginate-encapsulated human islet cell implants in the peritoneal cavity of mice leading to a pilot study in a type 1 diabetic patient. Diabetologia. 2013;56(7):1605–14.
82. Jaroch DB, Lu J, Madangopal R, Stull ND, Stensberg M, Shi J, et al. Mouse and human islets survive and function after coating by biosilicification. Am J Physiol Endocrinol Metab. 2013; 305(10):E1230–40.
83. Kakabadze Z, Gupta S, Pileggi A, Molano RD, Ricordi C, Shatirishvili G, et al. Correction of diabetes mellitus by transplanting minimal mass of syngeneic islets into vascularized small intestinal segment. Am J Transplant. 2013;13(10):2550–7.
84. Santamaria X, Massasa EE, Feng Y, Wolff E, Taylor HS. Derivation of insulin producing cells from human endometrial stromal stem cells and use in the treatment of murine diabetes. Mol Ther. 2011;19(11):2065–71.
85. Takita M, Matsumoto S, Shimoda M, Chujo D, Itoh T, Sorelle JA, et al. Safety and tolerability of the T-cell depletion protocol coupled with anakinra and etanercept for clinical islet cell transplantation. Clin Transplant. 2012;26(5):E471–84.
86. Cooper DK. A brief history of cross-species organ transplantation. Proc (Bayl Univ Med Cent). 2012;25(1):49–57.
87. Reemtsma K. Xenotransplantation: a historical perspective. ILAR J. 1995;37(1):9–12.
88. Deschamps JY, Roux FA, Sai P, Gouin E. History of xenotransplantation. Xenotransplantation. 2005;12(2):91–109.
89. O'Connell PJ, Cowan PJ, Hawthorne WJ, Yi S, Lew AM. Transplantation of xenogeneic islets: are we there yet? Curr Diab Rep. 2013;13(5):687–94.
90. Nagaraju S, Bottino R, Wijkstrom M, Hara H, Trucco M, Cooper DK. Islet xenotransplantation from genetically engineered pigs. Curr Opin Organ Transplant. 2013;18(6): 695–702.
91. Ashkenazi E, Baranovski BM, Shahaf G, Lewis EC. Pancreatic islet xenograft survival in mice is extended by a combination of alpha-1-antitrypsin and single-dose anti-CD4/CD8 therapy. PLoS One. 2013;8(5):e63625.
92. Picher MM, Kupcu S, Huang CJ, Dostalek J, Pum D, Sleytr UB, et al. Nanobiotechnology advanced antifouling surfaces for the continuous electrochemical monitoring of glucose in whole blood using a lab-on-a-chip. Lab Chip. 2013;13(9): 1780–9.
93. Carrara S, Ghoreishizadeh S, Olivo J, Taurino I, Baj-Rossi C, Cavallini A, et al. Fully integrated biochip platforms for advanced healthcare. Sensors (Basel). 2012;12(8):11013–60.
94. Yu Y, Zhang Y, Martin JA, Ozbolat IT. Evaluation of cell viability and functionality in vessel-like bioprintable cell-laden tubular channels. J Biomech Eng. 2013;135(9):91011.
95. Soman P, Chung PH, Zhang AP, Chen S. Digital microfabrication of user-defined 3D microstructures in cell-laden hydrogels. Biotechnol Bioeng. 2013;110(11):3038–47.
96. Li JL, Cai YL, Guo YL, Fuh JY, Sun J, Hong GS, et al. Fabrication of three-dimensional porous scaffolds with controlled filament orientation and large pore size via an improved E-jetting technique. J Biomed Mater Res B Appl Biomater. Oct. 24 2013.
97. Sekiya S, Shimizu T, Yamato M, Okano T. Hormone supplying renal cell sheet in vivo produced by tissue engineering technology. Biores Open Access. 2013;2(1):12–9.
98. Chung S, King MW. Design concepts and strategies for tissue engineering scaffolds. Biotechnol Appl Biochem. 2011;58(6):423–38.
99. Fotino C, Molano RD, Ricordi C, Pileggi A. Transdisciplinary approach to restore pancreatic islet function. Immunol Res. 2013; 57:210–21.
100. Ellis CE, Suuronen E, Yeung T, Seeberger K, Korbutt GS. Bioengineering a highly vascularized matrix for the ectopic transplantation of islets. Islets. 2013;5(5):216–225.
101. Michels AW, Eisenbarth GS. Immune intervention in type 1 diabetes. Semin Immunol. 2011;23(3):214–9.
102. Diabetes overview. NIH Publication No. 09–3873. November 2008. http://www.diabetes.niddk.nih.gov
103. Stuckey MI, Shapiro S, Gill DP, Petrella RJ. A lifestyle intervention supported by mobile health technologies to improve the cardiometabolic risk profile of individuals at risk for cardiovascular disease and type 2 diabetes: study rationale and protocol. BMC Public Health. 2013;13(1):1051.
104. Sagarra R, Costa B, Cabre JJ, Sola-Morales O, Barrio F, el Grupo de Investigacion D-P-CP. Lifestyle interventions for diabetes mellitus type 2 prevention. Rev Clin Esp. 2014:214(2):59–68.
105. Penn L, White M, Lindstrom J, den Boer AT, Blaak E, Eriksson JG, et al. Importance of weight loss maintenance and risk prediction in the prevention of type 2 diabetes: analysis of European Diabetes Prevention Study RCT. PLoS One. 2013;8(2):e57143.
106. Lakerveld J, Bot SD, Chinapaw MJ, van Tulder MW, van Oppen P, Dekker JM, et al. Primary prevention of diabetes mellitus type 2 and cardiovascular diseases using a cognitive behavior program aimed at lifestyle changes in people at risk: design of a randomized controlled trial. BMC Endocr Disord. 2008;8:6.
107. Tuomilehto J, Lindstrom J, Eriksson JG, Valle TT, Hamalainen H, Ilanne-Parikka P, et al. Prevention of type 2 diabetes mellitus by changes in lifestyle among subjects with impaired glucose tolerance. N Engl J Med. 2001;344(18):1343–50.

Index

E.V. Lerma and V. Batuman (eds.), *Diabetes and Kidney Disease*,
DOI 10.1007/978-1-4939-0793-9, © Springer Science+Business Media New York 2014

Printed by Printforce, the Netherlands